Chronic Liver Diseases: Diagnosis and Treatment

Chronic Liver Diseases: Diagnosis and Treatment

Editor: Alexandra Culliford

AMERICAN
MEDICAL PUBLISHERS
www.americanmedicalpublishers.com

AMERICAN
MEDICAL PUBLISHERS
www.americanmedicalpublishers.com

Cataloging-in-Publication Data

Chronic liver diseases : diagnosis and treatment / edited by Alexandra Culliford.
p. cm.
Includes bibliographical references and index.
ISBN 978-1-63927-981-4
1. Liver--Diseases. 2. Liver--Diseases--Diagnosis. 3. Liver--Diseases--Treatment.
4. Biliary tract--Diseases. 5. Chronic diseases. I. Culliford, Alexandra.
RC845 .C474 2023
616.362--dc23

American Medical Publishers,
41 Flatbush Avenue,
1st Floor, New York,
NY 11217, USA

ISBN 978-1-63927-981-4 (Hardback)

Contents

Preface

A progressive deterioration of the liver functions for more than six months is referred to as chronic liver disease (CLD). The function of liver includes production of clotting factors and other proteins, detoxification of toxic substances of metabolism, and excretion of bile. The continuous process of CLD that includes inflammation, destruction, and regeneration of liver parenchyma results in fibrosis and cirrhosis. Diagnosis and treatment of CLD focuses on stopping the disease progression through a multidisciplinary approach. Abdominal ultrasound, CT scan, fibro scan, hepatic wedge pressure, endoscopy, EEG, TIPS, triphasic CT, and Doppler scan are some of the radiologic investigations that can be used to diagnose and evaluate CLD. Ultrasound of abdomen is the most common imaging tool used for CLD. Computed Tomography (CT) scan is used to detect a lesion in the liver whereas triphasic CT detects hepatocellular carcinoma. The management of CLD involves underlying cause correction, portal hypertension management, and specific treatments for individual diseases. The topics included in this book with respect to the diagnosis and treatments of chronic liver diseases are of utmost significance and bound to provide incredible insights to readers. It is appropriate for students seeking detailed information on these diseases as well as for experts.

Significant researches are present in this book. Intensive efforts have been employed by authors to make this book an outstanding discourse. This book contains the enlightening chapters which have been written on the basis of significant researches done by the experts.

Finally, I would also like to thank all the members involved in this book for being a team and meeting all the deadlines for the submission of their respective works. I would also like to thank my friends and family for being supportive in my efforts.

Editor

1

New Therapeutic Targets in Autoimmune Cholangiopathies

*Alessio Gerussi[1,2], Martina Lucà[1,2], Laura Cristoferi[1,2], Vincenzo Ronca[1,2,3], Clara Mancuso[1,2], Chiara Milani[1,2], Daphne D'Amato[1,2], Sarah Elizabeth O'Donnell[1,2], Marco Carbone[1,2] and Pietro Invernizzi[1,2]**

[1] Division of Gastroenterology and Center for Autoimmune Liver Diseases, Department of Medicine and Surgery, University of Milano-Bicocca, Monza, Italy, [2] European Reference Network on Hepatological Diseases (ERN RARE-LIVER), San Gerardo Hospital, Monza, Italy, [3] National Institute of Health Research Liver Biomedical Research Centre Birmingham, Centre for Liver Research, Institute of Immunology and Immunotherapy, University of Birmingham, Birmingham, United Kingdom

***Correspondence:**
Pietro Invernizzi
pietro.invernizzi@unimib.it

Primary biliary cholangitis (PBC) and primary sclerosing cholangitis (PSC) are autoimmune cholangiopathies characterized by limited treatment options. A more accurate understanding of the several pathways involved in these diseases has fostered the development of novel and promising targeted drugs. For PBC, the characterization of the role of farnesoid X receptor (FXR) and perixosome-proliferator activated receptor (PPAR) has paved the way to several clinical trials including different molecules with choleretic and antinflammatory action. Conversely, different pathogenetic models have been proposed in PSC such as the "leaky gut" hypothesis, a dysbiotic microbiota or a defect in mechanisms protecting against bile acid toxicity. Along these theories, new treatment approaches have been developed, ranging from drugs interfering with trafficking of lymphocytes from the gut to the liver, fecal microbiota transplantation or new biliary acids with possible immunomodulatory potential. Finally, for both diseases, antifibrotic agents are under investigation. In this review, we will illustrate current understanding of molecular mechanisms in PBC and PSC, focusing on actionable biological pathways for which novel treatments are being developed.

Keywords: primary biliary cholangitis, primary sclerosing cholangitis, liver, FXR agonists, fibrates, microbiome, gut-liver axis

INTRODUCTION

Autoimmune diseases of the biliary tract include primary biliary cholangitis (PBC) and primary sclerosing cholangitis (PSC). PBC and PSC are rare diseases of unknown etiology, immune-mediated pathogenesis and limited treatment options. Recently, there has been an increasing attention toward these rare diseases and novel agents are under investigation in clinical trials.

This review outlines the most promising novel agents for the treatment of PBC and PSC, adopting a target-driven approach: the biological target of each class of molecules is briefly summarized in the context of the pathogenesis of the disease and then preclinical and clinical results are presented (**Figure 1** and **Table 1**).

FARNESOID X RECEPTOR AGONISTS

Hepatocytes generate bile acids, i.e., cholic acid and chenodeoxycholic acid, from cholesterol through two pathways: most of the BAs are produced by the classical pathway, which involves

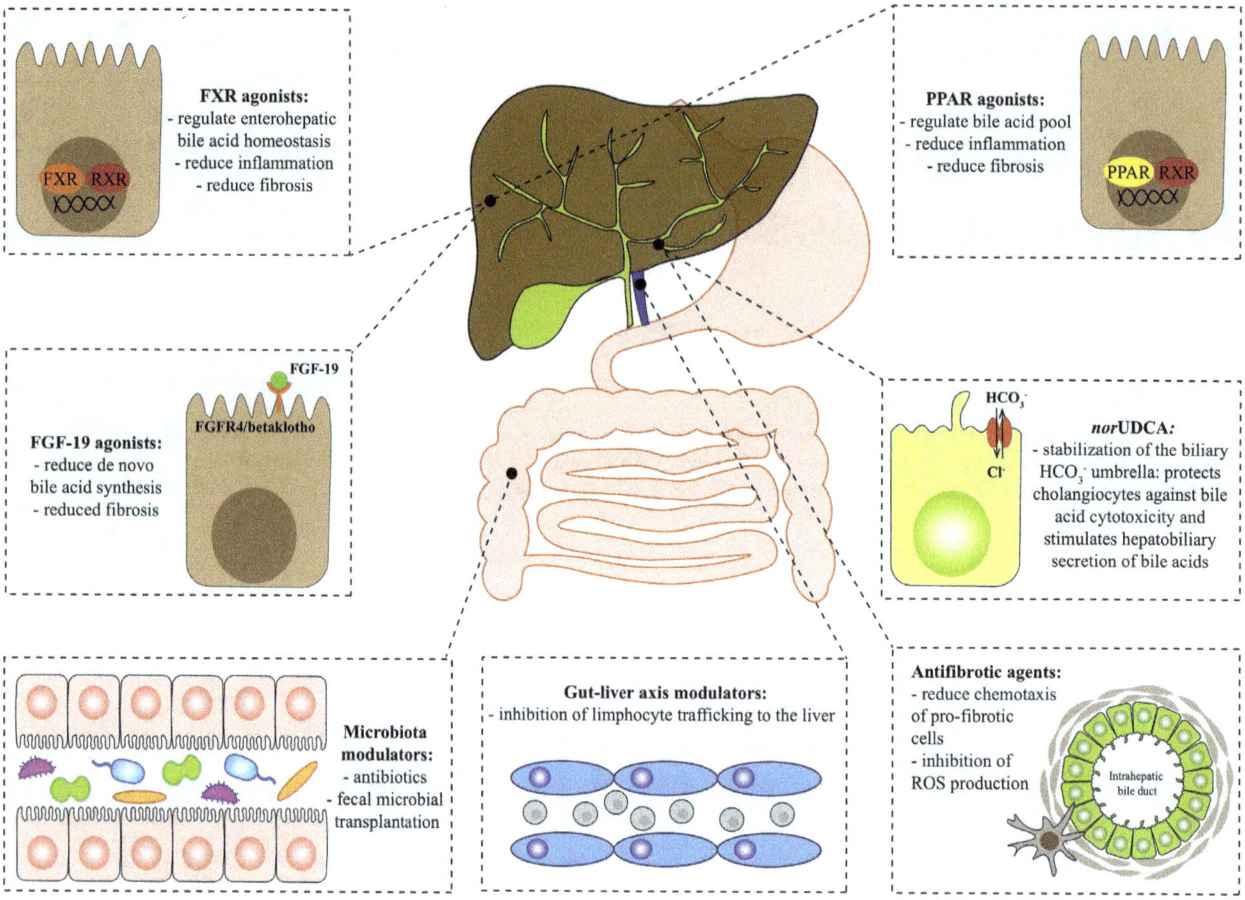

FIGURE 1 | Therapeutical targets in autoimmune cholangiopathies. FGF-19, fibroblast growth factor 19; FGFR4, fibroblast growth factor receptor 4; FXR, farnesoid X receptor; HCO_3^-, bicarbonate; norUDCA, norursodeoxycholic acid; PPAR, Peroxisome proliferator-activated receptor; ROS, reactive oxygen species; RXR, retinoid x receptor.

the rate-limiting cholesterol 7alphahydroxylase (CYP7A1); the cytochrome (CYP) P450 27 alpha hydroxylase (CYP27A1) generates the remaining fractions. More recently, it has been reported that bile acids can also be generated by gut microbiota: these new bile acids are the phenylalanocholic acid, tyrosocholic acid and leucocholic acid (1).

Bile acids can exert different activities by binding to nuclear receptors, such as the farnesoid X receptor (FXR; NR1H4), pregnane X receptor, vitamin D receptor and Takeda G-protein-coupled receptor 5 (TGR5). FXR acts as transcription factor binding to FXR response elements in the DNA; it can operate as a monomer or together with retinoid X receptor (RXR; NR2B1) (2). FXR is mainly expressed in the liver and the gut, but can also be found in the kidney and adrenal gland, and its action exerts effects on the metabolism of bile acids, carbohydrates and lipids.

In the liver, FXR regulates bile acid synthesis, preventing their toxic accumulation. The bile salt export pump (BSEP) is expressed on the canalicular membranes of hepatocytes and promotes biliary excretion of bile acids. Its expression is dependent on FXR, while other transporters [e.g., multidrug resistance-associated protein (MRP) 3 and MRP4] are independent from FXR.

OSTα-OSTβ (*SLC51A* and *SLC51B*) is an heteromeric transporter expressed mainly in the distal portions of the gut and bile ducts, localized to the basolateral membrane of ileal enterocytes and biliary epithelial cells, respectively. Its main role is to transport bile acids across the membrane, but OSTα-OSTβ is also involved in steroids transport (3–5). FXR controls gene expression of OSTα-OSTβ, as proven by the marked reduction in OSTα and OSTβ expression in the ileum of Fxr-/- mice (6).

FXR induces the expression of the small heterodimer protein (SHP), also known as NR0B2 nuclear receptor subfamily 0, group B, member 2. SHP acts as transcription factor despite lacking a DNA binding domain, and inhibits CYP7A1 thanks to the recruitment of other proteins (mSin3A-Swi/Snf complex, G9a methyltransferase, the corepressor subunit GPS2) (7–10). CYP7A1 inhibition translates into a negative feedback inhibition of bile acid synthesis (2).

TABLE 1 | Novel pharmacological agents in autoimmune cholangiopathies.

	Primary Biliary Cholangitis	Primary Sclerosing Cholangitis
FXR agonists		
Bile acid		
- Obeticholic acid	✓	✓
Non bile acid		
- Tropifexor	✓	
- Cilofexor	✓	✓
- EDP-503	✓	
FGF-19 agonists		
- NGM-282	✓	✓
PPAR agonists		
- *PPAR-α/(γ)-* Bezafibrate/Fenofibrate	✓	✓
- PPAR-α/δ - Elafibranor	✓	✓
- PPAR-δ-Seladelpar	✓(*)	
24-*nor*ursodeoxycholic (*nor*-UDCA)		✓
Antifibrotic agents		
- Cenicriviroc		✓
- Setanaxib	✓	
Immunological Agents		
- Rituximab	✓	
- Ustekimumab	✓	
- Abatacept	✓	
- Baricitinib	✓(**)	
Gut-Liver axis		
- Vedolizumab		✓
- Antibiotics (Metronidazole, Vancomicin)		✓
- Timolumab		✓
- Fecal Microbial Transplantation		✓

(*)Trial closed for adverse event.
(**)Trial closed in august 2019.
FXR, farnesoid X receptor; FGF-19, fibroblast growth factor 19; PPAR, Peroxisome proliferator-activated receptor; HCO_3^-, bicarbonate; norUDCA, norursodeoxycholic acid.

In pre-clinical setting, the activation of hepatic FXR is beneficial in reducing hepatic fibrosis, since it prevents toxicity due to accumulation of bile acids (11).

Among the FXR-agonists the main distinction is based on whether they are steroidal (i.e., bile acids) or non-steroidal agents. Limitations of steroidal agents are due to the intrinsic lipophilicity of FXR ligand binding site, which reduces solubility and bioavailability. Moreover, one of the most common side effects of steroidal FXR agonists is pruritus, which depends on the TGR5 agonistic properties (12). Nonetheless, also non-steroidal agents have shown mild pruritogen action despite not binding the TGR5 receptor. Interestingly, there is preliminary evidence that support the concept that non-steroidal FXR-agonists might have more anti-fibrotic effects (13).

Obeticholic acid (OCA) belongs to the class of steroidal FXR agonists and is a semi-synthetic bile acid. Currently, OCA is the only registered option for patients with PBC and incomplete response after 12 months of treatment with UDCA or intolerant to UDCA (14). The main side effect is itching, which is typically mild and seldom requires treatment withdrawal. Another side effect of OCA is the increase in low-density lipoprotein (LDL) cholesterol; the long-term significance of this side effect on cardiovascular risk is still unknown. OCA has been tested also in patients with PSC (AESOP trial), however final results are still waited.

Non-bile Acid FXR Agonists

Tropifexor has been evaluated in a double-blind, randomized, placebo-controlled, phase 2 study in PBC, but only the interim analysis is available. Interestingly, to avoid confounding due to the possible FXR-mediated alkaline phosphatase (ALP) gene induction, gamma glutamyl transpeptidase (GGT) reduction was chosen instead of ALP reduction as primary endpoint of this trial.

The non-steroidal FXR agonist **Cilofexor** has been tested in PSC in a randomized, double-blind, placebo-controlled phase 2 trial, and although the primary endpoint was safety, it can be noticed that it significantly reduced ALP levels, especially in the 100 mg arm (15). A randomized, double-blind, placebo-controlled phase 2 trial in PBC and a phase 3 trial in PSC are currently undergoing.

EDP-305 is another non-steroidal FXR agonist being evaluated in a randomized, double-blind, placebo-controlled phase 2 trial in PBC. In murine models of fibrosis EDP-305 reduced the extent of fibrotic areas assessed by morphometric quantification (16).

FIBROBLAST GROWTH FACTOR 19 AGONISTS

During cholestasis, high levels of bile acids favor fibroblast growth factor 19 (FGF-19) expression. The increased concentration of FGF-19 in the gut stimulates activation of the FGFR4/betaklotho receptor in the liver. FGF19 then migrates to the liver where reduces CYP7A1 gene expression (7, 17). FGFR4 and betaklotho forms a cell surface receptor complex and represent the effectors of the liver activity of FGF19. FGF19 is also induced by FXR activation in the enterocytes.

Preclinical data have shown a higher risk of hepatocellular carcinoma (HCC) in transgenic mice with ectopic expression of FGF19 in the skeletal muscle of transgenic mice (18). Furthermore, 15% of human HCC cancers show co-amplification of FGF19 and cyclin D1 on 11q13.3 (19).

A synthetic analog **NGM282** was developed without carcinogenic potential and its safety and efficacy is under investigation in clinical trials. NGM282 has been tested in two randomized, double-blind, placebo-controlled trials in PBC and PSC, showing conflicting results. The PBC study lasted for 28 days while the design of the PSC study scheduled treatment for 12 weeks.

In PBC, NGM282 achieved a reduction of >15% of ALP levels in 50% of patients treated compared to 7% of the placebo group. Similar proportions were found between the 0.3 mg and the 3 mg arms. Main side effect was non severe diarrhea (20).

Conversely, in the PSC study of NGM282, ALP levels did not significantly drop in the 1 and 3 mg arms compared to placebo

(21). We do acknowledge that the clinical significance of ALP in PBC and PSC is different, considering that PBC has a fairly stable and slowly progressing disease course where ALP is a good prognostic marker, compared to the erratic disease course of PSC, where ALP levels can intermittently rise and fall due to episodic cholangitis (22).

Interestingly, in both studies, NGM282 decreased the α-Hydroxy-4-cholesten-3-one (C4) levels in treatment groups confirming that this drug acts by directly inhibiting the *de-novo* bile acid synthesis through the classical pathway.

PEROXISOME PROLIFERATOR-ACTIVATED RECEPTORS AGONISTS

Peroxisome proliferator-activated receptors (PPARs) are nuclear receptors of a family containing three isotypes: PPARα (NR1C1), PPARβ/δ (NR1C2) and PPARγ (NR1C3). After engagement with their ligand, PPARs form a heterodimer with the retinoid X receptor, binding to specific DNA sequences in the regulatory regions of target genes.

PPARα is highly expressed in tissues with marked fatty acid oxidation activity, including liver, heart and skeletal muscle, brown adipose tissue and kidney. Beyond its ability to regulate fatty acid catabolism in different conditions of food intake and starvation, animal models of atherosclerosis and non-alcoholic steatohepatitis have shown that PPARα has also anti-inflammatory properties. Moreover, PPARα agonism determines inhibition of bile acids synthesis by acting on CYP7A1 and cytochrome sterol 27-hydroxylase (CYP27A1). There is also evidence that PPAR-α abrogates the uptake of bile acids in hepatocytes through the inhibition of the basolateral transporter sodium-taurocholate-cotransporting polypeptide and up-regulates expression of human *MDR3* gene favoring canalicular export of phospholipids (23).

PPARβ/δ is expressed in hepatocytes, cholangiocytes, and non-parenchymal cells (Kuppfer cells, hepatic stellate cells). PPARδ is utilized by biliary epithelial cells to control bile components transporters (24) and favors the timely removal of apoptotic cells by Kuppfer cells, in order to prevent potential autoimmune phenomena to arise (25). PPAR-γ expression is mostly restricted to Kupffer cells (25). In cultured human biliary epithelial cells from patients with PBC there is a down-regulation of PPAR-γ and the activation of PPAR-γ is associated with reduced inflammation (26). A PPAR-γ agonist reduced portal inflammation in murine models of PBC (27).

Natural ligands of PPAR-α are derivatives of fatty acids generated during lipolysis, lipogenesis or fatty acids catabolism. Synthetic PPAR-α agonists belong to the group of fibrates, derivatives of fibric acid: Gemfibrozil, Fenofibrate, Ciprofibrate and Bezafibrate (**Figure 2**). They are typically used in treatment of isolated hypertriglyceridemia or mixed dyslipidemia. Fenofibrate is 10-fold more specific for the α- isoform compared to the γ- one, while Bezafibrate is considered a pan-PPAR-agonist due to its similar affinity for the three isoforms. Most of their actions are derived from their PPARα agonism.

There is growing evidence of the therapeutic efficacy of fibrates in PBC, while evidence is still limited for PSC. **Bezafibrate** has been evaluated in a 24 months, double-blind, randomized, placebo-controlled, phase 3 trial (BEZURSO trial), at the dosage of 400 mg per day in patients with incomplete biochemical response after 12 months of UDCA. The rate of ALP normalization was 67% in the treatment arm, compared to the 2% in placebo group. In addition, Bezafibrate did not worsen pruritus, which was even improved in a subset of cases, which is in line with available literature (28). The results from BEZURSO trial endorse the concept that fibrates reduce the production of bile acids in hepatocytes since patients in the 400 mg arm experienced a 70% drop in C4 serum levels, whereas patients in the placebo arm did not show any significant change. Conversely, experience on **Fenofibrate** in PBC derive from smaller cohorts (29–33). Both Bezafibrate and Fenofibrate show side effects typical of their pharmacological class, namely myalgias, transaminitis and increase in creatine kinase and creatinine. The long-term safety of these agents during treatment for cholestatic diseases is still to be ascertained. Since safety and efficacy profile of Bezafibrate and Fenofibrate seems to be similar, but Bezafibrate is supported by a randomized controlled trial, it would be reasonable to choose Bezafibrate as the fibrate of choice in PBC until new data are available.

There are now new molecules in the pipeline which show more selective PPAR-δ activity. Seladelpar is a selective PPAR-δ agonist (34), while Elafibranor is PPARα/δ.

Based on the safety information derived from two phase 2 trials (35), the potential efficacy of **Seladelpar** has been evaluated in the ENHANCE trial, a 52-week, double-blind, placebo-controlled, randomized, Phase 3 study. However, in November 2019, the ENHANCE trial was put on hold following the unexpected histological findings observed in the Phase 2b study of Seladelpar in subjects with non-alcoholic steatohepatitis (NASH). Atypical histological findings, including interface hepatitis and biliary injury were found in the planned interval biopsies.

Elafibranor has been recently evaluated in a multicenter randomized double-blind placebo-controlled phase 2 Study in PBC.

Literature supporting the use of fibrates in PSC is scanty. At the time of writing, no randomized controlled trials have been published, and retrospective case series come mostly from Japan (36, 37).

A French-Spanish retrospective study showed a 40% reduction in the levels of ALP after 12 weeks of treatment with fibrates [either Fenofibrate (200 mg/day) or Bezafibrate (400 mg/day)]. There were no major safety issues and authors cautiously support further studies. To us, it is conceivable to further investigate the potential benefit of fibrates in PSC, based on their inherent anticholestatic and anti-inflammatory properties.

24-*NOR*URSODEOXYCHOLIC AND THE BILIARY HCO_3^- UMBRELLA

The HCO_3^- umbrella hypothesis asserts that bicarbonate (HCO_3^-) ions, secreted by cholangiocytes and hepatocytes, form a defensive barrier on the apical side of the hepatocytes

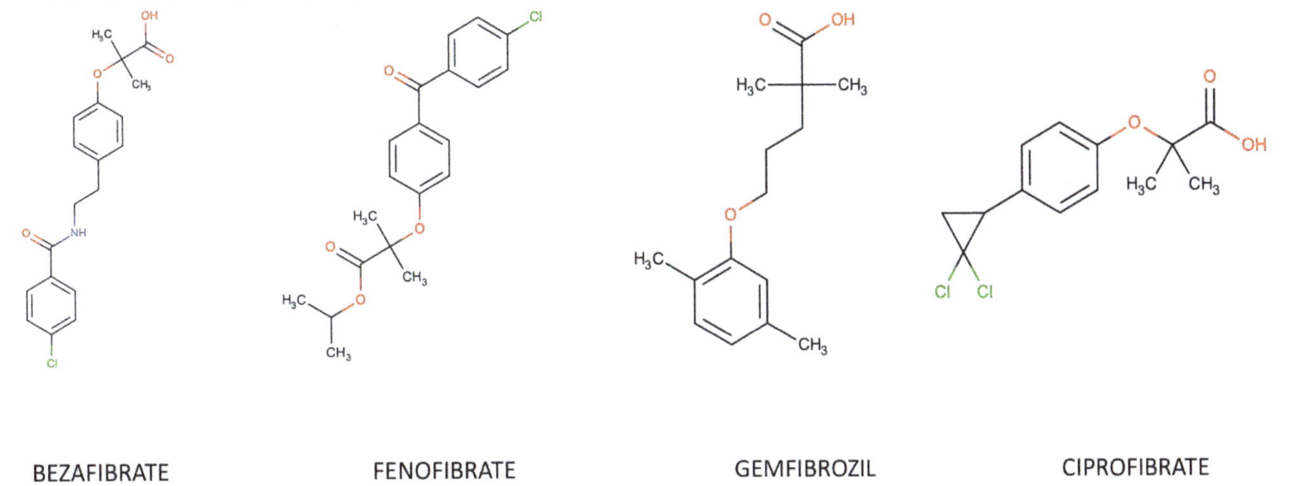

FIGURE 2 | Chemical structure of most common fibrates.

(38). When this system is malfunctioning, glycine-conjugated bile acids become able to cross the cholangiocyte membrane, bypassing membrane transporters. This phenomenon leads to cholangiocyte apoptosis and senescence (39). There is evidence supporting the concept that in cholangiopathies like PBC and PSC the biliary HCO_3^- umbrella is defective (40, 41).

The biliary HCO_3^- umbrella can be stabilized through **24-norursodeoxycholic (nor-UDCA),** mainly thank to its ability of undergoing cholehepatic shunting. *Nor*-UDCA is relatively resistant to *N*-acyl-amidation with taurine or glycine, so that cholangiocytes can reabsorb it and it can be re-secreted into bile after getting through periductular capillary plexus and hepatocytes. The importance of this process is the ability to cause a profound stimulus to bicarbonate secretion from cholangiocytes, strengthening the impaired HCO_3^- umbrella of cholangiopathies.

Mdr2-/- mice are typically considered a surrogate *in vivo* model of PSC (42). The lack of *Mdr2*-encoded membrane protein, which is a canalicular transporter deputed to transport phospholipids from hepatocytes to the bile, causes a cholangiocyte injury, due to bile acid toxicity from increased concentration of free non-micellar bile acids. In this model *nor*-UDCA increases the hydrophilicity of bile acids, stimulates bile flow and induces biliary transporters and detoxification enzymes (43).

A double-blind, randomized, placebo-controlled, phase 2 study evaluating *nor*-UDCA in patients with PSC has shown promising results in terms of safety of the molecule and reduction of serum alkaline phosphatase after 12 weeks of treatment (44). This trial assessed three different treatment regimens (*nor*-UDCA 500, 1,000 mg/day, and 1,500 mg/day) compared to a four arm with placebo. All doses showed a significant reduction in ALP levels, in a dose-dependent manner, and similar results were achieved for transaminases and gamma-glutamyl transferase levels. Pruritus did not occur more frequently in the treatment arms, and *nor*-UDCA showed a good safety profile.

A phase 3 clinical study is currently ongoing.

IMMUNOLOGICAL TARGETS

PBC and PSC are both included in the group of autoimmune diseases of the biliary tract; however, while PBC is much closer to a typical autoimmune condition, PSC is a complex disease with aspects also typical of fibrotic and preneoplastic conditions. Aside from the classificatory debate, the immune system takes part of many pathogenetic processes of both PBC and PSC. Nevertheless, many strategies targeting immune cells have failed so far (45–53). Biological agents, like **Rituximab** (54, 55), **Ustekinumab** (56), and **Abatacept** (57) were studied in PBC, based on preclinical promising data (rituximab and abatacept) or stimulated by results from genome-wide association studies (ustekinumab), but conflicting results have been produced and these molecules are not part of the therapeutic armamentarium.

Among the novel agents under investigation, there is **Baricitinib**, a small molecule which is a reversible inhibitor of Janus kinase (JAK) 1 and 2. In mammals, different receptors are bound by members of the JAK family (JAK 1-3). The receptor-ligand binding determines a cascade of activation and modifications leading to the generation of docking sites for the SH2 domain of the cytoplasmic transcription factors termed signal transducers and activators of transcription (STATs). Several downstream signals are regulated by JAK and STAT proteins, comprising interleukins (ILs), interferons (IFNs), and the switch toward T helper (Th) 1, 2, or 17 of naïve T cells is finely regulated by a JAK-mediated signaling (58). Baricitinib is already included in the available registered drugs for the treatment of rheumatoid arthritis (59), and was supposed to be evaluated in a randomized double-blind, placebo-controlled, phase 2, study in patients with PBC and partial response to UDCA. Unexpectedly, in August 2019 Lilly, the company that developed the molecule, decided to terminate the trial.

ANTIFIBROTIC AGENTS

Inflammation, cholestasis and fibrosis are tightly connected to determine the vicious cycle toward cirrhosis (60).

Cholangiopathies show a biliary-type of fibrosis which usually spreads from the portal tract to the lobule (61). None of the registered therapies for PBC are inherently antifibrotic, but halt progression of the fibrotic process through antagonism of inflammation and/or cholestasis. However, specific antifibrotic therapies are urgently needed to potentially achieve fibrosis reversal, considered that a not negligible proportion of patients do progress despite effective treatment (62).

A novel agent located at the crossroad between inflammation and fibrosis is **Cenicriviroc**. Cenicriviroc targets C-C motif chemokine receptor (CCR) types 2 and 5, which are typically expressed by monocytes, Kupffer cells and hepatic stellate cells. There is mounting evidence that, upon liver injury, CCR2 and CCR5 together with their ligands favor macrophage recruitment infiltration and stellate cells activation (63, 64). In Bile-duct ligated and Mdr2-/- mice Cenicriviroc, together with another agent (all-trans retinoic acid), reduced bile acids, plasma liver enzymes and histological markers of necrosis and fibrosis (65). A randomized, double-blind, multinational, phase 2b enrolling patients with Non-alcoholic fatty liver steatohepatitis (NASH) revealed the antifibrotic capacity of Cenicriviroc, which halted fibrosis progression more frequently than placebo, without improving NASH-related liver inflammation (66). Cenicriviroc is currently under evaluation in PSC.

Setanaxib is another promising antifibrotic agent characterized by a completely novel molecular target and potentially representing a first-in-class molecule for the treatment of PBC and PSC. The main targets of Setanaxib are NADPH oxidase (NOX) proteins (67), which are enzymes over-induced in conditions of chronic stress, like chronic inflammatory and fibrosing diseases (68, 69). Activation of stellate cells to myofibroblasts is promoted by NOX1, NOX2, and NOX4 isoforms (70, 71).

In bile-duct ligation and NASH murine models, Setanaxib reduced histological markers of fibrosis through NOX-inhibition. Setanaxib has been recently evaluated in a multicenter, randomized, double-blind, placebo-controlled, phase 2 study in patients with PBC and incomplete response to UDCA. The primary endpoint was reduction in the levels of GGT, which is considered a more accurate marker of oxidative stress in the liver (72).

MODULATION OF THE MICROBIOTA AND GUT-LIVER AXIS

While PBC is classically limited to the small bile ducts of the liver, PSC also involves large ducts and is often associated with inflammatory bowel disease (IBD) (53). The involvement of the distal part of the biliary tree and the frequent co-existence of IBD have suggested that PSC may derive from the disruption of some physiological process in the gut. The focus has been put onto two players: the microbiota and the gut-liver axis.

There is a rising interest in the study of microbiota changes in pathological conditions (73–76). Dysbiosis, i.e., the abnormal composition of gut microbiota, has been described in patients across several diseases, included cirrhosis (77), PBC (78), and PSC (79). Dysbiosis in the gut can also involve viral and fungal species, as recently proved in IBD (80) and PSC (81). Germ-free Mdr2-/- mice show increased hepatitis and cholestatic injury compared to conventionally-housed Mdr2-/- mice (82). Nevertheless, it is still under debate whether dysbiosis has a causal relationship with these pathological findings in humans.

From a therapeutic point of view, modulation of microbiota in PSC represents a fascinating option, since some data suggest that the progression of the disease might be due to a vicious cycle of inflammation and fibrosis driven by translocation of pathobionts from the gut to the liver (83). It is likely that tackling this process could be of benefit, and there is some clinical evidence to support this concept. The use of antibiotics (e.g., **Metronidazole**, **Vancomycin**) in patients with PSC can reduce blood markers of liver injury and cholestasis, despite data on long-term benefit are lacking (84–86).

Recently, the provoking concept that non-communicable diseases (i.e., those not caused by infectious microbes) might be communicable via the transfer of microbiota has been proposed (87). This challenging theory is supported by several line of experimental data showing that if a dysbiotic microbiota is transferred from diseased animals to healthy mice the latter will develop the disease (88). Conversely, there is also evidence that **Fecal Microbial Transplantation (FMT)** may be of benefit for many diseases (89, 90), in addition to the established indication for recurrent Clostridium Difficile infection (91). Indeed, a seminal open-label study has shown the capacity of FMT to augment microbiota diversity in patients with PSC. In a subset of individuals FMT improved biochemical markers of cholestasis; however the small number of individuals included in this pilot study (i.e., 10 patients) obviously prevents solid conclusions on efficacy (92).

Regarding gut-liver axis, the anatomical link between gut and liver translates also in an intimate interconnection at the molecular level, with several substances flowing to the liver through the portal vein system. When intestinal permeability is higher than normal, bacterial byproducts reaching the liver are potential drivers of inflammation and fibrogenesis. Two main barriers control this process: the epithelial barrier and the gut-vascular barrier (93). Under physiological conditions, mucosal addressin cell adhesion molecule (MAdCAM)-1 is expressed on gut endothelium and is not expressed in the liver, avoiding recruitment of T cells in the liver (94). In PSC there is evidence of aberrant expression of MAdCAM-1 in the liver (95). Despite theoretically promising, the use of **Vedolizumab**, which antagonize MAdCAM-1 and its receptor $\alpha 4\beta 7$ and it is approved for IBD treatment, did not show efficacy in patients with PSC and IBD (a phase 3 trial was retired in 2018). A retrospective study on Vedolizumab in patients with PSC and IBD also failed to reveal a positive signal (96).

The increased expression of MAdCAM-1 in the liver is mainly due to the activation of vascular adhesion protein (VAP)-1, which is an enzyme involved in amine oxidation. Intrahepatic and circulating levels of VAP-1 are increased in patients with

PSC compared to non-PSC individuals, and a single-arm, open-label, multi-center trial evaluating the efficacy of an anti-VAP-1 molecule, **Timolumab**, is currently ongoing (97).

CONCLUSIONS

Many novel drugs are currently under investigation for PBC and PSC. The potential future availability of many novel agents opens the challenge for the identification of the right candidate for each specific drug or combination of drugs based on the mechanism of action and safety profile.

It is key the improvement of risk stratification strategies for this purpose (98), which will require deep, longitudinal phenotyping of individuals by means of multi-omics analysis including the exposome, along with the microbiome, genome, metabolome, among the others (99–104). Then, we need to implement algorithms to proficiently integrate these big data to cluster patients across different phenotypes and trajectories of the disease (105, 106); for this, the collaboration with data science professionals and experts in artificial intelligence will be fundamental (107, 108). The last part of this process will be to put in practice clinical trials with different, multimodal treatment strategies (109).

AUTHOR CONTRIBUTIONS

This work was done in full by AG. ML has contributed to a part of the contents. CMi and DD'A have created and processed the image. LC has created the table. All authors contributed to manuscript revision, read, and approved the submitted version.

ACKNOWLEDGMENTS

The authors of this publication are members of the European Reference Network on Hepatological Diseases (ERN RARE-LIVER).

REFERENCES

1. Quinn RA, Melnik A V, Vrbanac A, Fu T, Patras KA, Christy MP, et al. Global chemical effects of the microbiome include new bile-acid conjugations. *Nature.* (2020) 579:123–9. doi: 10.1038/s41586-020-2047-9
2. Han YC. Update on FXR biology: promising therapeutic target? *Int J Mol Sci.* (2018) 19:E2069. doi: 10.3390/ijms19072069
3. Ashley EA. Towards precision medicine. *Nat Rev Genet.* (2016) 17:507–22. doi: 10.1038/nrg.2016.86
4. Boyer JL, Trauner M, Mennone A, Soroka CJ, Cai S-Y, Moustafa T, et al. Upregulation of a basolateral FXR-dependent bile acid efflux transporter OSTα-OSTβ in cholestasis in humans and rodents. *Am J Physiol Liver Physiol.* (2006) 290:G1124–30. doi: 10.1152/ajpgi.00539.2005
5. Boyer JL. OSTα-OSTβ guards the ileal enterocyte from the accumulation of toxic levels of bile acids. *Cell Mol Gastroenterol Hepatol.* (2018) 5:649–50. doi: 10.1016/j.jcmgh.2018.01.015
6. Zollner G, Wagner M, Moustafa T, Fickert P, Silbert D, Gumhold J, et al. Coordinated induction of bile acid detoxification and alternative elimination in mice: role of FXR-regulated organic solute transporter-alpha/beta in the adaptive response to bile acids. *Am J Physiol Gastrointest Liver Physiol.* (2006) 290:G923–32. doi: 10.1152/ajpgi.00490.2005
7. Kliewer SA, Mangelsdorf DJ. Bile acids as hormones: the FXR-FGF15/19 pathway. *Dig Dis.* (2015) 33:327–31. doi: 10.1159/000371670
8. Fang S, Miao J, Xiang L, Ponugoti B, Treuter E, Kemper JK. Coordinated recruitment of histone methyltransferase G9a and other chromatin-modifying enzymes in SHP-mediated regulation of hepatic bile acid metabolism. *Mol Cell Biol.* (2007) 27:1407–24. doi: 10.1128/MCB.00944-06
9. Kemper JK, Kim H, Miao J, Bhalla S, Bae Y. Role of an mSin3A-Swi/Snf chromatin remodeling complex in the feedback repression of bile acid biosynthesis by SHP. *Mol Cell Biol.* (2004) 24:7707–19. doi: 10.1128/MCB.24.17.7707-7719.2004
10. Sanyal S, Båvner A, Haroniti A, Nilsson L-M, Lundåsen T, Rehnmark S, et al. Involvement of corepressor complex subunit GPS2 in transcriptional pathways governing human bile acid biosynthesis. *Proc Natl Acad Sci USA.* (2007) 104:15665–70. doi: 10.1073/pnas.0706736104
11. Chávez-Talavera O, Tailleux A, Lefebvre P, Staels B. Bile acid control of metabolism and inflammation in obesity, type 2 diabetes, dyslipidemia, and nonalcoholic fatty liver disease. *Gastroenterology.* (2017) 152:1679–94. doi: 10.1053/j.gastro.2017.01.055
12. Alemi F, Kwon E, Poole DP, Lieu T, Lyo V, Cattaruzza F, et al. The TGR5 receptor mediates bile acid-induced itch and analgesia. *J Clin Invest.* (2013) 123:1513–30. doi: 10.1172/JCI64551
13. Verbeke L, Nevens F, Laleman W. Steroidal or non-steroidal FXR agonists - Is that the question? *J Hepatol.* (2017) 66:680–1. doi: 10.1016/j.jhep.2017.01.013
14. Nevens F, Andreone P, Mazzella G, Strasser SI, Bowlus C, Invernizzi P, et al. A placebo-controlled trial of obeticholic acid in primary biliary cholangitis. *N Engl J Med.* (2016) 375:631–43. doi: 10.1056/NEJMoa1509840
15. Trauner M, Gulamhusein A, Hameed B, Caldwell S, Shiffman ML, Landis C, et al. The nonsteroidal farnesoid x receptor agonist cilofexor (GS-9674) improves markers of cholestasis and liver injury in patients with primary sclerosing cholangitis. *Hepatology.* (2019) 70:788–801. doi: 10.1002/hep.30509
16. Erstad DJ, Farrar CT, Masia R, Ferreira DDS, Wei L, Choi J-K, et al. A novel farnesoid X receptor agonist: EDP-305, reduces fibrosis progression in animal models of fibrosis. *J Hepatol.* (2017) 66:S165. doi: 10.1016/S0168-8278(17)30608-6
17. Degirolamo C, Sabbà C, Moschetta A. Therapeutic potential of the endocrine fibroblast growth factors FGF19, FGF21 and FGF23. *Nat Rev Drug Discov.* (2016) 15:51–69. doi: 10.1038/nrd.2015.9
18. Nicholes K, Guillet S, Tomlinson E, Hillan K, Wright B, Frantz GD, et al. A mouse model of hepatocellular carcinoma: ectopic expression of fibroblast growth factor 19 in skeletal muscle of transgenic mice. *Am J Pathol.* (2002) 160:2295–307. doi: 10.1016/S0002-9440(10)61177-7
19. Sawey ET, Chanrion M, Cai C, Wu G, Zhang J, Zender L, et al. Identification of a therapeutic strategy targeting amplified FGF19 in liver cancer by oncogenomic screening. *Cancer Cell.* (2011) 19:347–58. doi: 10.1016/j.ccr.2011.01.040
20. Mayo MJ, Wigg AJ, Leggett BA, Arnold H, Thompson AJ, Weltman M, et al. NGM282 for treatment of patients with primary biliary cholangitis: a multicenter, randomized, double-blind, placebo-controlled trial. *Hepatol Commun.* (2018) 2:1037–50. doi: 10.1002/hep4.1209
21. Hirschfield GM, Chazouillères O, Drenth JP, Thorburn D, Harrison SA, Landis CS, et al. Effect of NGM282, an FGF19 analogue,

in primary sclerosing cholangitis: a multicenter, randomized, double-blind, placebo-controlled phase II trial. *J Hepatol.* (2019) 70:483–93. doi: 10.1016/j.jhep.2018.10.035
22. Gerussi A, Invernizzi P. Better end points needed in primary sclerosing cholangitis trials. *Nat Rev Gastroenterol Hepatol.* (2019) 16:143–4. doi: 10.1038/s41575-019-0110-5
23. Ghonem NS, Assis DN, Boyer JL. Fibrates and cholestasis. *Hepatology.* (2015) 62:635–43. doi: 10.1002/hep.27744
24. Xia X, Jung D, Webb P, Zhang A, Zhang B, Li L, et al. Liver X receptor β and peroxisome proliferator-activated receptor δ regulate cholesterol transport in murine cholangiocytes. *Hepatology.* (2012) 56:2288–96. doi: 10.1002/hep.25919
25. Mukundan L, Odegaard JI, Morel CR, Heredia JE, Mwangi JW, Ricardo-Gonzalez RR, et al. PPAR-δ senses and orchestrates clearance of apoptotic cells to promote tolerance. *Nat Med.* (2009) 15:1266–72. doi: 10.1038/nm.2048
26. Harada K, Isse K, Kamihira T, Shimoda S, Nakanuma Y. Th1 cytokine-induced downregulation of PPARγ in human biliary cells relates to cholangitis in primary biliary cirrhosis. *Hepatology.* (2005) 41:1329–38. doi: 10.1002/hep.20705
27. Nozaki Y, Harada K, Sanzen T, Nakanuma Y. PPARγ ligand attenuates portal inflammation in the MRL-lpr mouse: a new strategy to restrain cholangiopathy in primary biliary cirrhosis. *Med Mol Morphol.* (2013) 46:153–9. doi: 10.1007/s00795-013-0017-0
28. Reig A, Sesé P, Parés A. Effects of bezafibrate on outcome and pruritus in primary biliary cholangitis with suboptimal ursodeoxycholic acid response. *Am J Gastroenterol.* (2018) 113:49–55. doi: 10.1038/ajg.2017.287
29. Hegade VS, Khanna A, Walker LJ, Wong L-L, Dyson JK, Jones DEJ. Long-term fenofibrate treatment in primary biliary cholangitis improves biochemistry but not the UK-PBC risk score. *Dig Dis Sci.* (2016) 61:3037–44. doi: 10.1007/s10620-016-4250-y
30. Han XF, Wang QX, Liu Y, You ZR, Bian ZL, Qiu DK, et al. Efficacy of fenofibrate in Chinese patients with primary biliary cirrhosis partially responding to ursodeoxycholic acid therapy. *J Dig Dis.* (2012) 13:219–24. doi: 10.1111/j.1751-2980.2012.00574.x
31. Liberopoulos EN, Florentin M, Elisaf MS, Mikhailidis DP, Tsianos E. Fenofibrate in primary biliary cirrhosis: a pilot study. *Open Cardiovasc Med J.* (2010) 4:120–6. doi: 10.2174/1874192401004010120
32. Cheung AC, Lapointe-Shaw L, Kowgier M, Meza-Cardona J, Hirschfield GM, Janssen HLA, et al. Combined ursodeoxycholic acid (UDCA) and fenofibrate in primary biliary cholangitis patients with incomplete UDCA response may improve outcomes. *Aliment Pharmacol Ther.* (2016) 43:283–93. doi: 10.1111/apt.13465
33. Levy C, Peter JA, Nelson DR, Keach J, Petz J, Cabrera R, et al. Pilot study: fenofibrate for patients with primary biliary cirrhosis and an incomplete response to ursodeoxycholic acid. *Aliment Pharmacol Ther.* (2011) 33:235–42. doi: 10.1111/j.1365-2036.2010.04512.x
34. Haczeyni F, Wang H, Barn V, Mridha AR, Yeh MM, Haigh WG, et al. The selective peroxisome proliferator-activated receptor-delta agonist seladelpar reverses nonalcoholic steatohepatitis pathology by abrogating lipotoxicity in diabetic obese mice. *Hepatol Commun.* (2017) 1:663–74. doi: 10.1002/hep4.1072
35. Jones D, Boudes PF, Swain MG, Bowlus CL, Galambos MR, Bacon BR, et al. Seladelpar (MBX-8025), a selective PPAR-δ agonist, in patients with primary biliary cholangitis with an inadequate response to ursodeoxycholic acid: a double-blind, randomised, placebo-controlled, phase 2, proof-of-concept study. *Lancet Gastroenterol Hepatol.* (2017) 2:716–26. doi: 10.1016/S2468-1253(17)30246-7
36. Mizuno S, Hirano K, Isayama H, Watanabe T, Yamamoto N, Nakai Y, et al. Prospective study of bezafibrate for the treatment of primary sclerosing cholangitis. *J Hepatobiliary Pancreat Sci.* (2015) 22:766–70. doi: 10.1002/jhbp.281
37. Mizuno S, Hirano K, Tada M, Yamamoto K, Yashima Y, Yagioka H, et al. Bezafibrate for the treatment of primary sclerosing cholangitis. *J Gastroenterol.* (2010) 45:758–62. doi: 10.1007/s00535-010-0204-x
38. Beuers U, Hohenester S, de Buy Wenniger LJM, Kremer AE, Jansen PLM, Elferink RPJO. The biliary HCO_3^- umbrella: a unifying hypothesis on pathogenetic and therapeutic aspects of fibrosing cholangiopathies. *Hepatology.* (2010) 52:1489–96. doi: 10.1002/hep.23810
39. Hohenester S, Maillette de Buy Wenniger L, Paulusma CC, van Vliet SJ, Jefferson DM, Oude Elferink RP, et al. A biliary HCO3− umbrella constitutes a protective mechanism against bile acid-induced injury in human cholangiocytes. *Hepatology.* (2012) 55:173–83. doi: 10.1002/hep.24691
40. Banales JM, Sáez E, Úriz M, Sarvide S, Urribarri AD, Splinter P, Tietz Bogert PS, et al. Up-regulation of microRNA 506 leads to decreased Cl−/HCO3− anion exchanger 2 expression in biliary epithelium of patients with primary biliary cirrhosis. *Hepatology.* (2012) 56:687–97. doi: 10.1002/hep.25691
41. Rodrigues PM, Perugorria MJ, Santos-Laso A, Bujanda L, Beuers U, Banales JM. Primary biliary cholangitis: a tale of epigenetically-induced secretory failure? *J Hepatol.* (2018) 69:1371–83. doi: 10.1016/j.jhep.2018.08.020
42. Fickert P, Fuchsbichler A, Wagner M, Zollner G, Kaser A, Tilg H, et al. Regurgitation of bile acids from leaky bile ducts causes sclerosing cholangitis in Mdr2 (Abcb4) knockout mice. *Gastroenterology.* (2004) 127:261–74. doi: 10.1053/j.gastro.2004.04.009
43. Fickert P, Wagner M, Marschall HU, Fuchsbichler A, Zollner G, Tsybrovskyy O, et al. 24-norUrsodeoxycholic acid is superior to ursodeoxycholic acid in the treatment of sclerosing cholangitis in Mdr2 (Abcb4) knockout mice. *Gastroenterology.* (2006) 130:465–81. doi: 10.1053/j.gastro.2005.10.018
44. Fickert P, Hirschfield GM, Denk G, Marschall HU, Altorjay I, Färkkilä M, et al. norUrsodeoxycholic acid improves cholestasis in primary sclerosing cholangitis. *J Hepatol.* (2017) 67:549–58. doi: 10.1016/j.jhep.2017.05.009
45. Gong Y, Christensen E, Gluud C. Azathioprine for primary biliary cirrhosis. *Cochrane Database Syst Rev.* (2007) 18:CD006000. doi: 10.1002/14651858.CD006000.pub2
46. Wolfhagen FHJ, van Hoogstraten HJF, Buuren HR va., van Berge-Henegouwen GP, ten Kate FJW, Hop WCJ, et al. Triple therapy with ursodeoxycholic acid, prednisone and azathioprine in primary biliary cirrhosis: a 1-year randomized, placebo-controlled study. *J Hepatol.* (1998) 29:736–42. doi: 10.1016/S0168-8278(98)80254-7
47. Treiber G, Malfertheiner P. Mycophenolate mofetil for the treatment of primary biliary cirrhosis in patients with an incomplete response to ursodeoxycholic acid. *J Clin Gastroenterol.* (2005) 39:168–71. doi: 10.1097/01.mcg.0000177235.36640.21
48. Wiesner RH, Ludwig J, Lindor KD, Jorgensen RA, Baldus WP, Homburger HA, et al. A controlled trial of cyclosporine in the treatment of primary biliary cirrhosis. *N Engl J Med.* (1990) 322:1419–24. doi: 10.1056/NEJM199005173222003
49. Combes B, Emerson SS, Flye NL, Munoz SJ, Luketic VA, Mayo MJ, et al. Methotrexate (MTX) plus ursodeoxycholic acid (UDCA) in the treatment of primary biliary cirrhosis. *Hepatology.* (2005) 42:1184–93. doi: 10.1002/hep.20897
50. Leuschner M, Maier K, Schlichting J, Strahl S, Herrmann G, Dahm HH, et al. Oral budesonide and ursodeoxycholic acid for treatment of primary biliary cirrhosis: results of a prospective double-blind trial. *Gastroenterology.* (1999) 117:918–25. doi: 10.1016/S0016-5085(99)70351-3
51. Rautiainen H, Kärkkäinen P, Karvonen A-L, Nurmi H, Pikkarainen P, Nuutinen H, et al. Budesonide combined with UDCA to improve liver histology in primary biliary cirrhosis: A three-year randomized trial. *Hepatology.* (2005) 41:747–52. doi: 10.1002/hep.20646
52. Angulo P, Jorgensen RA, Keach JC, Dickson ER, Smith C, Lindor KD. Oral budesonide in the treatment of patients with primary biliary cirrhosis with a suboptimal response to ursodeoxycholic acid. *Hepatology.* (2000) 31:318–23. doi: 10.1002/hep.510310209
53. Karlsen TH, Folseraas T, Thorburn D, Vesterhus M. Primary sclerosing cholangitis - a comprehensive review. *J Hepatol.* (2017) 67:1298–323. doi: 10.1016/j.jhep.2017.07.022
54. Tsuda M, Moritoki Y, Lian ZX, Zhang W, Yoshida K, Wakabayashi K, et al. Biochemical and immunologic effects of rituximab in patients with primary biliary cirrhosis and an incomplete response to ursodeoxycholic acid. *Hepatology.* (2012) 55:512–21. doi: 10.1002/hep.24748
55. Myers RP, Swain MG, Lee SS, Shaheen AAM, Burak KW. B-cell depletion with rituximab in patients with primary biliary cirrhosis refractory to ursodeoxycholic acid. *Am J Gastroenterol.* (2013) 108:933–41. doi: 10.1038/ajg.2013.51

56. Hirschfield GM, Gershwin ME, Strauss R, Mayo MJ, Levy C, Zou B, et al. Ustekinumab for patients with primary biliary cholangitis who have an inadequate response to ursodeoxycholic acid: a proof-of-concept study. *Hepatology.* (2016) 64:189–99. doi: 10.1002/hep.28359
57. Bowlus CL, Yang G-X, Liu CH, Johnson CR, Dhaliwal SS, Frank D, et al. Therapeutic trials of biologics in primary biliary cholangitis: an open label study of abatacept and review of the literature. *J Autoimmun.* (2019) 101:26–34. doi: 10.1016/j.jaut.2019.04.005
58. Villarino A V, Kanno Y, O'Shea JJ. Mechanisms and consequences of Jak-STAT signaling in the immune system. *Nat Immunol.* (2017) 18:374–84. doi: 10.1038/ni.3691
59. Smolen JS, Landewé R, Breedveld FC, Buch M, Burmester G, Dougados M, et al. EULAR recommendations for the management of rheumatoid arthritis with synthetic and biological disease-modifying antirheumatic drugs: 2013 update. *Ann Rheum Dis.* (2014) 73:492–509. doi: 10.1136/annrheumdis-2013-204573
60. Koyama Y, Brenner DA. Liver inflammation and fibrosis. *J Clin Invest.* (2017) 127:55–64. doi: 10.1172/JCI88881
61. Pinzani M, Luong TV. Pathogenesis of biliary fibrosis. *Biochim Biophys Acta Mol Basis Dis.* (2018) 1864:1279–83. doi: 10.1016/j.bbadis.2017.07.026
62. Schuppan D, Ashfaq-Khan M, Yang AT, Kim YO. Liver fibrosis: direct antifibrotic agents and targeted therapies. *Matrix Biol.* (2018) 68–9:435–51. doi: 10.1016/j.matbio.2018.04.006
63. Miura K, Yang L, van Rooijen N, Ohnishi H, Seki E. Hepatic recruitment of macrophages promotes nonalcoholic steatohepatitis through CCR2. *Am J Physiol Gastrointest Liver Physiol.* (2012) 302:G1310–21. doi: 10.1152/ajpgi.00365.2011
64. Berres M-L, Koenen RR, Rueland A, Zaldivar MM, Heinrichs D, Sahin H, et al. Antagonism of the chemokine Ccl5 ameliorates experimental liver fibrosis in mice. *J Clin Invest.* (2010) 120:4129–40. doi: 10.1172/JCI41732
65. Yu D, Cai S-Y, Mennone A, Vig P, Boyer JL. Cenicriviroc, a cytokine receptor antagonist, potentiates all-trans retinoic acid in reducing liver injury in cholestatic rodents. *Liver Int.* (2018) 38:1128–38. doi: 10.1111/liv.13698
66. Friedman SL, Ratziu V, Harrison SA, Abdelmalek MF, Aithal GP, Caballeria J, et al. A randomized, placebo-controlled trial of cenicriviroc for treatment of nonalcoholic steatohepatitis with fibrosis. *Hepatology.* (2018) 67:1754–67. doi: 10.1002/hep.29477
67. Lambeth JD. NOX enzymes and the biology of reactive oxygen. *Nat Rev Immunol.* (2004) 4:181–9. doi: 10.1038/nri1312
68. Campbell EL, Colgan SP. Control and dysregulation of redox signalling in the gastrointestinal tract. *Nat Rev Gastroenterol Hepatol.* (2018) 16:106–20. doi: 10.1038/s41575-018-0079-5
69. Barnes JL, Gorin Y. Myofibroblast differentiation during fibrosis: role of NAD(P)H oxidases. *Kidney Int.* (2011) 79:944–56. doi: 10.1038/ki.2010.516
70. Cui W, Matsuno K, Iwata K, Ibi M, Matsumoto M, Zhang J, et al. NOX1/nicotinamide adenine dinucleotide phosphate, reduced form (NADPH) oxidase promotes proliferation of stellate cells and aggravates liver fibrosis induced by bile duct ligation. *Hepatology.* (2011) 54:949–58. doi: 10.1002/hep.24465
71. Jiang JX, Chen X, Serizawa N, Szyndralewiez C, Page P, Schröder K, et al. Liver fibrosis and hepatocyte apoptosis are attenuated by GKT137831, a novel NOX4/NOX1 inhibitor *in vivo*. *Free Radic Biol Med.* (2012) 53:289–96. doi: 10.1016/j.freeradbiomed.2012.05.007
72. Kunutsor SK. Gamma-glutamyltransferase-friend or foe within? *Liver Int.* (2016) 36:1723–34. doi: 10.1111/liv.13221
73. Lynch S V, Pedersen O. The human intestinal microbiome in health and disease. *N Engl J Med.* (2016) 375:2369–79. doi: 10.1056/NEJMra1600266
74. Zmora N, Suez J, Elinav E. You are what you eat: diet, health and the gut microbiota. *Nat Rev Gastroenterol Hepatol.* (2018) 16: 35–56. doi: 10.1038/s41575-018-0061-2
75. Clemente JC, Manasson J, Scher JU. The role of the gut microbiome in systemic inflammatory disease. *BMJ.* (2018) 360:j5145. doi: 10.1136/bmj.j5145
76. Tripathi A, Debelius J, Brenner DA, Karin M, Loomba R, Schnabl B, et al. Erratum to: the gut-liver axis and the intersection with the microbiome (Nature Reviews Gastroenterology & Hepatology, (2018), 15, 7, (397-411), 10.1038/s41575-018-0011-z). *Nat Rev Gastroenterol Hepatol.* (2018) 15:785. doi: 10.1038/s41575-018-0011-z
77. Woodhouse CA, Patel VC, Singanayagam A, Shawcross DL. Review article: the gut microbiome as a therapeutic target in the pathogenesis and treatment of chronic liver disease. *Aliment Pharmacol Ther.* (2018) 47:192–202. doi: 10.1111/apt.14397
78. Tang R, Wei Y, Li Y, Chen W, Chen H, Wang Q, et al. Gut microbial profile is altered in primary biliary cholangitis and partially restored after UDCA therapy. *Gut.* (2018) 67:534–41. doi: 10.1136/gutjnl-2016-313332
79. Sabino J, Vieira-Silva S, Machiels K, Joossens M, Falony G, Ballet V, et al. Primary sclerosing cholangitis is characterised by intestinal dysbiosis independent from IBD. *Gut.* (2016) 65:1681–9. doi: 10.1136/gutjnl-2015-311004
80. Ungaro F, Massimino L, D'Alessio S, Danese S. The gut virome in inflammatory bowel disease pathogenesis: from metagenomics to novel therapeutic approaches. *United Eur Gastroenterol J.* (2019) 7:999–1007. doi: 10.1177/2050640619876787
81. Lemoinne S, Kemgang A, Ben Belkacem K, Straube M, Jegou S, Corpechot C, et al. Fungi participate in the dysbiosis of gut microbiota in patients with primary sclerosing cholangitis. *Gut.* (2019) 69:92–102. doi: 10.1136/gutjnl-2018-317791
82. Tabibian JH, O'Hara SP, Trussoni CE, Tietz PS, Splinter PL, Mounajjed T, et al. Absence of the intestinal microbiota exacerbates hepatobiliary disease in a murine model of primary sclerosing cholangitis. *Hepatology.* (2016) 63:185–96. doi: 10.1002/hep.27927
83. Hov J, Karlsen T. The microbiome in primary sclerosing cholangitis: current evidence and potential concepts. *Semin Liver Dis.* (2017) 37:314–31. doi: 10.1055/s-0037-1608801
84. Tabibian JH, Weeding E, Jorgensen RA, Petz JL, Keach JC, Talwalkar JA, et al. Randomised clinical trial: vancomycin or metronidazole in patients with primary sclerosing cholangitis - a pilot study. *Aliment Pharmacol Ther.* (2013) 37:604–12. doi: 10.1111/apt.12232
85. Silveira MG, Torok NJ, Gossard AA, Keach JC, Jorgensen RA, Petz JL, et al. Minocycline in the treatment of patients with primary sclerosing cholangitis: results of a pilot study. *Am J Gastroenterol.* (2009) 104:83–8. doi: 10.1038/ajg.2008.14
86. Rahimpour S, Nasiri-Toosi M, Khalili H, Daryani NE, Taromlou MKN, Azizi Z. A triple blinded, randomized, placebo-controlled clinical trial to evaluate the efficacy and safety of oral vancomycin in primary sclerosing cholangitis: a pilot study. *J Gastrointest Liver Dis.* (2016) 25:457–64. doi: 10.15403/jgld.2014.1121.254.rah
87. Finlay BB. Are noncommunicable diseases communicable? *Science (80-).* (2020) 367:250–1. doi: 10.1126/science.aaz3834
88. Elinav E, Strowig T, Kau AL, Henao-Mejia J, Thaiss CA, Booth CJ, et al. NLRP6 inflammasome regulates colonic microbial ecology and risk for colitis. *Cell.* (2011) 145:745–57. doi: 10.1016/j.cell.2011.04.022
89. Wang Y, Wiesnoski DH, Helmink BA, Gopalakrishnan V, Choi K, DuPont HL, et al. Fecal microbiota transplantation for refractory immune checkpoint inhibitor-associated colitis. *Nat Med.* (2018) 24:1804–8. doi: 10.1038/s41591-018-0238-9
90. D'Haens GR, Jobin C. Fecal microbial transplantation for diseases beyond recurrent clostridium difficile infection. *Gastroenterology.* (2019) 157:624–36. doi: 10.1053/j.gastro.2019.04.053
91. Hvas CL, Dahl Jørgensen SM, Jørgensen SP, Storgaard M, Lemming L, Hansen MM, et al. Fecal microbiota transplantation is superior to fidaxomicin for treatment of recurrent clostridium difficile infection. *Gastroenterology.* (2019) 156:1324–32.e3. doi: 10.1053/j.gastro.2018.12.019
92. Allegretti JR, Kassam Z, Carrellas M, Mullish BH, Marchesi JR, Pechlivanis A, et al. Fecal microbiota transplantation in patients with primary sclerosing cholangitis: a pilot clinical trial. *Am J Gastroenterol.* (2019) 114:1071–9. doi: 10.14309/ajg.0000000000000115
93. Spadoni I, Zagato E, Bertocchi A, Paolinelli R, Hot E, Di Sabatino A, et al. A gut-vascular barrier controls the systemic dissemination of bacteria. *Science (80-).* (2015) 350:830–4. doi: 10.1126/science.aad0135
94. Habtezion A, Nguyen LP, Hadeiba H, Butcher EC. Leukocyte trafficking to the small intestine and colon. *Gastroenterology.* (2016) 150:340–54. doi: 10.1053/j.gastro.2015.10.046

95. Grant AJ, Lalor PF, Hübscher SG, Briskin M, Adams DH. MAdCAM-1 expressed in chronic inflammatory liver disease supports mucosal lymphocyte adhesion to hepatic endothelium (MAdCAM-1 in chronic inflammatory liver disease). *Hepatology.* (2001) 33:1065–72. doi: 10.1053/jhep.2001.24231
96. Lynch KD, Chapman RW, Keshav S, Montano-Loza AJ, Mason AL, Kremer AE, et al. Effects of vedolizumab in patients with primary sclerosing cholangitis and inflammatory bowel diseases. *Clin Gastroenterol Hepatol.* (2019) 18:179–87.e6. doi: 10.1016/j.cgh.2019.05.013
97. Trivedi PJ, Tickle J, Vesterhus MN, Eddowes PJ, Bruns T, Vainio J, et al. Vascular adhesion protein-1 is elevated in primary sclerosing cholangitis, is predictive of clinical outcome and facilitates recruitment of gut-tropic lymphocytes to liver in a substrate-dependent manner. *Gut.* (2018) 67:1135–45. doi: 10.1136/gutjnl-2016-312354
98. Bossen L, Gerussi A, Lygoura V, Mells GF, Carbone M, Invernizzi P. Support of precision medicine through risk-stratification in autoimmune liver diseases - histology, scoring systems, and non-invasive markers. *Autoimmun Rev.* (2018) 17:854–65. doi: 10.1016/j.autrev.2018.02.013
99. Karczewski KJ, Snyder MP. Integrative omics for health and disease. *Nat Rev Genet.* (2018) 19:299–310. doi: 10.1038/nrg.2018.4
100. Sia D, Llovet JM. Liver cancer: translating "-omics" results into precision medicine for hepatocellular carcinoma. *Nat Rev Gastroenterol Hepatol.* (2017) 14:571–2. doi: 10.1038/nrgastro.2017.103
101. Schüssler-Fiorenza Rose SM, Contrepois K, Moneghetti KJ, Zhou W, Mishra T, Mataraso S, et al. A longitudinal big data approach for precision health. *Nat Med.* (2019) 25:792–804. doi: 10.1038/s41591-019-0414-6
102. Menche J, Guney E, Sharma A, Branigan PJ, Loza MJ, Baribaud F, et al. Integrating personalized gene expression profiles into predictive disease-associated gene pools. *NPJ Syst Biol Appl.* (2017) 3:10. doi: 10.1038/s41540-017-0009-0
103. Zhou W, Sailani MR, Contrepois K, Zhou Y, Ahadi S, Leopold SR, et al. Longitudinal multi-omics of host-microbe dynamics in prediabetes. *Nature.* (2019) 569:663–71. doi: 10.1038/s41586-019-1236-x
104. Chen R, Mias GI, Li-Pook-Than J, Jiang L, Lam HYK, Chen R, et al. Personal omics profiling reveals dynamic molecular and medical phenotypes. *Cell.* (2012) 148:1293–307. doi: 10.1016/j.cell.2012.02.009
105. Seymour CW, Kennedy JN, Wang S, Chang CH, Elliott CF, Xu Z, et al. Derivation, validation, and potential treatment implications of novel clinical phenotypes for sepsis. *JAMA.* (2019) 321:2003–17. doi: 10.1001/jama.2019.5791
106. Ahlqvist E, Storm P, Käräjämäki A, Martinell M, Dorkhan M, Carlsson A, et al. Novel subgroups of adult-onset diabetes and their association with outcomes: a data-driven cluster analysis of six variables. *Lancet Diabetes Endocrinol.* (2018) 6:361–9. doi: 10.1016/S2213-8587(18)30051-2
107. Topol EJ. High-performance medicine: the convergence of human and artificial intelligence. *Nat Med.* (2019) 25:44–56. doi: 10.1038/s41591-018-0300-7
108. Littmann M, Selig K, Cohen-Lavi L, Frank Y, Hönigschmid P, Kataka E, et al. Validity of machine learning in biology and medicine increased through collaborations across fields of expertise. *Nat Mach Intell.* (2020) 38:991–4. doi: 10.1038/s42256-019-0139-8
109. Wagner M, Fickert P. Time for the dawn of multimodal therapies and the dusk for mono-therapeutic trials for cholestatic liver diseases? *Liver Int.* (2018) 38:991–4. doi: 10.1111/liv.13744

2

Liver Failure of Wilson's Disease With Manifestations Similar to Porphyria and Uncommon *ATP7B* Gene Mutation

Ju Zou [1,2†], *Ying-Hao Wang* [3†], *Ling Wang* [1,2] *and Ruo-Chan Chen* [1,2*]

[1] *Department of Infectious Disease, Xiangya Hospital, Central South University, Changsha, China,* [2] *Hunan Key Laboratory of Viral Hepatitis, Xiangya Hospital, Central South University, Changsha, China,* [3] *Department of Ophthalmology, The Second Xiangya Hospital, Central South University, Changsha, China*

***Correspondence:**
Ruo-Chan Chen
84172332@qq.com

† *These authors have contributed equally to this work and share first authorship*

Background: Wilson's disease (WD) is a rare condition; its diagnosis is challenging owing to a wide spectrum of *ATP7B* genotypes and variable clinical phenotypes, along with environmental factors. Few cases of WD with presentation of skin lesions and acute neurovisceral symptoms have been reported in the literature. To our knowledge, this is the first reported case of WD with an uncommon *ATP7B* gene mutation and rare symptoms of photosensitivity, sensation abnormality, and skin eruption occurring in a 19-year-old woman.

Case presentation: We report the case of a 19-year-old woman with WD presenting with liver failure, skin manifestations, and acute neurovisceral symptoms.The rare mutation in intron 1 of ATP7B (c.51+2T > G) was further confirmed by gene sequencing. The patients' symptoms improved after administration of penicillamine and zinc therapy combined with plasma exchange. She received long-term penicillamine treatment, and her liver function was within the normal range at 1 year after discharge. However, she underwent liver transplantation at 1.5 years after discharge.

Conclusions: We present a case of WD with a novel *ATP7B* gene mutation that may serve as a reference to generalists and specialists in hepatology or neurology of the rare clinical characteristics of WD, to prevent misdiagnosis and aid in the early diagnosis and treatment of the condition.

Keywords: ATP7B, copper storage disease, liver failure, porphyria, Wilson's disease

INTRODUCTION

Wilson's disease (WD), also termed hepatolenticular degeneration, was first reported by Kinnear Wilson in 1912. WD is an autosomal recessive inherited disease, which is caused by a dysfunction of the *ATP7B* gene located on chromosome 13q14.3 (~80 kb). The *ATP7B* gene is composed of 21 exons and 20 introns encoding a copper-transporting P-type ATPase containing 1,465 amino acids that comprise six copper binding domains, eight transmembrane domains, and one ATP loop (1). It plays a key role in transforming apoceruloplasmin into ceruloplasmin and evacuating excessive copper into biliary canaliculi. Defects of ATP7B will result in an overdose of copper accumulation in many vital organs, primarily in the liver and brain (2). The incidence of WD is between 1 in 30,000 and 1 in 100,000 people worldwide (3). However, reports of the disease occurring in the Chinese population have been increasing (4).

Additionally, patients with WD present with variable clinical manifestations, including hepatic abnormality and neurological and psychiatric disturbances. Liver damage includes decompensated chronic liver disease, chronic hepatitis, and fulminant hepatic failure, leading to severe coagulopathy, infections, hepatorenal syndrome, and hepatic encephalopathy. However, less common clinical features include renal disease, osteoarthritis (5), and pancreatitis (6). Some reports have shown that different *ATP7B* mutation genotypes cause distinctive clinical phenotypes (7). Consequently, WD is easily misdiagnosed as other diseases owing to the heterogeneity of its clinical presentations and loci mutations.

Porphyria, a term for a group of metabolic diseases, leads to an overload of porphyrins and their precursors. Acute intermittent porphyria (AIP) is characterized by acute neurovisceral symptoms and abdominal pain predominantly (8), while porphyria cutanea tarda (PCT) is characterized by the development of blisters and sores after light exposure (9). WD presenting originally as skin lesions and acute neurovisceral symptoms similar to AIP or PCT has been rarely reported.

Here, we report a case of a young Chinese woman with WD and an uncommon *ATP7B* gene defect, similar to porphyria.The patient presented with photosensitivity of rash, paresthesia, acute neurovisceral symptoms of stomachache, and exacerbation of liver failure. Additionally, we present relevant literature to discuss our conclusions.

CASE PRESENTATION

A 19-year-old woman was admitted to the Department of Infectious Diseases, Xiangya Hospital of Central South University on September 14, 2019, with the chief complaint of body numbness for 9 days and stomachache with jaundice for 5 days. She developed acute burning sensations on the skin of the forehead, face, neck, and palms of both hands that progressed into numbness, especially in the proximal joints on September 5, 2019. The above symptoms progressively worsened, with blisters and pruritus on sun-exposed areas. She experienced paroxysmal colic in the upper right abdomen, with no nausea, vomiting, fever and diarrhea on September 11, 2019, and presented with jaundice gradually. After a series of treatments, including anti-inflammatory, antispasmodic, liver protective, and rehydration medications at the local hospital, the symptoms of abdominal pain were relieved, jaundice was intensified and the total bilirubin level continued to rise (36.67 mg/dL). She was then referred to our hospital for further treatment.

During her pregnancy in February, 2019, the patient was diagnosed with abnormal liver function and took ursodeoxycholic acid (0.25 mg TID) irregularly, resulting in the continued increase of her aspartate aminotransferase (AST) and alanine aminotransferase (ALT) levels. In July, 2019, cesarean delivery was performed on the primigravida at 36 weeks and 5 days of gestation because of misdiagnosis of intrahepatic cholestasis of pregnancy at a local hospital. The baby boy's weight was 2.7 kg, with an Apgar score of 10. The patient had no history of drug abuse or known allergies, and had never smoked or drank alcohol. She had no history of liver disease or similar symptoms in her families. Notable examination findings included anemia, severe jaundice, liver palms, hepatosplenomegaly, belly bulge, and shifting dullness. Remarkably, some scattered skin rashes with pigmentation were present on her scalp and forehead.

After the patient was admitted, laboratory findings revealed mild erythropenia, moderate hypochromia, and significantly elevated total bilirubin (27.13 mg/dL) and aminotransferase (AST > ALT) levels. Poor hepatic synthetic function revealed low levels of total protein (58.5 g/L) and albumin (32.9 g/L). Additionally, prothrombin time was prolonged and prothrombin activity was severely decreased to 34.44% (**Table 1**). Severe and prominent liver damage was observed in this patient, whereas hepatitis B virus, autoimmune hepatitis-related antibodies, and Budd-Chiari syndrome were ruled out, and the patient had no history of alcohol and use of drugs as treatment for liver lesions. Inherited metabolic diseases were considered first because of the young age of onset with obvious liver enlargement and cirrhosis on abdominal ultrasound examination. Porphyria was suspected based on the initial symptoms of photosensitivity, acute stomachache, and pink urine under Wood's lamp illumination. However, genetic sequencing without porphyria-associated gene mutations excluded the diagnosis.

The diagnosis of WD was established based on the presence of Coombs negative hemolytic anemia, Kayser-Fleischer rings on slit lamp examination (**Figure 1**), low level of serum ceruloplasmin, and obviously elevated levels of 24-h urine copper (3,804 μg/24 h) (**Table 1**). The whole exon region (about 20,000 genes) in the human genome sequencing was performed on the Illumina MiSeq next-generation sequencing (NGS) and Sanger sequencing. The former presented a possible loss of heterozygosity in the area of chr13q14.3 (52158814-53624916) with a length of 1.47 Mb. The latter revealed a novel heterozygote splicing mutation c.51+2T>G within intron 1 of the ATP7B (13q14.3|NM_000053.3) (**Figure 1A**), which was evaluated as likely pathogenic according to the American College of Medical Genetics and Genomics (ACMG) (10) criteria. The evidence of pathogenicity of the this mutation is PVS1+PM2+PP3+PP5.According to the scoring system developed at the 8th International Meeting on Wilson's disease, Leipzig 2001 (11), the patient received a score of 8 points in total, which further confirmed the diagnosis of WD.

Treatments included ornithine aspartate for preventing hepatic encephalopathy and albumin infusion combined with hydragogue for reducing ascites. Non-biological artificial liver treatment (plasmapheresis) was used to remove harmful substances and relieve hemolytic crisis and hepatic failure. For WD, the patient was treated with oral penicillamine (increased to 0.9 g/d) and zinc (0.15 mg/d). Plasmapheresis combined with chelation therapy was effective, because the ceruloplasmin level returned to the normal range and serum bilirubin and

TABLE 1 | Laboratory results of the patient at the first day of admission and 1.5 years after discharge and a data comparison of another WD patient with a different mutation.

Laboratory tests	The patient of this case		The control patient
	First day of admission	1.5 years after discharge (recently)	First day of admission
WBC (× 10^9/L) (3.5–9.5)	6.6	9.24	1.9
N (× 10^9/L) (1.8–6.3)	5.0	4.86	1.4
RBC (× 10^{12}/L) (3.80–5.10)	2.55	5.15	4.36
Hb (g/L) (115–150)	89	145	127
PLT (× 10^9/L) (125–350)	174	288	17
ALT (U/L) (7–40)	42.5	24.7	17.6
AST (U/L) (13–35)	61.7	19.6	26
Γ-GGT (U/L) (7–45)	157.6	52.3	104.7
TB (μmol/L) (1.7–17.1)	464.0	9.6	8
CB (μmol/L) (0–6.8)	255.8	2.9	4.7
TP (g/L) (65–85)	58.5	71	63.1
Alb (g/L) (40–55)	32.9	45.2	40.1
PT (s) (10–16)	23.7	12.4	14.4
PTA (%) (70–140)	34.44	119	82
INR (0.8–1.2)	1.91	0.91	1.15
APTT (s) (20–43)	70.9	36.5	39.7
Fibrinogen (g/L) (2–4)	1.47	2.88	2.1
C3 (mg/L) (790–1,520)	254	n.a.	612
C4 (mg/L) (100–400)	79.8	n.a.	142
Ceruloplasmin (mg/L) (210–530)	66.1	n.a.	33.2
24-H urine copper (μg/24 h) (15–30)	3,804	n.a.	2,899
Coombs test (–)	–	n.a.	n.a.

n.a., not available; WBC, white blood cells; N, neutrophils; RBC, red blood cells; Hb, hemoglobin; PLT, platelets; ALT, alanine aminotransferase; AST, aspartate transaminase; γ-GGT, gamma-glutamyltransferase; TB, total bilirubin; CB, conjugated bilirubin; TP, total protein; Alb, albumin; PT, prothrombin time; PTA, prothrombin activity; INR, international standard ratio; APTT, activated partial thromboplastin time.

hemoglobin levels were normal on the day of her discharge. Notably, the patient's abdominal pain was relieved and the scattered papules on the scalp and forehead disappeared after a comprehensive treatment, which possibly suggested that photosensitivity and stomachache were symptoms of WD. However, the treatment of WD is life-long and should be continued after discharge to maintain normal liver functioning.

The patient had normal liver functioning during follow-up at 1 year after discharge, which was maintained by treatment with oral penicillamine (0.25 g). However, her liver function deteriorated after drug withdrawal without the authorization of her attending physicians at the latest follow-up; thus, she had to undergo liver transplantation. At the time of writing, specifically at 1.5 years after discharge, she is in a good condition (**Table 1**).

DISCUSSION

Prominent cirrhosis and hepatomegaly in this young patient on abdominal ultrasound suggested a long course of illness. Porphyria was considered first based on her outstanding symptoms of skin damage and stomachache. Porphyria, caused by the absence of enzyme activity in the heme biosynthetic pathway, leads to the increased concentration of porphyrin or its precursors (12). Some patients may present with chronic liver damage and cholelithiasis because of the excessive release of protoporphyrin into the biliary tract (13). Therefore, porphyrin accumulation in the liver and biliary tract leads to liver damage, ranging from minor liver biochemical abnormalities of elevated levels of bilirubin and transaminase to liver carcinoma (14). In addition, acute hepatic porphyrias present with episodic and acute neurovisceral symptoms (8), while photosensitivity may occur mainly in cutaneous porphyria (9). The clinical manifestations of porphyria hepatica are atypical and diversified. Specific diagnostic tests are few, and most of them show negative results. Therefore, the clinical misdiagnosis rate of WD is high. In this case, the diagnosis of porphyria was excluded using gene sequencing. However, attention must be given to such confounding manifestations to avoid misdiagnosis.

Studies focusing on characterizing mutations within the *ATP7B* gene have soared recently. Approximately 1019 different mutations have been reported in the *ATP7B* gene from the Human Genome Organization database (http://www.hgmd.cf.ac.uk/ac/index.php), updated in April, 2019. Among them, single-nucleotide missense/nonsense mutations are the most common, followed by insertions/deletions, and a few of splice site mutations. WD gene mutations are with significant geographic variations. The p.His1069Gln is found mostly in Northern America (15) and Europe (16), while the p.Arg778Leu is the most common in East Asians (17, 18). WD presents multiple phenotypic manifestations due to the combined action of genotype, diet, and environment (19). Multiple previous studies on the association between genotypes and clinical features showed that p.Arg778Leu is associated with a young age of onset and low levels of ceruloplasmin and serum copper, and both p.Arg919Gly and p.Thr935Met indicate high levels of ceruloplasmin (20). Another research suggested that a p.H1069Q variant is related to late onset and neurologic presentation of WD (21).

In the present case, the pathogenic mutation c.51 + 2T > G and loss of heterozygosity are compound heterozygotes on the two chromosomes of the proband, inherited from her father and new mutation of her own. The mutation c.51 + 2T > G is a new mutation that was first identified in 2019. The mutation is located in intron one, which predicted results in exon skipping, leading to a disorder of the encoded protein and loss of its normal function (22). As a result, *ATP7B* ATPase cannot be encoded, and copper accumulates. Hence, it could be classified as "pathogenic variants" of WD according to ACMG Standards and Guidelines (10). It has been confirmed previously that splice variants can alter the order of intron removal, thereby leading to exon skipping (23). One study had found that a splice mutation (c.561-3T>C) of intron 6, in the *POC1B* gene, in which exon 6 is partly skipped (24). Based on the findings reported in the literature (25) and those of our case, mRNA sequencing analysis revealed that deep intron deletion on both sides of the affected

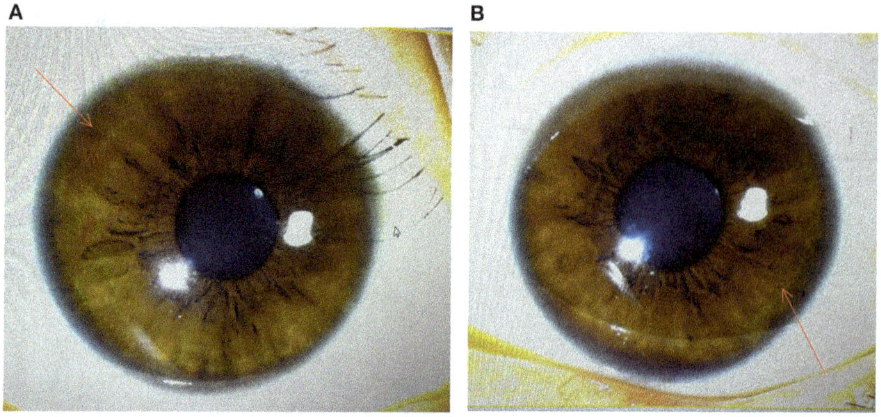

FIGURE 1 | Image obtained during slit lamp examination showing characteristic Kayser–Fleischer (K–F) ring (arrowhead) at the margin of the cornea and scler. **(A)** the image of the left eye; **(B)** the image of the right eye.

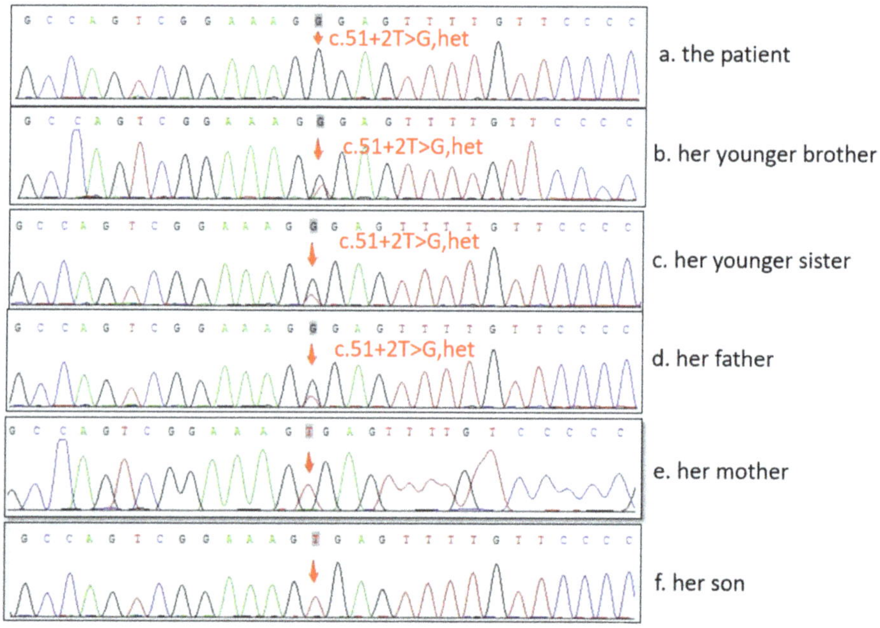

FIGURE 2 | Sequence analysis of *ATP7B* gene in the family.

exon can cause exon jumping, intron retention, or sequence insertion of other genes in mRNA, and intron deletion may be a pathogenic mutation.

In addition, this patient showed special symptoms of skin damage, photosensitivity, and acute neurovisceral manifestations, which may be a special phenotype of the gene mutation (c.51 + 2T > G). For nonspecific skin changes, some features of hyperpigmentation, xerosis, acanthosis nigricans, and dermatomyositis have been reported in patients with WD (26). In a study involving children aged 4–17 years, Muammer et al. found that xerosis was common (45.7%) in relatively newly diagnosed children with WD, followed by keratosis pilaris (10.8%) and spider angioma (10.8%) (27). In an early study, hyperpigmentation was known to be related to WD. Histologically, it was found that hyperpigmentation of the skin was due to excessive melanin deposition rather than the presence of copper or iron (28). It had been confirmed that the skin changes are caused by the treatment with penicillamine, as its cutaneous side-effects include degenerative dermatoses, including cutis laxa, anetoderma, elastosis perforans serpiginosa, and lymphangiectasis (29, 30). Obviously, the skin lesion of this patient was not caused by adverse drug reactions, because of the first diagnosis. Most of the patients with WD have copper metabolic abnormalities with liver dysfunction. It seems likely that the liver abnormality plays an important role in the development of skin pigmentation in patients with WD. Thus,

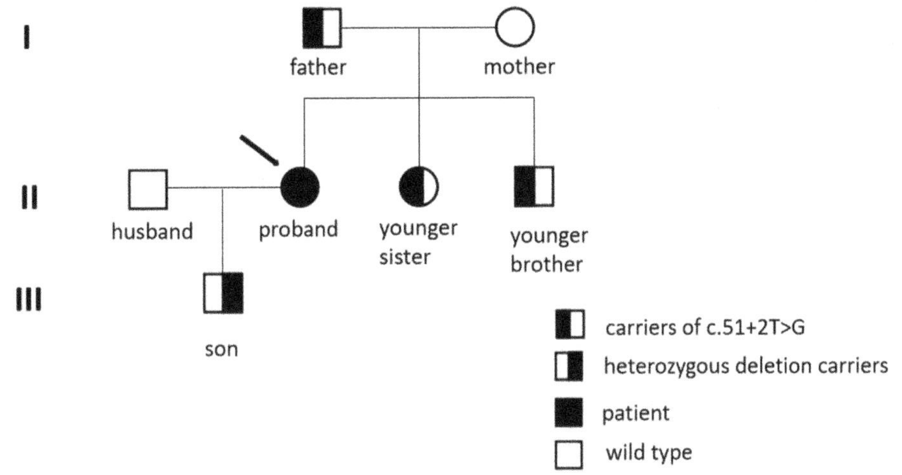

FIGURE 3 | Family pedigree of the mutation in c.51+2T>G and heterozygous deletion.

far, the exact pathophysiological mechanism of varied skin lesions in WD is not clear. Additionally, for acute neurovisceral manifestation, one patient presented with mild pancreatitis, which was attributed to copper deposition in the pancreas (31). The pigmented gallstone pancreatitis and cholangitis with concomitant obstructive jaundice have also been reported as the features of WD (6). A study involving 10 WD patients with different causes included three cases showed that acute pancreatitis is a complication of massive hemolysis, with a prevalence of ~25% (32). The cause of WD presenting as pancreatitis, thus, was presumed to be copper deposition or hemolysis. Therefore, further investigation is still needed to verify the causality between genotype and phenotype, especially the novel mutation c.51 + 2T > G and skin manifestations and acute neurovisceral symptoms. Unfortunately, few studies have reported a splice site variant of c.51 + 2T > G.

First-degree relatives of the proband must be screened for WD; a higher (4.08%) than expected (0.5%) frequency of WD among their subsequent generations was detected (33). The parents, younger sister, and baby boy of the patient all underwent genetic testing, as shown in **Figure 2**. The c.51 + 2T > G variant located on intron one was detected in both the father and younger sister of the patient, and the same heterozygous deletion in the chr13q14.3 (52158814-53624916) region was located in her son. In this case, the pathogenic gene of the splicing mutation c.51 + 2T > G in intron one came from her father, while the new heterozygosity deletion originated from herself, which led to the formation of complex heterozygotes. Based on the phenotype of their families, we mapped the family pedigree, as shown in **Figure 3**. Although, none of her first-degree relatives had any pathognomonic physical sign of the disease, a study showed that prophylactic therapy was effective in WD, whereas a long period must elapse before the illness could be prevented in these asymptomatic families (34). We suggest that her family should regularly undergo liver function tests and should note any neuropsychiatric symptoms of WD. A low-copper diet and zinc therapy have been used successfully in asymptomatic or presymptomatic individuals (3).

The limitations in our report are quite obvious. It was not a controlled study, and only one patient with WD with splicing variants of c.51 + 2T > G in the *ATP7B* gene was involved. Thus, our findings may not be generalizable to other patients with WD. However, we have added a data comparison with a WD patient with other mutation (p.R778L) in **Table 1**. Although this mutation has been reported previous studies, more animal experiments with greater scientific rigor are needed to confirm the relationship between genotype and phenotype.

CONCLUSION

In this case, the diagnosis of porphyria was excluded using gene sequencing. However, attention must be given to such confounding manifestations to avoid misdiagnosis. In this case report, we identified the rare splicing variants of c.51 + 2T > G in the *ATP7B* gene that may be involved in the pathogenesis of WD.The patient developed skin changes and stomachache, which have never been reported in WD populations. We hope that our case report may serve as a useful reference for generalists and specialists in hepatology or neurology in diagnosing the rare clinical characteristics of WD, to prevent misdiagnosis and for the early diagnosis and treatment of the condition.

ETHICS STATEMENT

Written informed consent was obtained from the individuals for the publication of any potentially identifiable images or data included in this article.

AUTHOR CONTRIBUTIONS

JZ and Y-HW contributed to the design of this case report, recorded the medical information, and drafted the article. LW and R-CC analyzed the data and made revisions of the manuscript. All authors contributed to the critical revision and provided final approval of the submitted version of this article.

82070613) and Innovation-Driven Project of Central South University (No. 2020CX044).

ACKNOWLEDGMENTS

The authors would like to thank the patient for agreeing and providing her case history.

REFERENCES

1. Terada K, Schilsky LM, Miura N, Sugiyama T. Molecules in focus ATP7B (WND) protein. *Int J Biochem Cell Bio.* (1998) 30:1063–7. doi: 10.1016/S1357-2725(98)00073-9
2. Menkes JH. Menkes disease and Wilson disease: two sides of the same copper coin Part II: Wilson disease. *Eur J Paediatr.* (1999) 3:245–53. doi: 10.1016/S1090-3798(99)90979-0
3. Ala A, Walker AP, Ashkan K, Dooley JS, Schilsky ML. Wilson's disease. *Lancet.* (2007) 369:397–408. doi: 10.1016/S0140-6736(07)60196-2
4. Xie J-J, Wu Z-Y. Wilson's Disease in China. *Neurosci Bull.* (2017) 33:323–30. doi: 10.1007/s12264-017-0107-4
5. Kapoor N, Cherian KE, Sajith KG, Thomas M, Eapen CE, Thomas N, et al. Renal tubular function, bone health and body composition in Wilson's disease: a cross-sectional study from India. *Calcif Tissue Int.* (2019) 105:459–65. doi: 10.1007/s00223-019-00588-z
6. Nussinson E, Shahbari A, Shibli F, Chervinsky E, Trougouboff P, Markel A. Diagnostic challenges of Wilson's disease presenting as acute pancreatitis, cholangitis, and jaundice. *World J Hepatol.* (2013) 5:649–53. doi: 10.4254/wjh.v5.i11.649
7. Zhu Q, Zhu K, Wang J, Bian W, Lu J. Relationship between genetic mutations and clinical phenotypes in patients with Wilson disease. *Medicine.* (2019) 98:e18284. doi: 10.1097/MD.0000000000018284
8. Wang B, Rudnick S, Cengia B, Bonkovsky HL. Acute hepatic porphyrias: review and recent progress. *Hepatol Commun.* (2019) 3:193–206. doi: 10.1002/hep4.1297
9. Christiansen AL, Aagaard L, Krag A,Rasmussen LM, Bygum A. Cutaneous porphyrias: causes, symptoms, treatments and the danish incidence 1989-2013. *Acta Derm Venereol.* (2016) 96:868–72. doi: 10.2340/00015555-2444
10. Richards S, Aziz N, Bale S, Bick D, Das S, Gastier-Foster J, et al. Standards and guidelines for the interpretation of sequence variants: a joint consensus recommendation of the American college of medical genetics and genomics and the association for molecular pathology. *Genet Med.* (2015) 17:405–24. doi: 10.1038/gim.2015.30
11. Heathcote EJ, Marcellin P, Buti M, Gane E, De Man RA, Krastev Z. European association for study of the liver. EASL clinical practice guidelines: Wilson's disease. *J Hepatol.* (2012) 56:671–85. doi: 10.1016/j.jhep.2011.11.007
12. Puy H, Gouya L, Deybach J-C. Porphyrias. *Lancet.* (2010) 375:924–37. doi: 10.1016/S0140-6736(09)61925-5
13. Baravelli CM, Sandberg S, Aarsand AK, Tollanes MC. Porphyria cutanea tarda increases risk of hepatocellular carcinoma and premature death: a nationwide cohort study. *Orphanet J Rare Dis.* (2019) 14:77. doi: 10.1186/s13023-019-1051-3
14. Singal AK. Porphyria cutanea tarda: recent update. *Mol Genet Metab.* (2019) 128:271–81. doi: 10.1016/j.ymgme.2019.01.004
15. Shah AB, Chernov I, Zhang HT, Ross BM, Das K, Lutsenko S, et al. Identification and analysis of mutations in the Wilson disease gene (ATP7B): population frequencies, genotype-phenotype correlation, and functional analyses. *Am J Hum Genet.* (1997) 61:317–28. doi: 10.1086/514864
16. Ferenci P. Regional distribution of mutations of the ATP7B gene in patients with Wilson disease: impact on genetic testing. *Hum Genet.* (2006) 120:151–9. doi: 10.1007/s00439-006-0202-5
17. Dong Y, Ni W, Chen W-J, Wan B, Zhao G-X, Shi Z-Q. Spectrum and classification of ATP7B variants in a large cohort of chinese patients with Wilson's disease guides genetic diagnosis. *Theranostics.* (2016) 6:638–49. doi: 10.7150/thno.14596
18. Tatsumi Y, Hattori A, Hayashi H, Ikoma J, Kaito M, Imoto M. Current state of Wilson disease patients in central Japan. *Intern Med.* (2010) 49:809–15. doi: 10.2169/internalmedicine.49.2931
19. Czlonkowska A, Gromadzka G, Chabik G. Monozygotic female twins discordant for phenotype of Wilson's disease. *Mov Disord.* (2009) 24:1066–88. doi: 10.1002/mds.22474
20. Cheng N, Wang H, Wu W, Yang R,Liu L, Han Y, et al. Spectrum of ATP7B mutations and genotype-phenotype correlation in large-scale chinese patients with Wilson disease. *Clin Genet.* (2017) 92:69–79. doi: 10.1111/cge.12951
21. Stapelbroek JM, Bollen CW, van Amstel JK, van Erpecum KJ, van Hattum J, van den Berg LH, et al. The H1069Q mutation in ATP7B is associated with late and neurologic presentation in Wilson disease: results of a meta-analysis. *J Hepatol.* (2004) 41:758–63. doi: 10.1016/j.jhep.2004.07.017
22. Chen Y-C, Yu H, Wang R-M, Xie J-J, Ni W, Zhang Y, et al. Contribution of intragenic deletions to mutation spectrum in chinese patients with Wilson's disease and possible mechanism underlying ATP7B gross deletions. *Parkinsonism Relat Disord.* (2019) 62:128–33. doi: 10.1016/j.parkreldis.2019.01.001
23. Takahara K, Schwarze U, Imamura Y, Hoffman GG, Toriello H, Smith LT, et al. Order of intron removal influences multiple splice outcomes, including a two-exon skip, in a COL5A1 acceptor-site mutation that results in abnormal pro-alpha1(V) N-propeptides and Ehlers-Danlos syndrome type I. *Am J Hum Genet.* (2002) 71:451–65. doi: 10.1086/342099
24. Weisschuh N, Mazzola P, Bertrand M, Haack TB, Wissinger B, Kohl S, et al. Clinical characteristics of POC1B-associated retinopathy and assignment of pathogenicity to novel deep intronic and non-canonical splice site variants. *Int J Mol Sci.* (2021) 22:5396. doi: 10.3390/ijms22105396
25. Baskin B, Gibson WT, Ray PN. Duchenne muscular dystrophy caused by a complex rearrangement between intron 43 of the DMD gene and chromosome 4. *Neuromuscul Disord.* (2011) 21:178–82. doi: 10.1016/j.nmd.2010.11.008
26. Czlonkowska A, Litwin T, Dusek P, Ferenci P, Lutsenko S, Medici V, et al. Wilson disease. *Nat Rev Dis Primers.* (2018) 4:21. doi: 10.1038/s41572-018-0018-3
27. Seyhan M, Erdem T, Selimoglu MA, Ertekin V. Dermatological signs in Wilson's disease. *Pediatr Int.* (2009) 51:395–8. doi: 10.1111/j.1442-200X.2008.02766.x
28. Leu ML, Strickland GT, Wang CC, Chen TSN. Skin pigmentation in Wilson's disease. *JAMA.* (1970) 211:1542–3. doi: 10.1001/jama.1970.03170090058016
29. Na SY, Choi M, Kim MJ, Lee JH, Cho S. Penicillamine-induced elastosis perforans serpiginosa and cutis laxa in Wilson's disease. *Bri J Dermatol.* (2000) 142:560–91. doi: 10.1046/j.1365-2133.2000.03379.x
30. Goldstein JB, McNutt NS, Hambrick GW, Hsu A. Penicillamine dermatopathy with lymphangiectases. *Arch Dermatol.* (1989) 125:92–7. doi: 10.1001/archderm.1989.01670130094014
31. Weizman Z, Picard E, Barki Y, Moses S. Wilson's disease associated with pancreatitis. *J Pediatr Gastroenterol Nutr.* (1988) 7:931–3. doi: 10.1097/00005176-198811000-00024

32. Druml W, Laggner AN, Lenz K, Grimm G, Schneewei B. Pancreatitis in acute hemolysis. *Ann Hematol.* (1991) 63:39–41. doi: 10.1007/BF01714959
33. Dziezyc K, Litwin T, Chabik G, Gramza K, Czlonkowska A. Families with Wilson's disease in subsequent generations: clinical and genetic analysis. *Mov Disord.* (2014) 29:1828–32. doi: 10.1002/mds.26057
34. Sternlieb I, Scheinberg IH. Prevention of Wilson's disease in asymptomatic patients. *New Eng J Med.* (1968) 278:352–9. doi: 10.1056/NEJM196802152780702

3

The Application of Induced Pluripotent Stem Cells Against Liver Diseases

Lei Zhang[1,2,3†], Ke Pu[4,5†], Xiaojun Liu[6], Sarah Da Won Bae[7], Romario Nguyen[7], Suyang Bai[4,5], Yi Li[4,5] and Liang Qiao[7]*

[1] The First Clinical Medical College, Lanzhou University, Lanzhou, China, [2] Department of General Surgery, The First Hospital of Lanzhou University, Lanzhou, China, [3] Key Laboratory of Biological Therapy and Regenerative Medicine Transformation Gansu Province, Lanzhou, China, [4] Department of Gastroenterology, The First Hospital of Lanzhou University, Lanzhou, China, [5] Key Laboratory for Gastrointestinal Diseases of Gansu Province, Lanzhou University, Lanzhou, China, [6] Department of Medical Oncology, The First Hospital of Lanzhou University, Lanzhou, China, [7] Storr Liver Centre, Westmead Institute for Medical Research, University of Sydney at Westmead Clinical School, Westmead, NSW, Australia

***Correspondence:**
Liang Qiao
liang.qiao@sydney.edu.au

† These authors have contributed equally to this work

Liver diseases are a major health concern globally, and are associated with poor survival and prognosis of patients. This creates the need for patients to accept the main alternative treatment of liver transplantation to prevent progression to end-stage liver disease. Investigation of the molecular mechanisms underpinning complex liver diseases and their pathology is an emerging goal of stem cell scope. Human induced pluripotent stem cells (hiPSCs) derived from somatic cells are a promising alternative approach to the treatment of liver disease, and a prospective model for studying complex liver diseases. Here, we review hiPSC technology of cell reprogramming and differentiation, and discuss the potential application of hiPSC-derived liver cells, such as hepatocytes and cholangiocytes, in refractory liver-disease modeling and treatment, and drug screening and toxicity testing. We also consider hiPSC safety in clinical applications, based on genomic and epigenetic alterations, tumorigenicity, and immunogenicity.

Keywords: HLCs, primary human hepatocytes, liver disease, clinical application, IPS cell

INTRODUCTION

Liver disease causes ~2 million deaths annually worldwide. Cirrhosis-related complications account for 50% of deaths, and viral hepatitis and hepatocellular carcinoma (HCC) together account for the other 50% of deaths annually worldwide. Cirrhosis is currently the 11th most common cause of death globally, and liver cancer is the 16th leading cause of death. Cirrhosis and HCC together account for 3.5% of all deaths worldwide (1). Currently, liver transplantation is the most effective treatment option for patients with end-stage liver disease (ESLD). However, <10% of global liver transplantation needs are met (2). The shortage of donor organs and transplant costs are the major limiting factors (3). In addition, the recipient's immune system may reject the transplanted organ (4). Therefore, the development of alternative therapeutic strategies for patients with chronic liver disease is of utmost importance.

Human induced pluripotent stem cells (hiPSCs) are pluripotent stem cells that are induced and reprogrammed from adult cells into undifferentiated cells by exposure to specific mediators. They have the capacity for self-renewal and differentiation into a variety of somatic cells, such as embryonic stem cells (5). HiPSC-derived hepatocyte-like cells (hiPSC-HLCs) exhibit morphological and phenotypic characteristics of primary human hepatocytes (PHHs) (6). hiPSC-HLCs should be incorporated into future studies of liver diseases to solve the problems of organ shortage and prevent recipient immunorejection of PHHs. hiPSC-HLCs can be considered as an ideal source of hepatocytes. In addition, these cells may enable cell-based therapy, exploration of liver disease models, *in vitro* models for pharmacology and toxicology studies (7) and ESLD treatment.

In this review article, we aimed to provide a perspective on the current organization and provision of transplant services based on specific challenges and environmental settings. We review how these specific requirements are addressed by the existing cell culture systems for the generation of hiPSC-derived hepatocytes, describe their applications for modeling hepatic disorders, and discuss future directions for the use of hiPSCs in the study and treatment of liver diseases.

RECENT DEVELOPMENTS IN THE iPSC REPROGRAMMING METHODOLOGY

Protocols for somatic cells transformed into induced pluripotent stem cells are widely used for iPSC reprogramming method. The key to the success of these protocols is the ability to efficiently induce pluripotent cells to adopt a definitive endoderm fate. Earlier studies have shown that mouse fibroblasts can be reprogrammed to develop embryonic stem cell (ESC)-like features, and grow in the presence of four factors: Oct3/4, Sox2, c-Myc, and Klf4 (8). These induced cells were named iPSCs. These insights opened the door to further refinements in the cell differentiation methodology and enabled the derivation of visceral, endodermal-derived tissues. The same protocol was used to successfully generate iPSCs from adult human skin cells (9). In addition, human somatic cells were transformed into PSCs by inducing the expression of a new set of four factors: Oct4, Sox2, Nanog, and Lin28 (10). Many optimization steps have been devised to improve the efficiency of reprogramming factors, such as the use of integration-free methods (8, 11). Episomal vectors, Sendai viruses, and synthetic mRNAs are among the most commonly used methods for generating hiPSCs (12–14) without modifying the host genome, which could interfere with disease modeling or experimental outcomes.

Abbreviations: iPSCs, induced pluripotent stem cell; HLC, hepatic like cell; PHH, primary human hepatocytes; confidence interval; ESLD, end-stage liver disease; ESC, embryonic stem cells; IMD, metabolic disorder of liver; HCC, Hepatocellular carcinoma; NAFLD, non-alcoholic fatty liver disease; NASH, Non-alcoholic steatohepatitis; HBV, hepatitis B virus; HCV, hepatitis C virus; AATD, α1-antitrypsin deficiency; FH, familial hypercholesterolemia; EVs, extracellular vesicles; HSC, hepatic stellate cell; CSC, cancer stem cells; XCI, X-chromosome inactivation; CNV, copy number variations; SNV, single-nucleotide variations.

CURRENT APPROACHES FOR GENERATION OF hiPSC-HLCs AND CHOLANGIOCYTE-LIKE CELLS

In 2009, hiPSCs were induced to differentiate into hepatic cells for the first time, via a timed administration of various growth factors. The expression of hepatocyte markers and liver-related functions in hiPSC-HLCs was monitored and compared with those in differentiated human ESCs and PHHs (15). This revealed that hepatic cells could be generated from iPSCs but the process took more than 20 d. To overcome this, the differentiation step was revised to a more efficient three-step protocol, allowing rapid generation of HLCs from hiPSCs (**Figure 1**) (16). Hepatic progenitor-like cells derived from hiPSCs possess the potential for bipotent differentiation into HLCs and cholangiocyte-like cells (17).

For clinical applications, differentiated cells should be assessed by comparing them with primary liver-derived cells, to verify their morphology and expression of liver-specific proteins, such as alpha-fetoprotein (AFP) and albumin. However, neither ESCs nor iPSCs can differentiate into fully mature hepatocytes *in vitro*. As a consequence of an emerging interest in using iPSCs in regenerative medicine to treat liver diseases, many researchers are focused on developing the most efficient and reproducible approaches for the derivation of high-quality hiPSC-HLCs. Currently, the differentiation strategies for obtaining hiPSC-HLCs generally require a stepwise induction of definitive endoderm, hepatocyte specification, and hepatoblast expansion into mature HLCs. Activin A, Wnt3a (18)and fibroblast growth factor 2 (FGF) signaling (19) play important roles in hiPSC differentiation toward hepatic endoderm, whereas hepatocyte growth factor (HGF) promotes the growth of hepatoblast cells (20, 21). Another factor, the interleukin (IL) 6 family cytokine oncostatin M (OSM), combined with the glucocorticoid dexamethasone (DEX), accelerates the maturation of hepatocytes. Meanwhile, many protocols for iPSC differentiation to hepatocytes have been reported, which involve the use of various growth factors and cytokines, plating techniques, and transduction of key liver-specific transcription factors (22).

Other studies have reported strategies for the generation of cholangiocyte-like cells from hiPSCs. The first differentiation of cholangiocyte-like cells from hiPSC hepatoblasts was induced in the presence of growth hormone, epidermal growth factor (EGF), IL-6, and sodium taurocholate (23). Subsequently, efficient differentiation of cholangiocytes from iPSCs was improved by 3D co-culture of hepatoblasts and OP9 stromal cells in the presence of HGF, EGF, and TGF-β (24), and by stimulating cholangiocyte progenitor specification using FGF10, activin A, and retinoic acid (25). Yet another stepwise cholangiocyte differentiation approach involves a definitive endoderm–hepatic specification–hepatic progenitor–cholangiocyte procedure, with Jagged1 and TGF-β supplementation being key for the promotion of iPSC-cholangiocyte formation (26). These cells were subsequently characterized *in vitro* and *in vivo*. Induced-cholangiocytes show mature markers, such as SOX9, CK7, CK19, CFTR,

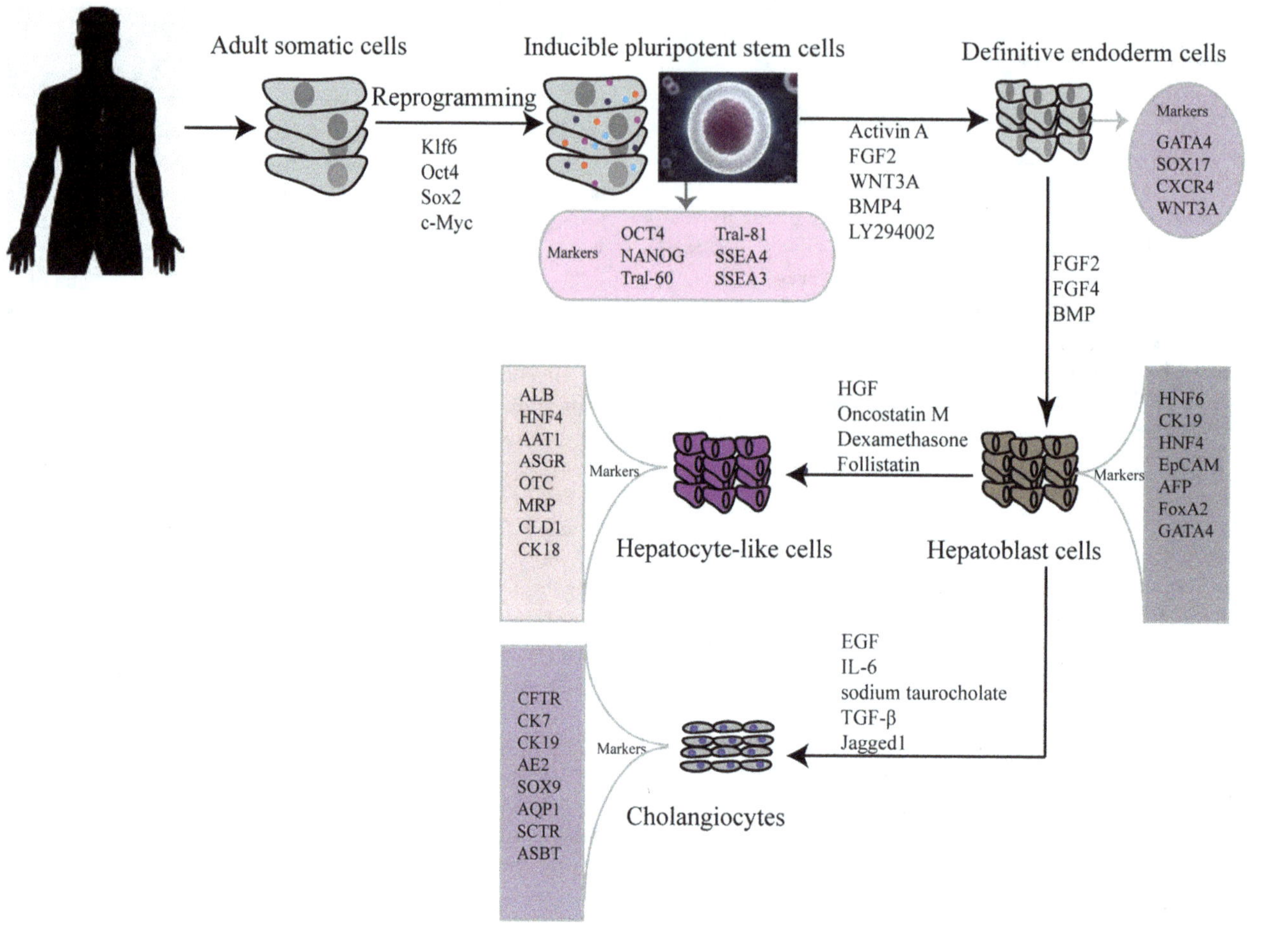

FIGURE 1 | Flow diagram showing typical protocol for iPSCs reprogramming and hepatic differentiation of human into hepatocyte-like cells *in vitro*. OCT 4, octamer binding transcription factor 3/4; SSEA, stage-specific embryonic antigen; TRA, Tumor resistance antigen 1-60; SOX2 sex determining region Y box 2; KLF4 (Kruppel-like factor 4); GATA4, GATA binding protein 4; CXCR4, C-X-C chemokine receptor type 4; FGF, fibroblast growth factor; HGF, hepatocyte growth factor; BMP, bone morphogenetic protein; HNF6, Hepatocyte nuclear factor 6; CK, cytokeratin; EpCAM, Epithelial cell adhesion molecule; AFP, alpha-fetoprotein; AAT1, α1-anti-tripsin; ALB, albumin; ASGR, asialoglycoprotein receptor; MRP, multidrug resistance protein; CLD, claudin; EGF, epidermal growth factor; IL-6, interleukin 6; TGF-β, transforming growth factor beta; CK7, cytokeratin 7; CK19, cytokeratin 19; AE2, chloride/bicarbonate anion exchanger 2; ASBT, apical sodium-dependent bile acid transporter; CFTR, cystic fibrosis transmembrane conductance regulator; AQP1, aquaporin-1; SOX9, SRY-box 9; SCTR, secretin receptor.

AE2, ASBT, AQP1, and SCTR and they are negative for the hepatocyte marker HNF4a.

FEATURES AND FUNCTIONS OF hiPSC-HLCs

The liver performs a wide range of fundamental functions, including metabolic, nutrient storage, and detoxification functions. Hence, each protocol for an efficient maturation of iPSCs into HLCs needs to incorporate a thorough and critical evaluation of the hepato-specific transcriptome and enzymatic activities of the obtained cells. Drug metabolizing capacity, urea cycle activity, or bile acid and lipoprotein synthesis and excretion need to be evaluated to ascertain HLC maturation (**Figure 2**). By contrast, most of the current reports on HLC generation show that HLCs express genes at levels that are characteristic for the fetal liver and display a fetal-like phenotype. According to one study (26), HLC mitochondria display specific morphological changes, such as elongation, swollen cristae, dense matrix, and cytoplasmic migration, with an increased expression of mitochondrial DNA transcription and replication-related genes, and increased oxygen consumption. Following differentiation, HLCs express liver-specific proteins, including albumin and hepatocyte nuclear factor 4 alpha, and show intrinsic hepatocyte functions, including CYP450 activity. However, HLCs also express high levels of AFP, suggesting a persistent immature phenotype or inability to turn off early-stage genes. Furthermore, albumin production, urea production, CYP450 activity, and mitochondrial function of HLCs are significantly lower than those of primary human hepatocytes. Functional indicators, urea synthesis, glycogen synthesis, lipid storage, indocyanine green intake, and low-density lipoprotein intake, are also used to evaluate the function of HLCs (27–31)

(**Table 1**). Liver function after HLC transplantation in disease-specific models in mouse is assessed using glycogen content synthesis, low-density lipoprotein, and indocyanine green intake (32).

Hepatocyte isolation is not easy to perform, and requires expertise and access to primary human liver tissue. An alternative strategy for the acquisition of hepatocytes may grant the researchers access to important control material, thanks to commercially available cryopreserved hepatocytes, or as an alternative to using human liver tissue. Recently, an important and detailed report describing the expression of more than 60 hepatic, pluripotency, and developmental genes has been published to map their changes during liver cell isolation and stem cell maturation into HLC (33). In this report, the specific traits of iPSC-HLC were compared with those of adult liver and fetal liver cells, proving that several hepatic enzymes, whose expression is limited during the fetal period and absent at the postnatal stage, are highly expressed in iPSC-HLCs. In the study, *CYP3A4* and *CYP3A7* genes were used for a convenient and quick evaluation of hepatic maturation.

hiPSC-HLCs FOR THE TREATMENT OF ESLD

At present, some promising stem cell-based transportation treatments for ESLD have been reported. Several studies have demonstrated the restoration of liver function in hematopoietic stem cells (HSCs), mesenchymal stem cells (MSCs), and endothelial progenitor cells (EPCs) in acute liver failure (34–37). Although alleviation of liver dysfunction was observed in patients who have received these treatments in clinical trials, the safety and short-term efficacy of stem cell-based transplantation were not explored in detail and should be further evaluated in large-scale prospective cohort studies (38). In fact, stem cell transplantation as an alternative treatment for ESLD cannot be used for remodeling injured hepatic structure. In theory, iPSC-HLCs can be regarded as the optimal cell replacement treatment for acute liver failure (ALF) and ESLD. Meanwhile, HLCs derived from patient-specific iPSCs are an unlimited source of hepatocytes to treat liver failure.

To date, the application of iPSCs in ALF and liver failure has been tested in animal models. Indeed, iPSC-HLC transplantation improves the general condition in a mouse model of CCl_4-induced liver injury (39). Further, the survival rate of immunodeficient mice with ALF significantly increased and liver fibrosis levels in mice with chronic liver injury significantly decreased after hiPSC-HLC transplantation (40). According to another study, hiPSC-HLCs rescue drug-induced ALF in rodents, and hiPSC-HLCs have functional and proliferative potential for liver regeneration after transplantation in an ALF model (41, 42). These studies indicated the potential of these cells in regenerative medicine for future clinical applications. Of note, the aforementioned studies only focused on rodent models rather than primates. To date, no studies have illustrated the application of iPSC-HLCs in human liver failure.

The first transplantation of hiPSCs in regenerative medicine took place in 2014, and was performed to treat a 77-year-old female patient with polypoidal choroidal vasculopathy in both eyes. Autologous iPSCs were generated from the patient's skin fibroblasts, differentiated into retinal pigment epithelium, and then transplanted into the eye. Immune response to autologous transplantation was observed 18 months postoperatively, and the results indicated no complications. The retinal pigment epithelial sheet that had been transplanted survived well, and the corrected visual acuity of the treated eye did not improve or worsen.

Unfortunately, not all cases are as successful as the autologous transplant discussed above. Another clinical trial involving three patients with age-related macular degeneration involved intravitreal administration of stem cells derived from autologous adipose tissue. Post-treatment observation revealed vision loss associated with ocular hypertension, hemorrhagic retinopathy, vitreous hemorrhage, combined traction and rhegmatogenous retinal detachment, or lens dislocation (43).

The above trials demonstrate the need for further investigation of stem cell therapy and, more specifically, the use of hiPSCs in regenerative medicine to treat ESLD.

hiPSC-HLC MODELING OF LIVER DISEASE DEVELOPMENT

Infectious Liver Diseases

Hepatitis B virus (HBV) and hepatitis C virus (HCV) are the most prevalent agents of infectious liver diseases. Approximately 520 million people suffer from infections caused by one of these viruses worldwide, including 170 million people with HBV and 350 million people with HCV infections (44). The infected population will develop virus-related cirrhosis and liver cancer (45). At present, the interaction between these viruses and host hepatocytes remains unclear because of the absence of viral culture models to reflect the infection process and reproduce the molecular events within an infected host cell.

PHHs are the gold standard for studying the physiopathology of liver infections. However, low cell viability and yield caused by a rapid loss of hepatic phenotype upon isolation from the liver microenvironment are the main limitations of their application. As an alternative to overcome these limitations, iPSC-HLCs could be used to study the viral infection process and virus–host interactions, as well as the viral life cycle, to ultimately identify efficacious drugs for infectious liver diseases.

In the past, iPSC-HLCs have been successfully used as an *in vitro* system for modeling hepatitis virus infections and virus–host interactions. When HCV entry and genomic replication is stimulated, iPSC-HLCs more commonly express HCV receptors and show increased susceptibility to HCV infection than PHHs (46). Further, HCV entry inhibitor (CD81 antibody) and HCV genomic replication inhibitor (interferon) attenuate HCV pseudovirus entry and HCV sub-genomic replication, respectively, in iPSC-HLCs. It has been reported that hiPSC-HLCs support the entire life cycle of HCV, including the

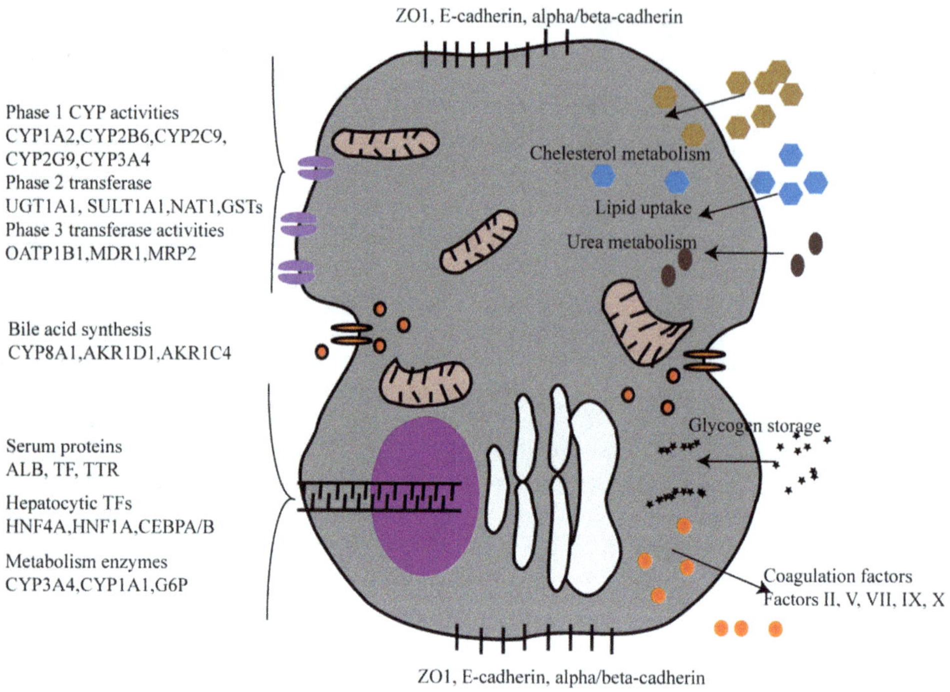

FIGURE 2 | The phenotypic characterization of Hepatocyte-like cells derived from iPSCs. CYP, CYPs cytochromes P450; UGT, UDP glucuronosyltransferase. SULT1A1, Sulfotransferase Family 1A Member 1; NAT1, N-Acetyltransferase 1; GSTs, Glutathione S-Transferase; OATP, organic anion-transporting polypeptide; MDR, Multiple drug resistance; MRP2:multidrug resistance protein 2; AKR1D1, aldo-keto reductase family 1 member D1, AKR1C4, aldo-keto reductase family 1 member C4, TTR:Transthyretin, TP, Total protein, ALB, Albumin, HNF, Hepatocyte nuclear factor, CEBPA/B, CCAAT Enhancer Binding Protein Alpha/Beta, G6P, Glucose-6-Phosphatase.

inflammatory response to infection and host genetics impacting viral pathogenesis (31). Furthermore, iPSC-HLCs that show an appropriate antiviral response produce interferon (47, 48) and survive *in vitro* for up to 1 week after inoculation with HCV (47), comprising a superior model for observing hepatocyte function during a relatively long-term infection. Detailed molecular mechanisms allowing viral infection can also be investigated using this model (49).

The above observations suggest that iPSC-HLCs can act as a promising cell model for analyzing hepatocyte responses to viral infection, as well as an ideal platform for drug target discovery for HCV therapy. However, some limitations should be considered. For example, some studies have reported lower virus titers in culture supernatants of HBV-infected iPSC-HLCs than those in PHHs (50), and suggested lack of functional maturation of iPSC-HLCs obtained using various differentiation protocols. Finally, it is necessary to increase the diversity of hiPSC lines used in similar such analyses to assess the impact of the host genetic background on the cellular response and efficiency of infection.

Inherited Metabolic Disorders of the Liver (IMDs)

The liver is vital for metabolic homeostasis. Approximately 70% of patients with IMDs are affected by liver tissue damage. α1-Antitrypsin deficiency (AATD) and familial hypercholesterolemia (FH) are common IMDs that have been extensively studied. AATD results from a single base-pair mutation (leading to Glu342Lys substitution in the protein product), known as the Z mutation, in the *SERPINA1* gene. The substitution causes the protein to misfold and be retained in the endoplasmic reticulum (ER), with the formed protein polymers inducing hepatocyte death (51). By contrast, FH is an autosomal dominant hypercholesterolemia caused by mutations in a gene for the low-density lipoprotein receptor (LDLR) or LDLR-related genes. FH is characterized by elevated serum levels of low-density lipoprotein (LDL)-cholesterol (C), which lead to xanthoma formation and premature cardiovascular disease (52, 53).

The use of iPSC-HLCs as a novel model of the above monogenic diseases and iPSC-HLC application for a gene correction therapy for the generation of disease-free autologous cells are attracting increasing attention. For instance, accumulation of A1AT variant polymers in the endoplasmic reticulum of iPSC-HLCs was observed when iPSCs from AATD patients were differentiated into HLCs (54). Further, biochemical features and morphological manifestations of iPSC-HLC models generated from cells from AATD patients with and without severe liver disease (SLD) were explored (55). The analysis of individual disease phenotypes of AATD patients revealed rapid degradation of misfolded α1-antitrypsin Z (ATZ) and

TABLE 1 | Functional features of hepatocyte-like cells (HLCs) derived from human induced pluripotent stem cells.

Function features	hiPSC-HLCs	PHHs
Phase I CYP activities		
CYP1A2 (28, 31)	−	+
CYP2B6 (28, 31)	−	+
CYP3A4 (31)	−	+
CYP3A7 (31)	+	−
Phase II transferase (27)	+	+
UGT1A1	+	+
SULT1A1	+	+
NAT1	+	+
GSTs	+	+
Phase III transferase (27)	+	+
OATP1B1	+	+
MDR1	+	+
MRP2	+	+
Hepatocytic TFs	+	+
HNF4A (29, 30)	+	+
AFP (27, 29)	+	−
Bile acid synthesis	+	+
Albumin synthesis (29, 30)	+	+
Glycogen storage (30)	+	+
LDL uptake (29, 30)	+	+
Urea metabolism (30)	+	+
Cholesterol metabolism (29)	+	+

no globular inclusions in cells from patients in which the liver disease had been ameliorated (55). Similar, the main pathological characteristic of FH was recapitulated by inducing iPSCs obtained from patients with FH to form HLCs (54). In addition, analysis of iPSC-HLCs obtained from an FH patient with a mutation in the *LDLR* gene demonstrated that FH-derived iPSC-HLCs are unable to take up LDL-C, and secrete more apolipoprotein B-100 than the controls (56). Furthermore, these HLCs do not respond to statin treatment (56). Together, these observations demonstrate that IMD-hiPSCs effectively model the pathological features of IMD.

Animal models have been used to assess the efficacy of iPSC-HLC therapy in IMDs (57). The first reported targeted gene correction of AATD in iPSCs was achieved by bi-allelic correction of mutated loci by using zinc finger nucleases (ZFNs) and PB technology to correct the *A1AT* gene in hiPSCs (58). Genetic correction of iPSC-HLCs restored the normal structure and function of the A1AT protein *in vitro* and *in vivo*. Gene correction for AATD has been also successfully attempted using the TALEN approach, which is more efficient than ZEN (59). In addition, the use of CRISPR/Cas9 gene editing technology to correct point mutations in specific genes has been reported (60) and experimental data have highlighted the advantages of using the CRISPR/Cas9 system for allele-specific genome targeting and for gene disruption mediated by non-homologous end joining. Indeed, CRISPR/Cas9 genome editing was used to permanently correct a 3-bp homozygous deletion in *LDLR* exon 4 in patient-derived homozygous FH (HoFH)-iPSCs (61). This genetic correction restored LDLR-mediated endocytosis in FH-HLCs and is a proof-of-principle that CRISPR-mediated genetic modification can be successfully used to normalize HoFH cholesterol metabolism deficiency at the cellular level. The above findings clearly demonstrate that genome-editing technology can be used to achieve functional correction of patient-derived iPSC-HLCs.

Non-alcoholic Fatty Liver Disease (NAFLD)

NAFLD is becoming a serious clinical concern because of its severe morbidity and potential progression to ESLD, such as liver cirrhosis and HCC (62). The current global prevalence of NAFLD is estimated to be 25.24% (63) and NAFLD is the second most common cause of liver transplantation (64). The disease develops when chronic hepatic lipid accumulation stimulates an overload of metabolic alterations, including mitochondrial dysfunction, endoplasmic reticulum stress, and hepatic insulin resistance, and induces an inflammatory response (65–68). It is not possible to predict the progression of NAFLD because of adverse events and sampling variability of the currently used invasive diagnostic methods (liver biopsy) (69).

Several studies have reported cell models of NAFLD that use HCC cell lines or immortalized primary hepatocytes (70, 71) Differences in cell function and gene expression between the two have been demonstrated. However, the main limitation of these models is that cultivation of liver biopsy-derived primary hepatocytes for NAFLD modeling takes several days. Hence, using iPSC-HLCs to model NAFLD and non-alcoholic steatohepatitis (NASH) would facilitate research on molecular diagnosis and prognosis, disease progression, and drug development for NAFLD. hiPSC-HLCs have been used as an *in vitro* model to first demonstrate intracellular lipid accumulation in NAFLD (72). Major changes in the expression of metabolism-associated genes and upregulation of the lipid droplet-coating protein Perilipin2 (PLIN2) were detected in the model. Upregulation of the expression of numerous genes of the peroxisome proliferator-activated receptor (PPAR) pathway, constituting a regulatory hub for metabolic processes, was also detected. Taking previous studies into consideration, an iPSC-HLCs model with the *PNPLA3* genotype that is closely associated with hepatic steatosis in moderate (30–40% fatty changes) and severe (70% fatty changes) NAFLD patients was established and characterized (73, 74). Other studies, on the association between endoplasmic reticulum stress response and hepatocyte metabolism disorders in hiPSC-HLCs have been published (75). ER stress pathways play an important role in lipid metabolism, and ER stress enhances lipid accumulation ~5-fold in hiPSC-HLCs compared to their respective controls (71).

Taken together, the hiPSC-HLC model of NAFLD can be used to characterize some of the metabolic features of NAFLD. However, the pathological progression of lipotoxicity in NAFLD involves not only lipid accumulation but also a complex pathophysiological response, such as inflammation and the immune response. Future studies should highlight the applicability of hiPSC-HLCs as a discovery platform for the exploration of molecular events and aid in drug development for NAFLD.

Liver Cirrhosis

Liver cirrhosis is characterized by the presence of diffuse, chronic necro-inflammatory, and fibrogenetic hepatocytes, ultimately leading to the development of features of chronic liver injury, such as structurally abnormal nodules, dense fibrotic septa, concomitant parenchymal exhaustion, and collapse of the liver tissue (76). Chronic liver injury remains one of the most common causes of death in the Western world (77). Currently, modeling liver cirrhosis *in vitro* to unveil the intricate cellular interactions underlying its pathological development is challenging. Traditional approaches involve treatment of cell culture models with toxic drugs or compounds that are often not specific to liver disease (78). Meanwhile, 3D models of primary hepatocyte co-culture with stellate cells are limited by the availability of tissue samples (79). 3D-Organoid cell culture models using iPSC-HLCs, stromal cells, and Kupffer cells (80, 81) can be an excellent approach to study the cellular interactions underlying the pathophysiology of liver cirrhosis. However, some chronic liver injuries, such as cardiac cirrhosis, are difficult to study in an *in vitro* setting and require major advances in 3D co-culture systems.

Previous studies have demonstrated enhanced liver regeneration in mouse model (42), reduced murine liver fibrosis (82) and stabilization of chronic liver disease (39) following iPSC-HLC administration, highlighting its potential as a therapeutic strategy for liver cirrhosis. Recently, the anti-fibrotic properties of iPSCs were demonstrated. Namely, iPSC-derived extracellular vesicles (EVs) were shown to regulate hepatic stellate cell activation and have anti-fibrotic effects (83). Consequently, the use of iPSC-EVs is regarded as a novel anti-fibrotic approach that may reduce or reverse liver fibrosis in patients with chronic liver disease. Furthermore, the therapeutic potential of iPSC-HLCs in liver fibrosis was explored by generation of iPSC-HLCs from mouse embryonic fibroblasts by using a reprogramming technology, and migrating iPSC-HLCs cluster to the intra-spleen and the liver (84). Transplantation of iPSC-HLCs significantly attenuated liver fibrosis induced by CCL4 (80); hence, iPSC-HLCs may be used as a novel therapeutic strategy for the treatment of liver fibrosis. However, while a cell-based therapy for cirrhosis can temporarily relieve cellular hepatocyte injury, it cannot eliminate collagen deposits or restore the original liver structure. Further detailed studies could bring about a novel method by which fibrogenic cells can be reprogrammed into hepatic parenchymal cells in the cirrhotic liver (85).

Liver Cancer

HCC is the third leading cause of cancer-related deaths worldwide and the sixth most common malignancy (86, 87). Liver cancer research mainly focuses on the molecular pathways and treatments for HCC. Within the cancer stem cell (CSC) research, previous reports have explored the possibility of generating liver CSCs by the induction of reprogramming-related factors, such as Oct4 or Nanog (88, 89). However, the induction of HCC cells into liver CSCs using pluripotency-related transcription factors has not yet been widely studied. According to one report, reprogramming can be achieved in tumor cells by retroviral induction of reprograming-associated genes (76). Interestingly, the reprogrammed pluripotent cancer cells (iPCs) were very different from the original cancer cells in terms of colony shape and gene expression of tumor markers. Further, the induction of pluripotent liver cancer cells is correlated with the p53 status, suggesting that varying the gene expression level of p53 may affect the reprogramming process.

In one study, potential tumorigenicity of hiPSC-HLCs during differential induction from hiPSCs to HLC was observed after knockdown of p21 (90). The authors of that study also investigated whether hepatoma-like cells derived from hiPSCs of HCC patients can be transformed into normal hepatocyte cells upon treatment with acyclic retinoid and AKR1B10 inhibitor (tolestat). Combining acyclic retinoid (10 μM) with tolestat (10 μM) is considered to be an appropriate regimen for inducing differentiation of hepatoma-like cells into hepatocytes. The efficacy and toxicity of this combination therapy for individual patients with HCC will be evaluated in the near future.

Previously, iPSCs have been used to treat HCC. More specifically, the therapeutic effect of IPS cell-derived myeloid lineage cells (iPS-ML) and their ability to produce interferon (IFN) β in primary and metastatic liver cancer were reported in mice xenograft model of liver metastasis (91). Further, iPS-ML producing IFN-β injection hindered cancer progression and increased the survival rate in a mouse model.

In summary, at present, the applicability of iPSC technology for HCC treatment mainly focuses on cell reprogramming from HCC to CSCs, and the search for novel HCC treatments. The above studies provide valuable insights for studying and treating HCC.

hiPSC-Cholangiocyte Modeling of Cholangiocyte Disease Development

Cystic fibrosis (CF) is a single-gene inherited disease characterized by mutations in the cystic fibrosis transmembrane conductance regulator gene (*CFTR*), affecting the function of chloride ion channels, with intrahepatic bile stasis. The iPSC-cholangiocytes are superior to other cells from the perspective of the exploration of these diseases and drug discovery. In 2015, two studies reported generation of cholangiocyte organoids from CF patient-iPSCs using their iPSC-cholangiocytes protocols (24, 92). The disease phenotype was modeled in these studies by exploring non-functional CFTR proteins, with subsequent chloride channel impairment and the inability of fluid secretion to form cysts. The effects of the drug VX809 on CF were also tested, demonstrating a functional rescue of impaired CFTR proteins. Both disease models illustrate valid applications of iPSCs, not only as a proof of pathophysiological interactions, but also for biliary-specific pharmacological screening.

Currently, no other types of cholangiopathy have been modeled using iPSC-cholangiocytes, modeling these disease-types rely on animal models of a deficiency or mutation of disease-specific genes. It may be easier to characterize disease

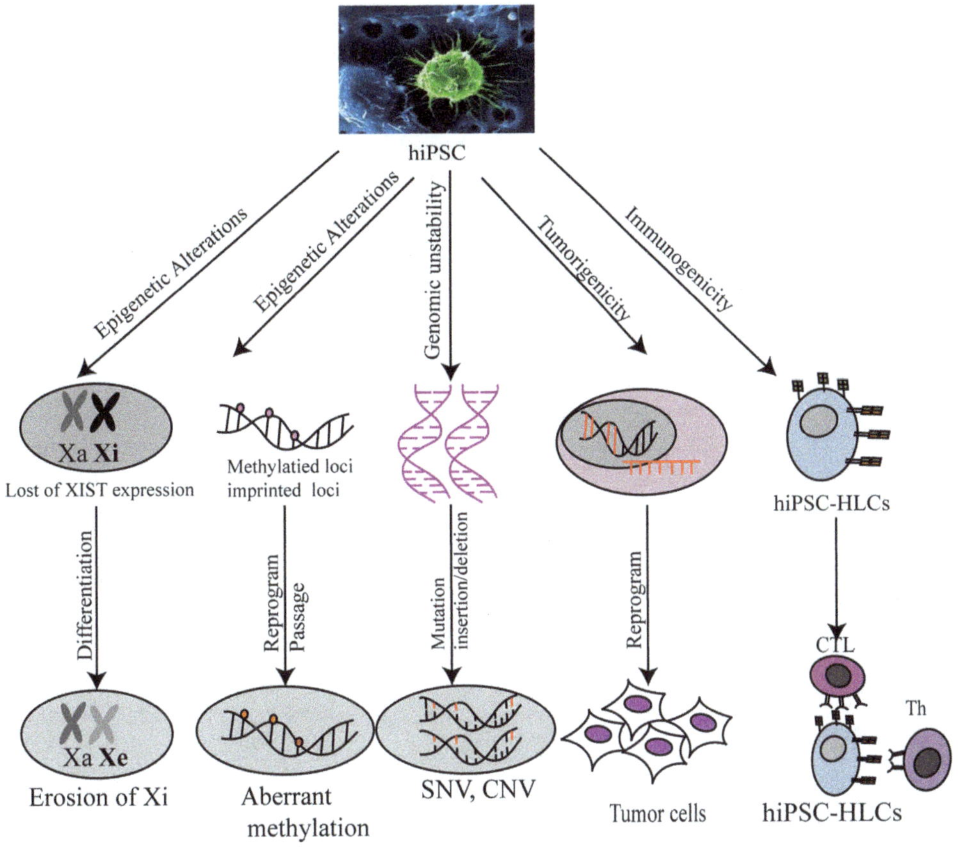

FIGURE 3 | Safety evaluation of hiPSC-HLC in various applications. Xa, X chromosome activity; Xi, X chromosome inactivity; XIST, X-inactive specific transcripts; CNV, copy number variation; SNP, single nucleotide polymorphism.

pathophysiology and obtain detailed drug test information if cholangiocytes derived from patient-related iPSC have direct disease-specific genes information. The etiology of biliary atresia, primary biliary cholangitis, primary sclerosing cholangitis, and cholangiocarcinoma is still unknown because of the intricate interaction between the environment and the genes. Therefore, iPSC cholangiocytes derived from disease-specific cases can be studied to confirm the etiological hypotheses and identify potential therapeutic targets.

DRUG DISCOVERY AND TOXICITY TESTING

Another important application of iPSCs is assessing the therapeutic effect and toxicity of drugs, as has been reported in many studies (93, 94). The effect of drugs is influenced by the genetic background and other complex factors. It is easier to screen drugs using iPSCs than via pharmacological testing of animals. Consequently, organoids, as an innovative technique for drug screening and toxicity assessment, have been extensively researched. However, iPSC-derived organoids in 2D culture cannot be used for drug screening because iPSCs in such culture receive similar stimuli as those in monolayer and cannot be used to model the physiological microenvironment. By contrast, 3D culture models the *in vivo* microenvironment and approximates the physiological conditions. Many studies have reported high-throughput screening of small molecule libraries for drug development and toxicity assessment for liver diseases using iPSC-hepatocytes (59, 95, 96). Generation of organoids in several liver cell co-cultures yields a more sensitive cellular model than that constructed using single cell type. Recently, Broutier et al. (97) developed organoids representing the tumor structure and reflecting the expression profile of hepatocellular carcinoma, cholangiocarcinoma, and hepatocellular cholangiocarcinoma. These organoids open up new opportunities for drug testing and personalized medicine, and can be used for the generation of tumor bio-banks to be used as screening platforms (98). Additionally, "liver-on-a-chip" as a platform for drug development and toxicology testing can be used in pharmacokinetic and pharmacodynamic studies. In one study, liver organoids were generated using hepatocytes and cholangiocytes on a perfusable microcapillary chip (99). These organoids were then used to test the dose- and time-dependent hepatotoxic effects of acetaminophen. Thus, "organ-on-a-chip" represents a novel and valid platform for drug testing.

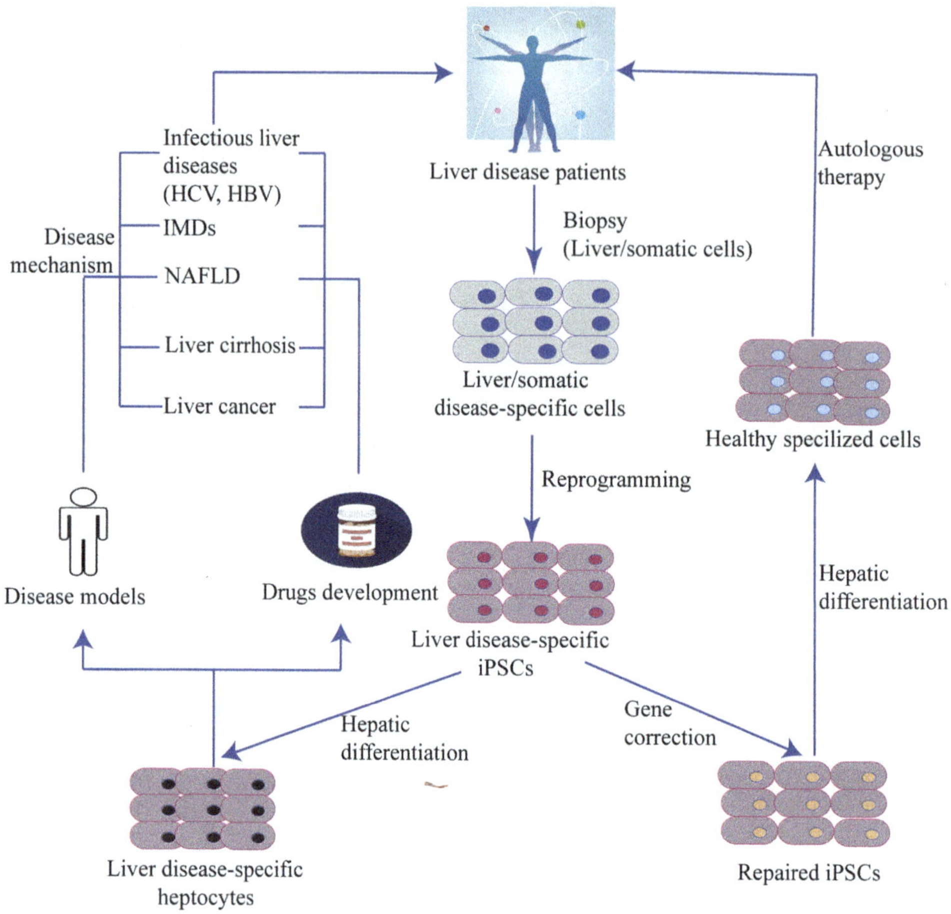

FIGURE 4 | Generation of liver cells from iPSC and their applications. The scheme illustrates an overview of iPSC and organoid technology in relation to liver diseases. Disease specific iPSCs are generated by reprogramming technology from a biopsy of patients. One hand, iPSCs with disease-related gene mutation can be corrected by genome editing and then differentiated into functional disease-specific liver cells *in vitro*. These corrected cells are used to autologous cell therapy. Another hand, Non-corrected iPSC-derived disease-specific liver cells can be remodeled liver disease phenotypes, pathogenesis, and drug testing. IMD, Inherit metabolism disease; NAFLD, Non-alcoholic fatty liver disease.

SAFETY EVALUATION OF hiPSC-HLCs IN VARIOUS APPLICATIONS

While iPSCs have considerable applications in regenerative medicine, the genomic stability of these cells, such as the occurrence of genomic and epigenetic aberrations, copy number variation (CNV), and single-nucleotide polymorphisms (SNPs), is a matter of concern. Genomic aberrations in human PSCs (hPSCs) include abnormal karyotypes, such as recurrent trisomy of chromosomes 12, 17, or X, and aneuploidies of sub-chromosomal regions, such as duplications of the 12p, 17q, or 20q11.21 loci (100). Some studies have demonstrated that iPSCs, unlike somatic cells, contain regions of uniparental disomy (UPD), sharing the equivalent chromosomal and sub-chromosomal characteristics (101). These abnormalities may confer a selective advantage to certain genes during prolonged culturing.

In addition to genomic aberrations, other studies have focused on epigenetic aberrations, but the possibility of hiPSC application for complex diseases remains unknown (102). Epigenetic variations are often observed in different iPSC lines, and prolonged periods of culture (103) may affect disease modeling and clinical applications. For example, reactivating X-chromosome inactivation (XCI) and erosion of inactive X chromosome (Xi) silencing in female hiPSCs during iPSC reprogramming may trigger phenotypic and epigenetic changes in iPSCs, reducing their differentiation potential and increasing their tumorigenicity (104). Furthermore, local epigenetic variations in iPSCs, such as cellular memory and aberrant methylation loci, have been noted. Cellular memory leads to incomplete reprogramming, as DNA hypomethylation and histone modification at specific loci render iPSCs remain similar to the source cell. Further, iPSCs with cellular memory are susceptible to preferential differentiation into the cell type that they had been derived from (105–108). The iPSC-associated methylated loci contain certain imprinted loci and other genomic regions. Some alteration of genomic imprinted loci occurs during cell reprogramming or long-term culture (109–112). For instance, aberrant silencing of the *D1K1-Dio3* imprinted locus is functionally associated with the failure to generate iPSCs in mouse during reprogramming (113, 114). Methylome profiling has been used to detect differentially methylated regions (DMRs) in hESCs and hiPSCs (115). In the study, all hypermethylated CG DMRs in hiPSCs were recognized as reprogramming-induced aberrancies.

CNVs and SNVs can be introduced into iPSCs as they may already exist in source cell lines or be acquired during the reprogramming process. hiPSCs contain more CNVs than hESCs, source cells, and somatic cells (116). Therefore, it is possible that iPSCs are more susceptible to CNV generation during cell reprogramming. However, sequencing-based findings suggest the occurrence of few or no detectable *de novo* CNVs in iPSCs (117–121). By contrast, low-grade genetic mosaicism of CNVs in source cells was tracked to iPSC derivation. Hence, it is possible that low-grade genetic mosaicism of somatic cells is the major source of CNVs in iPSCs. In addition, several studies have discussed the potential relationship between SNVs and iPSC generation. Most studies revealed no specific functional enrichment of genes with SNVs in iPSCs (117, 120, 122, 123). Most iPSC-manifested SNVs appear to be randomly distributed in the genome and are functionally irrelevant to iPSC generation. Therefore, the safety of iPSCs for use in regenerative medicine still faces many challenges.

Another safety concern has been raised regarding immunogenicity and tumorigenicity of the iPSC technology. Both genetic and epigenetic instability arising from iPSC reprogramming increases the risk of immunogenicity and tumorigenicity *in vivo* during iPSC-derived hepatic cell-associated therapy. Theoretically, the recipients of autologous iPSC-HLC transplants should not reject the transplants (124). However, in a teratoma mouse model, immune rejection in recipients was observed after iPSC transplantation (125). Undifferentiated PSCs, which possess the privilege property of immune tolerance because of low MHC-I antigen expression and the absence of MCH-II antigen expression, are expected to be less immunogenic than iPSCs (126–129). However, abnormal epigenetic differences between iPSCs and PSCs could contribute to the expression of immunogenic antigens during iPSC differentiation (128). Further, iPSC tumorigenicity poses a challenge for the development of individualized iPSC-HLC therapy. Pluripotency acquired by somatic cells upon reprogramming methods can increase genomic instability on the chromosomal and sub-chromosomal levels, contributing to the risk of tumorigenic transformation (130). Therefore, before the clinical development of iPSCs, current reprogramming technologies need to be optimized to minimize the occurrence of immunogenicity and tumorigenicity (**Figure 3**).

CONCLUSION

Together with the burgeoning application of stem cell-based techniques, iPSC technology has been incorporated into new approaches such as -omics–related research, nuclear reprogramming, gene-editing technology, RNAi, tissue engineering, medical devices, high-throughput screens (HTS), and humanized chimeric animal models. iPSCs provide promising opportunities to study novel therapies for liver diseases using cell properties of self-renewal and differentiation for the generation of HLCs. Recent studies have demonstrated that iPSC-derived hepatocytes are applicable for *in vitro* studies of complex liver disorders, such as viral hepatitis, inherited metabolic disorders, non-alcoholic liver diseases, cirrhosis, and HCC (**Figure 4**). HLCs can also be used as cell therapy to repair and regenerate liver mass to treat liver disease and prolong patient survival. The genetic and molecular mechanisms underlying liver disorders are an emerging area of research. By studying iPSC-HLCs as a possible treatment option, researchers are able to gain valuable insight into *in vitro* disease modeling and personalized medicine.

Nevertheless, several limitations still exist that prevent the clinical application of iPSC technology. The protocols for reprogramming and differentiation of hiPSCs into HLCs should be optimized and standardized to increase the efficiency of inducibility and promote HLC maturation. The risk of potential tumorigenicity associated with genomic and epigenetic variations should also be assessed. In addition, to commercialize iPSCs for clinical applications, further investigation into the limitations and challenges of using iPSCs is needed. Very few scientific reports have tested HLC injection/transplantation in life-threatening models of congenital diseases. To the best of our knowledge, to date, no single study has been able to demonstrate correction of amino acid or neurotransmitter abnormalities by injecting iPSC-HLCs. Nonetheless, with rapid technological advances in stem cell therapy, hiPSCs are likely to become effective and safe treatment of liver diseases in the future.

AUTHOR CONTRIBUTIONS

LQ provided the concept of this manuscript and prepared the figures. LZ, KP, and XL drafted this manuscript and prepared the figures. SDWB, RN, SB, and YL revised the manuscript. All authors contributed to the article and approved the submitted version.

REFERENCES

1. Asrani SK, Devarbhavi H, Eaton J, Kamath PS. Burden of liver diseases in the world. *J Hepatol.* (2019) 70:151–71. doi: 10.1016/j.jhep.2018.09.014
2. *Global Observatory on Donation and Transplantation* (2019). Available online at: http://www.transplant-observatory.org/
3. Trotter JF, Cardenas A. Liver transplantation around the world. *Liver Transpl.* (2016) 22:1059–61. doi: 10.1002/lt.24508
4. Soltys KA, Setoyama K, Tafaleng EN, Soto Gutierrez A, Fong J, Fukumitsu K, et al. Host conditioning and rejection monitoring in hepatocyte transplantation in humans. *J Hepatol.* (2017) 66:987–1000. doi: 10.1016/j.jhep.2016.12.017
5. Sampaziotis F, Segeritz CP, Vallier L. Potential of human induced pluripotent stem cells in studies of liver disease. *Hepatology.* (2015) 62:303–11. doi: 10.1002/hep.27651
6. Nakamori D, Takayama K, Nagamoto Y, Mitani S, Sakurai F, Tachibana M, et al. Hepatic maturation of human iPS cell-derived hepatocyte-like cells by ATF5, c/EBPalpha, and PROX1 transduction. *Biochem Biophys Res Commun.* (2016) 469:424–9. doi: 10.1016/j.bbrc.2015.12.007
7. Schwartz RE, Fleming HE, Khetani SR, Bhatia SN. Pluripotent stem cell-derived hepatocyte-like cells. *Biotechnol Adv.* (2014) 32:504–13. doi: 10.1016/j.biotechadv.2014.01.003
8. Takahashi K, Yamanaka S. Induction of pluripotent stem cells from mouse embryonic and adult fibroblast cultures by defined factors. *Cell.* (2006) 126:663–76. doi: 10.1016/j.cell.2006.07.024
9. Takahashi K, Tanabe K, Ohnuki M, Narita M, Ichisaka T, Tomoda K, et al. Induction of pluripotent stem cells from adult human fibroblasts by defined factors. *Cell.* (2007) 131:861–72. doi: 10.1016/j.cell.2007.11.019
10. Yu J, Vodyanik MA, Smuga-Otto K, Antosiewicz-Bourget J, Frane JL, Tian S, et al. Induced pluripotent stem cell lines derived from human somatic cells. *Science.* (2007) 318:1917–20. doi: 10.1126/science.1151526
11. Takahashi K, Yamanaka S. A decade of transcription factor-mediated reprogramming to pluripotency. *Nat Rev Mol Cell Biol.* (2016) 17:183–93. doi: 10.1038/nrm.2016.8
12. Fusaki N, Ban H, Nishiyama A, Saeki K, Hasegawa M. Efficient induction of transgene-free human pluripotent stem cells using a vector based on Sendai virus, an RNA virus that does not integrate into the host genome. *Proc Jpn Acad Ser B Phys Biol Sci.* (2009) 85:348–62. doi: 10.2183/pjab.85.348
13. Okita K, Matsumura Y, Sato Y, Okada A, Morizane A, Okamoto S, et al. A more efficient method to generate integration-free human iPS cells. *Nat Methods.* (2011) 8:409–12. doi: 10.1038/nmeth.1591
14. Warren L, Manos PD, Ahfeldt T, Loh YH, Li H, Lau F, et al. Highly efficient reprogramming to pluripotency and directed differentiation of human cells with synthetic modified mRNA. *Cell Stem Cell.* (2010) 7:618–30. doi: 10.1016/j.stem.2010.08.012
15. Song Z, Cai J, Liu Y, Zhao D, Yong J, Duo S, et al. Efficient generation of hepatocyte-like cells from human induced pluripotent stem cells. *Cell Res.* (2009) 19:1233–42. doi: 10.1038/cr.2009.107
16. Chen YF, Tseng CY, Wang HW, Kuo HC, Yang VW, Lee OK. Rapid generation of mature hepatocyte-like cells from human induced pluripotent stem cells by an efficient three-step protocol. *Hepatology.* (2012) 55:1193–203. doi: 10.1002/hep.24790
17. Yanagida A, Ito K, Chikada H, Nakauchi H, Kamiya A. An *in vitro* expansion system for generation of human iPS cell-derived hepatic progenitor-like cells exhibiting a bipotent differentiation potential. *PLoS ONE.* (2013) 8:e67541. doi: 10.1371/journal.pone.0067541
18. Hay DC, Fletcher J, Payne C, Terrace JD, Gallagher RC, Snoeys J, et al. Highly efficient differentiation of hESCs to functional hepatic endoderm requires ActivinA and Wnt3a signaling. *Proc Natl Acad Sci USA.* (2008) 105:12301–6. doi: 10.1073/pnas.0806522105
19. Morrison GM, Oikonomopoulou I, Migueles RP, Soneji S, Livigni A, Enver T, et al. Anterior definitive endoderm from ESCs reveals a role for FGF signaling. *Cell Stem Cell.* (2008) 3:402–15. doi: 10.1016/j.stem.2008.07.021
20. Zaret KS. Regulatory phases of early liver development: paradigms of organogenesis. *Nat Rev Genet.* (2002) 3:499–512. doi: 10.1038/nrg837
21. Schmidt C, Bladt F, Goedecke S, Brinkmann V, Zschiesche W, Sharpe M, et al. Scatter factor/hepatocyte growth factor is essential for liver development. *Nature.* (1995) 373:699–702. doi: 10.1038/373699a0
22. Hansel MC, Davila JC, Vosough M, Gramignoli R, Skvorak KJ, Dorko K, et al. The use of induced pluripotent stem cells for the study and treatment of liver diseases. *Curr Protoc Toxicol.* (2016) 67:14.13.1–14.13.27. doi: 10.1002/0471140856.tx1413s67
23. Dianat N, Dubois-Pot-Schneider H, Steichen C, Desterke C, Leclerc P, Raveux A, et al. Generation of functional cholangiocyte-like cells from human pluripotent stem cells and HepaRG cells. *Hepatology.* (2014) 60:700–14. doi: 10.1002/hep.27165
24. Ogawa M, Ogawa S, Bear CE, Ahmadi S, Chin S, Li B, et al. Directed differentiation of cholangiocytes from human pluripotent stem cells. *Nat Biotechnol.* (2015) 33:853–61. doi: 10.1038/nbt.3294
25. Sampaziotis F, de Brito MC, Madrigal P, Bertero A, Saeb-Parsy K, Soares FAC, et al. Cholangiocytes derived from human induced pluripotent stem cells for disease modeling and drug validation. *Nat Biotechnol.* (2015) 33:845–52. doi: 10.1038/nbt.3275
26. Yu Y, Liu H, Ikeda Y, Amiot BP, Rinaldo P, Duncan SA, et al. Hepatocyte-like cells differentiated from human induced pluripotent stem cells: relevance to cellular therapies. *Stem Cell Res.* (2012) 9:196–207. doi: 10.1016/j.scr.2012.06.004
27. Roy-Chowdhury N, Wang X, Guha C, Roy-Chowdhury J. Hepatocyte-like cells derived from induced pluripotent stem cells. *Hepatol Int.* (2017) 11:54–69. doi: 10.1007/s12072-016-9757-y
28. Lu J, Einhorn S, Venkatarangan L, Miller M, Mann DA, Watkins PB, et al. Morphological and functional characterization and assessment of ipsc-derived hepatocytes for *in vitro* toxicity testing. *Toxicol Sci.* (2015) 147:39–54. doi: 10.1093/toxsci/kfv117
29. Larsen LE, Smith MA, Abbey D, Korn A, Reeskamp LF, Hand NJ, et al. Hepatocyte-like cells derived from induced pluripotent stem cells: A versatile tool to understand lipid disorders. *Atherosclerosis.* (2020) 303:8–14. doi: 10.1016/j.atherosclerosis.2020.03.014
30. Grandy R, Tomaz RA, Vallier L. Modeling disease with human inducible pluripotent stem cells. *Annu Rev Pathol.* (2019) 14:449–68. doi: 10.1146/annurev-pathol-020117-043634
31. Gao X, Liu Y. A transcriptomic study suggesting human iPSC-derived hepatocytes potentially offer a better *in vitro* model of hepatotoxicity than most hepatoma cell lines. *Cell Biol Toxicol.* (2017) 33:407–21. doi: 10.1007/s10565-017-9383-z
32. Chen Y, Li Y, Wang X, Zhang W, Sauer V, Chang CJ, et al. Amelioration of hyperbilirubinemia in gunn rats after transplantation of human induced pluripotent stem cell-derived hepatocytes. *Stem Cell Rep.* (2015) 5:22–30. doi: 10.1016/j.stemcr.2015.04.017
33. Zabulica M, Srinivasan RC, Vosough M, Hammarstedt C, Wu T, Gramignoli R, et al. Guide to the assessment of mature liver gene expression in stem cell-derived hepatocytes. *Stem Cells Dev.* (2019) 28:907–19. doi: 10.1089/scd.2019.0064
34. Nakamura T, Torimura T, Sakamoto M, Hashimoto O, Taniguchi E, Inoue K, et al. Significance and therapeutic potential of endothelial progenitor cell transplantation in a cirrhotic liver rat model. *Gastroenterology.* (2007) 133:91–107. doi: 10.1053/j.gastro.2007.03.110
35. Fang B, Shi M, Liao L, Yang S, Liu Y, Zhao RC. Systemic infusion of FLK1(+) mesenchymal stem cells ameliorate carbon tetrachloride-induced liver fibrosis in mice. *Transplantation.* (2004) 78:83–8. doi: 10.1097/01.TP.0000128326.95294.14
36. Aziz MTA, Atta HM, Mahfouz S, Fouad HH, Roshdy NK, Ahmed HH, et al. Therapeutic potential of bone marrow-derived mesenchymal stem cells on experimental liver fibrosis. *Clin Biochem.* (2007) 40:893–9. doi: 10.1016/j.clinbiochem.2007.04.017
37. Sakaida I, Terai S, Yamamoto N, Aoyama K, Ishikawa T, Nishina H, et al. Transplantation of bone marrow cells reduces CCl4-induced liver fibrosis in mice. *Hepatology.* (2004) 40:1304–11. doi: 10.1002/hep.20452
38. Amer MEM, El-Sayed SZ, El-Kheir WA, Gabr H, Gomaa AA, El-Noomani N, et al. Clinical and laboratory evaluation of patients

with end-stage liver cell failure injected with bone marrow-derived hepatocyte-like cells. *Eur J Gastroenterol Hepatol.* (2011) 23:936–41. doi: 10.1097/MEG.0b013e3283488b00

39. Asgari S, Moslem M, Bagheri-Lankarani K, Pournasr B, Miryounesi M, Baharvand H. Differentiation and transplantation of human induced pluripotent stem cell-derived hepatocyte-like cells. *Stem Cell Rev Rep.* (2013) 9:493–504. doi: 10.1007/s12015-011-9330-y
40. Takayama K, Akita N, Mimura N, Akahira R, Taniguchi Y, Ikeda M, et al. Generation of safe and therapeutically effective human induced pluripotent stem cell-derived hepatocyte-like cells for regenerative medicine. *Hepatol Commun.* (2017) 1:1058–69. doi: 10.1002/hep4.1111
41. Isobe K, Cheng Z, Ito S, Nishio N. Aging in the mouse and perspectives of rejuvenation through induced pluripotent stem cells (iPSCs). *Results Probl Cell Differ.* (2012) 55:413–27. doi: 10.1007/978-3-642-30406-4_21
42. Espejel S, Roll GR, McLaughlin KJ, Lee AY, Zhang JY, Laird DJ, et al. Induced pluripotent stem cell-derived hepatocytes have the functional and proliferative capabilities needed for liver regeneration in mice. *J Clin Invest.* (2010) 120:3120–6. doi: 10.1172/JCI 43267
43. Kuriyan AE, Albini TA, Townsend JH, Rodriguez M, Pandya HK, Leonard RE, et al. Vision loss after intravitreal injection of autologous "Stem Cells" for AMD. *N Engl J Med.* (2017) 376:1047–53. doi: 10.1056/NEJMoa1609583
44. Evans AA, London WT, Gish RG, Cohen C, Block TM. Chronic HBV infection outside treatment guidelines: is treatment needed? *Antivir Ther.* (2013) 18:229–35. doi: 10.3851/IMP2325
45. Yang JD, Roberts LR. Hepatocellular carcinoma: a global view. *Nat Rev Gastroenterol Hepatol.* (2010) 7:448–58. doi: 10.1038/nrgastro.2010.100
46. Yoshida T, Takayama K, Kondoh M, Sakurai F, Tani H, Sakamoto N, et al. Use of human hepatocyte-like cells derived from induced pluripotent stem cells as a model for hepatocytes in hepatitis C virus infection. *Biochem Biophys Res Commun.* (2011) 416:119–24. doi: 10.1016/j.bbrc.2011.11.007
47. Liu H, Ye Z, Kim Y, Sharkis S, Jang YY. Generation of endoderm-derived human induced pluripotent stem cells from primary hepatocytes. *Hepatology.* (2010) 51:1810–9. doi: 10.1002/hep.23626
48. Furuyama K, Kawaguchi Y, Akiyama H, Horiguchi M, Kodama S, Kuhara T, et al. Continuous cell supply from a Sox9-expressing progenitor zone in adult liver, exocrine pancreas and intestine. *Nat Genet.* (2011) 43:34–41. doi: 10.1038/ng.722
49. Si-Tayeb K, Noto FK, Nagaoka M, Li J, Battle MA, Duris C, et al. Highly efficient generation of human hepatocyte-like cells from induced pluripotent stem cells. *Hepatology.* (2010) 51:297–305. doi: 10.1002/hep.23354
50. Sakurai F, Mitani S, Yamamoto T, Takayama K, Tachibana M, Watashi K, et al. Human induced-pluripotent stem cell-derived hepatocyte-like cells as an *in vitro* model of human hepatitis B virus infection. *Sci Rep.* (2017) 7:45698. doi: 10.1038/srep45698
51. Kaserman JE, Wilson AA. Patient-derived induced pluripotent stem cells for alpha-1 antitrypsin deficiency disease modeling and therapeutic discovery. *Chronic Obstr Pulm Dis.* (2018) 5:258–66. doi: 10.15326/jcopdf.5.4.2017.0179
52. Rader DJ, Cohen J, Hobbs HH. Monogenic hypercholesterolemia: new insights in pathogenesis and treatment. *J Clin Invest.* (2003) 111:1795–803. doi: 10.1172/JCI200318925
53. Harada-Shiba M, Arai H, Ishigaki Y, Ishibashi S, Okamura T, Ogura M, et al. Guidelines for diagnosis and treatment of familial hypercholesterolemia 2017. *J Atheroscler Thromb.* (2018) 25:751–70. doi: 10.5551/jat.CR003
54. Rashid ST, Corbineau S, Hannan N, Marciniak SJ, Miranda E, Alexander G, et al. Modeling inherited metabolic disorders of the liver using human induced pluripotent stem cells. *J Clin Invest.* (2010) 120:3127–36. doi: 10.1172/JCI43122
55. Tafaleng EN, Chakraborty S, Han B, Hale P, Wu W, Soto-Gutierrez A, et al. Induced pluripotent stem cells model personalized variations in liver disease resulting from alpha1-antitrypsin deficiency. *Hepatology.* (2015) 62:147–57. doi: 10.1002/hep.27753
56. Cayo MA, Cai J, DeLaForest A, Noto FK, Nagaoka M, Clark BS, et al. JD induced pluripotent stem cell-derived hepatocytes faithfully recapitulate the pathophysiology of familial hypercholesterolemia. *Hepatology.* (2012) 56:2163–71. doi: 10.1002/hep.25871
57. Chun YS, Chaudhari P, Jang YY. Applications of patient-specific induced pluripotent stem cells; focused on disease modeling, drug screening and therapeutic potentials for liver disease. *Int J Biol Sci.* (2010) 6:796–805. doi: 10.7150/ijbs.6.796
58. Yusa K, Rashid ST, Strick-Marchand H, Varela I, Liu PQ, Paschon DE, et al. Targeted gene correction of alpha1-antitrypsin deficiency in induced pluripotent stem cells. *Nature.* (2011) 478:391–4. doi: 10.1038/nature10424
59. Choi SM, Kim Y, Shim JS, Park JT, Wang RH, Leach SD, et al. Efficient drug screening and gene correction for treating liver disease using patient-specific stem cells. *Hepatology.* (2013) 57:2458–68. doi: 10.1002/hep.26237
60. Smith C, Abalde-Atristain L, He C, Brodsky BR, Braunstein EM, Chaudhari P, et al. Efficient and allele-specific genome editing of disease loci in human iPSCs. *Mol Ther.* (2015) 23:570–7. doi: 10.1038/mt.2014.226
61. Omer L, Hudson EA, Zheng S, Hoying JB, Shan Y, Boyd NL. CRISPR correction of a homozygous low-density lipoprotein receptor mutation in familial hypercholesterolemia induced pluripotent stem cells. *Hepatol Commun.* (2017) 1:886–98. doi: 10.1002/hep4.1110
62. Starley BQ, Calcagno CJ, Harrison SA. Nonalcoholic fatty liver disease and hepatocellular carcinoma: a weighty connection. *Hepatology.* (2010) 51:1820–32. doi: 10.1002/hep.23594
63. Younossi ZM, Koenig AB, Abdelatif D, Fazel Y, Henry L, Wymer M. Global epidemiology of nonalcoholic fatty liver disease-meta-analytic assessment of prevalence, incidence, and outcomes. *Hepatology.* (2016) 64:73–84. doi: 10.1002/hep.28431
64. Wong RJ, Aguilar M, Cheung R, Perumpail RB, Harrison SA, Younossi ZM, et al. Nonalcoholic steatohepatitis is the second leading etiology of liver disease among adults awaiting liver transplantation in the United States. *Gastroenterology.* (2015) 148:547–55. doi: 10.1053/j.gastro.2014.11.039
65. Fon Tacer K, Rozman D. Nonalcoholic Fatty liver disease: focus on lipoprotein and lipid deregulation. *J Lipids.* (2011) 2011:783976. doi: 10.1155/2011/783976
66. Grochowski CM, Loomes KM, Spinner NB. Jagged1 (JAG1): structure, expression, and disease associations. *Gene.* (2016) 576:381–4. doi: 10.1016/j.gene.2015.10.065
67. Guegan K, Stals K, Day M, Turnpenny P, Ellard S. JAG1 mutations are found in approximately one third of patients presenting with only one or two clinical features of Alagille syndrome. *Clin Genet.* (2012) 82:33–40. doi: 10.1111/j.1399-0004.2011.01749.x
68. Tiniakos DG, Vos MB, Brunt EM. Nonalcoholic fatty liver disease: pathology and pathogenesis. *Annu Rev Pathol.* (2010) 5:145–71. doi: 10.1146/annurev-pathol-121808-102132
69. Pu K, Wang Y, Bai S, Wei H, Zhou Y, Fan J, et al. Diagnostic accuracy of controlled attenuation parameter (CAP) as a non-invasive test for steatosis in suspected non-alcoholic fatty liver disease: a systematic review and meta-analysis. *BMC Gastroenterol.* (2019) 19:51. doi: 10.1186/s12876-019-0961-9
70. De Gottardi A, Vinciguerra M, Sgroi A, Moukil M, Ravier-Dall'Antonia F, Pazienza V, et al. Microarray analyses and molecular profiling of steatosis induction in immortalized human hepatocytes. *Lab Invest.* (2007) 87:792–806. doi: 10.1038/labinvest.3700590
71. Ricchi M, Odoardi MR, Carulli L, Anzivino C, Ballestri S, Pinetti A, et al. Differential effect of oleic and palmitic acid on lipid accumulation and apoptosis in cultured hepatocytes. *J Gastroenterol Hepatol.* (2009) 24:830–40. doi: 10.1111/j.1440-1746.2008.05733.x
72. Graffmann N, Ring S, Kawala MA, Wruck W, Ncube A, Trompeter HI, et al. Modeling nonalcoholic fatty liver disease with human pluripotent stem cell-derived immature hepatocyte-like cells reveals activation of PLIN2 and confirms regulatory functions of peroxisome proliferator-activated receptor alpha. *Stem Cells Dev.* (2016) 25:1119–33. doi: 10.1089/scd.2015.0383
73. Graffmann N, Bohndorf M, Ncube A, Kawala MA, Wruck W, Kashofer K, et al. Establishment and characterization of an iPSC line from a 35years old high grade patient with nonalcoholic fatty liver disease (30-40% steatosis) with homozygous wildtype PNPLA3 genotype. *Stem Cell Res.* (2018) 31:113–6. doi: 10.1016/j.scr.2018.07.015
74. Graffmann N, Bohndorf M, Ncube A, Wruck W, Kashofer K, Zatloukal K, et al. Establishment and characterization of an iPSC line from a 58years old high grade patient with nonalcoholic fatty liver disease (70% steatosis) with homozygous wildtype PNPLA3 genotype. *Stem Cell Res.* (2018) 31:131–4. doi: 10.1016/j.scr.2018.07.011

75. Parafati M, Kirby RJ, Khorasanizadeh S, Rastinejad F, Malany S. A nonalcoholic fatty liver disease model in human induced pluripotent stem cell-derived hepatocytes, created by endoplasmic reticulum stress-induced steatosis. *Dis Model Mech.* (2018) 11:33530. doi: 10.1242/dmm.033530
76. Romanelli RG, Stasi C. Recent advancements in diagnosis and therapy of liver cirrhosis. *Curr Drug Targets.* (2016) 17:1804–17. doi: 10.2174/1389450117666160613101413
77. Murray KF, Carithers RL, Jr., Aasld. AASLD practice guidelines: evaluation of the patient for liver transplantation. *Hepatology.* (2005) 41:1407–32. doi: 10.1002/hep.20704
78. Van de Bovenkamp M, Groothuis GM, Meijer DK, Olinga P. Liver fibrosis *in vitro*: cell culture models and precision-cut liver slices. *Toxicol In Vitro.* (2007) 21:545–57. doi: 10.1016/j.tiv.2006.12.009
79. Guyot C, Lepreux S, Combe C, Doudnikoff E, Bioulac-Sage P, Balabaud C, et al. Hepatic fibrosis and cirrhosis: the (myo)fibroblastic cell subpopulations involved. *Int J Biochem Cell Biol.* (2006) 38:135–51. doi: 10.1016/j.biocel.2005.08.021
80. Bhatia SN, Balis UJ, Yarmush ML, Toner M. Effect of cell-cell interactions in preservation of cellular phenotype: cocultivation of hepatocytes and nonparenchymal cells. *FASEB J.* (1999) 13:1883–900. doi: 10.1096/fasebj.13.14.1883
81. Takebe T, Sekine K, Enomura M, Koike H, Kimura M, Ogaeri T, et al. Vascularized and functional human liver from an iPSC-derived organ bud transplant. *Nature.* (2013) 499:481–4. doi: 10.1038/nature12271
82. Chen Z, Qi LZ, Zeng R, Li HY, Dai LJ. Stem cells and hepatic cirrhosis. *Panminerva Med.* (2010) 52:149–65.
83. Povero D, Pinatel EM, Leszczynska A, Goyal NP, Nishio T, Kim J, et al. Human induced pluripotent stem cell-derived extracellular vesicles reduce hepatic stellate cell activation and liver fibrosis. *JCI Insight.* (2019) 5:e125652. doi: 10.1172/jci.insight.125652
84. Park S, In Hwang S, Kim J, Hwang S, Kang S, Yang S, et al. The therapeutic potential of induced hepatocyte-like cells generated by direct reprogramming on hepatic fibrosis. *Stem Cell Res Ther.* (2019) 10:21. doi: 10.1186/s13287-018-1127-3
85. Choi SM, Kim Y, Liu H, Chaudhari P, Ye Z, Jang YY. Liver engraftment potential of hepatic cells derived from patient-specific induced pluripotent stem cells. *Cell Cycle.* (2011) 10:2423–7. doi: 10.4161/cc.10.15.16869
86. Ferlay J, Shin HR, Bray F, Forman D, Mathers C, Parkin DM. Estimates of worldwide burden of cancer in 2008: GLOBOCAN (2008). *Int J Cancer.* (2010) 127:2893–917. doi: 10.1002/ijc.25516
87. Forner A, Bruix J. Biomarkers for early diagnosis of hepatocellular carcinoma. *Lancet Oncol.* (2012) 13:750–1. doi: 10.1016/S1470-2045(12)70271-1
88. Sun C, Liu YK. Induced pluripotent cancer cells: progress and application. *J Cancer Res Clin Oncol.* (2011) 137:1–8. doi: 10.1007/s00432-010-0955-z
89. Zheng YW, Nie YZ, Taniguchi H. Cellular reprogramming and hepatocellular carcinoma development. *World J Gastroenterol.* (2013) 19:8850–60. doi: 10.3748/wjg.v19.i47.8850
90. Moriguchi H, Chung RT, Sato C. An identification of novel therapy for human hepatocellular carcinoma by using human induced pluripotent stem cells. *Hepatology.* (2010) 51:1090–1. doi: 10.1002/hep.23418
91. Sakisaka M, Haruta M, Komohara Y, Umemoto S, Matsumura K, Ikeda T, et al. Therapy of primary and metastatic liver cancer by human iPS cell-derived myeloid cells producing interferon-beta. *J Hepatobiliary Pancreat Sci.* (2017) 24:109–19. doi: 10.1002/jhbp.422
92. Sampaziotis F, de Brito MC, Geti I, Bertero A, Hannan NR, Vallier L. Directed differentiation of human induced pluripotent stem cells into functional cholangiocyte-like cells. *Nat Protoc.* (2017) 12:814–27. doi: 10.1038/nprot.2017.011
93. Sayed N, Liu C, Wu JC. Translation of human-induced pluripotent stem cells: from clinical trial in a dish to precision medicine. *J Am Coll Cardiol.* (2016) 67:2161–76. doi: 10.1016/j.jacc.2016.01.083
94. Shi Y, Inoue H, Wu JC, Yamanaka S. Induced pluripotent stem cell technology: a decade of progress. *Nat Rev Drug Discovery.* (2017) 16:115–30. doi: 10.1038/nrd.2016.245
95. Cayo MA, Mallanna SK, Di Furio F, Jing R, Tolliver LB, Bures M, et al. A drug screen using human iPSC-derived hepatocyte-like cells reveals cardiac glycosides as a potential treatment for hypercholesterolemia. *Cell Stem Cell.* (2017) 20:478–89. doi: 10.1016/j.stem.2017.01.011
96. Jing R, Corbett JL, Cai J, Beeson GC, Beeson CC, Chan SS, et al. A screen using iPSC-derived hepatocytes reveals NAD(+) as a potential treatment for mtDNA depletion syndrome. *Cell Rep.* (2018) 25:1469–84. doi: 10.1016/j.celrep.2018.10.036
97. Broutier L, Mastrogiovanni G, Verstegen MM, Francies HE, Gavarró LM, Bradshaw CR, et al. Human primary liver cancer-derived organoid cultures for disease modeling and drug screening. *Nat Med.* (2017) 23:1424–35. doi: 10.1038/nm.4438
98. Artegiani B, Clevers H. Use and application of 3D-organoid technology. *Human Mol Genet.* (2018) 27:R99–107. doi: 10.1093/hmg/ddy187
99. Wang Y, Wang H, Deng P, Chen W, Guo Y, Tao T, et al. *In situ* differentiation and generation of functional liver organoids from human iPSCs in a 3D perfusable chip system. *Lab Chip.* (2018) 18:3606–16. doi: 10.1039/C8LC00869H
100. Draper JS, Smith K, Gokhale P, Moore HD, Maltby E, Johnson J, et al. Recurrent gain of chromosomes 17q and 12 in cultured human embryonic stem cells. *Nat Biotechnol.* (2004) 22:53–4. doi: 10.1038/nbt922
101. Hannoun Z, Steichen C, Dianat N, Weber A, Dubart-Kupperschmitt A. The potential of induced pluripotent stem cell derived hepatocytes. *J Hepatol.* (2016) 65:182–99. doi: 10.1016/j.jhep.2016.02.025
102. Panopoulos AD, Ruiz S, Izpisua Belmonte JC. iPSCs: induced back to controversy. *Cell Stem Cell.* (2011) 8:347–8. doi: 10.1016/j.stem.2011.03.003
103. Liang G, Zhang Y. Genetic and epigenetic variations in iPSCs: potential causes and implications for application. *Cell Stem Cell.* (2013) 13:149–59. doi: 10.1016/j.stem.2013.07.001
104. Anguera MC, Sadreyev R, Zhang Z, Szanto A, Payer B, Sheridan SD, et al. Molecular signatures of human induced pluripotent stem cells highlight sex differences and cancer genes. *Cell Stem Cell.* (2012) 11:75–90. doi: 10.1016/j.stem.2012.03.008
105. Polo JM, Liu S, Figueroa ME, Kulalert W, Eminli S, Tan KY, et al. Cell type of origin influences the molecular and functional properties of mouse induced pluripotent stem cells. *Nat Biotechnol.* (2010) 28:848–55. doi: 10.1038/nbt.1667
106. Kim K, Zhao R, Doi A, Ng K, Unternaehrer J, Cahan P, et al. Donor cell type can influence the epigenome and differentiation potential of human induced pluripotent stem cells. *Nat Biotechnol.* (2011) 29:1117–9. doi: 10.1038/nbt.2052
107. Kim K, Doi A, Wen B, Ng K, Zhao R, Cahan P, et al. Epigenetic memory in induced pluripotent stem cells. *Nature.* (2010) 467:285–90. doi: 10.1038/nature09342
108. Bar-Nur O, Russ HA, Efrat S, Benvenisty N. Epigenetic memory and preferential lineage-specific differentiation in induced pluripotent stem cells derived from human pancreatic islet beta cells. *Cell Stem Cell.* (2011) 9:17–23. doi: 10.1016/j.stem.2011.06.007
109. Pick M, Stelzer Y, Bar-Nur O, Mayshar Y, Eden A, Benvenisty N. Clone- and gene-specific aberrations of parental imprinting in human induced pluripotent stem cells. *Stem Cells.* (2009) 27:2686–90. doi: 10.1002/stem.205
110. Nishino K, Toyoda M, Yamazaki-Inoue M, Fukawatase Y, Chikazawa E, Sakaguchi H, et al. DNA methylation dynamics in human induced pluripotent stem cells over time. *PLoS Genet.* (2011) 7:e1002085. doi: 10.1371/journal.pgen.1002085
111. Nazor KL, Altun G, Lynch C, Tran H, Harness JV, Slavin I, et al. Recurrent variations in DNA methylation in human pluripotent stem cells and their differentiated derivatives. *Cell Stem Cell.* (2012) 10:620–34. doi: 10.1016/j.stem.2012.02.013
112. Chamberlain SJ, Chen PF, Ng KY, Bourgois-Rocha F, Lemtiri-Chlieh F, Levine ES, et al. Induced pluripotent stem cell models of the genomic imprinting disorders Angelman and Prader-Willi syndromes. *Proc Natl Acad Sci USA.* (2010) 107:17668–73. doi: 10.1073/pnas.1004487107
113. Stadtfeld M, Apostolou E, Akutsu H, Fukuda A, Follett P, Natesan S, et al. Aberrant silencing of imprinted genes on chromosome 12qF1 in mouse induced pluripotent stem cells. *Nature.* (2010) 465:175–81. doi: 10.1038/nature09017
114. Liu L, Luo GZ, Yang W, Zhao X, Zheng Q, Lv Z, et al. Activation of the imprinted Dlk1-Dio3 region correlates with pluripotency levels of mouse stem cells. *J Biol Chem.* (2010) 285:19483–90. doi: 10.1074/jbc.M110.131995

115. Lister R, Pelizzola M, Kida YS, Hawkins RD, Nery JR, Hon G, et al. Hotspots of aberrant epigenomic reprogramming in human induced pluripotent stem cells. *Nature.* (2011) 471:68–73. doi: 10.1038/nature09798
116. Hussein SM, Batada NN, Vuoristo S, Ching RW, Autio R, Narva E, et al. Copy number variation and selection during reprogramming to pluripotency. *Nature.* (2011) 471:58–62. doi: 10.1038/nature09871
117. Young MA, Larson DE, Sun CW, George DR, Ding L, Miller CA, et al. Background mutations in parental cells account for most of the genetic heterogeneity of induced pluripotent stem cells. *Cell Stem Cell.* (2012) 10:570–82. doi: 10.1016/j.stem.2012.03.002
118. Quinlan AR, Boland MJ, Leibowitz ML, Shumilina S, Pehrson SM, Baldwin KK, et al. Genome sequencing of mouse induced pluripotent stem cells reveals retroelement stability and infrequent DNA rearrangement during reprogramming. *Cell Stem Cell.* (2011) 9:366–73. doi: 10.1016/j.stem.2011.07.018
119. Gore A, Li Z, Fung HL, Young JE, Agarwal S, Antosiewicz-Bourget J, et al. Somatic coding mutations in human induced pluripotent stem cells. *Nature.* (2011) 471:63–7. doi: 10.1038/nature 09805
120. Cheng L, Hansen NF, Zhao L, Du Y, Zou C, Donovan FX, et al. Low incidence of DNA sequence variation in human induced pluripotent stem cells generated by nonintegrating plasmid expression. *Cell Stem Cell.* (2012) 10:337–44. doi: 10.1016/j.stem.2012.01.005
121. Abyzov A, Mariani J, Palejev D, Zhang Y, Haney MS, Tomasini L, et al. Somatic copy number mosaicism in human skin revealed by induced pluripotent stem cells. *Nature.* (2012) 492:438–42. doi: 10.1038/nature 11629
122. Ruiz S, Gore A, Li Z, Panopoulos AD, Montserrat N, Fung HL, et al. Analysis of protein-coding mutations in hiPSCs and their possible role during somatic cell reprogramming. *Nat Commun.* (2013) 4:1382. doi: 10.1038/ncomms 2381
123. Ji J, Ng SH, Sharma V, Neculai D, Hussein S, Sam M, et al. Elevated coding mutation rate during the reprogramming of human somatic cells into induced pluripotent stem cells. *Stem Cells.* (2012) 30:435–40. doi: 10.1002/stem.1011
124. Araki R, Uda M, Hoki Y, Sunayama M, Nakamura M, Ando S, et al. Negligible immunogenicity of terminally differentiated cells derived from induced pluripotent or embryonic stem cells. *Nature.* (2013) 494:100–4. doi: 10.1038/nature 11807
125. Zhao T, Zhang ZN, Rong Z, Xu Y. Immunogenicity of induced pluripotent stem cells. *Nature.* (2011) 474:212–5. doi: 10.1038/nature 10135
126. Tan Y, Ooi S, Wang L. Immunogenicity and tumorigenicity of pluripotent stem cells and their derivatives: genetic and epigenetic perspectives. *Curr Stem Cell Res Ther.* (2014) 9:63–72. doi: 10.2174/1574888X1130866 60068
127. Säljö K, Barone A, Mölne J, Rydberg L, Teneberg S, Breimer ME. HLA and histo-blood group antigen expression in human pluripotent stem cells and their derivatives. *Sci Rep.* (2017) 7:13072. doi: 10.1038/s41598-017-12231-8
128. Zhao T, Zhang ZN, Westenskow PD, Todorova D, Hu Z, Lin T, et al. Humanized mice reveal differential immunogenicity of cells derived from autologous induced pluripotent stem cells. *Cell Stem Cell.* (2015) 17:353–9. doi: 10.1016/j.stem.2015.07.021
129. Chen HF, Yu CY, Chen MJ, Chou SH, Chiang MS, Chou WH, et al. Characteristic expression of major histocompatibility complex and immune privilege genes in human pluripotent stem cells and their derivatives. *Cell Transplant.* (2015) 24:845–64. doi: 10.3727/096368913X674639
130. Laurent LC, Ulitsky I, Slavin I, Tran H, Schork A, Morey R, et al. Dynamic changes in the copy number of pluripotency and cell proliferation genes in human ESCs and iPSCs during reprogramming and time in culture. *Cell Stem Cell.* (2011) 8:106–18. doi: 10.1016/j.stem.2010.12.003

4

Attenuation of the Hepatoprotective Effects of Ileal Apical Sodium Dependent Bile Acid Transporter (ASBT) Inhibition in Choline-Deficient L-Amino Acid-Defined (CDAA) Diet-Fed Mice

*Anuradha Rao[1], Ivo P. van de Peppel[2], Sanjeev Gumber[3], Saul J. Karpen[1] and Paul A. Dawson[1]**

[1] Department of Pediatrics, Emory University School of Medicine, Atlanta, GA, United States, [2] Section of Molecular Metabolism and Nutrition, Department of Pediatrics, University Medical Center Groningen, University of Groningen, Groningen, Netherlands, [3] Division of Pathology, Yerkes National Primate Research Center, Emory University, Atlanta, GA, United States

***Correspondence:**
Paul A. Dawson
paul.dawson@emory.edu

Non-alcoholic fatty liver disease (NAFLD) is a major growing worldwide health problem. We previously reported that interruption of the enterohepatic circulation of bile acids using a non-absorbable apical sodium-dependent bile acid transporter inhibitor (ASBTi; SC-435) reduced the development of NAFLD in high fat diet fed mice. However, the ability of ASBTi treatment to impact the progression of NAFLD to non-alcoholic steatohepatitis (NASH) and fibrosis in a diet-induced mouse model remains untested. In the current study, we assessed whether ASBTi treatment is hepatoprotective in the choline-deficient, L-amino acid-defined (CDAA) diet model of NASH-induced fibrosis.

Methods: Male C57Bl/6 mice were fed with: (A) choline-sufficient L-amino acid-defined diet (CSAA) (31 kcal% fat), (B) CSAA diet plus ASBTi (SC-435; 60 ppm), (C) CDAA diet, or (D) CDAA diet plus ASBTi. Body weight and food intake were monitored. After 22 weeks on diet, liver histology, cholesterol and triglyceride levels, and gene expression were measured. Fecal bile acid and fat excretion were measured, and intestinal fat absorption was determined using the sucrose polybehenate method.

Results: ASBTi treatment reduced bodyweight gain in mice fed either the CSAA or CDAA diet, and prevented the increase in liver to body weight ratio observed in CDAA-fed mice. ASBTi significantly reduced hepatic total cholesterol levels in both CSAA and CDAA-fed mice. ASBTi-associated significant reductions in hepatic triglyceride levels and histological scoring for NAFLD activity were observed in CSAA but not CDAA-fed mice. These changes correlated with measurements of intestinal fat absorption, which was significantly reduced in ASBTi-treated mice fed the CSAA (85 vs. 94%, $P < 0.001$) but not CDAA diet (93 vs. 93%). As scored by Ishak staging of Sirius red stained liver sections, no hepatic fibrosis was evident in the CSAA diet mice. The CDAA diet-fed mice developed hepatic fibrosis, which was increased by the ASBTi.

Conclusions: ASBT inhibition reduced intestinal fat absorption, bodyweight gain and hepatic steatosis in CSAA diet-fed mice. The effects of the ASBTi on steatosis and fat absorption were attenuated in the context of dietary choline-deficiency. Inhibition of intestinal absorption of fatty acids may be involved in the therapeutic effects of ASBTi treatment.

Keywords: liver, triglyceride, fibrosis, fat absorption, cholesterol

INTRODUCTION

Parallel to the global rise in obesity, the disease burden related to non-alcoholic fatty liver disease (NAFLD) is emerging as a major worldwide problem. The number of adults and children with NAFLD is steadily increasing and the current global prevalence is estimated at 24% (1, 2). NAFLD comprises a spectrum of disease states, from non-symptomatic hepatic steatosis to non-alcoholic steatohepatitis (NASH) and liver fibrosis. NAFLD also increases the morbidity and mortality associated with type 2 diabetes mellitus, cardiovascular disease, and chronic kidney disease (3). Unfortunately, an incomplete understanding and lack of experimental NAFLD/NASH animal models that faithfully reproduce the human pathophysiology has slowed the development of new therapies (4). Recently, bile acid-related pathways have emerged as an important therapeutic target for disorders of glucose and lipid metabolism (5). Under physiological conditions, bile acid synthesis and enterohepatic cycling are tightly regulated to maintain a relatively constant whole-body bile acid pool size and restrict the systemic distribution of bile acids. After their secretion along with bile into the duodenum, about 95% of the bile acids are reabsorbed by the apical sodium-dependent bile acid transporter (ASBT; also called the ileal bile acid transporter, IBAT) in the distal small intestine, thereby limiting their flux into the colon. This system is tightly controlled in part by bile acid signaling via the farnesoid-X receptor (FXR) in the liver and intestine. The intestinal microbiota harbor enzymes to deconjugate and convert primary bile acids into secondary bile acids, changing the bile acid pool size, composition, and physicochemical properties (6). These changes alter signaling through FXR and other bile acid-activated receptors, and modulates the metabolic response to bile acids (7).

Several bile acid-based approaches are currently under investigation as potential therapies for liver diseases, including NAFLD. Obeticholic acid, a derivative of the naturally occurring FXR agonist chenodeoxycholic acid (CDCA), improved liver biochemistry and histology scores in NASH patients (8, 9). In addition, we have shown that interruption of the bile acid enterohepatic circulation by an ASBT inhibitor (ASBTi), SC-435, prevented hepatic lipid accumulation and improved markers of NAFLD in mice fed a high fat diet (10). Although these results and similar findings in high fat diet-fed Ldlr$^{-/-}$. Leiden mice demonstrated a robust effect of ASBT inhibition on hepatic lipid accumulation, the effects of ASBT inhibition on the progression from hepatic steatosis to steatohepatitis and fibrosis remain unclear (10, 11). Feeding a Western-type diet (high fat, sucrose, and cholesterol) to mice typically models aspects of the human condition including successfully inducing hepatic lipid accumulation. However, progression from steatosis to NASH and fibrosis is generally limited and highly variable (12–14). Therefore, other dietary, genetic or toxic interventions, or combinations thereof, are required to induce development of NASH in animal models. One widely used intervention for dietary induction of NASH and subsequent fibrosis is the methionine/choline-deficient (MCD) diet. Depriving mice of dietary choline impairs hepatic secretion of very low density lipoproteins (VLDL) and results in hepatic steatosis, oxidative stress, cell death, and increases in cytokine levels (15). Combined with methionine deficiency, the mice develop extensive inflammation after 2 weeks and significant fibrosis after 6 weeks (12). However, MCD diet-fed mice generally lose considerable bodyweight and show no insulin resistance (or even increased sensitivity), conditions that poorly correlate with development of NASH in humans (16, 17). In this current study we assessed the effects of ASBTi treatment on development of NAFLD and fibrosis using a choline-deficient L-amino acid-defined (CDAA) diet, which has been shown to successfully induce hepatic steatosis and subsequent fibrosis after 22 weeks without bodyweight loss (18, 19).

MATERIALS AND METHODS

Animals

Male C57Bl/6J mice aged 10 weeks were obtained from Jackson Laboratories. Animals were group-housed with 4 mice per ventilated cage (Super Mouse 750 Microisolator System; Lab Products) containing bedding (1/8" Bed-O-Cobbs; Andersons Lab Bedding Products) in the same temperature (22° C) and light/dark cycle (12-h; 7 AM to 7 PM) controlled room of the animal facility to minimize environmental differences. Mice were fed *ad libitum* for 22 weeks with either a choline-sufficient L-amino acid-defined control diet (CSAA, Catalog # 518754; Dyets Inc., Bethlehem, PA, USA) or choline-deficient L-amino acid-defined diet (CDAA, Catalog # 518753; Dyets Inc., Bethlehem,

---

Abbreviations: ASBT, Apical sodium-dependent bile acid transporter; ASBTi, Apical sodium-dependent bile acid transporter inhibitor; BW, bodyweight; CA, cholic acid; CDAA, choline-deficient, L-amino acid-defined; CSAA, choline-sufficient L-amino acid-defined; DCA, deoxycholic acid; FXR, farnesoid-X receptor; GC, gas chromatography; HCA, hyodeoxycholic acid; IBAT, ileal bile acid transporter; LCA, lithocholic acid; MCA, muricholic acid; MCD, methionine/choline-deficient; NAFLD, non-alcoholic fatty liver disease; NAS, NAFLD Activity Score; NASH, non-alcoholic steatohepatitis; PC, phosphatidylcholine; VLDL, very low density lipoprotein.

PA, USA) with or without 0.006% (w/w) of the ASBTi (SC-435). This amount of ASBTi in the diet provides a dose of ~11 mg/kg/day of SC-435 (10). The CSAA and CDAA diets contain 31% of calories as fat (in the form of corn oil and partially hydrogenated vegetable oil; fatty acid composition: 23.4% saturated, 52.1% monounsaturated, 24.5% polyunsaturated) and have no added cholesterol. Food consumption was measured by weighing new and remaining food two times weekly. Calorie intake was calculated by multiplying the weight of the food consumed by their caloric density. During the final week on diet, the mice were individually housed to measure fat absorption and fecal bile acid and neutral sterol excretion.

Animal Experiments

During the final week of CSAA and CDAA (+/− ASBTi) diet feeding, mice received powdered diet containing 0.7% sucrose polybehenate (w/w) (20). Sucrose polybehenate is not absorbed in the intestine. Therefore, by comparing the ratio of behenic acid to total fatty acids in the diet and feces, the fractional fat absorption can be calculated without being reliant on food intake measurements. Powdered diet was placed in a feeding jar in the cage and replaced every 2–3 days. Feces were collected for individual mice during the final 3 days of the experiment and used for fatty acid, neutral sterol and bile acid measurements. After, mice were sacrificed and tissues collected for further analysis. Mice were anesthetized using isoflurane. Blood was obtained via cardiac puncture, centrifuged and the plasma was stored at −80°C. Livers were excised, weighed and pieces collected for subsequent histology analysis. Remaining liver tissue was snap frozen in liquid nitrogen. The small intestines were excised, measured, cut into five equal length segments, flushed with ice cold phosphate buffered solution (PBS) and snap frozen in liquid nitrogen. The length of the colon was measured, divided into proximal (60%) and distal (40%) segments, flushed with ice cold PBS and immediately snap frozen in liquid nitrogen.

Fatty Acid Measurements

Weighed samples of the synthetic diet and feces were saponified with methanolic NaOH, extracted with hexane, and converted to methyl esters. Samples were analyzed using gas chromatography (GC) to quantitate the fatty acid methyl esters and determine the amount of behenic acid (C22:0), saturated (14:0, 16:0, 18:0), monounsaturated (C18:1), and polyunsaturated (18:1, 18:2, 18:3ω3, 20:5ω3, 22:6ω3) fatty acids as previously described (21, 22). Each chromatogram was examined to verify the identification of constituent fatty acids and for quality control.

Histology

The livers were removed, weighed, and a portion was fixed in 10% neutral buffered formalin, embedded in paraffin, sectioned at 5 µm, and stained with hematoxylin and eosin. Sirius red staining was performed using the paraffin-embedded liver sections (method adapted from Picrosirius Red Stain Kit, Polysciences, Inc., Warrington, PA, USA). The liver histology was assessed in a blinded fashion by a veterinary pathologist (S.G.) for steatosis, lobular inflammation, and hepatocellular ballooning to derive the NAFLD Activity Score (NAS) as described (23). Sirius red stained sections were blindly assessed by S.G. for Ishak Stage using the scores adapted from Ishak et al. (24).

Hepatic and Jejunal Lipids

Hepatic lipids were extracted according to a protocol based on the Folch method (25). Briefly, lipids were extracted from ~60 mg of tissue using 3 ml of chloroform:methanol (2:1) and incubated at 55°C for at least 2 h. Phases were split by adding 0.05% (v/v) sulfuric acid in water and centrifugation at 1,500 rpm for 15 min. Part of the bottom layer was transferred, dried under nitrogen and dissolved in 2% (v/v) Triton X-100 in water. Hepatic concentrations of total cholesterol (Pointe Scientific, C7510-01-906), free cholesterol (Fujifilm Wako Diagnostics, Cat# 993-02501), and triglyceride (Fujifilm Wako Diagnostics, Cat# 994-02891 and Cat# 990-02991) were subsequently measured by enzymatic assays.

Gene Expression

Total RNA was isolated from proximal colon and liver using a miRNeasy kit (Qiagen, Cat# 74106). Reverse transcriptase polymerase chain reaction (RT-PCR) was performed with 1 µg RNA using a high capacity cDNA reverse transcription kit (Applied Biosystems, Cat# 4368814). Real-time quantitative PCR was performed with a Sybr Green master mix (Applied Biosystems, Cat# 4309155) using a StepOne Plus real time PCR system (Applied Biosystems). The mRNA expression levels were calculated based on the ΔΔ-CT method; values are means of triplicate determinations and expression was normalized using cyclophilin. The sequences of the primers used has been published previously (26).

Fecal Bile Acids and Neutral Sterols

Fecal pellets were sorted, air-dried, weighed and mechanically homogenized. Neutral sterols and bile acids were extracted from 50 mg of feces or diet as described (27). Briefly, samples were heated for 2 h at 80°C with a mixture of 1 M sodium hydroxide and methanol (3:1). Neutral sterols were then extracted twice with 2 ml petroleum ether and derivatized with *N*, *O*-Bis(trimethylsilyl)trifluoroacetamide (BSTFA)-pyridine-trimethylchlorosilane (TMCS) (5:5:0.1). Bile acids were quantitatively extracted from feces, isolated on Sep-Pak C-18 columns, methylated with methanol/acetyl chloride (20:1) and derivatized with BSTFA-pyridine-TMCS (5:5:0.1) (27). Both neutral sterols and bile acids were measured by gas chromatography (GC) (28). The total amount of bile acids or neutral sterols was calculated as the sum of the individual species.

Statistical Analyses

Data are presented as means ± standard deviation (SD), unless stated otherwise. Statistical analyses were performed and graphs were created using GraphPad Prism 8 (GraphPad Software, La Jolla, CA, USA). Differences between groups were assessed by one-way ANOVA with Tukey's *post-hoc* test except for Ishak Stage, which was tested using a Chi-Squared test. Different lowercase letters indicate statistically significant differences ($P < 0.05$) between groups.

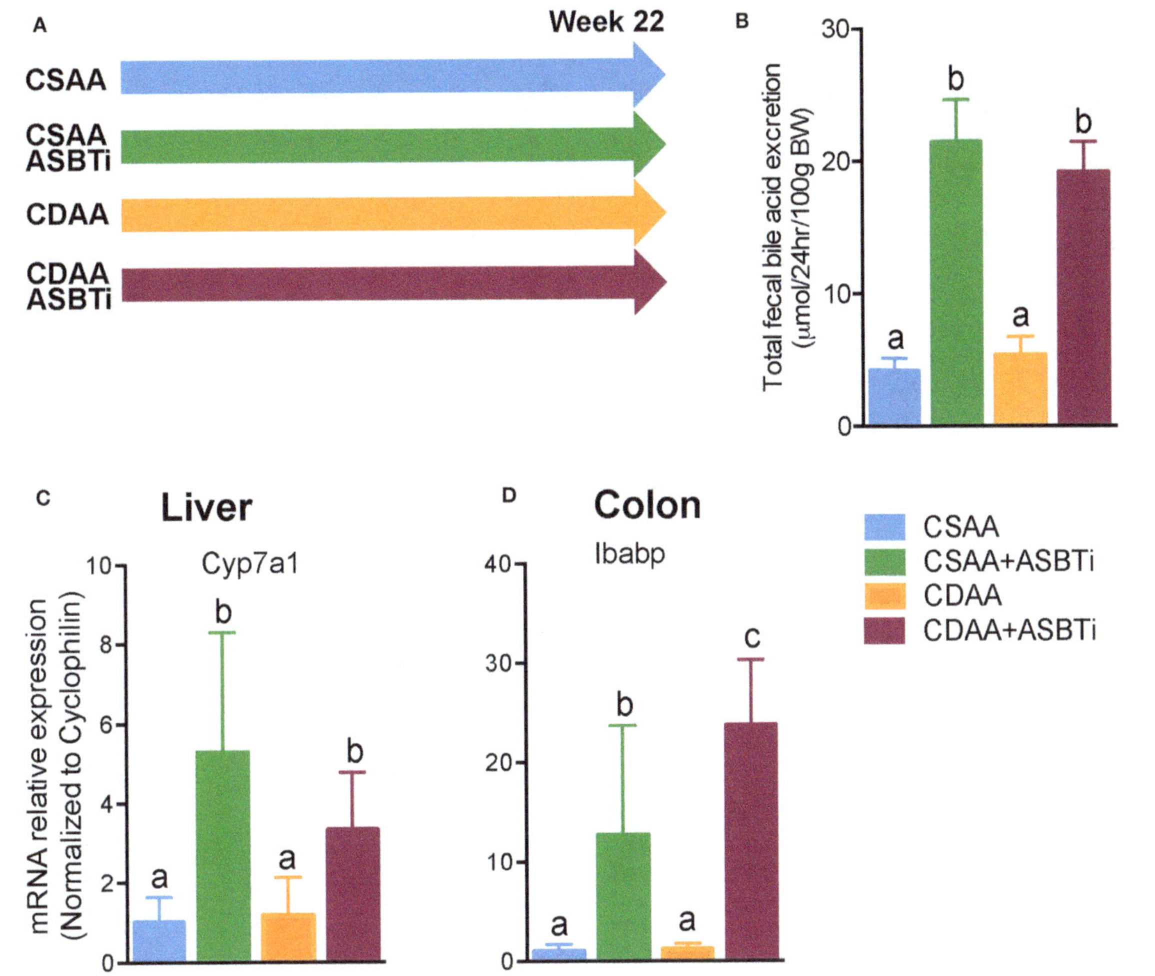

FIGURE 1 | ASBTi treatment increases fecal bile acid excretion and bile acid synthesis in mice fed a CSAA and CDAA diet. **(A)** Study design showing the four experimental groups, **(B)** Total fecal bile acid excretion, **(C)** Hepatic Cyp7a1 gene expression, **(D)** Colonic Ibabp gene expression. Means ± SD are shown. Distinct lowercase letters indicate significant differences between groups. $P < 0.05$; $n = 9$–12 per group.

RESULTS

ASBT Inhibitor Treatment Reduces Bodyweight Gain in CSAA and CDAA Diet-Fed Mice

To determine whether ASBT inhibition can prevent development of NASH and fibrosis in mice, male C57Bl/6J mice were fed a choline-deficient L-amino-defined diet (CDAA) or a choline-sufficient control diet (CSAA) with or without an ASBTi for 22 weeks (**Figure 1A**). ASBTi treatment increased total fecal bile acid excretion by approximately 5-fold in CSAA (4.1 vs. 21.4 μmol/24 h/100 g BW, $P < 0.001$) and 4-fold in CDAA diet-fed mice (5.3 vs. 19.1 μmol/24 h/100 g BW, $P < 0.001$) (**Figure 1B**). Interruption of the enterohepatic circulation of bile acids was confirmed by gene expression measurements, with increases in hepatic cholesterol 7alpha-hydroxylase (*Cyp7a1*) mRNA as a marker of bile acid synthesis, and colonic intestinal bile acid-binding protein (*Ibabp*) mRNA as a marker of colon bile acid exposure (**Figures 1C,D**) in both the CSAA and CDAA diet-fed mice.

Inhibiting the ASBT in mice has been shown to increase the proportion of cholic acid (CA) plus its bacterial dehydroxylation product deoxycholic acid (DCA) and to reduce the proportion of 6-hydroxylated bile acid species, including alpha-muricholic acid (αMCA), beta-muricholic acid (βMCA), and the bacterial product omega-muricholic acid (ωMCA) (10, 11, 29). To determine if the CDAA diet alters the effect of ASBT inhibition on bile acid composition, the fecal bile acid profiles were determined using quantitative three-day fecal collections performed for individually-housed mice (**Figure 2**). The mass of feces excreted per day per unit body weight (g dry feces/24 h/100 g BW, mean ± SD, $n = 9$–12/group) was similar for the CSAA vs. CDAA diet-fed mice, showed a trend toward an increase in ASBTi-treated CSAA diet-fed mice, and was significantly decreased in ASBTi-treated CDAA diet-fed mice (CSAA: 1.100 ± 0.266 vs. CSAA plus ASBTi: 1.326 ± 0.169, $P = 0.088$; CDAA: 1.157 ± 0.230

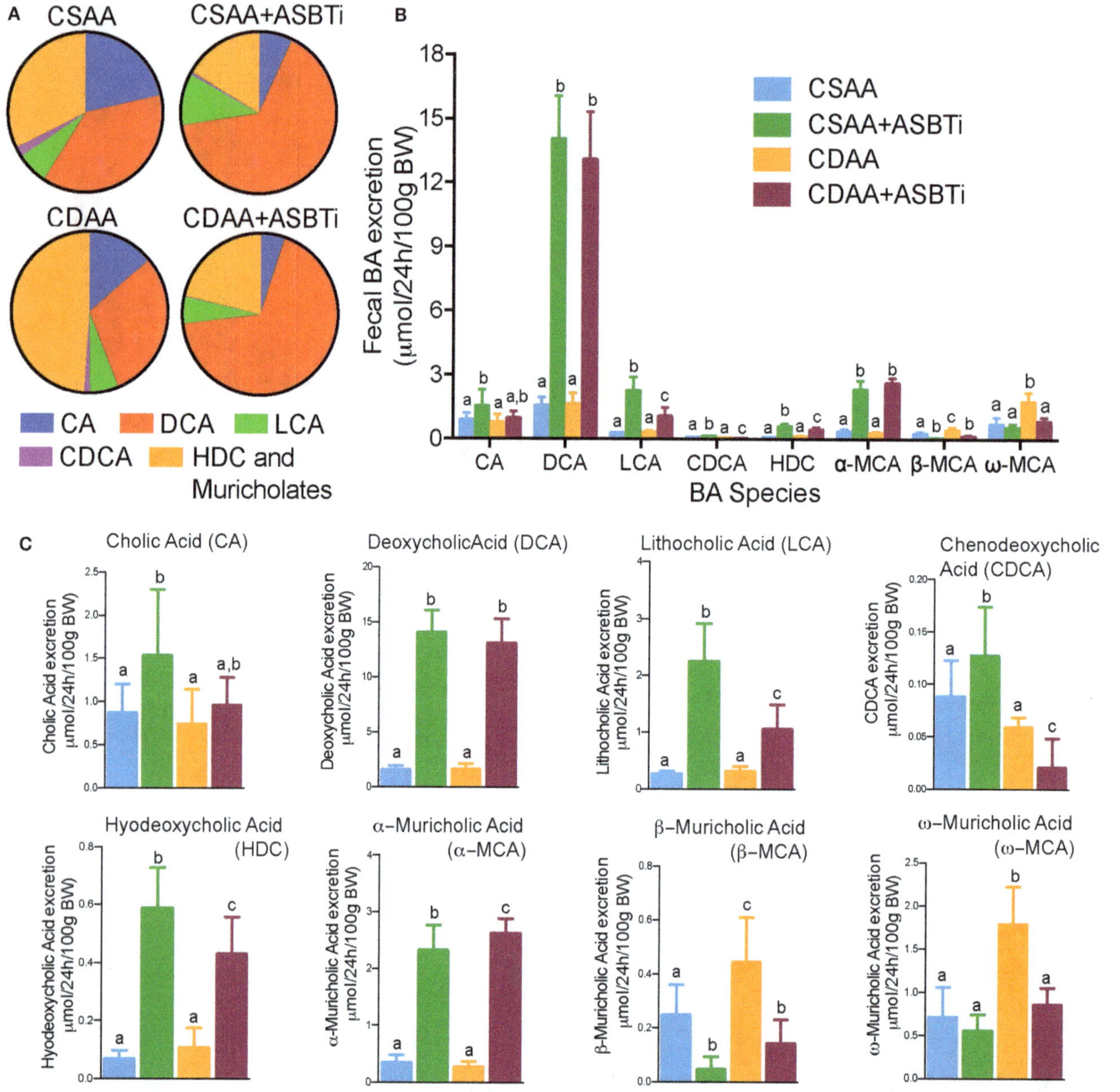

FIGURE 2 | The effects of ASBTi treatment on the fecal bile acid species profile. ASBTi treatment increased excretion of the secondary bile acids, deoxycholic acid (DCA) and lithocholic acid (LCA), and the primary bile acid, α-muricholic acid (MCA). **(A)** Pie charts for the fecal bile acid profiles. **(B)** Mass of bile acid species excreted into the feces per day. **(C)** Individual species of BA excreted in feces. Means ± SD are shown. Distinct lowercase letters indicate significant differences between groups. $P < 0.05$; $n = 8$–12 per group.

vs. CDAA plus ASBTi: 0.908 ± 0.071, $P = 0.02$). The fecal bile acid results are expressed as a proportion of the total amount of bile acid excreted per day per unit body weight (**Figure 2A**) and as the mass of individual bile acid species excreted per day per unit body weight (**Figures 2B,C**). For the fecal bile acid profiles, the proportion of βMCA and its bacterial product ωMCA were increased and the proportion of CA and its bacterial product DCA decreased in the CDAA vs. CSAA diet-fed mice. Following administration of the ASBTi, the fecal bile acid species distribution became remarkably similar in the CSAA and CDAA diet-fed mice (**Figure 2A**). Increases were observed in excretion of the primary bile acid αMCA and secondary bile acids DCA, lithocholic acid (LCA), and hyodeoxycholic acid (HCA). The differences in fecal excretion of βMCA and ωMCA between the CSAA and CDAA-fed mice were lost after ASBTi treatment (**Figures 2B,C**). In addition, DCA becomes the major fecal bile acid, likely reflecting increases in bacterial 7α-dehydroxylation and possibly decreased hepatic rehydroxylation of DCA to CA

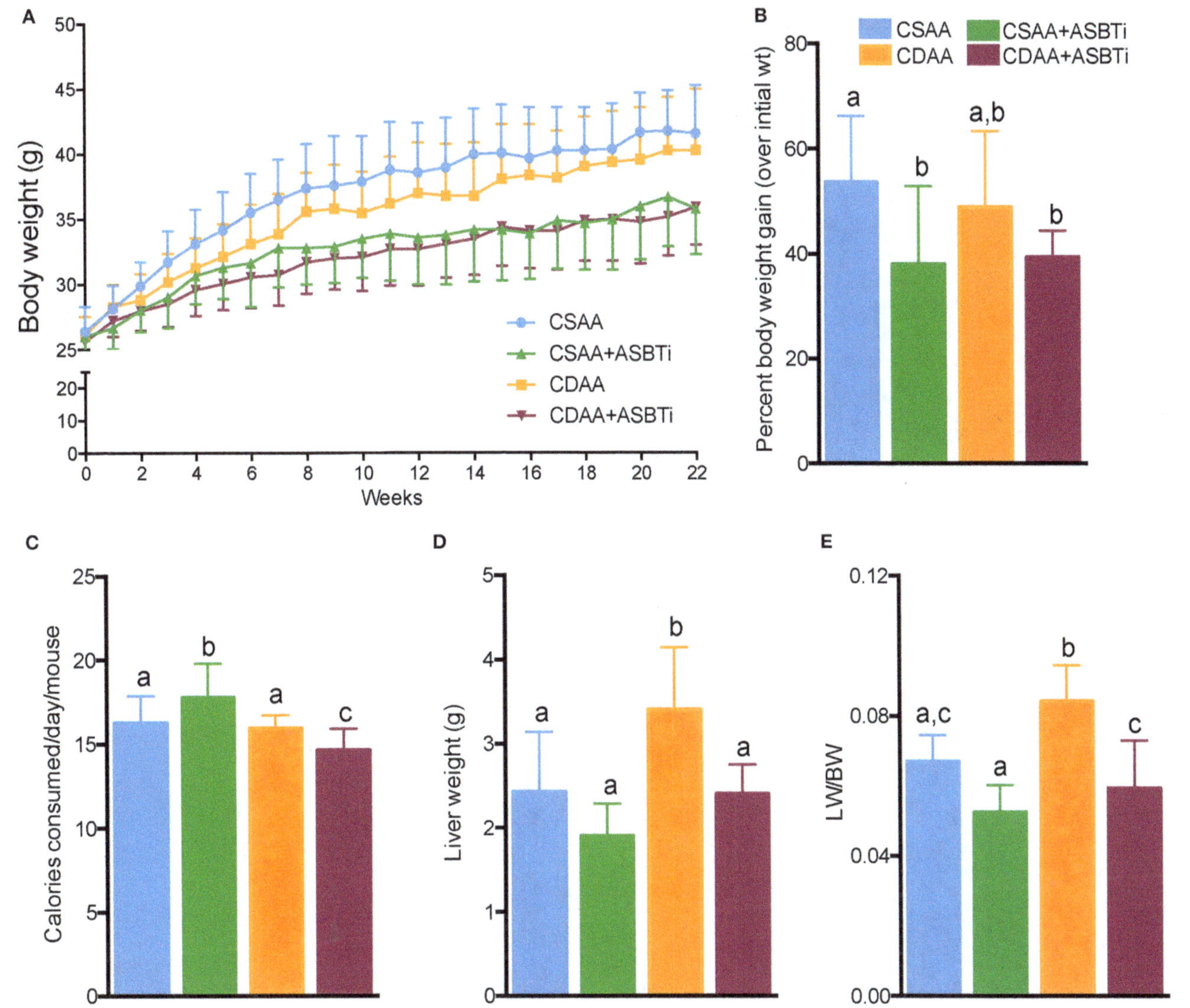

FIGURE 3 | ASBTi treatment decreases bodyweight gain in CSAA and CDAA diet-fed mice and reduces liver weight in CDAA diet-fed mice. **(A)** Bodyweight gain over time in *ad libitum* fed mice, **(B)** Bodyweight gain as percentage of initial bodyweight after 22 weeks, **(C)** Calories consumed per mouse per day, **(D)** Absolute liver weights after 22 weeks, **(E)** Liver to bodyweight ratio; Means ± SD are shown. Distinct lowercase letters indicate significant differences between groups. $P < 0.05$; $n = 9$–12 per group.

by the enzyme Cyp2a12 (30), and this was not affected by feeding a choline-deficient diet.

To assess whether dietary choline deficiency and/or ASBTi treatment affected body mass, we recorded bodyweight each week (**Figure 3A**). Bodyweight gain was similar for mice fed the CSAA and the CDAA diets. After 22 weeks, the increase in bodyweight was 54% and 49% ($P = 0.8$, **Figure 3B**) in the CSAA and CDAA diet-fed mice, respectively. The ASBTi treated groups gained less weight over the course of 22 weeks, irrespective of the diet, significantly reducing bodyweight gain by ~38 and 39% in the CSAA and CDAA diet-fed mice. The caloric intake was slightly higher in the ASBTi-treated CSAA group (17.8 vs. 16.3 kcal/24 h/mouse in the untreated CDAA group, $P = 0.006$) and slightly lower in the ASBTi-treated CDAA group (14.6 vs. 16 kcal/24 h/mouse in the untreated CDAA group, $P = 0.013$, **Figure 3C**). Hepatomegaly due to steatosis and inflammation is a common feature of NAFLD. After 22 weeks, both absolute liver weight (2.4 vs. 3.4 g, $P = 0.001$, **Figure 3D**) and liver to bodyweight ratio (0.06 vs. 0.08, $P < 0.001$, **Figure 3E**) was increased in mice on the CDAA vs. CSAA diet. On the CSAA diet, there was a trend toward a reduced liver weight (1.9 vs. 2.4 g, $P = 0.2$, **Figure 3D**) and liver to bodyweight ratio (0.052 vs. 0.067, $P = 0.45$) with ASBTi treatment (**Figure 3E**). On the CDAA diet, liver weight (2.4 vs. 3.4, $P = 0.001$, **Figure 3D**) and liver to bodyweight ratio (0.059 vs. 0.084, $P = 0.001$, **Figure 3E**) were significantly lower with ASBTi treatment, and decreased to values similar to that in CSAA diet-fed mice.

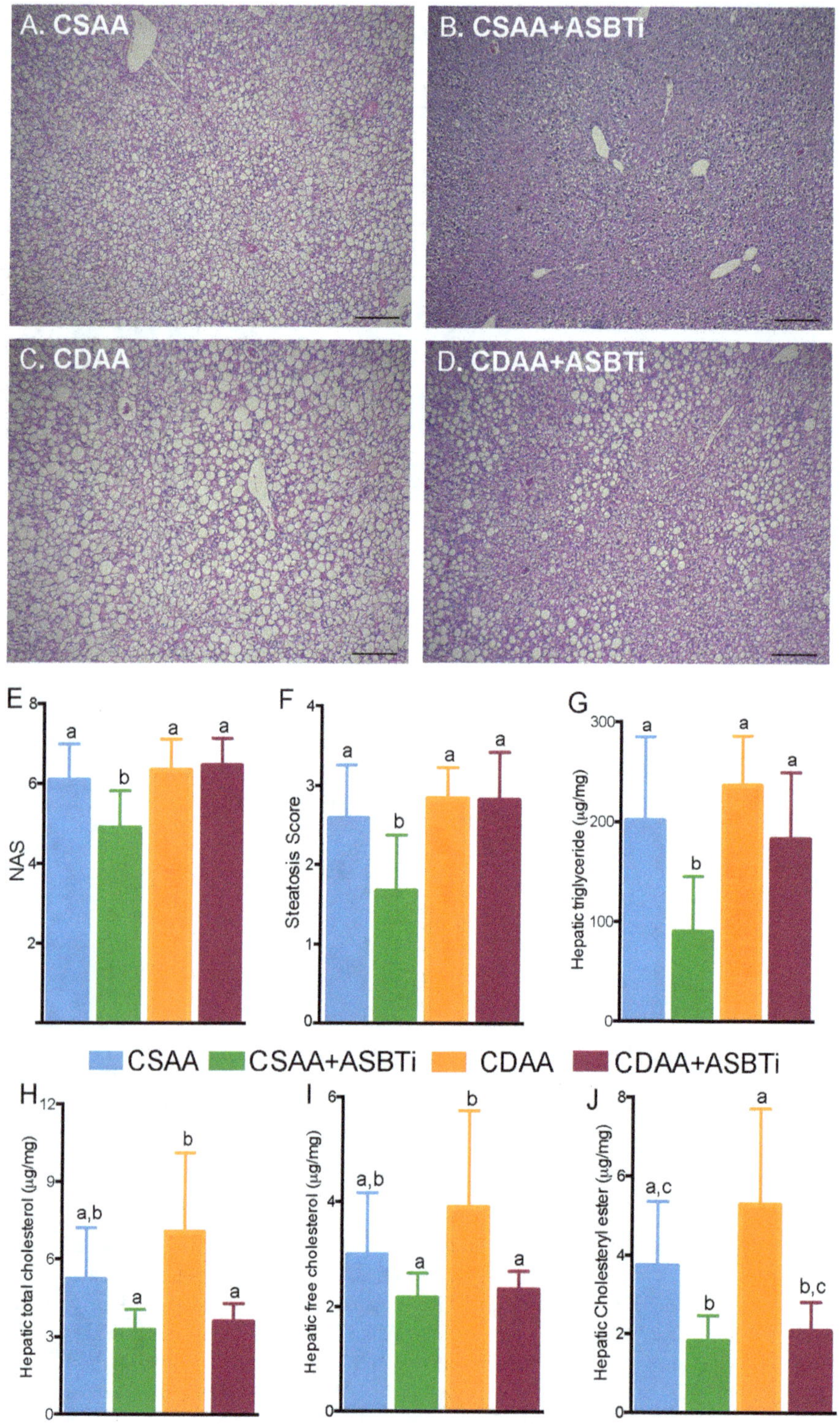

FIGURE 4 | ASBTi treatment reduces hepatic steatosis in CSAA but not CDAA diet-fed mice. Hemotoxylin and eosin stained liver sections from **(A)** CSAA, **(B)** CSAA+ASBTi, **(C)** CDAA, and **(D)** CDAA+ASBTi fed mice after 22 weeks; Scale bars = 100 μm, representative samples; **(E)** Non-alcoholic fatty liver disease Activity Score (NAS), **(F)** Steatosis score, **(G)** Hepatic triglyceride content, **(H)** Hepatic total cholesterol content, **(I)** Hepatic free cholesterol content, **(J)** Hepatic cholesteryl ester content. Means ± SD are shown. Distinct lowercase letters indicate significant differences between groups. $P < 0.05$; $n = 9$–12 per group.

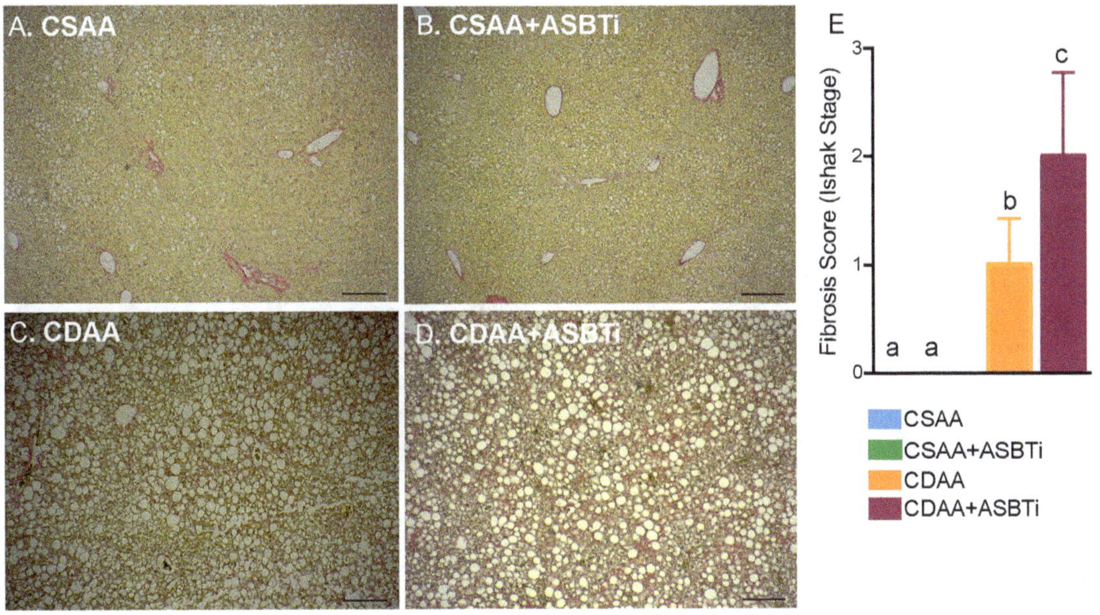

FIGURE 5 | ASBTi treatment increases hepatic fibrosis in CDAA diet-fed mice. Sirius red stained liver sections from **(A)** CSAA, **(B)** CSAA+ASBTi, **(C)** CDAA, and **(D)** CDAA+ASBTi fed mice after 22 weeks; Scale bars=100 μm, representative samples; **(E)** Fibrosis score (Ishak stage). Means ± SD are shown. Distinct lowercase letters indicate significant differences between groups. $P < 0.05$; $n = 9$–12 per group.

ASBT Inhibitor Treatment Reduces Hepatic Steatosis in CSAA but Not CDAA Diet-Fed Mice

To assess key features of the pathophysiology and progression of NAFLD, we examined the liver histology of the CSAA and CDAA diet-fed mice. Untreated mice fed the CSAA or CDAA diet showed clear features of NAFLD, including steatosis, lobular inflammation and hepatocyte ballooning (**Figures 4A,C**). Treatment with the ASBTi reduced visible lipid accumulation in mice fed the CSAA diet (**Figure 4B**) whereas the effects on lipid accumulation were attenuated in mice fed the CDAA diet (**Figure 4D**). Slides were assessed by a certified veterinary pathologist (author S.G.), who was blinded to the 4 groups, to determine NAFLD activity (NAS) and steatosis scores (**Figures 4E,F**). NAFLD activity (6.1 vs. 6.3, $P = 0.9$, **Figure 4E**) and steatosis scores (2.6 vs. 2.8, $P = 0.7$, **Figure 4F**) were similar for mice fed the CSAA and CDAA diets. ASBTi treatment significantly reduced the NAS and steatosis in mice fed the CSAA but not CDAA diet. To quantify hepatic lipid accumulation, we measured hepatic triglyceride and cholesterol content biochemically. In agreement with the NAS assessment, hepatic triglyceride levels were similar in mice fed the CSAA and CDAA diets (201 vs. 236 μg/mg liver wet weight, $P = 0.6$, **Figure 4G**). ASBTi treatment significantly reduced hepatic triglyceride accumulation for mice fed the CSAA diet (90 vs. 201 μg/mg liver wet weight, $P = 0.002$, **Figure 4G**), but the ASBTi-associated reduction in hepatic triglyceride was attenuated in mice fed the CDAA diet (183 vs. 236 μg/mg liver wet weight, $P = 0.2$, **Figure 4G**). Total hepatic cholesterol content in the liver was similar between the mice fed the low cholesterol-containing CSAA and CDAA diets (5.2 vs. 7.0 μg/mg liver wet weight, $P = 0.1$, **Figure 4H**). Upon ASBTi treatment, hepatic total (3.6 vs. 7.0 μg/mg liver wet weight, $P < 0.001$) and free cholesterol (2.3 vs. 3.9 μg/mg liver wet weight, $P = 0.01$) levels in the CDAA diet-fed mice were reduced and a similar trend was observed for the CSAA diet (**Figures 4H,I**). Cholesteryl esters were significantly reduced upon ASBTi treatment for both CSAA and CDAA-fed mice (**Figure 4J**). Altogether, these show that ASBTi treatment reduces hepatic steatosis on the CSAA diet, in agreement with previous observations (10, 11). However, choline deficiency in the CDAA diet attenuated these effects.

ASBT Inhibitor Treatment Worsens Hepatic Fibrosis in CDAA Diet-Fed Mice

The CDAA diet has been shown to successfully induce fibrosis after feeding for 22 weeks (18, 19, 31). To visualize fibrosis on histology, collagen was stained with Sirius Red. The CSAA diet did not induce visually evident fibrosis, and treatment with the ASBTi had no visual impact on histologic Sirius Red staining (**Figures 5A,B**). For the CDAA diet, hepatic fibrosis was readily apparent irrespective of ASBTi treatment (**Figures 5C,D**). To quantify the degree of fibrosis, slides were analyzed and scored by a certified veterinary pathologist (author S.G., blinded to diet and treatment groups) using the Ishak Scoring system (24, 32). Livers of mice on the CSAA diet with or without ASBTi did not show any signs of fibrosis and received an Ishak score of 0. Mice on the CDAA diet had significantly higher fibrosis compared to the CSAA diet and received an average Ishak score of 1 (**Figure 5E**,

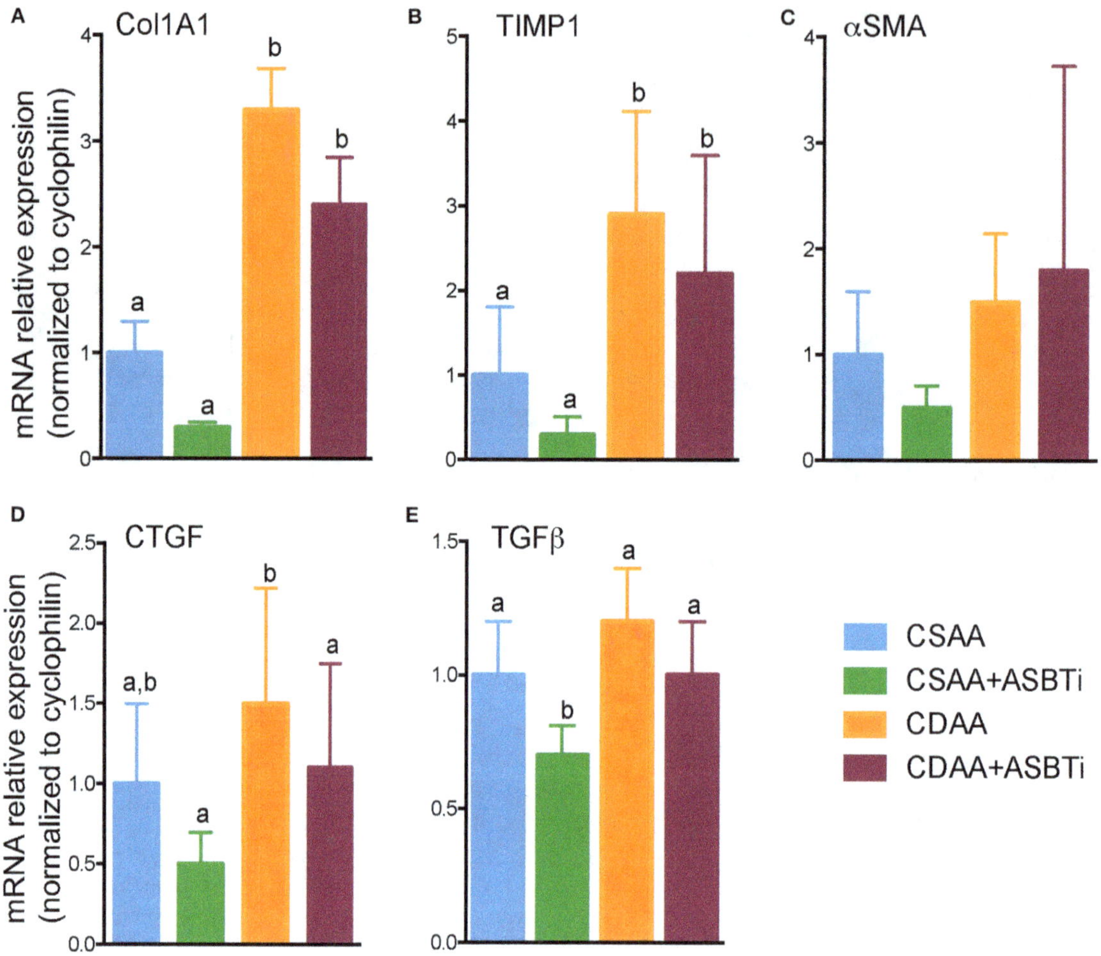

FIGURE 6 | Effect of ASBTi treatment on hepatic gene expression related to fibrosis in mice fed a CSAA and CDAA diet. **(A–E)** Relative hepatic mRNA expression of genes related to fibrosis, normalized to cyclophilin. Distinct lowercase letters indicate significant differences between groups. Means ± SD are shown. $P < 0.05$; $n = 9$–12 per group.

$P < 0.001$), which corresponds to a Sirius Red stained proportion of 3.0% and fibrous expansion of *some* of the portal areas with or without fibrous septa. ASBTi treatment of the CDAA diet-fed mice resulted in a significantly higher Ishak score of 2 (**Figure 5E**, $P = 0.02$), which corresponds to a Sirius Red stained proportion of 3.6% and fibrous expansion to *most* of the portal areas with or without short fibrous septa.

Hepatic mRNA expression of a panel of fibrosis related genes, shown previously to be upregulated by feeding the CDAA diet (31), was measured to assess whether the histological changes were reflected by the gene expression. Collagen type I alpha 1 (*Col1a1*), encoding the main component of collagen type 1 fibers, was upregulated in the CDAA diet and unaffected by ASBTi treatment (**Figure 6A**). Hepatic mRNA expression of tissue inhibitor of metalloproteinase-1 (*TIMP-1*), a protein involved in degradation of extracellular matrix and promoting proliferation, was similarly increased in the mice fed the CDAA diet and CDAA diet plus the ASBTi (**Figure 6B**). Interestingly, alpha-smooth muscle actin (α-*SMA*) mRNA, a marker used for hepatic stellate cell activation (33), was unaffected by diet or treatment (**Figure 6C**). Connective tissue growth factor (CTGF) and transforming growth factor beta (TGFβ) play important roles in fibrogenesis. Hepatic *CTGF* mRNA showed a trend toward increased expression in the CDAA vs. CSAA diet-fed mice, and was significantly decreased with ASBTi treatment in the CDAA diet-fed mice (**Figure 6D**). *TGFβ* was similar between the CSAA and CDAA diets (**Figure 6E**). ASBTi treatment significantly lowered hepatic *TGFβ* expression for the CSAA but not on the CDAA diet-fed mice.

As progression of liver steatosis to fibrosis generally involves inflammation, we measured hepatic gene expression of several important inflammatory genes. Expression of the proinflammatory genes tumor necrosis factor α (*TNFα*), inducible nitric oxide synthase (*iNOS*), and monocyte chemoattractant protein 1 (*MCP1*) were upregulated in the CDAA vs. CSAA diet-fed mice and unaffected by ASBTi treatment (**Figures 7A–C**). Hepatic cell damage and increases in inflammation are often paired with oxidative stress. Therefore,

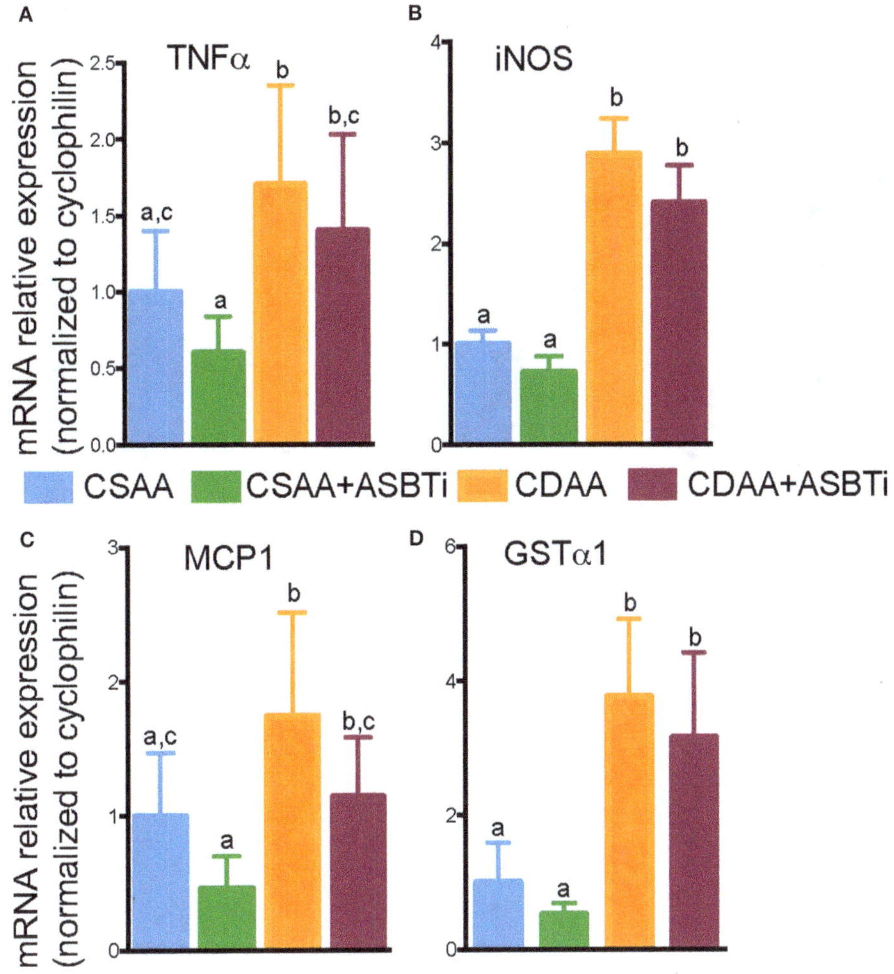

FIGURE 7 | Effect of ASBTi treatment on hepatic gene expression related to inflammation in mice fed a CSAA and CDAA diet. **(A–D)** Relative hepatic mRNA expression of genes related to inflammation, normalized to cyclophilin. Means ± SD are shown. Distinct lowercase letters indicate significant differences between groups. $P < 0.05$; $n = 9$–12 per group.

we measured glutathione S-transferase A1 (*GSTα1*) expression, the gene encoding a key enzyme in the anti-oxidative glutathione pathway. *GSTα1* expression was increased upon feeding the CDAA vs. CSAA diet but unaffected by ASBTi treatment (**Figure 7D**). Altogether, these data suggest that the ASBTi treatment was not able to prevent inflammation, oxidative stress or fibrosis in this dietary choline deficiency mouse model of NAFLD/NASH.

ASBT Inhibitor Treatment Reduces Intestinal Fat Absorption in CSAA but Not CDAA Diet-Fed Mice

We previously reported that genetic ASBT knockout in mice reduces intestinal fat and cholesterol absorption (29, 34, 35). In order to determine if the ASBTi treatment had similar effects in the CSAA and CDAA diet-fed mice, we measured fat absorption using the sucrose polybehenate method (20). For mice on the CSAA diet, ASBTi treatment reduced total fatty acid absorption by almost 10% (85.3 vs. 94.6%, $P < 0.001$, **Figure 8A**). The ASBTi treatment-associated decrease in fat absorption in the CSAA diet-fed mice was greater for the saturated fatty acids myristic acid (C14:0), palmitic acid (C16:0), margaric acid (C17:0), and stearic acid (C18:0) followed by the *trans* saturated fatty acid, elaidic acid (C18:1 ω9) (**Figure 8B**). For the group of saturated fatty acids, the ASBTi treatment effect on absorption increased with fatty acid acyl chain length, which corresponds to greater hydrophobicity and correlates with increased bile acid requirement for efficient micellar solubilization (36). The ASBTi treatment-associated decreases in fat absorption in the CSAA diet-fed mice for the mono- and polyunsaturated fatty acids oleic acid (C18:1ω9), vaccenic acid (C18:1ω7), and linoleic acid (C18:2ω6) were also statistically significant but the absolute differences were smaller (**Figure 8B**). We found no difference in total fat absorption between the mice fed the CSAA and the CDAA diets (94.6 vs. 93.6%, $P = 0.9$, **Figure 8A**). However, in contrast to mice

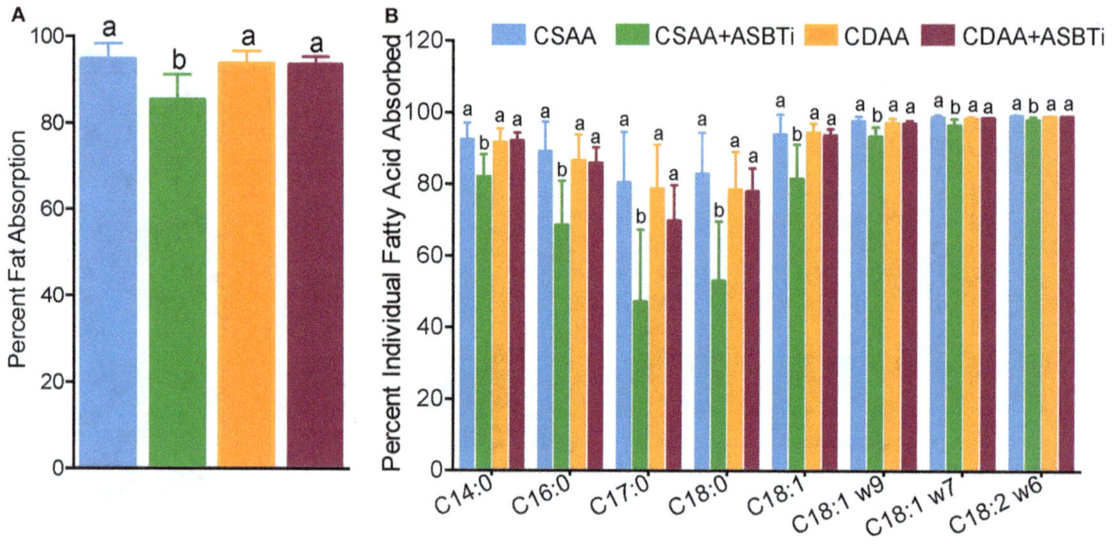

FIGURE 8 | ASBTi treatment reduces intestinal fat absorption in mice fed a CSAA but not CDAA diet. **(A)** Percentage of total intestinal fat absorption, **(B)** Percentage of intestinal absorption of individual fatty acid. Distinct lowercase letters indicate significant differences between groups. Distinct lowercase letters indicate significant differences between groups. $P < 0.05$; $n = 9$–12 per group.

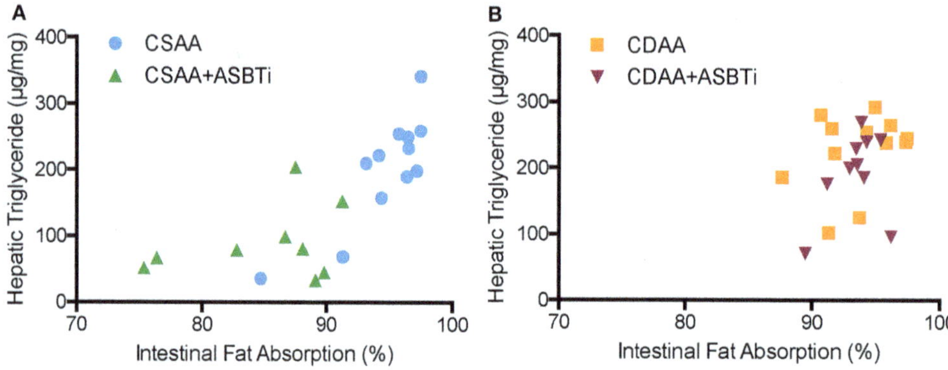

FIGURE 9 | Correlation of hepatic triglyceride content to intestinal fat absorption. **(A)** Hepatic triglyceride content correlated to intestinal fatty acid absorption in CSAA and CSAA+ASBTi fed mice (Spearman $R = 0.75$, $P < 0.0001$) **(B)** Hepatic triglyceride content did not correlate to intestinal fatty acid absorption in CDAA and CDAA+ASBTi fed mice (Spearman $R = 0.32$, $P = 0.13$ $n = 9$–12 per group).

fed the CSAA diet, absorption of neither total fat (93.5 vs. 93.6%, $P = 1.0$, **Figure 8A**) or the individual fatty acids were affected by ASBTi treatment of CDAA diet-fed mice. Correlation analysis showed that the hepatic triglyceride content is highly correlated to intestinal fatty acid absorption in mice fed the CSAA (Spearman $R = 0.75$, $P < 0.001$, **Figure 9A**) but not CDAA diet (Spearman $R = 0.32$, $P = 0.9$, **Figure 9B**).

Although we did not directly assess cholesterol absorption in the current study, we measured fecal excretion of neutral sterols, cholesterol and its fecal metabolites. Fecal neutral excretion (µmol/24 h/100 g BW, mean ± SD, $n = 9$–12 per group) was significantly higher in CSAA mice treated with an ASBTi compared to CSAA control mice (CSAA plus ASBTi: 12.0 ± 4.8 vs. CSAA: 7.5 ± 3.3, $P = 0.02$). On the CDAA diet, fecal neutral sterol excretion was comparable to the CSAA diet (CDAA: 9.7 ± 3.2 vs. CSAA:7.5 ± 3.3, $P = 0.4$). However, in contrast to the CSAA diet, ASBTi treatment did not significantly increase fecal neutral sterol excretion in mice fed the CDAA diet (CDAA plus ASBTi: 8.0 ± 1.2 vs. 9.7 ± 3.2, $P = 0.6$). Previous studies have suggested that feeding a choline-deficient diet can promote triglyceride accumulation in enterocytes as a result of impaired chylomicron secretion (37, 38). In this study, there was a trend toward increased jejunal tissue triglyceride in CDAA vs. CSAA diet-fed mice, but the differences were not statistically significant ($P > 0.05$) and there was no effect of ASBTi treatment on the jejunal tissue triglyceride (µg per g tissue, mean ± SD, $n = 9$–12 per group; CSAA: 23.2 ± 10.5; CSAA plus ASBTi: 22.8 ± 9.2; CDAA: 29.8 ± 9.2; CDAA plus ASBTi: 33.01 ± 10.7). The jejunal tissue total cholesterol content (µg per g tissue, mean ± SD, $n = 9$–12 per group) was also not different ($P > 0.05$) between the different groups (CSAA: 2.5 ± 0.2; CSAA plus ASBTi: 2.31 ± 0.23; CDAA: 2.27 ± 0.28; CDAA plus ASBTi: 2.22 ± 0.39).

DISCUSSION

In the current study, we showed that treatment with an ASBTi did not prevent development of hepatic fibrosis in a CDAA diet-fed mouse model. Additionally, under dietary choline-deficient conditions, previously reported effects of ASBT inhibition on fat and cholesterol absorption were nullified, possibly contributing to the phenotype. Dietary interventions in mouse models to reproducibly induce NASH and fibrosis are limited. The CDAA diet was used in the current study because, contrary to the MCD diet, the CDAA diet was shown to successfully induce hepatic fibrosis without significantly lowering bodyweight and plasma glucose levels (18, 19). Approximately 95% of the choline in animal tissues is present as phosphatidylcholine (PC), a major component of membranes (39). The primary mechanism believed to be involved in the effects of choline deficiency on hepatic steatosis is impairment of VLDL secretion due to insufficient PC (15). Interestingly, bile acid sequestrants act similar to ASBT inhibition by interrupting the enterohepatic circulation of bile acids, and have been shown to increase plasma VLDL and triglyceride levels (40–42). Therefore, one of the mechanisms contributing to the anti-steatotic actions of ASBTi treatment may be increasing hepatic VLDL secretion and triglyceride export from the liver, which is attenuated under choline-deficient conditions.

In addition to affecting VLDL secretion, choline deficiency alters mitochondrial function (43), fatty acid beta-oxidation (44), and changes epigenetic marking (45). Choline deficiency also alters the intestinal microbiota, which may be involved in the development of NAFLD (46). Treatment with the ASBTi induces similar changes in the fecal bile acid profile for the CSAA and CDAA diet-fed mice, such that the fecal bile acid composition including the microbiota-derived secondary bile acids is almost identical for the two ASBTi-treated groups. Changes in the gut microbiota composition associated with feeding the choline-deficient amino acid-defined diet have been reported previously (47). However, the almost identical fecal secondary bile acid profiles suggests that at least this aspect (bile acid biotransformation) of the gut microbiome actions does not appear to account for the differential response of the CSAA and CDAA diet-fed mice to the ASBTi. It was previously shown that treatment of high fat diet-fed mice with the ASBTi for 16 weeks shifted the hepatic bile acid composition shifted toward a more hydrophobic and thus potentially cytotoxic profile (10). *In vitro* studies have shown that PC protects hepatocytes from bile acid-induced cytotoxicity (48, 49). Although not injurious when hepatic PC synthesis is intact, the ASBTi-induced shift to a more hydrophobic bile acid pool may be injurious under PC-deficient conditions. The absence of beneficial effects in the CDAA model has been noted for other therapeutic interventions such as FXR agonism with obeticholic acid (50). Moreover, feeding a choline-deficient, iron-supplemented L-amino acid-defined diet to rats has been shown to induce a persistent fibrosis, potentially secondary to increased oxidative stress (51). This later observation is particularly important since it has recently been shown that interrupting the enterohepatic circulation of bile acids in mice decreases hepatic glutathione levels and impairs glutathione regenerating capacity (52). This is due in part to increased expression of cysteine dioxygenase type 1, in order to shunt cysteine toward taurine biosynthesis to meet the increased demand for synthesis of taurine-conjugated bile acids. A decrease in hepatic cysteine and glutathione levels combined with choline deficiency may underlie the increase in fibrosis observed in the ASBTi-treated CDAA diet-fed mice. However, these results should be interpreted with caution in regard to human NAFLD/NASH pathophysiology, as this rarely involves choline deficiency (53) and humans preferentially use glycine vs. taurine for bile acid conjugation (54). Future studies using different models are needed for understand the potential impact of ASBTi treatment on NASH and fibrosis. Fortunately, several recently developed murine NAFLD models have shown promising results in mimicking human NAFLD/NASH pathophysiology (55, 56).

Anti-steatotic effects of ASBT pharmacological inhibition have been a consistent finding in high fat diet-fed mouse models, including the CSAA diet-fed mice in this study (10, 11), and we previously observed inhibitory effects of ASBT genetic inactivation on intestinal cholesterol and fat absorption (29, 34, 35). In our current study, ASBTi treatment lowered fatty acid absorption and intestinal fat absorption positively correlated with hepatic triglyceride levels in the CSAA diet-fed mice. By contrast in the choline-deficient CDAA diet-fed mice, ASBTi-treatment had no effect on intestinal fat absorption and the hepatic anti-steatotic effects were attenuated. The mechanisms underlying our observations in the CDAA-fed mice remain unclear. Intestinal intraluminal PC concentrations contribute to mixed micelle formation, lipid transport across the unstirred water layer, and subsequent lipid translocation to the brush border membrane (57). In rats, dietary choline deficiency was shown to decrease chylomicron secretion and alter intestinal cell morphology and physiology, resulting in impairments of dietary fat absorption (37, 38). One could speculate that intestinal adaptations present in the choline-deficient CDAA diet-fed mice to compensate for decreased biliary PC affect lipolytic and post-lipolytic events related to intestinal lipid absorption. The absence of a protective effect on hepatic steatosis for interventions that act via reduced intestinal fat absorption has been observed previously in dietary choline-deficient models. For example, intestine-specific knockout of the zinc finger transcription factor GATA4 reduces intestinal lipid absorption and was protective against hepatic steatosis induced by feeding a high fat but not MCD diet (58).

In conclusion, this study showed that ASBTi treatment did not affect intestinal fat absorption and was not protective against hepatic fibrosis in a choline-deficient mouse model of NASH. Nevertheless, these findings add to our understanding of the uses and limitations of dietary choline-deficient mouse and the potential mechanisms by which interrupting the enterohepatic circulation of bile acids may impact development of NAFLD and NASH. Indirectly modulating intestinal fat absorption via ASBTi treatment is an interesting potential therapeutic target. Future studies using different models for NASH are warranted to further understand the relationship between bile acids and the progression of hepatic steatosis to NASH and fibrosis.

ETHICS STATEMENT

The animal study was reviewed and approved by Emory University Institutional Animal Care and Use Committee.

AUTHOR CONTRIBUTIONS

AR, IP, and SG performed the experiments and collected and analyzed the data. AR managed the study. AR, SK, and PD designed the study and conceived the experiments. PD, IP, AR, and SK wrote the paper.

ACKNOWLEDGMENTS

We thank Lumena/Shire for the research gift of the ASBTi (SC-435), Dr. D. Shayakhmetov (Emory University School of Medicine) for assistance with the microscopy, Matthew Davis (Lipoprotein Analysis Laboratory at Wake Forest University School of Medicine) for fatty acid analysis, the Children's Healthcare of Atlanta pathology Services for processing tissues for histology, and the Yerkes Nonhuman Primate Molecular Pathology Core for assistance with Sirius Red staining. We also thank Kim Pachura for assistance with the mouse necropsies. Portions of this work were presented at the Annual Meeting of the American Gastroenterology Association in San Diego, CA, 18–21 May 2019 and have appeared in abstract form Gastroenterology. 156 (6), Supplement 1, S-1296 (Su1556). Portions of this work are also included in an author's doctoral thesis in accordance with the author's University policy (59).

REFERENCES

1. Estes C, Anstee QM, Arias-Loste MT, Bantel H, Bellentani S, Caballeria J, et al. Modeling NAFLD disease burden in China, France, Germany, Italy, Japan, Spain, United Kingdom, and United States for the period 2016-2030. *J Hepatol.* (2018) 69:896–904. doi: 10.1016/j.jhep.2018.05.036
2. Younossi Z, Anstee QM, Marietti M, Hardy T, Henry L, Eslam M, et al. Global burden of NAFLD and NASH: trends, predictions, risk factors and prevention. *Nat Rev Gastroenterol Hepatol.* (2018) 15:11–20. doi: 10.1038/nrgastro.2017.109
3. Byrne CD, Targher G. NAFLD: a multisystem disease. *J Hepatol.* (2015) 62:S47–64. doi: 10.1016/j.jhep.2014.12.012
4. Friedman SL, Neuschwander-Tetri BA, Rinella M, Sanyal AJ. Mechanisms of NAFLD development and therapeutic strategies. *Nat Med.* (2018) 24:908–22. doi: 10.1038/s41591-018-0104-9
5. Chavez-Talavera O, Tailleux A, Lefebvre P, Staels B. Bile acid control of metabolism and inflammation in obesity, type 2 diabetes, dyslipidemia, and nonalcoholic fatty liver disease. *Gastroenterology.* (2017) 152:1679–94.e3. doi: 10.1053/j.gastro.2017.01.055
6. Ridlon JM, Harris SC, Bhowmik S, Kang DJ, Hylemon PB. Consequences of bile salt biotransformations by intestinal bacteria. *Gut Microbes.* (2016) 7:22–39. doi: 10.1080/19490976.2015.1127483
7. Wahlstrom A, Sayin SI, Marschall HU, Backhed F. Intestinal crosstalk between bile acids and microbiota and its impact on host metabolism. *Cell Metab.* (2016) 24:41–50. doi: 10.1016/j.cmet.2016.05.005
8. Mudaliar S, Henry RR, Sanyal AJ, Morrow L, Marschall HU, Kipnes M, et al. Efficacy and safety of the farnesoid X receptor agonist obeticholic acid in patients with type 2 diabetes and nonalcoholic fatty liver disease. *Gastroenterology.* (2013) 145:574–82.e1. doi: 10.1053/j.gastro.2013.05.042
9. Neuschwander-Tetri BA, Loomba R, Sanyal AJ, Lavine JE, Van Natta ML, Abdelmalek MF, et al. Farnesoid X nuclear receptor ligand obeticholic acid for non-cirrhotic, non-alcoholic steatohepatitis (FLINT): a multicentre, randomised, placebo-controlled trial. *Lancet.* (2015) 385:956–65. doi: 10.1016/S0140-6736(14)61933-4
10. Rao A, Kosters A, Mells JE, Zhang W, Setchell KD, Amanso AM, et al. Inhibition of ileal bile acid uptake protects against nonalcoholic fatty liver disease in high-fat diet-fed mice. *Sci Transl Med.* (2016) 8:357ra122. doi: 10.1126/scitranslmed.aaf4823
11. Salic K, Kleemann R, Wilkins-Port C, McNulty J, Verschuren L, Palmer M. Apical sodium-dependent bile acid transporter inhibition with volixibat improves metabolic aspects and components of non-alcoholic steatohepatitis in Ldlr-/-.Leiden mice. *PLoS ONE.* (2019) 14:e0218459. doi: 10.1371/journal.pone.0218459
12. Lau JK, Zhang X, Yu J. Animal models of non-alcoholic fatty liver disease: current perspectives and recent advances. *J Pathol.* (2017) 241:36–44. doi: 10.1002/path.4829
13. Denk H, Abuja PM, Zatloukal K. Animal models of NAFLD from the pathologist's point of view. *Biochim Biophys Acta Mol Basis Dis.* (2019) 1865:929–42. doi: 10.1016/j.bbadis.2018.04.024
14. Jahn D, Kircher S, Hermanns HM, Geier A. Animal models of NAFLD from a hepatologist's point of view. *Biochim Biophys Acta Mol Basis Dis.* (2019) 1865:943–53. doi: 10.1016/j.bbadis.2018.06.023
15. Corbin KD, Zeisel SH. Choline metabolism provides novel insights into nonalcoholic fatty liver disease and its progression. *Curr Opin Gastroenterol.* (2012) 28:159–65. doi: 10.1097/MOG.0b013e32834e7b4b
16. Rinella ME, Green RM. The methionine-choline deficient dietary model of steatohepatitis does not exhibit insulin resistance. *J Hepatol.* (2004) 40:47–51. doi: 10.1016/j.jhep.2003.09.020
17. Machado MV, Michelotti GA, Xie G, Almeida Pereira T, Boursier J, Bohnic B, et al. Mouse models of diet-induced nonalcoholic steatohepatitis reproduce the heterogeneity of the human disease. *PLoS ONE.* (2015) 10:e0127991. doi: 10.1371/journal.pone.0127991
18. Miura K, Kodama Y, Inokuchi S, Schnabl B, Aoyama T, Ohnishi H, et al. Toll-like receptor 9 promotes steatohepatitis by induction of interleukin-1beta in mice. *Gastroenterology.* (2010). 139:323–34.e7. doi: 10.1053/j.gastro.2010.03.052
19. Pizarro M, Solis N, Quintero P, Barrera F, Cabrera D, Rojas-de Santiago P, et al. Beneficial effects of mineralocorticoid receptor blockade in experimental non-alcoholic steatohepatitis. *Liver Int.* (2015) 35:2129–38. doi: 10.1111/liv.12794
20. Jandacek RJ, Heubi JE, Tso P. A novel, noninvasive method for the measurement of intestinal fat absorption. *Gastroenterology.* (2004) 127:139–44. doi: 10.1053/j.gastro.2004.04.007
21. Simon T, Cook VR, Rao A, Weinberg RB. Impact of murine intestinal apolipoprotein A-IV expression on regional lipid absorption, gene expression, and growth. *J Lipid Res.* (2011) 52:1984–94. doi: 10.1194/jlr.M0 17418
22. Sun H, Hu Y, Gu Z, Wilson MD, Chen YQ, Rudel LL, et al. Endogenous synthesis of n-3 polyunsaturated fatty acids in Fat-1 mice is associated with increased mammary gland and liver syndecan-1. *PLoS ONE.* (2011) 6:e20502. doi: 10.1371/journal.pone.0020502
23. Kleiner DE, Brunt EM, Van Natta M, Behling C, Contos MJ, Cummings OW, et al. Design and validation of a histological scoring system for nonalcoholic fatty liver disease. *Hepatology.* (2005) 41:1313–21. doi: 10.1002/hep.20701
24. Ishak K, Baptista A, Bianchi L, Callea F, De Groote J, Gudat F, et al. Histological grading and staging of chronic hepatitis. *J Hepatol.* (1995) 22:696–9. doi: 10.1016/0168-8278(95)80226-6

25. Folch J, Lees M, Sloane Stanley GH. A simple method for the isolation and purification of total lipides from animal tissues. *J Biol Chem.* (1957) 226:497–509.
26. Rao A, Haywood J, Craddock AL, Belinsky MG, Kruh GD, Dawson PA. The organic solute transporter alpha-beta, Ostalpha-Ostbeta, is essential for intestinal bile acid transport and homeostasis. *Proc Natl Acad Sci USA.* (2008) 105:3891–6. doi: 10.1073/pnas.0712328105
27. van Meer H, Boehm G, Stellaard F, Vriesema A, Knol J, Havinga R, et al. Prebiotic oligosaccharides and the enterohepatic circulation of bile salts in rats. *Am J Physiol Gastrointest Liver Physiol.* (2008) 294:G540–7. doi: 10.1152/ajpgi.00396.2007
28. Gamble W, Vaughan M, Kruth HS, Avigan J. Procedure for determination of free and total cholesterol in micro- or nanogram amounts suitable for studies with cultured cells. *J Lipid Res.* (1978) 19:1068–70.
29. van de Peppel IP, Bertolini A, van Dijk TH, Groen AK, Jonker JW, Verkade HJ. Efficient reabsorption of transintestinally excreted cholesterol is a strong determinant for cholesterol disposal in mice. *J Lipid Res.* (2019) 60:1562–72. doi: 10.1194/jlr.M094607
30. Honda A, Miyazaki T, Iwamoto J, Hirayama T, Morishita Y, Monma T, et al. Regulation of bile acid metabolism in mouse models with hydrophobic bile acid composition. *J Lipid Res.* (2020) 61:54–69. doi: 10.1194/jlr.RA119000395
31. Cabrera D, Wree A, Povero D, Solis N, Hernandez A, Pizarro M, et al. Andrographolide ameliorates inflammation and fibrogenesis and attenuates inflammasome activation in experimental non-alcoholic steatohepatitis. *Sci Rep.* (2017) 7:3491. doi: 10.1038/s41598-017-03675-z
32. Standish RA, Cholongitas E, Dhillon A, Burroughs AK, Dhillon AP. An appraisal of the histopathological assessment of liver fibrosis. *Gut.* (2006) 55:569–78. doi: 10.1136/gut.2005.084475
33. Carpino G, Morini S, Ginanni Corradini S, Franchitto A, Merli M, Siciliano M, et al. Alpha-SMA expression in hepatic stellate cells and quantitative analysis of hepatic fibrosis in cirrhosis and in recurrent chronic hepatitis after liver transplantation. *Dig Liver Dis.* (2005) 37:349–56. doi: 10.1016/j.dld.2004.11.009
34. Dawson PA, Haywood J, Craddock AL, Wilson M, Tietjen M, Kluckman K, et al. Targeted deletion of the ileal bile acid transporter eliminates enterohepatic cycling of bile acids in mice. *J Biol Chem.* (2003) 278:33920–7. doi: 10.1074/jbc.M306370200
35. Dawson PA. Impact of inhibiting ileal apical versus basolateral bile acid transport on cholesterol metabolism and atherosclerosis in mice. *Dig Dis.* (2015) 33:382–7. doi: 10.1159/000371691
36. McKimmie RL, Easter L, Weinberg RB. Acyl chain length, saturation, and hydrophobicity modulate the efficiency of dietary fatty acid absorption in adult humans. *Am J Physiol Gastrointest Liver Physiol.* (2013) 305:G620–627. doi: 10.1152/ajpgi.00258.2013
37. Takahashi Y, Mizunuma T, Kishino Y. Effects of choline deficiency and phosphatidylcholine on fat absorption in rats. *J Nutr Sci Vitaminol.* (1982) 28:139–47. doi: 10.3177/jnsv.28.139
38. da Silva RP, Kelly KB, Lewis ED, Leonard KA, Goruk S, Curtis JM, et al. Choline deficiency impairs intestinal lipid metabolism in the lactating rat. *J Nutr Biochem.* (2015) 26:1077–83. doi: 10.1016/j.jnutbio.2015.04.015
39. Li Z, Vance DE. Phosphatidylcholine and choline homeostasis. *J Lipid Res.* (2008) 49:1187–94. doi: 10.1194/jlr.R700019-JLR200
40. Beil U, Crouse JR, Einarsson K, Grundy SM. Effects of interruption of the enterohepatic circulation of bile acids on the transport of very low density-lipoprotein triglycerides. *Metabolism.* (1982) 31:438–44. doi: 10.1016/0026-0495(82)90231-1
41. Watanabe M, Houten SM, Wang L, Moschetta A, Mangelsdorf DJ, Heyman RA, et al. Bile acids lower triglyceride levels via a pathway involving FXR, SHP, and SREBP-1c. *J Clin Invest.* (2004) 113:1408–18. doi: 10.1172/JCI21025
42. Mazidi M, Rezaie P, Karimi E, Kengne AP. The effects of bile acid sequestrants on lipid profile and blood glucose concentrations: a systematic review and meta-analysis of randomized controlled trials. *Int J Cardiol.* (2017) 227:850–7. doi: 10.1016/j.ijcard.2016.10.011
43. Teodoro JS, Rolo AP, Duarte FV, Simoes AM, Palmeira CM. Differential alterations in mitochondrial function induced by a choline-deficient diet: understanding fatty liver disease progression. *Mitochondrion.* (2008) 8:367–76. doi: 10.1016/j.mito.2008.07.008
44. Serviddio G, Giudetti AM, Bellanti F, Priore P, Rollo T, Tamborra R, et al. Oxidation of hepatic carnitine palmitoyl transferase-I (CPT-I) impairs fatty acid beta-oxidation in rats fed a methionine-choline deficient diet. *PLoS ONE.* (2011) 6:e24084. doi: 10.1371/journal.pone.0024084
45. Mehedint MG, Niculescu MD, Craciunescu CN, Zeisel SH. Choline deficiency alters global histone methylation and epigenetic marking at the Re1 site of the calbindin 1 gene. *FASEB J.* (2010) 24:184–95. doi: 10.1096/fj.09-140145
46. Tremaroli V, Backhed F. Functional interactions between the gut microbiota and host metabolism. *Nature.* (2012) 489:242–9. doi: 10.1038/nature11552
47. Ishioka M, Miura K, Minami S, Shimura Y, Ohnishi H. Altered gut microbiota composition and immune response in experimental steatohepatitis mouse models. *Dig Dis Sci.* (2017) 62:396–406. doi: 10.1007/s10620-016-4393-x
48. Ikeda Y, Morita SY, Terada T. Cholesterol attenuates cytoprotective effects of phosphatidylcholine against bile salts. *Sci Rep.* (2017) 7:306. doi: 10.1038/s41598-017-00476-2
49. Morita SY, Ikeda Y, Tsuji T, Terada T. Molecular mechanisms for protection of hepatocytes against bile salt cytotoxicity. *Chem Pharm Bull.* (2019) 67:333–40. doi: 10.1248/cpb.c18-01029
50. Tolbol KS, Stierstorfer B, Rippmann JF, Veidal SS, Rigbolt KTG, Schonberger T, et al. Disease progression and pharmacological intervention in a nutrient-deficient rat model of nonalcoholic steatohepatitis. *Dig Dis Sci.* (2019) 64:1238–56. doi: 10.1007/s10620-018-5395-7
51. Takeuchi-Yorimoto A, Noto T, Yamada A, Miyamae Y, Oishi Y, Matsumoto M. Persistent fibrosis in the liver of choline-deficient and iron-supplemented L-amino acid-defined diet-induced nonalcoholic steatohepatitis rat due to continuing oxidative stress after choline supplementation. *Toxicol Appl Pharmacol.* (2013) 268:264–77. doi: 10.1016/j.taap.2013.01.027
52. Wang Y, Li J, Matye D, Zhang Y, Dennis K, Ding WX, et al. Bile acids regulate cysteine catabolism and glutathione regeneration to modulate hepatic sensitivity to oxidative injury. *JCI Insight.* (2018) 3:e99676. doi: 10.1172/jci.insight.99676
53. Guerrerio AL, Colvin RM, Schwartz AK, Molleston JP, Murray KF, Diehl A, et al. Choline intake in a large cohort of patients with nonalcoholic fatty liver disease. *Am J Clin Nutr.* (2012) 95:892–900. doi: 10.3945/ajcn.111.020156
54. Li J, Dawson PA. Animal models to study bile acid metabolism. *Biochim Biophys Acta Mol Basis Dis.* (2019) 1865:895–911. doi: 10.1016/j.bbadis.2018.05.011
55. Hui ST, Kurt Z, Tuominen I, Norheim F, Davis RC, Pan C, et al. The genetic architecture of diet-induced hepatic fibrosis in mice. *Hepatology.* (2018) 68:2182–96. doi: 10.1002/hep.30113
56. Tsuchida T, Lee YA, Fujiwara N, Ybanez M, Allen B, Martins S, et al. A simple diet- and chemical-induced murine NASH model with rapid progression of steatohepatitis, fibrosis and liver cancer. *J Hepatol.* (2018) 69:385–95. doi: 10.1016/j.jhep.2018.03.011
57. Noh SK, Koo SI. Enteral infusion of phosphatidylcholine increases the lymphatic absorption of fat, but lowers alpha-tocopherol absorption in rats fed a low zinc diet. *J Nutr Biochem.* (2001) 12:330–7. doi: 10.1016/S0955-2863(01)00145-0
58. Patankar JV, Obrowsky S, Doddapattar P, Hoefler G, Battle M, Levak-Frank S, et al. Intestinal GATA4 deficiency protects from diet-induced hepatic steatosis. *J Hepatol.* (2012) 57:1061–8. doi: 10.1016/j.jhep.2012.06.028
59. van de Peppel IP. *Intestinal Bile Acid Reabsorption in Health and Disease.* Rijksuniversiteit Groningen (2019).

5

Advances in the Involvement of Gut Microbiota in Pathophysiology of NAFLD

Xiaofan Jiang[1], Juan Zheng[2,3], Shixiu Zhang[1], Baozhen Wang[1], Chaodong Wu[4] and Xin Guo[1]**

[1] Department of Nutrition and Food Hygiene, School of Public Health, Cheeloo College of Medicine, Shandong University, Jinan, China, [2] Department of Endocrinology, Union Hospital, Tongji Medical College, Huazhong University of Science and Technology, Wuhan, China, [3] Hubei Provincial Clinical Research Center for Diabetes and Metabolic Disorders, Wuhan, China, [4] Department of Nutrition, Texas A&M University, College Station, TX, United States

***Correspondence:**
Chaodong Wu
cdwu@tamu.edu
Xin Guo
xguo@sdu.edu.cn

Non-alcoholic fatty liver disease (NAFLD) is characterized by hepatic steatosis and progresses to non-steatohepatitis (NASH) when the liver displays overt inflammatory damage. Increasing evidence has implicated critical roles for dysbiosis and microbiota-host interactions in NAFLD pathophysiology. In particular, microbiota alter intestine absorption of nutrients and intestine permeability, whose dysregulation enhances the delivery of nutrients, endotoxin, and microbiota metabolites to the liver and exacerbates hepatic fat deposition and inflammation. While how altered composition of gut microbiota attributes to NAFLD remains to be elucidated, microbiota metabolites are shown to be involved in the regulation of hepatocyte fat metabolism and liver inflammatory responses. In addition, intestinal microbes and circadian coordinately adjust metabolic regulation in different stages of life. During aging, altered composition of gut microbiota, along with circadian clock dysregulation, appears to contribute to increased incidence and/or severity of NAFLD.

Keywords: circadian, microbiota, metabolic diseases, NAFLD, inflammation, reprogramming

INTRODUCTION

Non-alcoholic fatty liver disease (NAFLD) has become a leading cause of chronic liver disease worldwide. There are 25% of population in the world suffering from NAFLD, including children, adolescents, and elderly (1). NAFLD is characterized by hepatic steatosis. When exhibiting inflammatory damage and fibrosis in addition to steatosis, NAFLD progresses to non-alcoholic steatohepatitis (NASH), the advanced form of NAFLD. As supported by the results from various epidemiological and clinical studies, NASH is a causal factor of terminal liver diseases including liver cirrhosis and hepatocellular carcinoma. Unhealthy nutrition-related metabolic disorders, such as central obesity, insulin resistance, dyslipidemia, and hypertension are closely associated with NAFLD (2). Although the etiology and progression of NAFLD remain to be elucidated, growing studies indicate that, additional to insulin resistance and inflammation, gut microbiota, and circadian rhythmicity of hepatic metabolic genes are considered to play key roles in the pathogenesis of NAFLD (3, 4).

The gut microbiota is composed of huge numbers of microbes. Half century ago, it was discovered that the toxicity of *Escherichia coli's* endotoxin fatality rate was determined by the administering time of endotoxin (5). This phenomenal finding and others led to validation that the microbiota colonized within the gastrointestinal tract undergoes circadian oscillations, which influence the composition and function of gut microbiota (6, 7). For instance, the diurnal interaction between oscillating hosts and their gut microbiome affect the circadian clock activities in other tissues and organs (8, 9), which in turn critically regulate host's metabolic homeostasis (10).

It has been accepted that the intestine and the liver are closely linked. This link is manifested by that gut microbiota and its metabolites play critical roles in the pathogenesis of NAFLD. Also, circadian rhythm was reported to maintain hepatic glucose and lipid metabolic homeostasis through regulating gut microbiota balance. In this review, we focused on the regulation of gut microbiota in relation to hepatic lipid metabolism and liver function, the alterations of gut microbiota in NAFLD, and the effects of microbiota metabolites on the development of NAFLD. Furthermore, we evaluated the relationships among circadian clock, gut microbiota, and metabolic disease (in particular NAFLD). We also summarized the effects of intestinal microbes on regulating metabolism through reprogramming circadian clock. Lastly, we summarized the effects of the interplays between intestinal microbes and circadian on metabolism and NAFLD aspects in different stages of life.

GUT MICROBIOTA AND LIVER PATHOPHYSIOLOGY

Many studies have revealed that gut microbiota dysbiosis is linked to NAFLD (11, 12). The composition of gut microbiota varies from simple steatosis to NASH, fibrosis, and cirrhosis. Therefore, gut microbiota may be useful as predictors for NAFLD progression and severity (13, 14). Gut microbiota is capable of fermenting indigestible carbohydrates, resulting in important metabolites, such as short-chain fatty acids. The gut microbiota can also ferment tryptophan to generate other metabolites such as indole and indole derivatives. Animal studies and human studies have shown that these metabolites have beneficial effects on preventing against and/or alleviating obesity and NAFLD (15, 16). Understanding the mechanisms of how gut microbiota and metabolites are involved in NAFLD pathophysiology can inspire us to find out potential strategies to prevent or treat NAFLD/NASH. Recent advances in understanding the crosstalk between the gut and the liver pertinent to NAFLD pathophysiology is summarized in **Figure 1** and detailed below.

Influences of the Gut on Liver Metabolism

The intestine digests foods and absorbs nutrients. The liver receives nutrients from the intestine. As such, there are many metabolic events exhibiting the crosstalk between the gut and the liver. For instance, gut hormones participate in hepatic metabolism. In response to feeding, glucagon-like peptide 1 (GLP-1), which is secreted by the L cells of the small intestine, stimulates pancreatic β islet cells to produce insulin. Also, GLP-1 acts on GLP-1 receptor, present on human hepatocytes, to reduce hepatic glucose production and ameliorate hepatic fat deposition and insulin resistance (17). The release of intestinal GLP-1 enhances energy expenditure, which is associated with increases in the peripheral utilization of triglycerides (TG) for energy production, and reduces hepatic steatosis in mice fed a high-fat diet (HFD) (18, 19). Insulin-like peptide 5 (INSL5), which is also an L cell-derived gut hormone and regulated by gut microbiota, is reported to influence hepatic glucose production. Compared to that in conventionally raised (CONV-R) mice, the expression of INSL5 in the gut was 80-fold higher in germ-free (GF) mice and 20-fold higher in antibiotics-treated mice. The importance of INSL5 in regulating metabolism is further supported by the finding that $INSL5^{-/-}$ mice exhibited decreased hepatic glucose production due to, in part, decreased expression of gluconeogenic enzymes such as glucose-6-phosphatase (G6Pase) and phosphoenolpyruvate carboxykinase (PEPCK) (20). In addition, glucose-dependent insulinotropic polypeptide (GIP), another gut hormone that is released from K cells located in the duodenum and proximal jejunum, regulates glucose homeostasis and lipid metabolism (21). Indeed, GIP appears to inhibit glucagon-stimulated hepatic glucose production through an indirect way (22). There is evidence suggesting that GIP influences hepatic insulin resistance and steatosis via regulating myeloid-cell-derived S100A8/A9 (23). Fibroblast growth factor 15 and 19 (FGF15 and FGF 19), which are also from the gut, were reported to ameliorate HFD-induced hepatic fat accumulation and ER stress (24). In particular, FGF 19 promoted hepatic glycogen and protein synthesis (25), reduced inflammation and fibrosis in liver injury mouse model through downregulating the expression of cholesterol 7α-hydroxylase (CYP7A1) and sterol-27-hydroxylase (CYP27A1) and thereby inhibiting bile acid synthesis (26).

Additional to gut hormones that regulate hepatic metabolism and inflammation, gut microbiota is associated with the development of NAFLD (27). For instance, gut permeability and small intestinal bacterial overgrowth are increased in patients with NAFLD compared with those in health controls. In this case, the increased gut permeability caused by alteration of intercellular tight junction likely contributes to the development and progression of NAFLD (28–30). Inflammation promotes the development of simple steatosis into NASH. In NAFLD, impaired intestinal barrier caused by nutrition stress increases the translocation of microbes and their products into the blood, leading to hepatic inflammation and even fibrosis/cirrhosis (31). Gut-derived antigens in the circulation are considered as major causing factors of strong inflammatory responses in the liver. Although intestinal permeability is not the main cause of liver inflammation and fibrosis, due to increased intestinal permeability, the inflammatory responses to microbial antigen strongly influence the progression of the disease.

Gut-derived bacterial products, such as lipopolysaccharides (LPS) and unmethylated CpG DNA, activate the signaling pathways involved in liver inflammation and fibrogenesis through stimulating innate immune receptors, e.g., Toll-like receptors (TLRs). In NASH patients, hepatic and serum TLR4 is significantly increased. Thus, high serum levels of TLR4 are considered as a bio-marker for liver fibrosis development (32). In a study involving TLR4-mutant mice, the results indicated that TLR4 was required for fructose to induce NAFLD.

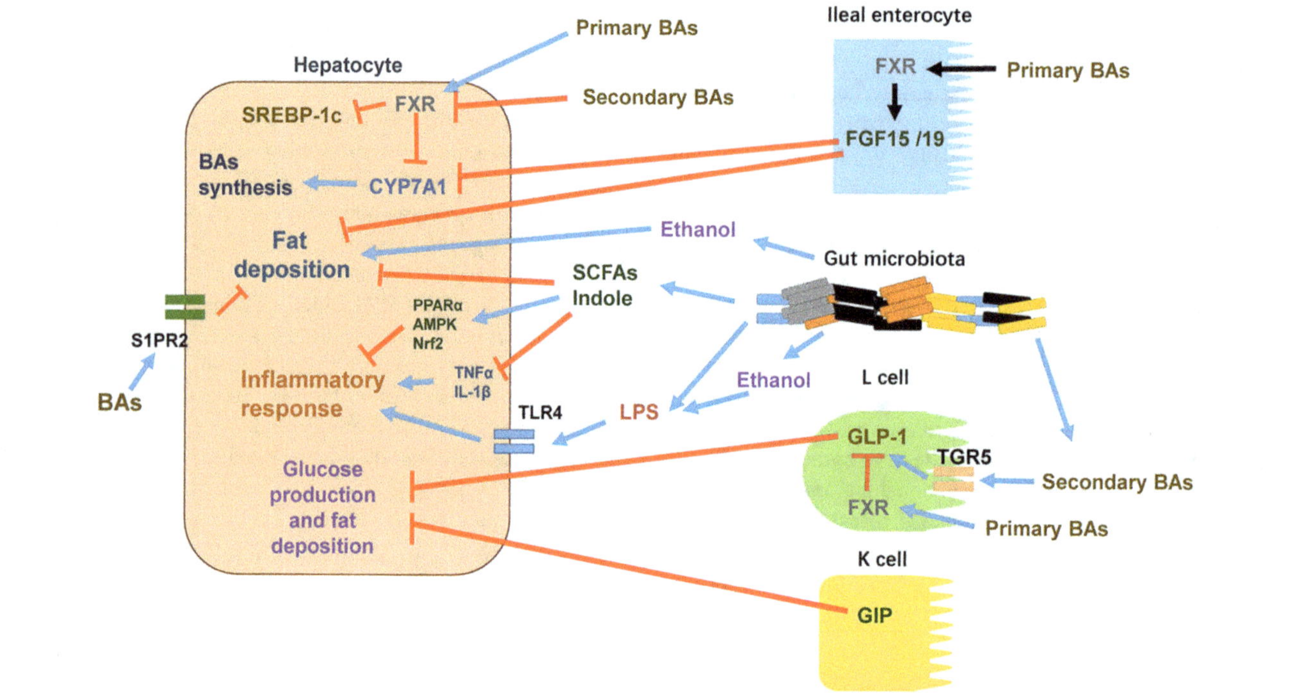

FIGURE 1 | The crosstalk between intestine and liver in the pathophysiology of NAFLD. Certain intestine hormones, e.g., GLP-1 and GIP, reduce hepatic glucose production and fat accumulation. In L cells, secondary BAs stimulate GLP-1 synthesis and release via TGR5 activation whereas primary BAs activate FXR to inhibit GLP-1 synthesis and release. Other intestine hormones, e.g., FGF15 and FGF19, decrease hepatic lipogenesis. BAs stimulate FXR in ileal enterocytes, leading to the release of FGF15/19 into circulation. After reaching to hepatocytes, FGF15/19 suppresses BA synthesis through inhibiting CYP7A1 expression. Increased gut permeability, altered composition of gut microbiota, and elevated levels of gut microbiota metabolites such as ethanol are shown to enhance hepatocyte fat deposition and increase the flow of LPS into the circulation to promote proinflammatory responses through activating TLR4 signaling pathway in target cells. In hepatocytes, certain primary BAs acts through activating FXR to suppress the activity of SREBP-1c and thus reduces the expressions of lipogenic genes. Primary BAs also inhibit CYP7A1 expression and thus reduces BAs synthesis. Certain secondary BAs inhibit the activation of hepatic FXR. In addition to activation of FXR, BAs are shown to regulate hepatic lipid and sterol metabolism through activating S1PR2. Certain gut microbiota metabolites such as SCFAs and indole reduce hepatocyte fat deposition and proinflammatory responses via decreasing TNFα and IL-1β and/or activating PPARα, AMPK, and Nrf2.

Compared with fructose-fed wild type mice, fructose-fed TLR4-mutant mice exhibited reduced hepatic fat accumulation, lipid peroxidation, inflammation, insulin resistance, and plasma ALT levels. This indicates the involvement of gut-derived endotoxin in the development of fructose-induced NAFLD (33). A similar study revealed that hepatic specific TLR4 deletion protected mice from fatty liver induced by 5% alcohol diet via decreasing the expression of hepatic inflammatory cytokines and endogenous lipogenesis (34). Saturated fatty acids (SFA) such as palmitate can activate proinflammatory signals through TLR4, inducing IL-1β and TNF-α production, as well as enhancing ROS production in hepatic infiltrating macrophages (35). Mechanistically, TLR4 promoting of the progression from simple steatosis to NASH involves in increases in ROS-dependent activation of X-box binding protein-1 (XBP-1) in Kupffer cells (36). TLR4 also is shown to induce transforming growth factor β (TGFβ) signaling pathway, activate hepatic stellate cell and increase extracellular matrix deposition, which all contribute to the progression of liver fibrosis (37). Moreover, gut microbiota and TLR4 appear to be required for the promotion of hepatocellular carcinoma (HCC), whose pathogenesis is enhanced by chronic liver inflammation and fibrosis (38).

More specific mechanisms of fat deposition and inflammation in the liver, caused by the alterations of gut permeability and barrier-induced infiltration of bacteria and bacteria products, involve increased signaling through nuclear factor kappa-light-chain-enhancer of activated B cells (NFκB) or c-Jun-N-terminal kinase (JNK), as well as increased levels of tumor necrosis factor alpha (TNFα) (39). Activation of NFκB in hepatocytes increased the production of cytokines and resulted in the recruitment and activation of Kupffer cells to mediate inflammation in the progression of NASH. Activation of NFκB induced the expression of TNFα, Fas ligand (FasL), and TGFβ, which contributed to fibrosis in NASH (40). Disruption of NFκB p65 in mice ameliorated HFD-induced hepatic steatosis and insulin resistance (41). JNK can be activated by diverse stimuli, such as cytokines, FFAs, reactive oxygen species (ROS), pathogens, and toxins. Activation of hepatic JNK decreased the expression of PPARα target genes and FGF21, up-regulated cytokines such as TNFα and interleukin-1 (IL-1), and promoted insulin resistance in liver (42).

Regulation of Gut Microbiota by Hepatic Bile Acids

Primary bile acids (BAs), produced in the liver from cholesterol, serve as an emulsifier for lipid digestion in the intestine. Primary BAs become secondary BAs after being metabolized by intestinal flora. BAs are associated with the establishment of the gut microbiota; given that bile salts have anti-bacteria effects and only bacteria that are resistant to bile salts can survive in the intestine (43, 44). The antimicrobial actions of BAs are likely attributable to that BAs cause bacterial cell membrane damage through dissolving membrane lipids and dissociating membrane proteins. BAs also disturb macromolecular stability, such as misfolding or denaturing protein and inducing DNA damage and oxidative stress (44). Moreover, in human, chenodeoxycholic acid (CDCA) and cholic acid (CA), which are primary bile acids, as well as deoxycholic (DCA) and lithocholic acid (LCA), which are the predominant forms of secondary bile acids, activate the nuclear receptor farnesoid X receptor (FXR) to induce the expression of genes that are responsible for inhibition of microbial overgrowth and intestinal mucosal damage (45). It is known that BAs play an important role in regulating the composition of gut microbiota in response to diet. When mice consumed a Western diet, the profiles of BAs were altered, which increased Firmicutes, decreased Bacteroidetes, and disturbed the ecological balance of microbes (46). A similar study using FXR-deficient mice upon HFD feeding also revealed that the abundance of Firmicutes was increased and the abundance of Bacteroidetes was reduced. The profiles of BAs were featured by increased levels of primary bile acids such as beta-muricholic acids (βMCA) and taurine-conjugated beta-muricholic acids (TβMCA) and decreased levels of secondary bile acids such as ωMCA, hyodeoxycholic acid (HDCA), and hyocholic acid (HCA) (47). A rapid increase in the gut BAs pool (35 out of 42 quantified BAs) was observed in mice upon HFD feeding within 12 h, and an alteration in gut microbiota composition occurred at 24 h. Treatment of chow diet-fed mice with glycine-conjugated cholic acid (GCA) and taurine-conjugated cholic acid (TCA) increased obesity-related microbial population and brought about obese phenotype. Inhibition hepatic BAs synthesis in HFD-fed mice ameliorated HFD-induced dysregulation of microbial composition (48). In NASH-HCC mouse model, HFD accelerated the incidence of liver tumors, which was accompanied with increased the levels of hepatic BAs, including GCA, TCA, and taurochenodeoxycholate (TCDCA). The changes in gut microbiota were correlated with altered levels of BAs in the liver, suggesting that high hepatic BAs are associated with the dysregulation of gut microbiota and the development of HCC (49). Compared with those in healthy controls, fecal total and secondary BAs (LCA and DCA) were lower while primary BAs (CA and CDCA) were higher in patients with advanced cirrhosis. Patients with advanced cirrhosis also exhibited higher levels of Enterobacteriaceae and lower levels of Lachonospiraceae, Ruminococcaceae, and Blautia. Therefore, the amounts of primary and secondary BAs are associated with the population of key gut microbiota during the pathogenesis of cirrhosis (50). There also is evidence indicating that feeding mice high-saturated fats (from milk), compared to polyunsaturated fats or chow diet, resulted in alterations of BAs composition with increased levels of TCA and changes in gut microbiota with enhanced the abundance of Bilophila wadsworthia (51). IL-$10^{-/-}$ mice on chow diet treated with TCA for a week exhibited higher abundance of Bilophila wadsworthia, which showed the similar results found in milk fat fed mice (52).

Modulation of Bile Acid Metabolism by Gut Microbiota

Gut microbiota regulates the metabolism of BA synthesis. Compared with GF mice, the BA pool (mainly for conjugated and unconjugated βMCA) in CONV-R mice was reduced by 71%. The composition of BAs between CONV-R and GF mice was quite different in the cecum and colon. In the liver, CONV-R mice had higher levels of TCA and TαMCA and lower levels of TβMCA, compared with GF mice. The expression and activity of CYP7A1, which is a rate-limiting enzyme in BA synthesis in the liver, were downregulated in CONV-R mice. Furthermore, in FXR-deficient CONV-R mice, the levels of CYP7A1 were not decreased in the liver. Treatment of GF mice with FXR agonist INT-747 reduced the level of hepatic CYP7A1. These findings suggest that gut microbiota suppresses CYP7A1 expression in the liver in an FXR-dependent manner. Ileum FGF15 was involved in the regulation of CYP7A1 expression through FXR signaling. Treatment of CONV-R mice with antibiotics (bacitracin, neomycin, and streptomycin) suppressed FGF15 expression in ileum and enhanced the expression of CYP7A1, thus increasing the levels of primary BAs (TCA and TβMCA) and decreasing the levels of secondary BAs (DCA and ωMCA) (53). Besides regulating CYP7A1, gut microbiota also affects other key enzymes in the alternative pathway of BA synthesis such as oxysterol 7α-hydroxylase (CYP7B1) and CYP27A1 (45). In addition, gut microbiota not only regulates BA synthesis, but also modulates BA conjugation and reabsorption. Bile acid acyl-CoA-synthetase (BACS), which catalyzes taurine conjugation in BAs in the liver and apical bile acid transporters in the ileum, were downregulated in CONV-R mice (53). In a human study for chronic hepatitis B, the levels of total and primary BAs (TCDCA, GCDCA, GCA, and TCA) were upregulated in hepatitis B patients with moderate/advanced fibrosis, accompanied with downregulation of gut microbiota (such as Bacteroides and Ruminococcus) responsible for BAs metabolism (54). Trimethylamine N-oxide (TMAO), which is a metabolite produced by gut microbiota from choline, stimulated the expression of CYP7A1 in the liver, increased the serum levels of BAs and promoted FXR-antagonistic BAs (55).

Altered Composition of Gut Microbiota During NAFLD

The composition of gut microbiota is altered during NAFLD. For instance, Lactobacillus species and some phylum Firmicutes such as Lachnospiraceae, genera, Dorea, Robinsoniella, and Roseburia were high in obese patients with NAFLD (56). Additionally, non-obese patients with NAFLD exhibited increased phylum Bacteroidetes and gram-negative bacteria and decreased Firmicutes including short-chain fatty acids-producing and 7α-dehydroxylating bacteria compared with healthy controls (57). When dietary choline was deficient, the levels of Gammaproteobacteria and Erysipelotrichi were correlated with the changes of fat accumulation in the liver. Gut microbiota such as Gammaproteobacteria and Erysipelotrichi can serve as a predictor for choline deficiency-induced fatty liver (58). Compared with that in NAFLD and healthy controls, higher abundance of Fusobacteria and Fusobacteriaceae was observed in NASH patients (59). Gut microbiota is related to advanced fibrosis in NAFLD. In both mild/moderate NAFLD and advanced fibrosis, the abundance of Firmicutes and Bacteroidetes is much higher. Proteobacteria is higher in advanced fibrosis, while Firmicutes is higher in mild/moderate NAFLD. Eubacterium rectale and Bacteroides vulgatu are rich in mild/moderate NAFLD, while *B. vulgatus* and *Escherichia coli* are rich in advanced fibrosis (60). Different steatosis in NAFLD patients exhibit differential compositions of gut microbiota. The abundance of Bacteroidetes is lower and the abundance of *C. coccoides* is higher during steatosis with inflammation and/or fibrosis, compared to simple steatosis (61). The composition of gut microbiota predicts the severity of NAFLD. Bacteroides is significantly higher in NASH and is independently associated with NASH, whereas Ruminococcus is higher in significant fibrosis (14).

Microbiota Metabolites in the Pathophysiology of NAFLD

In addition to gut microbiota, microbiota metabolites also influence the pathophysiology of NAFLD. As it is established, microbial products derived from fermentation of dietary fiber and protein can affect liver metabolism and the development of NAFLD (62). Microbial metabolites are different during the progression from NAFLD to fibrosis. In advanced fibrosis, 3-phenylpropanoate, generated from anaerobic bacteria, is the mostly increased metabolite (63). Further analyses of proteins and enzymes indicate that the enzymes related to lactate, acetate, and formate are enhanced in mild/moderate NAFLD whereas the enzymes associated with butyrate, D-lactate, propionate, and succinate are increased in advanced fibrosis (60). The following microbiota metabolites are investigated mostly and closely related to NAFLD.

Short Chain Fatty Acids

Indigestible carbohydrates are fermented by gut microbiota and generate short chain fatty acids (SCFAs) such as acetate, butyrate, and propionate. Pectin, which is one of the soluble dietary fibers, is reported to prevent NAFLD in HFD-fed mice. Pectin increases acetic acid and propionic acid, as well as the levels of Bacteroides, Parabacteroides, Olsenella, and Bifidobacterium in the gut of HFD-fed mice (64). Gut-derived SCFAs such as propionate and acetate are metabolized by the liver and alter hepatic glucose and lipid metabolism (16). Serum metabolomics reveals that the serum levels of butyric acid and propionic acid were decreased in patient with NAFLD (65). Also, down-regulation of SCFA-producing bacteria contributes to increased energy intake and HFD-induced hepatic steatosis (66). Butyrate is reported to maintain intestinal mucosal health, including serving as a fuel source and regulating the immune system (67). There is evidence suggesting that butyrate ameliorates HFD-induced NAFLD and NASH via restoring the dysbiosis of gut microbiota and improving gut barrier (68), activating peroxisome proliferator-activated receptor alpha (PPARα) in the liver, suppressing hepatic inflammation and enhancing GLP-1R expression (69, 70). Moreover, butyrate-producing probiotic reduces hepatic lipid accumulation and inflammatory responses and improves hepatic insulin resistance via activating AMP-activated protein kinase (AMPK), AKT, and the expression of nuclear factor erythroid 2-related factor 2 (Nrf2) in rats with NAFLD (71). As supported by the results from a study involving G protein-coupled receptor 41 (GPR41)-deficient and GF mice, SCFAs binding to GPR41 may account for the regulation of gut microbiota, thereby host fat accumulation (72). Another study indicated that SCFAs acted through downregulating the expression levels of NLPR3, apoptosis-associated speck like proteins (ASC), and Caspase-1 to decrease inflammation in a manner involving G protein-coupled receptor 43 (GPR43) (73). Also, supplementation of SCFAs reduces hepatic fat deposition and inflammation by decreasing the activities of fatty acids synthases, increasing lipid oxidation via activation of AMPK, and suppressing the expression hepatic inflammatory cytokines such as interleukin-6 and TNFα (74, 75). SCFAs may also act through stimulating the release of GLP-1 to bring about beneficial effects on reducing fat accumulation and increasing insulin resistance (76).

Ethanol

Gut microbiota dysbiosis increases intestinal ethanol levels, which is associated with the progression of NAFLD. In patients with NASH, elevated ethanol-producing bacteria increased blood ethanol concentrations that are considered to be the reason of enhanced oxidative stress and inflammation in the liver (77), through increasing gut permeability, decreasing gut barrier, and increasing the levels of LPS in the intestine. Similar mechanisms also lead to increased transportation of endotoxin to the liver (78). In addition, ethanol has a direct harmful effect on the liver, leading to steatosis, steatohepatitis, and fibrosis (79). Ethanol stimulation of hepatic fat accumulation is likely attributable to increased production of acetate, a substrate for the synthesis of fatty acids. In ob/ob mice, a model of obesity and NAFLD, the levels of intestinal bacteria-derived ethanol are increased. In addition, treatment of ob/ob mice with antibiotics ameliorates ethanol-induced fat deposition and inflammation in the liver (78). There are different microbes responsible for ethanol production responding to different carbohydrates from diet. Most of ethanol is produced by *S. cerevisiae*, *L. fermentum*, and *W. confusa* after consumption of glucose, whereas the highest amount of ethanol is produced by *S. cerevisiae* and *W. confusa* after consumption of fructose. Therefore, inhibition of these microbes may be a viable strategy to reduce ethanol production and, thereby preventing NAFLD, NASH, or fibrosis (80).

Bile Acids

Primary BAs are synthesized by the liver whereas secondary BAs are metabolized by gut microbiota. As such, BAs are also considered microbiota metabolites. After its metabolism by gut microbiota, BAs return to the liver via the enterohepatic circulation through transporters on ileal enterocytes and hepatocytes. BAs regulate BA homeostasis, glucose and lipid metabolism through FXR signaling in hepatocytes, ileal enterocytes, and colonic L cells. Primary BAs such as CDCA, CA, T(G)CDCA, and T(G)CA are FXR agonists. In the liver, FXR activation by BAs inhibits expression of the CYP7A1. In ileum, FXR activation induces the expression of FGF15/19, which goes to the liver and also inhibits the expression of CYP7A1 and suppresses BA synthesis. In colonic L cells, FXR activation suppresses the synthesis and release of GLP-1 (81). Some BAs are reported to be FXR antagonists, such as UDCA (secondary BAs in human) and Tα/βMCA (primary BAs in mice). Secondary BAs such as LCA and DCA act as signal molecules to regulate energy homeostasis, insulin signaling, and inflammation via Takeda G-protein-coupled receptor 5 (TGR5) in colon, adipose tissue, muscle, and bone marrow (12). A study revealed that TGR5 activation improved glucose tolerance, increased energy expenditure, and decreased hepatic steatosis in HFD-induced obese mice (18). Altering BA profiles via diet, probiotics, medication, or surgery is reported to reverse obese-related metabolic phenotypes such as NAFLD/NASH through modifying BA composition. The latter involves appropriate regulation of hepatic metabolism through FXR and metabolisms in other tissues through TGR5 (82). For example, TGR5 activation by secondary BAs (such as LCA and DCA) in colonic L cells stimulated the synthesis and release of GLP-1, which inhibited glucose production and fat accumulation in hepatocytes. In patients with NAFLD, the serum levels of primary and secondary BAs were high, which were accompanied with decreased activation of FXR, fibroblast growth factor receptor 4 (FGFR4)-mediated signaling and serum levels of FGF19. In addition, secondary BAs were increased in the intestine of patients with NAFLD via enhancing the metabolism of taurine and glycine (83). In patients with NASH, *de novo* biosynthesis of bile acids in the liver was increased compared with that in healthy controls. Furthermore, increased *de novo* biosynthesis of bile acids may be closely associated with gut microbiota dysbiosis in NASH (84). CA was reported to prevent hepatic lipid accumulation and VLDL secretion via activation of FXR to suppress the activity of SREBP-1c and thus downregulate the expression of lipogenic genes (85). In addition to activation of FXR, conjugated-BAs were shown to regulate hepatic lipid and sterol metabolism through activating sphingosine-1 phosphate receptor 2 (S1PR2) to trigger ERK1/2 signaling pathway, which directly or indirectly modulates transcription of many genes such as CYP7A1, SREBP1c, and ApoB-100 (86). S1PR2 activation was also associated with reducing macrophage infiltration, which is the characteristic in NASH and fibrosis (87). Of note, BAs and the gut microbiota closely interact with each other. On the one side, BAs directly suppress bacteria growth in the gut through the anti-bacterial effects of BAs. On the other side, certain intestinal bacterial such as *L. monocytogenes* encode bacterial bile salt hydrolase (BSH), which in turn degrades BAs and helps bacteria to resist BAs (44). Interestingly, up-regulating BSH in conventionally raised mice reduces weight gain, plasma cholesterol, and liver triglycerides by regulating the transcription of genes related to lipid and cholesterol metabolism such as peroxisome proliferator-activated receptor gamma (PPARγ), ANGPTL4, and ABCG5/8 (88). Therefore, reducing BAs by modulating gut microbiota appears to be a viable strategy to improve NAFLD.

Indole and Indole Derivatives

As a bacterial degradation product of tryptophan, indole exerts powerful anti-inflammatory effects on immune cells and enterocytes (89). Subsequently, there are studies that have explored the effects of several indole derivatives as it relates to NAFLD. In a mouse model with HFD-induced NAFLD, Choi et al. examined the effects of indole-3-carbinol (I3C) on NAFLD phenotypes and attributed the anti-steatotic effect of I3C, at least in part, to decreased expression of lipogenic genes (15, 89–91). Similarly, two recent studies have shown that treatment with indole-3-acetate (I3A) alleviated NAFLD phenotypes in mice (92, 93). At the cellular level, I3A decreased hepatocyte production of palmitate, which was weakened by inhibition of aryl hydrocarbon receptor (AhR, a proposed receptor that mediates indole actions) (92). Moreover, I3A decreased hepatocyte mRNA levels of fatty acid synthase (FAS) and SREBP1c, a key transcription factor of lipogenic gene expression (94, 95), implying that I3A has a suppressive effect on hepatic lipogenesis. Consistent with the anti-NAFLD effects of indole derivatives, indole, *per se*, has also been validated to ameliorate diet-induced NAFLD phenotype in mice. Specifically, treatment of HFD-fed mice with indole, via intraperitoneal injection, for 9 weeks caused significant decreases in HFD-induced insulin resistance, hepatic steatosis, and liver inflammation (93). The mechanisms underlying the beneficial effects of indole are attributable to that indole reduced HFD-induced expression of hepatic lipogenic genes such as SREBP-1, steraroyl coenzyme decarboxylase 1 (SCD1), PPARγ, acetyl-CoA carboxylasel (ACC1), and glycerol-3-phosphate acyltransferase, mitochondrial (GPAM), decreased the hepatic levels of reactive oxygen species (ROS) and lipid peroxidation product such as malonaldehyde, enhanced the activity of superoxide dismutase (SOD), and reduced hepatic macrophage infiltration, monocyte chemoattractant protein-1 (MCP1) and TNFα levels (93).

The relevance of indole to human NAFLD has been recently revealed, for the first time, in the study by Ma et al. In a cohort of 137 Chinese subjects, the circulating levels of indole were significantly lower than those in lean subjects and were reversely correlated with liver fat content (96). In parallel, the data from mice with diet-induced NAFLD further reveal that the hepatic levels of indole in HFD-fed mice were significantly lower than those in control mice. These two lines of evidence enabled the scientific premise for examining the effect of indole supplementation on alleviating NAFLD phenotype. As expected, oral supplementation of indole caused significant decreases in the severity of HFD-induced hepatic steatosis and inflammation. While gaining the mechanistic insights of indole actions, the study by Ma et al. also reveals that myeloid cell-specific disruption of PFKFB3, a master regulatory gene of glycolysis, nearly blunted the effects of indole on decreasing HFD-induced hepatic

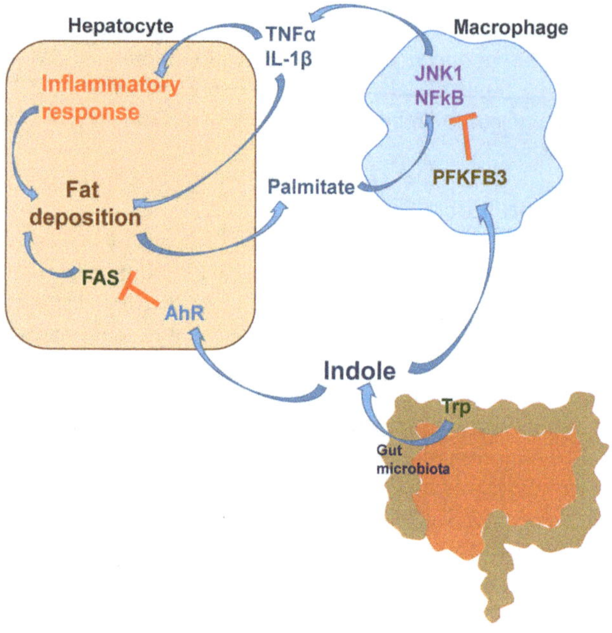

FIGURE 2 | The mechanistic scheme for indole alleviation of NAFLD. During NAFLD, hepatocytes release fat deposition-associated proinflammatory mediators and palmitate (hydrolysis product of very low-density lipoproteins), which act on macrophages to enhance the proinflammatory responses. Active macrophages release proinflammatory factors such as TNFα and IL-1β and act, via paracrine manners, to exacerbate the proinflammatory responses and fat accumulation in hepatocytes. Indole, a microbiota metabolite from tryptophan (Trp), acts to reduce hepatocyte fat deposition via suppressing the expression of FAS through a mechanism involving AhR activation. Moreover, indole reduces the inflammatory responses in both macrophages and hepatocytes and fat deposition in hepatocytes in a manner involving myeloid cell PFKFB3. *Modified based on Krishnan, S., et al. Cell Reports, 2018. 23(4): p. 1099-1111 and Zheng et al. Front Med 2015; 9: 173-186.*

steatosis and inflammation. PFKFB3 is the gene encoding inducible 6-phosphofructo-2-kinase (iPFK2) (97), whose product fructose-2,6-bisphosphate is the most potent activator of glycolytic enzyme 6-phosphofructo-1-kinase (98–100). In macrophages differentiated from bone marrow cells, indole displayed a suppressive effect on LPS-induced proinflammatory responses in a PFKFB3-dependent manner (**Figure 2**). Moreover, hepatocytes co-cultured with PFKFB3-disrupted macrophages displayed increases in palmitate-induced fat deposition and LPS-induced proinflammatory responses. Of note, treatment with indole did not alleviate these responses in hepatocytes co-cultured with PFKFB3-disrupted macrophages as did it in hepatocytes co-cultured with control macrophages. Clearly, indole exerts an anti-NAFLD effect in a manner involving myeloid cell PFKFB3.

The study by Ma et al. also revealed a number of significant and interesting findings (96). In particular, mice with HFD-induced NAFLD revealed altered composition of gut microbiota relative to that in mice fed a control low-fat diet (LFD). Moreover, treatment of HFD-fed mice with indole brought about changes in the composition of gut microbiota in a manner similar to that in LFD-fed mice. This validates that indole, as a microbiota metabolite, also alters the composition of gut microbiota. Another important finding from the pharmacokinetic study is that indole reached its peak levels in the liver at 6 h post a single oral dosing of indole. In addition, the levels of indole were significantly higher than those in the circulation. Because of this, the liver is considered a primary organ where indole is metabolized. As such, the liver appears to be primary target for indole-based therapeutic approaches. The mechanistic scheme for indole actions is summarized in **Figure 2**.

Clearly, the intestine plays an important role in the pathophysiology of NAFLD. Intestine hormones, intestine conditions (such as permeability and intercellular tight junction), gut microbiota composition and balance, and microbiota metabolites regulate glucose production, lipogenesis, inflammatory response and insulin resistance in the liver by directly or indirectly ways. These advances have significantly improved our understanding of how the crosstalk between intestine and liver critically regulates the pathogenesis of NAFLD.

Management of NAFLD/NASH via Modulating Gut Microbiota

As gut microbiota is considered to be a new therapeutic target for NAFLD/NASH, researchers are recently full of enthusiasm about looking for compounds to control NAFLD/NASH by altering gut microbiota. Probiotics are living microorganisms that can relieve intestinal diseases by restoring normal microbiota and provide health benefits to the host. A human study revealed that liver aminotransferases levels were improved in NAFLD patients treated with 500 million of *Lactobacillus bulgaricus* and *Streptococcus thermophiles* (101). MIYAIRI 588, a butyrate-producing probiotic from Japan, prevented hepatic steatosis from developing into liver cancer in a rat NAFLD model through activating of hepatic adenosine 5′-monophosphate-activated protein kinase (AMPK), AKT, nuclear factor erythoid 2-related factor 2 (Nrf2) and its targeted antioxidative enzymes (71). A probiotic mixture called VSL#3, which includes eight probiotic strains, has been proven to be very effective in the treatment of NAFLD. In obese children with NAFLD, supplementation with VSL#3 for 4 months decreased steatosis and BMI by enhancing the expression and the activity of GLP-1 (102, 103). Prebiotics, which are special form of dietary fibers, are fermented by gut microbiota to produce metabolites that promote the growth of beneficial intestinal flora. Alpha-galacto-oligosaccharides (alpha-GOS) from legumes was found to reduce food intake, improve fasting blood glucose, lower plasma non-esterified fatty acids, low-density lipoprotein (LDL), and total cholesterol in HFD-fed mice (104). Some phytochemicals also have prebiotic capacity and may become therapeutic compounds to prevent or treat NFALD. For instance, quercetin, which has antioxidant and anti-inflammatory properties, was reported to reduce hepatic fat accumulation, inflammation, and insulin resistance by increasing the population of Akkermansia genus in gut (105). Synbiotics, which are a combination of probiotics and prebiotics, was reported to provide more beneficial effects in NAFLD. Co-administering *Lactobacillus paracasei* N1115 and fructooligosaccharides in HFD-induced NAFLD mice reduced the levels of TNFα, insulin resistance and slowed the progression of cirrhosis (106). In lean patients with NAFLD, synbiotic (probiotics: 200 million bacteria of seven strains; prebiotic: 125 mg fructo-oligosaccharide) supplement significantly ameliorated fasting blood glucose, TG, and most inflammatory mediators (107).

SCFAs, which are metabolites from fermentation of dietary fiber by gut microbiota, have been used for preventing liver steatosis, inflammation, and fibrosis. Other metabolites such as BAs and indole-like molecules are potential therapeutic compounds to treat NAFLD/NASH. Antibiotics, such as neomycin and polymyxin B, can reduce fat accumulation in the liver by changing the gut microbiota and were found to be effective, to certain extent, for treating liver cirrhosis (108). After 90 days of solithromycin treatment, NASH patients showed reduction in liver steatosis and ALT levels (109). Gut-derived bacterial products and LPS increase hepatic inflammation in NAFLD through TLR4 signaling pathway. Blockage of TLR4 signaling pathway is considered as a potential therapy to alleviate hepatic inflammation and fibrosis. JKB-121, which is a TLR4 antagonist, was proved to reverse LPS-induced inflammation cytokine expressions, activation and proliferation of hepatic stellate cells, and collagen expression (110). Fecal microbiota transplantation (FMT) is an effective treatment for Clostridium difficile infection. There are some studies also suggesting that FMT may become a potential therapeutic strategy for NAFLD (111, 112). FMT from lean donors to obese recipients with metabolic syndrome for 6 weeks improved hepatic and systemic insulin sensitivity and increased butyrate-producing microbiota in obese recipients (113). A recent human study revealed that 6 weeks after allogenic FMT, small intestinal permeability in NAFLD patients was significantly reduced compared with that at baseline (114).

INTERPLAYS OF CIRCADIAN CLOCK AND GUT MICROBIOTA DURING NAFLD

There is evidence suggesting that circadian rhythms are related to gut microbiota, while gut microbiota also affects circadian rhythms (115). Both circadian and gut microbiota critically regulate metabolic homeostasis (116, 117) and are associated with the development of NAFLD (118, 119).

Circadian Dysregulation and Gut Microbiota Dysbiosis

While highly relevant to human health, microorganisms in the human body maintain a dynamic balance in the body. Also, the circadian rhythm and the intestinal microbes are closely linked (120). Indeed, gut microbiota itself exhibits diurnal compositional and functional oscillations (121, 122). More specifically, environmental factors such as disruption of feeding time and sleep pattern are shown to impair microbiota diurnal rhythmicity and cause microbiota dysbiosis (122, 123). There also are studies showing that circadian disruption alters microbiota configuration in gut. For instance, disruption of BMAL1 in mice abolished the circadian rhythms of fecal microbiota in both sexes, while changing microbiota composition in a sex-dependent manner (6). Also, circadian CLOCK mutant mice exhibited lower evenness and diversity of gut microbiota compared with wild type mice when fed a chow diet. When mice were fed an alcohol diet, gut microbiota taxonomic levels in circadian CLOCK mutant mice were significantly different from those in wild type mice, indicating that gut microbiota community structure is altered (10, 124). Moreover, the circadian clock also alters the function of the gut microbes. As supporting evidence, the bacterial adhesion oscillation in $PER1/2^{-/-}$ mice was remarkably disappeared (121). When combined with high-fat and high-sugar diets, mimicking rhythms disruption through frequent changes in light and darkness by reversing the light:dark cycle once weekly significantly changed the structure of microbial communities (124). Also, the microbe that impairs gut barrier integrity was increased and the microbe that improves the intestinal epithelial cell layer was decreased in mice exposed to constant 24 h light. Compared to that within normal light-dark cycles conditions, the diversity of rat's gut microbiota was significantly different in darkness or constant lighting conditions. The ratios of bacteria families such as Lactobacillus, Bacteroides, and Parabacteroides were altered in darkness or constant lighting conditions (125). In addition to the alterations of gut microbiota taxon, the expression of genes related to protective immune function was reduced whereas the expression of genes associated with gut inflammation was enhanced after circadian disruption. Specifically, the upregulated inflammatory genes include those for lipopolysaccharides (LPS) synthesis and transportation (126, 127).

Psychological factors also are shown to alter gut microbiota. A study reported that diurnal rhythm disorder caused by insomnia or a psychological and physiological pressure increased intestinal permeability and altered microbial composition (128). Also, in a study involving rhesus monkeys, stress was created by sound during pregnancy at night, and caused significant changes in intestinal microorganisms in the pregnant monkeys at 6 months before birth (129). The alteration of gut microbiota by stress includes reduced microorganism diversity and population of certain bacteria, such as Lactobacillus (130). Circadian rhythm disorder also can lead to the growth of some special intestinal microorganisms. In the first few days of sleep deprivation, mice revealed microbial invasion. At 20 days after sleep deprivation, the mice revealed 37 times more numbers of gram-negative bacteria in cecum relative to the control group (131). In a study involving human subjects, sleep deprivation increased Firmicutes in intestine, which usually found high relative abundance in obese population (132). The relative populations of Firmicutes, Lachnospiraceae, and Ruminococcaceae were increased and the relative populations of Bacteroidetes, Actinobacteria, Lactobacillmmaceae, and Bifidobacteriaceae were reduced in mice with 4 weeks of sleep fragmentation (133).

Involvement of Gut Microbiota Dysbiosis in Circadian Disruption-Related NAFLD

"Time difference phenomenon" has destructive power and increases the tendency of illness (122). Microbial dysregulation caused by circadian rhythm disorder leads to an increased probability of metabolic diseases such as obesity, insulin resistance, and NAFLD (134–136). There are studies showing that germ-free mice did not respond to HFD feeding whereas normal mice with microbiota became obese when fed with HFD (7). HFD-feeding altered the oscillations of gut microbiota composition and function, which were associated with disturbed host circadian rhythm and led to host metabolic dysregulation (7). This finding is similar to that observed in the human after weight loss surgery. The latter revealed that the energy intake was decreased and the numbers of bacteria were changed (such as increased levels of Prevotella and Bacteroides and decreased levels of Firmicutes) after gastric bypass surgery (137). In addition, chronic sleep restriction is associated with metabolic diseases including NAFLD. Workers with constant shift in schedules or individuals with frequent jet-lag exhibit alterations in gut microbiota, leading to increasing inflammatory responses and metabolic diseases (138). Mice under the treatment of inverted dark-light every 2 weeks for 8 weeks, which mimicked shift work, exhibited significantly increased intestine permeability and altered community of gut microbiota, systemic insulin resistance, dyslipidemia, and inflammation (139). Transplanting microbiota from circadian disrupted (such as jet-lagged) human to germ-free mice increased weight gain and blood glucose levels (122), which are associated a significant increase in the incidence of NAFLD.

In the pathogenesis of NAFLD or the progression to steatohepatitis, intestinal microbiota composition exhibits altered circadian oscillation, which enhances the permeability of intestinal endothelial barrier, leading to intestinal and hepatic inflammation (122, 140). Moreover, gut microbiota is involved in the regulation of the expression of circadian clock genes in the liver. This is significant because hepatic circadian disorder is associated with hepatic lipid accumulation, inflammation, and oxidative stress (141). In a study involving mice with diet-induced obesity and NAFLD, time-restricted feeding (feeding only for 8 h during dark phase) for HFD-fed mice, which consumed the same amount calories as that of HFD *ad libitum* mice, altered hepatic clock genes that are related to key enzymes for glucose and lipid metabolism in the liver, thus decreasing hepatic fat accumulation (142). Mice fed an *ad libitum* HFD displayed alterations in gut microbiome, luminal metabolomics, gut signaling, and hepatic gene expression, which resulted in metabolic dysregulation such as obesity, impaired glucose metabolism, insulin resistance, hepatic steatosis, and inflammation. However, mice with time-restricted HFD feeding revealed decreased obesogenic microbiota, increased obesity-protective microbiota, enhanced carbohydrate excretion, restored gut signaling and hepatic gene expression, which appeared to protect against obesity and metabolic dysregulation (136). Circadian disruption (mimicking shift work or jet-lag) in rats enhances the inflammatory responses when treated with LPS. In particular, Kupffer cells (KCs) isolated from circadian disrupted rats exhibited increased TNFα expression in response to LPS, indicating that liver immune cells are modulated by circadian rhythms (143). Furthermore, KCs itself showed circadian oscillation, indicated by the findings that the numbers of KCs varied during the circadian cycle and that some proteins in KCs have diurnal rhythmicity. The connection between immune response proteins of KCs and liver immune proteins is dominant during the daytime whereas the connection of metabolic proteins between KCs and liver is dominant during the nighttime (144). A study in which HFD-fed mice were under constant light revealed that melatonin ameliorated HFD- and circadian disruption-induced hepatic fat accumulation and insulin resistance and restored the gut microbiota. The latter was evidenced by that melatonin reversed the increased ratio of Firmicutes to Bacteroidetes (145).

GUT MICROBIOTA REGULATION OF NAFLD DURING AGING

Gut Microbes in Infants and Young Children

In an infant, the majority of bacterial strains comes from the mother. While most of the bacteria cannot be colonized for a long time (146), some intestinal strains always live with the host (146). It has been previously thought that baby's intestines are sterile. Numerous studies have now indicated that Staphylococcal and Enterococci are present in infant feces, verifying that microbial colonization has already occurred in the intestines (147). Compared with normal control, early intestinal microbiota in cesarean section infants is reduced and associated with T helper-1 (TH1) response (148). This in turn affects the weight of childhood; although the underlying mechanisms remain to be elucidated (149). In addition, premature infants with low birth weight exhibit altered intestinal microbes and increased risk of metabolic abnormalities (150). Accordingly, early control of multiple metabolic diseases, e.g., obesity (151) and diabetes (152), which both increase the incidence of NAFLD, may be achievable through breastfeeding. In severely malnourished children, microbes are lagging behind and cannot maintain optimal homeostasis, indicating that intestinal microbes play a role in metabolism (153). Gut microbes interplay with a variety of factors, including genetics and the environment (154). Congenital genetic materials can generate a significant impact on adults (155). Compared with those in normal mice, the numbers of gut microorganisms in the mice with congenital obesity have changed significantly (mainly Bactericides and Formicates) (156), and the alterations are also observed in human (157). Compared to healthy children, children with NAFLD have higher levels of Gammaproteobacteria and Prevotella, as well as higher levels of ethanol (158). In a similar study, the results indicate that children with NAFLD have higher levels of Actinobacteria and lower levels of Bacteroidetes compared with healthy controls. In addition, the levels of Bradyrhizobium, Anaerococcus, Peptoniphilus, Propionibacterium acnes, Dorea, and Ruminococcus are increased and the levels of

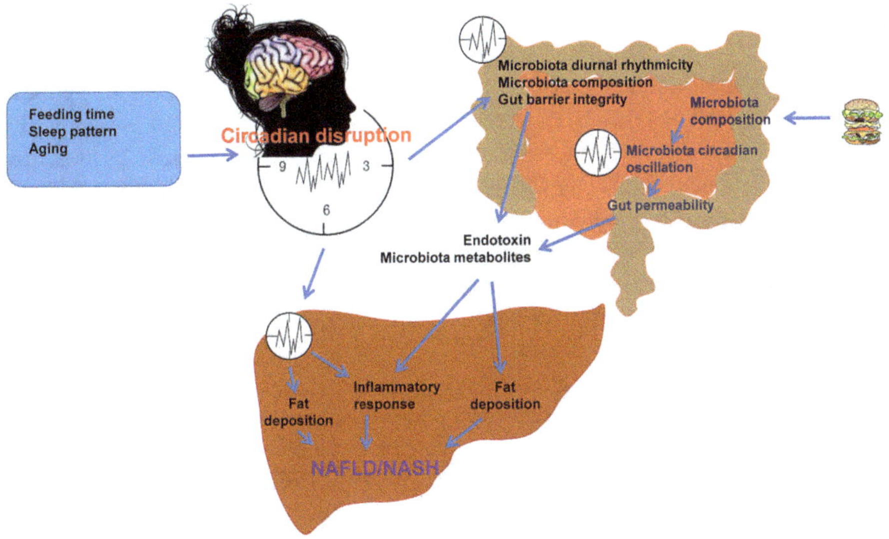

FIGURE 3 | Circadian rhythms and gut microbiota in the pathogenesis of NAFLD. Under normal physiological conditions, the central and peripheral clocks operate synchronously to maintain the normal operation of the body. Feeding time, sleep pattern, and aging cause circadian dysregulation, leading to alterations of microbiota diurnal rhythmicity, microbiota composition, and thus microbiota dysbiosis. Microbiota dysbiosis impairs gut barrier integrity and increases the gut permeability, which results in increased release of microbiota products such as endotoxin and microbiota metabolites into circulation. HFD or nutritional stress changes microbiota composition and circadian oscillation, increasing gut permeability and release of microbiota products. These microbiota products reach the liver and cause hepatic steatosis and inflammation, which are the features of NAFLD/NASH. Circadian disruption also directly causes dysregulation of liver metabolism, promoting NAFLD/NASH through increasing hepatic fat accumulation and inflammation.

Oscillospira and Rikenellaceae are reduced in children with NAFLD (159).

Both gut microbiota and circadian rhythms are linked to the metabolic homeostasis in infants and children and influence their health in the future. For instance, early microbial destruction induces metabolic dysregulation. Cho et al. found that treatment with antibiotics in early life in mice increased the levels of GIP, adiposity, and the expression of hepatic genes, which are involved in lipid metabolic processes. Although early antibiotics did not change the overall numbers of microbes, the composition of gut microbiota was altered in mice with antibiotics in early life, such as increased levels of Firmicutes (160). Of note, under a chow diet, limited antibiotics ameliorated hepatic accumulation of fat in early age in male mice (161). Mechanistically, LPS from gut microbiota is associated with the development of metabolic syndrome in children. A study indicates that sleep disruption contributes to gut bacteria dysbiosis and the increase in LPS levels, leading to inflammation and metabolic dysregulation (162). Child snoring disturbs sleeping pattern and is related to metabolic syndrome, neurocognitive, and behavioral problems. In the gut of children with snoring, the diversity of microbiota was reduced and pro-inflammatory bacteria population and the ratio of Firmicutes to Bacteroidetes were increased (163). Also, the results from a human study involving 40 children with NAFLD indicate that the serum levels of FGF21 were inversely associated with the severity of NAFLD in children at 8:00 am whereas more severe NAFLD revealed increased FGF21 levels at noon (164).

Gut Microbes Regulation of NAFLD During Aging

From colonization in early life, the body maintains the balance of microbes for decades and toward the end of life. For elders, their intestinal tract is fragile, their teeth are loose, and there are other factors affecting the intestinal microbes (165). In an epidemiological survey (166), the results obtained suggest that total proteobacteria are increased and stable within a limited time in people over 65 years old. However, there are some differences between the studies about whether the diversity of Bactericides is increased (167). Some studies suggest that the diversity of Bactericides is increased (167) whereas others showed the opposite results (168). Also, the gut microbial composition appears to be different in a sex-dependent way in elders. Obese male elders have lower levels of Bacteroidetes than obese female elders (169). Moreover, Clostridium levels are different between elders and young adults. The production of short chain fatty acids is reduced in elders, compared with young adults (170).

The circadian rhythm controls deep sleep and duration (171). In the conventional consciousness, the elders have less deep sleep (172) and more awakening (173). Through detecting body temperature and melatonin rhythm (174), the phase of rhythm is shifted forward (175), the amplitude of rhythm is reduced (176), and PER2 expression is impaired in elders (177, 178). These findings have been confirmed by many clinical studies. Indeed, chronic sleep disorders in old adults are associated with metabolic dysregulation. Also, in elders, diet has more effects on age-related dysbiosis in gut microbiota that affects circadian rhythm in the host and exacerbates metabolic disorders (7). The circadian rhythm gradually deteriorates in life (179), characterized by the shortening of sleep time, the loss of circadian amplitude (180), the reduction of neuronal synapses (181), and the increase in the proportion of silent cells (182). However, the results of a human study suggest that the risk of NAFLD is increased slightly in a middle-aged and elderly Chinese population with a long night time sleep duration (183). Similarly, young and old mice fed an HFD for 12 weeks revealed increased body weight, fat accumulation, insulin resistance, and NAFLD activity score regardless of sex. However, old mice exhibited exacerbation of NAFLD severity and gut microbiota dysbiosis (184). In elder people, the numbers of protective anaerobic bacteria are reduced, gastrointestinal function is declining, and the severity of hepatic steatosis and inflammation is greater in response to HFD. As such, the health status of the elders should be taken serious consideration (185).

CONCLUSION

Nutrition, lifestyle and environment (day and night cycle) influence metabolism, thereby the health, life quality, and life span. Individuals who are shift workers, frequently cross-continental traveler undergoing jet-lag, suffers of sleep disorders, and/or frequent consumers of high-fat and/or high-sugar diets have increased risks for metabolic diseases including NAFLD and NASH. Pathologically, dysregulation of circadian rhythms, along with dysfunctional composition of gut microbiota contribute to the development and progression of NAFLD, which has been summarized by this review (**Figure 3**). There exist circadian rhythms in intestinal microbes. The changes in intestinal microbes' oscillation are manifested by increased intestinal permeability, microbial composition, and increased inflammation. Intestinal microbe regulates metabolism via reprogramming circadian clock, in particular the liver circadian clocks. Aging and unhealthy diet, as well as dysfunctional intestinal microbes are factors that bring about rhythm disorders, leading to hepatic fat accumulation and inflammation. As such, a healthy diet and a clocklike lifestyle are of the effective ways to prevent NAFLD and maintain metabolic homeostasis, thereby keeping individuals healthy.

AUTHOR CONTRIBUTIONS

XJ and XG wrote most of this review. JZ, SZ, BW, and CW wrote some sections. CW and XG made the final editing. XG came up with the concept. All authors contributed to the article and approved the submitted version.

REFERENCES

1. Younossi Z, Tacke F, Arrese M, Chander Sharma B, Mostafa I, Bugianesi E, et al. Global perspectives on nonalcoholic fatty liver disease and nonalcoholic Steatohepatitis. *Hepatology.* (2019) 69:2672–82. doi: 10.1002/hep.30251
2. Younossi ZM. Non-alcoholic fatty liver disease - a global public health perspective. *J Hepatol.* (2019) 70:531–44. doi: 10.1016/j.jhep.2018.10.033
3. Sharpton SR, Ajmera V, Loomba R. Emerging role of the gut microbiome in nonalcoholic fatty liver disease: from composition to function. *Clin Gastroenterol Hepatol.* (2019) 17:296–306. doi: 10.1016/j.cgh.2018.08.065
4. Ponziani FR, Bhoori S, Castelli C, Putignani L, Rivoltini L, Del Chierico F, et al. Hepatocellular Carcinoma is associated with gut microbiota profile and inflammation in nonalcoholic fatty liver disease. *Hepatology.* (2019) 69:107–20. doi: 10.1002/hep.30036
5. Halberg F, Johnson EA, Brown BW, Bittner JJ. Susceptibility Rhythm to *E. coli* endotoxin and bioassay. *Proc Soc Exp Biol Med.* (1960) 103:142–4. doi: 10.3181/00379727-103-25439
6. Liang X, Bushman FD, FitzGerald GA. Rhythmicity of the intestinal microbiota is regulated by gender and the host circadian clock. *Proc Natl Acad Sci USA.* (2015) 112:10479–84. doi: 10.1073/pnas.1501305112
7. Leone V, Gibbons Sean M, Martinez K, Hutchison Alan L, Huang Edmond Y, Cham Candace M, et al. Effects of Diurnal variation of gut microbes and high-fat feeding on host circadian clock function and metabolism. *Cell Host Microbe.* (2015) 17:681–9. doi: 10.1016/j.chom.2015.03.006
8. Mukherji A, Kobiita A, Ye T, Chambon P. Homeostasis in intestinal epithelium is orchestrated by the circadian clock and microbiota cues transduced by TLRs. *Cell.* (2013) 153:812–27. doi: 10.1016/j.cell.2013.04.020
9. Zarrinpar A, Chaix A, Yooseph S, Panda S. Diet and feeding pattern affect the diurnal dynamics of the gut microbiome. *Cell Metab.* (2014) 20:1006–17. doi: 10.1016/j.cmet.2014.11.008
10. Voigt RM, Summa KC, Forsyth CB, Green SJ, Engen P, Naqib A, et al. The circadian clock mutation promotes intestinal dysbiosis. *Alcohol Clin Exp Res.* (2016) 40:335–47. doi: 10.1111/acer.12943
11. Canfora EE, Meex RCR, Venema K, Blaak EE. Gut microbial metabolites in obesity, NAFLD and T2DM. *Nat Rev Endocrinol.* (2019) 15:261–73. doi: 10.1038/s41574-019-0156-z
12. Kolodziejczyk AA, Zheng DP, Shibolet O, Elinav E. The role of the microbiome in NAFLD and NASH. *EMBO Mol Med.* (2019) 11:e9302. doi: 10.15252/emmm.201809302
13. Ren Z, Li A, Jiang J, Zhou L, Yu Z, Lu H, et al. Gut microbiome analysis as a tool towards targeted non-invasive biomarkers for early hepatocellular carcinoma. *Gut.* (2019) 68:1014–23. doi: 10.1136/gutjnl-2017-315084
14. Boursier J, Mueller O, Barret M, Machado M, Fizanne L, Araujo-Perez F, et al. The severity of nonalcoholic fatty liver disease is associated with gut dysbiosis and shift in the metabolic function of the gut microbiota. *Hepatology.* (2016) 63:764–75. doi: 10.1002/hep.28356
15. Whitfield-Cargile CM, Cohen ND, Chapkin RS, Weeks BR, Davidson LA, Goldsby JS, et al. The microbiota-derived metabolite indole decreases mucosal inflammation and injury in a murine model of NSAID enteropathy. *Gut Microbes.* (2016) 7:246–61. doi: 10.1080/19490976.2016.1156827
16. Chambers ES. Gut-derived short-chain fatty acids: a friend or foe for hepatic lipid metabolism? *Nutr Bull.* (2019) 44:154–9. doi: 10.1111/nbu.12377
17. Gupta NA, Mells J, Dunham RM, Grakoui A, Handy J, Saxena NK, et al. Glucagon-like peptide-1 receptor is present on human hepatocytes and has a direct role in decreasing hepatic steatosis *in vitro* by modulating elements of the insulin signaling pathway. *Hepatology.* (2010) 51:1584–92. doi: 10.1002/hep.23569
18. Thomas C, Gioiello A, Noriega L, Strehle A, Oury J, Rizzo G, et al. TGR5-mediated bile acid sensing controls glucose homeostasis. *Cell Metab.* (2009) 10:167–77. doi: 10.1016/j.cmet.2009.08.001

19. Tsimihodimos V, Elisaf M. Incretins and lipid metabolism. *Curr Med Chem.* (2018) 25:2133–9. doi: 10.2174/0929867324666170414164244
20. Lee YS, De Vadder F, Tremaroli V, Wichmann A, Mithieux G, Backhed F. Insulin-like peptide 5 is a microbially regulated peptide that promotes hepatic glucose production. *Mol Metab.* (2016) 5:263–70. doi: 10.1016/j.molmet.2016.01.007
21. Faure S. Incretins. *Actualites Pharm.* (2017) 56:13–7. doi: 10.1016/j.actpha.2017.09.020
22. Zarrinpar A, Loomba R. Review article: the emerging interplay among the gastrointestinal tract, bile acids and incretins in the pathogenesis of diabetes and non-alcoholic fatty liver disease. *Aliment Pharmacol Ther.* (2012) 36:909–21. doi: 10.1111/apt.12084
23. Mantelmacher FD, Zvibel I, Cohen K, Epshtein A, Pasmanik-Chor M, Vogl T, et al. GIP regulates inflammation and body weight by restraining myeloid-cell-derived S100A8/A9. *Nat Metab.* (2019) 1:58–69. doi: 10.1038/s42255-018-0001-z
24. Alvarez-Sola G, Uriarte I, Latasa MU, Fernandez-Barrena MG, Urtasun R, Elizalde M, et al. Fibroblast growth factor 15/19 (FGF15/19) protects from diet-induced hepatic steatosis: development of an FGF19-based chimeric molecule to promote fatty liver regeneration. *Gut.* (2017) 66:1818–28. doi: 10.1136/gutjnl-2016-312975
25. Kir S, Beddow SA, Samuel VT, Miller P, Previs SF, Suino-Powell K, et al. FGF19 as a postprandial, insulin-independent activator of hepatic protein and glycogen synthesis. *Science.* (2011) 331:1621–4. doi: 10.1126/science.1198363
26. Zhou M, Learned RM, Rossi SJ, dePaoli AM, Tian H, Ling L. Engineered fibroblast growth factor 19 reduces liver injury and resolves sclerosing cholangitis in Mdr2-Deficient mice. *Hepatology.* (2016) 63:914–29. doi: 10.1002/hep.28257
27. Schnabl B, Brenner DA. Interactions between the intestinal microbiome and liver diseases. *Gastroenterology.* (2014) 146:1513–24. doi: 10.1053/j.gastro.2014.01.020
28. Lam YY, Ha CWY, Campbell CR, Mitchell AJ, Dinudom A, Oscarsson J, et al. Increased gut permeability and microbiota change associate with mesenteric fat inflammation and metabolic dysfunction in diet-induced obese mice. *PLoS ONE.* (2012) 7:e34233. doi: 10.1371/journal.pone.0034233
29. Bashiardes S, Shapiro H, Rozin S, Shibolet O, Elinav E. Non-alcoholic fatty liver and the gut microbiota. *Mol Metab.* (2016) 5:782–94. doi: 10.1016/j.molmet.2016.06.003
30. Miele L, Valenza V, La Torre G, Montalto M, Cammarota G, Ricci R, et al. Increased intestinal permeability and tight junction alterations in nonalcoholic fatty liver disease. *Hepatology.* (2009) 49:1877–87. doi: 10.1002/hep.22848
31. Chen DS, Le TH, Shahidipour H, Read SA, Ahlenstiel G. The role of gut-derived microbial antigens on liver fibrosis initiation and progression. *Cells.* (2019) 8:1324. doi: 10.3390/cells8111324
32. Cengiz M, Ozenirler S, Elbeg S. Role of serum toll-like receptors 2 and 4 in non-alcoholic steatohepatitis and liver fibrosis. *J Gastroenterol Hepatol.* (2015) 30:1190–6. doi: 10.1111/jgh.12924
33. Spruss A, Kanuri G, Wagnerberger S, Haub S, Bischoff SC, Bergheim I. Toll-like receptor 4 is involved in the development of fructose-induced hepatic steatosis in mice. *Hepatology.* (2009) 50:1094–104. doi: 10.1002/hep.23122
34. Jia L, Chang XL, Qian SW, Liu C, Lord CC, Ahmed N, et al. Hepatocyte toll-like receptor 4 deficiency protects against alcohol-induced fatty liver disease. *Mol Metabol.* (2018) 14:121–9. doi: 10.1016/j.molmet.2018.05.015
35. Kim SY, Jeong JM, Kim SJ, Seo W, Kim MH, Choi WM, et al. Pro-inflammatory hepatic macrophages generate ROS through NADPH oxidase 2 via endocytosis of monomeric TLR4-MD2 complex. *Nat Commun.* (2017) 8:2247. doi: 10.1038/s41467-017-02325-2
36. Ye DW, Li FYL, Lam KSL, Li HT, Jia WP, Wang Y, et al. Toll-like receptor-4 mediates obesity-induced non-alcoholic steatohepatitis through activation of X-box binding protein-1 in mice. *Gut.* (2012) 61:1058–67. doi: 10.1136/gutjnl-2011-300269
37. Dattaroy D, Seth RK, Sarkar S, Kimono D, Albadrani M, Chandrashekaran V, et al. Sparstolonin B (SsnB) attenuates liver fibrosis via a parallel conjugate pathway involving P53-P21 axis, TGF-beta signaling and focal adhesion that is TLR4 dependent. *Eur J Pharmacol.* (2018) 841:33–48. doi: 10.1016/j.ejphar.2018.08.040
38. Dapito DH, Mencin A, Gwak G-Y, Pradere J-P, Jang M-K, Mederacke I, et al. Promotion of hepatocellular carcinoma by the intestinal microbiota and TLR4. *Cancer cell.* (2012) 21:504–16. doi: 10.1016/j.ccr.2012.02.007
39. Ding SL, Chi MM, Scull BP, Rigby R, Schwerbrock NMJ, Magness S, et al. High-fat diet: bacteria interactions promote intestinal inflammation which precedes and correlates with obesity and insulin resistance in mouse. *PLoS ONE.* (2010) 5:e12191. doi: 10.1371/journal.pone.0012191
40. Cobbina E, Akhlaghi F. Non-alcoholic fatty liver disease (NAFLD) - pathogenesis, classification, and effect on drug metabolizing enzymes and transporters. *Drug Metab Rev.* (2017) 49:197–211. doi: 10.1080/03602532.2017.1293683
41. Zeng TS, Zhou J, He LZ, Zheng J, Chen LL, Wu CD, et al. Blocking nuclear factor-Kappa B protects against diet-induced hepatic steatosis and insulin resistance in mice. *PLoS ONE.* (2016) 11:e0149677. doi: 10.1371/journal.pone.0149677
42. Potthoff MJ, Inagaki T, Satapati S, Ding XS, He TT, Goetz R, et al. FGF21 induces PGC-1 alpha and regulates carbohydrate and fatty acid metabolism during the adaptive starvation response. *Proc Natl Acad Sci USA.* (2009) 106:10853–10858. doi: 10.1073/pnas.0904187106
43. Ridlon JM, Kang DJ, Hylemon PB, Bajaj JS. Bile acids and the gut microbiome. *Curr Opin Gastroenterol.* (2014) 30:332–8. doi: 10.1097/MOG.0000000000000057
44. Begley M, Gahan CGM, Hill C. The interaction between bacteria and bile. *FEMS Microbiol Rev.* (2005) 29:625–51. doi: 10.1016/j.femsre.2004.09.003
45. Wahlstrom A, Sayin SI, Marschall HU, Backhed F. Intestinal crosstalk between bile acids and microbiota and its impact on host metabolism. *Cell Metabol.* (2016) 24:41–50. doi: 10.1016/j.cmet.2016.05.005
46. Murphy EF, Cotter PD, Healy S, Marques TM, O'Sullivan O, Fouhy F, et al. Composition and energy harvesting capacity of the gut microbiota: relationship to diet, obesity and time in mouse models. *Gut.* (2010) 59:1635–42. doi: 10.1136/gut.2010.215665
47. Parseus A, Sommer N, Sommer F, Caesar R, Molinaro A, Stahlman M, et al. Microbiota-induced obesity requires farnesoid X receptor. *Gut.* (2017) 66:429–37. doi: 10.1136/gutjnl-2015-310283
48. Zheng X, Huang F, Zhao A, Lei S, Zhang Y, Xie G, et al. Bile acid is a significant host factor shaping the gut microbiome of diet-induced obese mice. *BMC Biol.* (2017) 15:120. doi: 10.1186/s12915-017-0462-7
49. Xie G, Wang X, Huang F, Zhao A, Chen W, Yan J, et al. Dysregulated hepatic bile acids collaboratively promote liver carcinogenesis. *Int J Cancer.* (2016) 139:1764–75. doi: 10.1002/ijc.30219
50. Kakiyama G, Pandak WM, Gillevet PM, Hylemon PB, Heuman DM, Daita K, et al. Modulation of the fecal bile acid profile by gut microbiota in cirrhosis. *J Hepatol.* (2013) 58:949–55. doi: 10.1016/j.jhep.2013.01.003
51. Devkota S, Wang Y, Musch MW, Leone V, Fehlner-Peach H, Nadimpalli A, et al. Dietary-fat-induced taurocholic acid promotes pathobiont expansion and colitis in Il10$^{-/-}$ mice. *Nature.* (2012) 487:104–8. doi: 10.1038/nature11225
52. Devkota S, Chang EB. Interactions between diet, bile acid metabolism, gut microbiota, and inflammatory bowel diseases. *Digest Dis.* (2015) 33:351–6. doi: 10.1159/000371687
53. Sayin SI, Wahlstrom A, Felin J, Jantti S, Marschall HU, Bamberg K, et al. Gut microbiota regulates bile acid metabolism by reducing the levels of tauro-beta-muricholic acid, a naturally occurring FXR antagonist. *Cell Metab.* (2013) 17:225–35. doi: 10.1016/j.cmet.2013.01.003
54. Wang XL, Chen L, Wang H, Cai W, Xie Q. Modulation of bile acid profile by gut microbiota in chronic hepatitis B. *J Cell Mol Med.* (2020) 24:2573–81. doi: 10.1111/jcmm.14951
55. Tan XY, Liu Y, Long JG, Chen S, Liao GC, Wu SL, et al. Trimethylamine N-Oxide aggravates liver steatosis through modulation of bile acid metabolism and inhibition of Farnesoid X receptor signaling in nonalcoholic fatty liver disease. *Mol Nutr Food Res.* (2019) 63:e1900257. doi: 10.1002/mnfr.201900257
56. Raman M, Ahmed I, Gillevet PM, Probert CS, Ratcliffe NM, Smith S, et al. Fecal microbiome and volatile organic compound metabolome in obese humans with nonalcoholic fatty liver disease. *Clin Gastroenterol Hepatol.* (2013) 11:868–75.e753. doi: 10.1016/j.cgh.2013.02.015

57. Wang B, Jiang X, Cao M, Ge J, Bao Q, Tang L, et al. Altered fecal microbiota correlates with liver biochemistry in nonobese patients with non-alcoholic fatty liver disease. *Sci Rep.* (2016) 6:32002. doi: 10.1038/srep32002
58. Spencer MD, Hamp TJ, Reid RW, Fischer LM, Zeisel SH, Fodor AA. Association between composition of the human gastrointestinal microbiome and development of fatty liver with choline deficiency. *Gastroenterology.* (2011) 140:976–86. doi: 10.1053/j.gastro.2010.11.049
59. Rau M, Rehman A, Dittrich M, Groen AK, Hermanns HM, Seyfried F, et al. Fecal SCFAs and SCFA-producing bacteria in gut microbiome of human NAFLD as a putative link to systemic T-cell activation and advanced disease. *United Eur Gastroenterol J.* (2018) 6:1496–507. doi: 10.1177/2050640618804444
60. Loomba R, Seguritan V, Li W, Long T, Klitgord N, Bhatt A, et al. Gut microbiome-based metagenomic signature for non-invasive detection of advanced fibrosis in human nonalcoholic fatty liver disease. *Cell Metab.* (2017) 25:1054–62.e1055. doi: 10.1016/j.cmet.2017.04.001
61. Mouzaki M, Comelli EM, Arendt BM, Bonengel J, Fung SK, Fischer SE, et al. Intestinal microbiota in patients with nonalcoholic fatty liver disease. *Hepatology.* (2013) 58:120–7. doi: 10.1002/hep.26319
62. Chu H, Duan Y, Yang L, Schnabl B. Small metabolites, possible big changes: a microbiota-centered view of non-alcoholic fatty liver disease. *Gut.* (2019) 68:359–70. doi: 10.1136/gutjnl-2018-316307
63. Wikoff WR, Anfora AT, Liu J, Schultz PG, Lesley SA, Peters EC, et al. Metabolomics analysis reveals large effects of gut microflora on mammalian blood metabolites. *Proc Natl Acad Sci USA.* (2009) 106:3698–703. doi: 10.1073/pnas.0812874106
64. Li W, Zhang K, Yang H. Pectin alleviates high fat (lard) diet-induced nonalcoholic fatty liver disease in mice: possible role of short-chain fatty acids and gut microbiota regulated by pectin. *J Agric Food Chem.* (2018) 66:8015–25. doi: 10.1021/acs.jafc.8b02979
65. Chashmniam S, Ghafourpour M, Farimani AR, Gholami A, Ghoochani BFNM. Metabolomic biomarkers in the diagnosis of non-alcoholic fatty liver disease. *Hepatitis Monthly.* (2019) 19:e92244. doi: 10.5812/hepatmon.92244
66. Panasevich MR, Morris EM, Chintapalli SV, Wankhade U, Shankar K, Britton SL, et al. Reduced short-chain fatty acid producing microbiota are linked to increased energy intake and susceptibility to high fat diet induced hepatic steatosis in low aerobic capacity rats. *FASEB J.* (2016) 30:1252.1. doi: 10.1096/fasebj.30.1_supplement.1252.1
67. Jin CJ, Engstler AJ, Sellmann C, Ziegenhardt D, Landmann M, Kanuri G, et al. Sodium butyrate protects mice from the development of the early signs of non-alcoholic fatty liver disease: role of melatonin and lipid peroxidation. *Br J Nutr.* (2016) 1161:1–12. doi: 10.1017/S0007114516004025
68. Zhou D, Pan Q, Xin F-Z, Zhang R-N, He C-X, Chen G-Y, et al. Sodium butyrate attenuates high-fat diet-induced steatohepatitis in mice by improving gut microbiota and gastrointestinal barrier. *World J Gastroenterol.* (2017) 23:60–75. doi: 10.3748/wjg.v23.i1.60
69. Sun B, Jia Y, Hong J, Sun Q, Gao S, Hu Y, et al. Sodium butyrate ameliorates high-fat-diet-induced non-alcoholic fatty liver disease through peroxisome proliferator-activated receptor α-mediated activation of β oxidation and suppression of inflammation. *J Agric Food Chem.* (2018) 66:7633–42. doi: 10.1021/acs.jafc.8b01189
70. Zhou D, Chen Y-W, Zhao Z-H, Yang R-X, Xin F-Z, Liu X-L, et al. Sodium butyrate reduces high-fat diet-induced non-alcoholic steatohepatitis through upregulation of hepatic GLP-1R expression. *Exp Mol Med.* (2018) 50:1–12. doi: 10.1038/s12276-018-0183-1
71. Endo H, Niioka M, Kobayashi N, Tanaka M, Watanabe T. Butyrate-producing probiotics reduce nonalcoholic fatty liver disease progression in rats: new insight into the probiotics for the gut-liver axis. *PLoS ONE.* (2013) 8:e63388. doi: 10.1371/journal.pone.0063388
72. Samuel BS, Shaito A, Motoike T, Rey FE, Backhed F, Manchester JK, et al. Effects of the gut microbiota on host adiposity are modulated by the short-chain fatty-acid binding G protein-coupled receptor, Gpr41. *Proc Natl Acad Sci USA.* (2008) 105:16767–72. doi: 10.1073/pnas.0808567105
73. Liang YJ, Liang S, Zhang YP, Deng YJ, He YF, Chen YN, et al. Oral administration of compound probiotics ameliorates HFD-induced gut microbe dysbiosis and chronic metabolic inflammation via the G protein-coupled receptor 43 in non-alcoholic fatty liver disease rats. *Probiotics Antimicrob Proteins.* (2019) 11:175–85. doi: 10.1007/s12602-017-9378-3
74. Koh A, de Vadder F, Kovatcheva-Datchary P, Bäckhed F. From dietary fiber to host physiology: short-chain fatty acids as key bacterial metabolites. *Cell.* (2016) 165:1332–45. doi: 10.1016/j.cell.2016.05.041
75. Kondo T, Kishi M, Fushimi T, Kaga T. Acetic acid upregulates the expression of genes for fatty acid oxidation enzymes in liver to suppress body fat accumulation. *J Agric Food Chem.* (2009) 57:5982–6. doi: 10.1021/jf900470c
76. Marra F, Svegliati-Baroni G. Lipotoxicity and the gut-liver axis in NASH pathogenesis. *J Hepatol.* (2018) 68:280–95. doi: 10.1016/j.jhep.2017.11.014
77. Zhu L, Baker SS, Gill C, Liu W, Alkhouri R, Baker RD, et al. Characterization of gut microbiomes in nonalcoholic steatohepatitis (NASH) patients: a connection between endogenous alcohol and NASH. *Hepatology.* (2013) 57:601–9. doi: 10.1002/hep.26093
78. Abu-Shanab A, Quigley EMM. The role of the gut microbiota in nonalcoholic fatty liver disease. *Nat Rev Gastroenterol Hepatol.* (2010) 7:691–701. doi: 10.1038/nrgastro.2010.172
79. Leung C, Rivera L, Furness JB, Angus PW. The role of the gut microbiota in NAFLD. *Nat Rev Gastroenterol Hepatol.* (2016) 13:412–25. doi: 10.1038/nrgastro.2016.85
80. Elshaghabee FMF, Bockelmann W, Meske D, de Vrese M, Walte H-G, Schrezenmeir J, et al. Ethanol production by selected intestinal microorganisms and lactic acid bacteria growing under different nutritional conditions. *Front Microbiol.* (2016) 7:47. doi: 10.3389/fmicb.2016.00047
81. Arab JP, Karpen SJ, Dawson PA, Arrese M, Trauner M. Bile acids and nonalcoholic fatty liver disease: molecular insights and therapeutic perspectives. *Hepatology.* (2017) 65:350–62. doi: 10.1002/hep.28709
82. Tripathi A, Debelius J, Brenner DA, Karin M, Loomba R, Schnabl B, et al. The gut-liver axis and the intersection with the microbiome. *Nat Rev Gastroenterol Hepatol.* (2018) 15:397–411. doi: 10.1038/s41575-018-0011-z
83. Jiao N, Baker SS, Chapa-Rodriguez A, Liu W, Nugent CA, Tsompana M, et al. Suppressed hepatic bile acid signalling despite elevated production of primary and secondary bile acids in NAFLD. *Gut.* (2018) 67:1881–91. doi: 10.1136/gutjnl-2017-314307
84. Mouzaki M, Wang AY, Bandsma R, Comelli EM, Arendt BM, Zhang L, et al. Bile acids and dysbiosis in non-alcoholic fatty liver disease. *PLoS ONE.* (2016) 11:e0151829. doi: 10.1371/journal.pone.0151829
85. Watanabe M, Houten SM, Wang L, Moschetta A, Mangelsdorf DJ, Heyman RA, et al. Bile acids lower triglyceride levels via a pathway involving FXR, SHP, and SREBP-1c. *J Clin Invest.* (2004) 113:1408–18. doi: 10.1172/JCI21025
86. Kwong E, Li YZ, Hylemon PB, Zhou HP. Bile acids and sphingosine-1-phosphate receptor 2 in hepatic lipid metabolism. *Acta Pharm Sin B.* (2015) 5:151–7. doi: 10.1016/j.apsb.2014.12.009
87. Michaud J, Im DS, Hla T. Inhibitory role of sphingosine 1-phosphate receptor 2 in macrophage recruitment during inflammation. *J Immunol.* (2010) 184:1475–83. doi: 10.4049/jimmunol.0901586
88. Joyce SA, MacSharry J, Casey PG, Kinsella M, Murphy EF, Shanahan F, et al. Regulation of host weight gain and lipid metabolism by bacterial bile acid modification in the gut. *Proc Natl Acad Sci USA.* (2014) 111:7421–6. doi: 10.1073/pnas.1323599111
89. Bansal T, Alaniz RC, Wood TK, Jayaraman A. The bacterial signal indole increases epithelial-cell tight-junction resistance and attenuates indicators of inflammation. *Proc Natl Acad Sci USA.* (2010) 107:228–33. doi: 10.1073/pnas.0906112107
90. Cervantes-Barragan L, Chai JN, Tianero MD, Di Luccia B, Ahern PP, Merriman J, et al. Lactobacillus reuteri induces gut intraepithelial CD4(+)CD8 alpha alpha(+) T cells. *Science.* (2017) 357:806–10. doi: 10.1126/science.aah5825
91. Choi Y, Yanagawa Y, Kim S, Park T. Involvement of SIRT1-AMPK signaling in the protective action of indole-3-carbinol against hepatic steatosis in mice fed a high-fat diet. *J Nutr Biochem.* (2013) 24:1393–400. doi: 10.1016/j.jnutbio.2012.11.007
92. Krishnan S, Ding Y, Saedi N, Choi M, Sridharan GV, Sherr DH, et al. Gut microbiota-derived tryptophan metabolites modulate inflammatory response in hepatocytes and macrophages. *Cell Rep.* (2018) 23:1099–111. doi: 10.1016/j.celrep.2018.03.109
93. Ji Y, Gao Y, Chen H, Yin Y, Zhang W. Indole-3-Acetic acid alleviates nonalcoholic fatty liver disease in mice via attenuation of hepatic lipogenesis, and oxidative and inflammatory stress. *Nutrients.* (2019) 11:2062. doi: 10.3390/nu11092062

94. Azzout-Marniche D, Becard D, Guichard C, Foretz M, Ferre P, Foufelle F. Insulin effects on sterol regulatory-element-binding protein-1c (SREBP-1c) transcriptional activity in rat hepatocytes. *Biochem J.* (2000) 350:389–93. doi: 10.1042/bj3500389
95. Stoeckman AK, Towle HC. The role of SREBP-1c in nutritional regulation of lipogenic enzyme gene expression. *J Biol Chem.* (2002) 277:27029–35. doi: 10.1074/jbc.M202638200
96. Ma L, Li H, Hu J, Zheng J, Zhou J, Botchlett R, et al. Indole alleviates diet-induced hepatic steatosis and inflammation in a manner involving myeloid cell PFKFB3. *Hepatology.* (2020). doi: 10.1002/hep.31115. [Epub ahead of print].
97. Rider MH, Bertrand L, Vertommen D, Michels PA, Rousseau GG, Hue L. 6-phosphofructo-2-kinase/fructose-2,6-bisphosphatase: head-to-head with a bifunctional enzyme that controls glycolysis. *Biochem J.* (2004). 381:561–79. doi: 10.1042/BJ20040752
98. Atsumi T, Chesney J, Metz C, Leng L, Donnelly S, Makita Z, et al. High expression of inducible 6-phosphofructo-2-kinase/frctose-2,6-bisphosphatase (iPFK-2; PFKFB3) in human cancers. *Cancer Res.* (2002) 62:5881–7.
99. Kawaguchi T, Veech RL, Uyeda K. Regulation of energy metabolism in macrophages during hypoxia - roles of fructose 2,6-bisphosphate and ribose 1,5-bisphosphate. *J Biol Chem.* (2001) 276:28554–61. doi: 10.1074/jbc.M101396200
100. Marsin AS, Bouzin C, Bertrand L, Hue L. The stimulation of glycolysis by hypoxia in activated monocytes is mediated by AMP-activated protein kinase and inducible 6-phosphofructo-2-kinase. *J Biol Chem.* (2002) 277:30778–83. doi: 10.1074/jbc.M205213200
101. Aller R, de Luis DA, Izaola O, Conde R, Sagrado MG, Primo D, et al. Effect of a probiotic on liver aminotransferases in nonalcoholic fatty liver disease patients: a double blind randomized clinical trial. *Eur Rev Med Pharm Sci.* (2011) 15:1090–5.
102. Alisi A, Bedogni G, Baviera G, Giorgio V, Porro E, Paris C, et al. Randomised clinical trial: the beneficial effects of VSL# 3 in obese children with non-alcoholic steatohepatitis. *Aliment Pharm Ther.* (2014) 39:1276–85. doi: 10.1111/apt.12758
103. Mora D, Filardi R, Arioli S, Boeren S, Aalvink S, de Vos WM. Development of omics-based protocols for the microbiological characterization of multi-strain formulations marketed as probiotics: the case of VSL#3. *Microb Biotechnol.* (2019) 12:1371–86. doi: 10.1111/1751-7915.13476
104. Chappuis E, Morel-Depeisse F, Bariohay B, Roux J. Alpha-Galacto-Oligosaccharides at low dose improve liver steatosis in a high-fat diet mouse model. *Molecules.* (2017) 22:1725. doi: 10.3390/molecules22101725
105. Porras D, Nistal E, Martinez-Florez S, Olcoz JL, Jover R, Jorquera F, et al. Functional interactions between gut microbiota transplantation, quercetin, and high-fat diet determine non-alcoholic fatty liver disease development in germ-free mice. *Mol Nutr Food Res.* (2019) 63:e1800930. doi: 10.1002/mnfr.201800930
106. Yao FF, Jia RP, Huang H, Yu Y, Mei L, Bai LM, et al. Effect of Lactobacillus paracasei N1115 and fructooligosaccharides in nonalcoholic fatty liver disease. *Arch Med Sci.* (2019) 15:1336–44. doi: 10.5114/aoms.2019.86611
107. Mofidi F, Poustchi H, Yari Z, Nourinayyer B, Merat S, Sharafkhah M, et al. Synbiotic supplementation in lean patients with non-alcoholic fatty liver disease: a pilot, randomised, double-blind, placebo-controlled, clinical trial. *Br J Nutr.* (2017) 117:662–8. doi: 10.1017/S0007114517000204
108. Bergheim I, Weber S, Vos M, Kramer S, Volynets V, Kaserouni S, et al. Antibiotics protect against fructose-induced hepatic lipid accumulation in mice: role of endotoxin. *J Hepatol.* (2008) 48:983–92. doi: 10.1016/j.jhep.2008.01.035
109. Sumida Y, Yoneda M. Current and future pharmacological therapies for NAFLD/NASH. *J Gastroenterol.* (2018) 53:362–76. doi: 10.1007/s00535-017-1415-1
110. Diehl AM, Harrison S, Caldwell S, Rinella M, Paredes A, Moylan C, et al. JKB-121 in patients with nonalcoholic steatohepatitis: a phase 2 double blind randomized placebo control study. *J Hepatol.* (2018) 68:S103. doi: 10.1016/S0168-8278(18)30425-2
111. Delaune V, Orci LA, Lacotte S, Peloso A, Schrenzel J, Lazarevic V, et al. Fecal microbiota transplantation: a promising strategy in preventing the progression of non-alcoholic steatohepatitis and improving the anti-cancer immune response. *Expert Opin Biol Ther.* (2018) 18:1061–71. doi: 10.1080/14712598.2018.1518424
112. Lechner S, Yee M, Limketkai BN, Pham EA. Fecal microbiota transplantation for chronic liver diseases: current understanding and future direction. *Dig Dis Sci.* (2020) 65:897–905. doi: 10.1007/s10620-020-06100-0
113. Vrieze A, van Nood E, Holleman F, Salojarvi J, Kootte RS, Bartelsman J, et al. Transfer of intestinal microbiota from lean donors increases insulin sensitivity in individuals with metabolic syndrome. *Gastroenterology.* (2012) 143:913–6.e7. doi: 10.1053/j.gastro.2012.06.031
114. Craven L, Rahman A, Nair Parvathy S, Beaton M, Silverman J, Qumosani K, et al. Allogenic fecal microbiota transplantation in patients with nonalcoholic fatty liver disease improves abnormal small intestinal permeability: a randomized control trial. *Am J Gastroenterol.* (2020) 115:1055–65. doi: 10.14309/ajg.0000000000000661
115. Li Y, Hao Y, Fan F, Zhang B. The role of microbiome in insomnia, circadian disturbance and depression. *Front Psychiatry.* (2018) 9:669. doi: 10.3389/fpsyt.2018.00669
116. Parkar SG, Kalsbeek A, Cheeseman JF. Potential role for the gut microbiota in modulating host circadian rhythms and metabolic health. *Microorganisms.* (2019) 7:41. doi: 10.3390/microorganisms7020041
117. Voigt RM, Forsyth CB, Green SJ, Engen PA, Keshavarzian A. Chapter nine - circadian rhythm and the gut microbiome. In: Cryan JF, Clarke G, editors. *International Review of Neurobiology (Vol. 131).* San Diego, CA: Elsevier Academic Press Inc. (2016). p. 193–205. doi: 10.1016/bs.irn.2016.07.002
118. Rajani C, Jia W. Disruptions in gut microbial-host co-metabolism and the development of metabolic disorders. *Clin Sci.* (2018) 132:791–811. doi: 10.1042/CS20171328
119. Gnocchi D, Custodero C, Sabbà C, Mazzocca A. Circadian rhythms: a possible new player in non-alcoholic fatty liver disease pathophysiology. *J Mol Med.* (2019) 97:741–59. doi: 10.1007/s00109-019-01780-2
120. Ojeda P, Bobe A, Dolan K, Leone V, Martinez K. Nutritional modulation of gut microbiota - the impact on metabolic disease pathophysiology. *J Nutr Biochem.* (2016) 28:191–200. doi: 10.1016/j.jnutbio.2015.08.013
121. Thaiss CA, Levy M, Korem T, Dohnalová L, Shapiro H, Jaitin DA, et al. Microbiota diurnal rhythmicity programs host transcriptome oscillations. *Cell.* (2016) 167:1495–510.e1412. doi: 10.1016/j.cell.2016.11.003
122. Thaiss CA, Zeevi D, Levy M, Zilberman-Schapira G, Suez J, Tengeler AC, et al. Transkingdom control of microbiota diurnal oscillations promotes metabolic homeostasis. *Cell.* (2014) 159:514–29. doi: 10.1016/j.cell.2014.09.048
123. Trinder M, Bisanz JE, Burton JP, Reid G. Bacteria need “sleep” too?: microbiome circadian rhythmicity, metabolic disease, and beyond. *Univ Toronto Med J.* (2015) 92:52–5.
124. Voigt RM, Forsyth CB, Green SJ, Mutlu E, Engen P, Vitaterna MH, et al. Circadian disorganization alters intestinal microbiota. *PLoS ONE.* (2014) 9:e97500. doi: 10.1371/journal.pone.0097500
125. Klimina KM, Batotsyrenova EG, Yunes RA, Gilyaeva EH, Poluektova EU, Kostrova TA, et al. The effects of desynchronosis on the gut microbiota composition and physiological parameters of rats. *BMC Microbiol.* (2019) 19:160. doi: 10.1186/s12866-019-1535-2
126. Bubenik GA. Gastrointestinal melatonin: localization, function, and clinical relevance. *Dig Dis Sci.* (2002) 47:2336–48. doi: 10.1023/A:1020107915919
127. Deaver JA, Eum SY, Toborek M. Circadian disruption changes gut microbiome taxa and functional gene composition. *Front Microbiol.* (2018) 9:737. doi: 10.3389/fmicb.2018.00737
128. Dinan TG, Cryan JF. Regulation of the stress response by the gut microbiota: implications for psychoneuroendocrinology. *Psychoneuroendocrinology.* (2012) 37:1369–78. doi: 10.1016/j.psyneuen.2012.03.007
129. Bailey MT, Lubach GR, Coe CL. Prenatal stress alters bacterial colonization of the gut in infant monkeys. *J Pediatric Gastroenterol Nutr.* (2004) 38:414–21. doi: 10.1097/00005176-200404000-00009
130. Karl JP, Hatch AM, Arcidiacono SM, Pearce SC, Pantoja-Feliciano IG, Doherty LA, et al. Effects of psychological, environmental and physical stressors on the gut microbiota. *Front Microbiol.* (2018) 9:2013. doi: 10.3389/fmicb.2018.02013
131. Everson CA, Toth LA. Systemic bacterial invasion induced by sleep deprivation. *Am J Physiol Regul Integr Comp Physiol.* (2000) 278:R905–16. doi: 10.1152/ajpregu.2000.278.4.R905

132. Benedict C, Vogel H, Jonas W, Woting A, Blaut M, Schuermann A, et al. Gut microbiota and glucometabolic alterations in response to recurrent partial sleep deprivation in normal-weight young individuals. *Mol Metab.* (2016) 5:1175–86. doi: 10.1016/j.molmet.2016.10.003
133. Poroyko VA, Carreras A, Khalyfa A, Khalyfa AA, Leone V, Peris E, et al. Chronic sleep disruption alters gut microbiota, induces systemic and adipose tissue inflammation and insulin resistance in mice. *Sci Rep.* (2016) 6:35405. doi: 10.1038/srep35405
134. Asher G, Sassone-Corsi P. Time for food: the intimate interplay between nutrition, metabolism, and the circadian clock. *Cell.* (2015) 161:84–92. doi: 10.1016/j.cell.2015.03.015
135. Dabke K, Hendrick G, Devkota S. The gut microbiome and metabolic syndrome. *J Clin Invest.* (2019) 129:4050–57. doi: 10.1172/JCI129194
136. Frazier K, Chang EB. Intersection of the gut microbiome and circadian rhythms in metabolism. *Trends Endocrinol Metab.* (2020) 31:25–36. doi: 10.1016/j.tem.2019.08.013
137. Harakeh SM, Khan I, Kumosani T, Barbour E, Almasaudi SB, Bahijri SM, et al. Gut microbiota: a contributing factor to obesity. *Front Cell Infect Microbiol.* (2016) 6:95. doi: 10.3389/fcimb.2016.00095
138. Reynolds AC, Paterson JL, Ferguson SA, Stanley D, Wright KP, Jr., et al. The shift work and health research agenda: considering changes in gut microbiota as a pathway linking shift work, sleep loss and circadian misalignment, and metabolic disease. *Sleep Med Rev.* (2017) 34:3–9. doi: 10.1016/j.smrv.2016.06.009
139. Khalyfa A, Poroyko VA, Qiao Z, Gileles-Hillel A, Khalyfa AA, Akbarpour M, et al. Exosomes and metabolic functionin mice exposed to alternating dark-light cycles mimicking night shift work schedules. *Front Physiol.* (2017) 8:882. doi: 10.3389/fphys.2017.00882
140. Mazzoccoli G, De Cosmo S, Mazza T. The biological clock: a pivotal hub in non-alcoholic fatty liver disease pathogenesis. *Front Physiol.* (2018) 9:193. doi: 10.3389/fphys.2018.00193
141. Chen K, Ma J, Jia X, Ai W, Ma Z, Pan Q. Advancing the understanding of NAFLD to hepatocellular carcinoma development: from experimental models to humans. *Biochimica Et Biophysica Acta Rev Cancer.* (2019) 1871:117–25. doi: 10.1016/j.bbcan.2018.11.005
142. Hatori M, Vollmers C, Zarrinpar A, DiTacchio L, Bushong EA, Gill S, et al. Time-Restricted feeding without reducing caloric intake prevents metabolic diseases in mice fed a high-fat diet. *Cell Metab.* (2012) 15:848–60. doi: 10.1016/j.cmet.2012.04.019
143. Guerrero-Vargas NN, Guzmán-Ruiz M, Fuentes R, García J, Salgado-Delgado R, Basualdo MdC, et al. Shift work in rats results in increased inflammatory response after lipopolysaccharide administration: a role for food consumption. *J Biol Rhythms.* (2015) 30:318–30. doi: 10.1177/0748730415586482
144. Wang Y, Song L, Liu M, Ge R, Zhou Q, Liu W, et al. A proteomics landscape of circadian clock in mouse liver. *Nat Commun.* (2018) 9:1553. doi: 10.1038/s41467-018-03898-2
145. Hong F, Pan S, Xu P, Xue T, Wang J, Guo Y, et al. Melatonin orchestrates lipid homeostasis through the hepatointestinal circadian clock and microbiota during constant light exposure. *Cells.* (2020) 9:489. doi: 10.3390/cells9020489
146. Ferretti P, Pasolli E, Tett A, Asnicar F, Gorfer V, Fedi S, et al. Mother-to-infant microbial transmission from different body sites shapes the developing infant gut microbiome. *Cell Host Microbe.* (2018) 24:133–45.e5. doi: 10.1016/j.chom.2018.06.005
147. Moles L, Gomez M, Heilig H, Bustos G, Fuentes S, de Vos W, et al. Bacterial diversity in meconium of preterm neonates and evolution of their fecal microbiota during the first month of life. *PLoS ONE.* (2013) 8:e66986. doi: 10.1371/journal.pone.0066986
148. Jakobsson HE, Abrahamsson TR, Jenmalm MC, Harris K, Quince C, Jernberg C, et al. Decreased gut microbiota diversity, delayed Bacteroidetes colonisation and reduced Th1 responses in infants delivered by caesarean section. *Gut.* (2014) 63:559–66. doi: 10.1136/gutjnl-2012-303249
149. Lavin T, Preen DB. Investigating caesarean section birth as a risk factor for childhood overweight. *Child Obes.* (2018) 14:131–8. doi: 10.1089/chi.2017.0034
150. Unger S, Stintzi A, Shah P, Mack D, O'Connor DL. Gut microbiota of the very-low-birth-weight infant. *Pediatr Res.* (2015) 77:205–13. doi: 10.1038/pr.2014.162
151. Forbes JD, Azad MB, Vehling L, Tun HM, Konya TB, Guttman DS, et al. Association of exposure to formula in the hospital and subsequent infant feeding practices with gut microbiota and risk of overweight in the first year of life. *JAMA Pediatr.* (2018) 172:e181161. doi: 10.1001/jamapediatrics.2018.1161
152. Rosenbauer J, Herzig P, Giani G. Early infant feeding and risk of type 1 diabetes mellitus-a nationwide population-based case-control study in pre-school children. *Diabetes Metab Res Rev.* (2008) 24:211–22. doi: 10.1002/dmrr.791
153. Subramanian S, Huq S, Yatsunenko T, Haque R, Mahfuz M, Alam MA, et al. Persistent gut microbiota immaturity in malnourished Bangladeshi children. *Nature.* (2014) 510:417–21. doi: 10.1038/nature13421
154. Mohammadkhah AI, Simpson EB, Patterson SG, Ferguson JF. Development of the gut microbiome in children, and lifetime implications for obesity and cardiometabolic disease. *Children.* (2018) 5:160. doi: 10.3390/children5120160
155. Dietz WH. Critical periods in childhood for the development of obesity. *Am J Clin Nutr.* (1994) 59:955–9. doi: 10.1093/ajcn/59.5.955
156. Ley RE, Backhed F, Turnbaugh P, Lozupone CA, Knight RD, Gordon JI. Obesity alters gut microbial ecology. *Proc Natl Acad Sci USA.* (2005) 102:11070–75. doi: 10.1073/pnas.0504978102
157. Ley RE, Turnbaugh PJ, Klein S, Gordon JI. Microbial ecology - human gut microbes associated with obesity. *Nature.* (2006) 444:1022–3. doi: 10.1038/4441022a
158. Michail S, Lin M, Frey MR, Fanter R, Paliy O, Hilbush B, et al. Altered gut microbial energy and metabolism in children with non-alcoholic fatty liver disease. *FEMS Microbiol Ecol.* (2015) 91:1–9. doi: 10.1093/femsec/fiu002
159. Del Chierico F, Nobili V, Vernocchi P, Russo A, De Stefanis C, Gnani D, et al. Gut microbiota profiling of pediatric nonalcoholic fatty liver disease and obese patients unveiled by an integrated meta-omics-based approach. *Hepatology.* (2017) 65:451–64. doi: 10.1002/hep.28572
160. Cho I, Yamanishi S, Cox L, Methe BA, Zavadil J, Li K, et al. Antibiotics in early life alter the murine colonic microbiome and adiposity. *Nature.* (2012) 488:621–6. doi: 10.1038/nature11400
161. Cox LM, Yamanishi S, Sohn J, Alekseyenko AV, Leung JM, Cho I, et al. Altering the intestinal microbiota during a critical developmental window has lasting metabolic consequences. *Cell.* (2014) 158:705–21. doi: 10.1016/j.cell.2014.05.052
162. Kheirandish-Gozal L, Peris E, Wang Y, Kakazu MT, Khalyfa A, Carreras A, et al. Lipopolysaccharide-binding protein plasma levels in children: effects of obstructive sleep apnea and obesity. *J Clin Endocrinol Metab.* (2014) 99:656–63. doi: 10.1210/jc.2013-3327
163. Collado MC, Katila MK, Vuorela NM, Saarenpaa-Heikkila O, Salminen S, Isolauri E. Dysbiosis in snoring children: an interlink to comorbidities? *J Pediatr Gastroenterol Nutr.* (2019) 68:272–7. doi: 10.1097/MPG.0000000000002161
164. Crudele A, Mosca A, Corte CD, Panera N, Nobili V, Alisi A. Nocturnal increase of circulating fibroblast growth factor 21 is correlated with severity of non-alcoholic fatty liver disease in children. *J Hepatol.* (2016) 64:S475. doi: 10.1016/S0168-8278(16)00803-5
165. Jeffery IB, Lynch DB, O'Toole PW. Composition and temporal stability of the gut microbiota in older persons. *ISME J.* (2016) 10:170–82. doi: 10.1038/ismej.2015.88
166. Claesson MJ, Cusack S, O'Sullivan O, Greene-Diniz R, de Weerd H, Flannery E, et al. Composition, variability, and temporal stability of the intestinal microbiota of the elderly. *Proc Natl Acad Sci USA.* (2011) 108(Suppl. 1):4586–91. doi: 10.1073/pnas.1000097107
167. Hopkins MJ, Macfarlane GT. Changes in predominant bacterial populations in human faeces with age and with Clostridium difficile infection. *J Med Microbiol.* (2002) 51:448–54. doi: 10.1099/0022-1317-51-5-448
168. Woodmansey EJ, McMurdo MET, Macfarlane GT, Macfarlane S. Comparison of compositions and metabolic activities of fecal microbiotas in young adults and in antibiotic-treated and non-antibiotic-treated elderly subjects. *Appl Environ Microbiol.* (2004) 70:6113–22. doi: 10.1128/AEM.70.10.6113-6122.2004
169. Dominianni C, Sinha R, Goedert JJ, Pei Z, Yang L, Hayes RB, et al. Sex, body mass index, and dietary fiber intake influence the human gut microbiome. *PLoS ONE.* (2015) 10:e124599. doi: 10.1371/journal.pone.0124599

170. Biagi E, Nylund L, Candela M, Ostan R, Bucci L, Pini E, et al. Through ageing, and beyond: gut microbiota and inflammatory status in seniors and centenarians. *PLos One.* (2010) 5:e10667. doi: 10.1371/journal.pone.0010667
171. Dijk DJ, Czeisler CA. Contribution of the circadian pacemaker and the sleep homeostat to sleep propensity, sleep structure, electroencephalographic slow waves, and sleep spindle activity in humans. *J Neurosci.* (1995) 15:3526–38. doi: 10.1523/JNEUROSCI.15-05-03526.1995
172. Minors DS, Rabbitt PM, Worthington H, Waterhouse JM. Variation in meals and sleep-activity patterns in aged subjects; its relevance to circadian rhythm studies. *Chronobiol Int.* (1989) 6:139–46. doi: 10.3109/07420528909064624
173. Dijk DJ, Duffy JF, Czeisler CA. Age-related increase in awakenings: impaired consolidation of nonREM sleep at all circadian phases. *Sleep.* (2001) 24:565–77. doi: 10.1093/sleep/24.5.565
174. Duffy JF, Zitting K-M, Chinoy ED. Aging and circadian rhythms. *Sleep Med Clin.* (2015) 10:423–34. doi: 10.1016/j.jsmc.2015.08.002
175. Monk TH, Buysse DJ, Reynolds CF, Kupfer DJ, Houck PR. Circadian temperature rhythms of older people. *Exp Gerontol.* (1995) 30:455–74. doi: 10.1016/0531-5565(95)00007-4
176. Carrier J, Monk TH, Buysse DJ, Kupfer DJ. Amplitude reduction of the circadian temperature and sleep rhythms in the elderly. *Chronobiol Int.* (1996) 13:373–86. doi: 10.3109/07420529609012661
177. Weinert H, Weinert D, Schurov I, Maywood ES, Hastings MH. Impaired expression of the mPer2 circadian clock gene in the suprachiasmatic nuclei of aging mice. *Chronobiol Int.* (2001) 18:559–65. doi: 10.1081/CBI-100103976
178. Schroeder AM, Colwell CS. How to fix a broken clock. *Trends Pharm Sci.* (2013) 34:605–19. doi: 10.1016/j.tips.2013.09.002
179. Banks G, Nolan PM, Peirson SN. Reciprocal interactions between circadian clocks and aging. *Mamm Genome.* (2016) 27:332–40. doi: 10.1007/s00335-016-9639-6
180. Roenneberg T, Kuehnle T, Juda M, Kantermann T, Allebrandt K, Gordijn M, et al. Epidemiology of the human circadian clock. *Sleep Med Rev.* (2007) 11:429–38. doi: 10.1016/j.smrv.2007.07.005
181. Palomba M, Nygard M, Florenzano F, Bertini G, Kristensson K, Bentivoglio M. Decline of the presynaptic network, including GABAergic terminals, in the aging suprachiasmatic nucleus of the mouse. *J Biol Rhythms.* (2008) 23:220–31. doi: 10.1177/0748730408316998
182. Nygard M, Hill RH, Wikstrom MA, Kristensson K. Age-related changes in electrophysiological properties of the mouse suprachiasmatic nucleus *in vitro*. *Brain Res Bull.* (2005) 65:149–54. doi: 10.1016/j.brainresbull.2004.12.006
183. Liu C, Zhong R, Lou J, Pan A, Tang Y, Chang J, et al. Nighttime sleep duration and risk of nonalcoholic fatty liver disease: the Dongfeng-Tongji prospective study. *Ann Med.* (2016) 48:468–76. doi: 10.1080/07853890.2016.1193787
184. Liu C-Y, Chang C-W, Lee H-C, Chen Y-J, Tsai T-H, Chiau J-SC, et al. Metabolic damage presents differently in young and early-aged C57BL/6 mice fed a high-fat diet. *Int J Gerontol.* (2016) 10:105–11. doi: 10.1016/j.ijge.2015.10.004
185. Woodmansey EJ. Intestinal bacteria and ageing. *J Appl Microbiol.* (2007) 102:1178–86. doi: 10.1111/j.1365-2672.2007.03400.x

6

Pro- and Anti-fibrogenic Functions of Gram-Negative Bacterial Lipopolysaccharide in the Liver

Chandrashekhar R. Gandhi [1,2*]

[1] *Divisions of Gastroenterology, Hepatology and Nutrition, Department of Pediatrics, Cincinnati Children's Hospital Medical Center, Cincinnati, OH, United States,*
[2] *Cincinnati VA Medical Center, Cincinnati, OH, United States*

Correspondence:
Chandrashekhar R. Gandhi
chandrashekhar.gandhi@cchmc.org

Extensive research performed over several decades has identified cells participating in the initiation and progression of fibrosis, and the numerous underlying inter- and intra-cellular signaling pathways. However, liver fibrosis continues to be a major clinical challenge as the precise targets of treatment are still elusive. Activation of physiologically quiescent perisinusoidal hepatic stellate cells (HSCs) to a myofibroblastic proliferating, contractile and fibrogenic phenotype is a critical event in the pathogenesis of chronic liver disease. Thus, elucidation of the mechanisms of the reversal to quiescence or inhibition of activated HSCs, and/or their elimination via apoptosis has been the focus of intense investigation. Lipopolysaccharide (LPS), a gut-resident Gram-negative bacterial endotoxin, is a powerful pro-inflammatory molecule implicated in hepatic injury, inflammation and fibrosis. In both acute and chronic liver injury, portal venous levels of LPS are elevated due to increased intestinal permeability. LPS, via CD14 and Toll-like receptor 4 (TLR4) and its adapter molecules, stimulates macrophages, neutrophils and several other cell types to produce inflammatory mediators as well as factors that can activate HSCs and stimulate their fibrogenic activity. LPS also stimulates synthesis of pro- and anti-inflammatory cytokines/chemokines, growth mediators and molecules of immune regulation by HSCs. However, LPS was found to arrest proliferation of activated HSCs and to convert them into non-fibrogenic phenotype. Interestingly, LPS can elicit responses in HSCs independent of CD14 and TLR4. Identifying and/or developing non-inflammatory but anti-fibrogenic mimetics of LPS could be relevant for treating liver fibrosis.

Keywords: stellate cells, activation, fibrosis, endotoxin, LPS, reversal, inflammation

INTRODUCTION

Liver fibrosis is a repair response to injury caused by various noxious stimuli such as viral infection (hepatitis B [HBV] and C [HCV] virus), toxins and drugs, autoimmune hepatitis, biliary damage, and copper or iron accumulation. Although fibrosis is reversible, persistent presence of the injury stimulus leads to excessive accumulation of extracellular matrix (ECM), collagens I and III and fibronectin being the major components. This disrupts the hepatic architecture and blood supply to hepatocytes, the site of numerous essential metabolic functions. Ensuing irreversible liver cirrhosis is one of the principal leading causes of morbidity and mortality in the world with organ transplantation as the only option for survival (1–3). Major success has been achieved in treating HCV-induced fibrosis, the most common form of chronic liver disease, through clearance of the virus (4, 5). However, there is alarmingly increasing incidence of alcohol-induced and non-alcoholic (fatty) liver diseases that can remain undiagnosed and thus silently progress to fibrosis/cirrhosis in predisposed individuals (2). Distinct from these are chronic liver diseases originating from the portal tracts (primary biliary cholangitis and primary sclerosing cholangitis) with high morbidity and mortality. Remarkable advancements have been made in identifying the cell types that co-ordinate fibrogenesis as well as the underlying inter- and intra-cellular signaling mechanisms (6–9). Several animal models of liver fibrosis of various etiologies have been developed (10, 11), and mono- and co-culture systems established (8, 12, 13) to discover the mechanisms of cross-communication amongst the liver resident cells, infiltrating inflammatory cells and immune cells implicated in fibrosis at the organ and cellular/subcellular levels. However, fibrosis of the liver and other organs remains untreatable.

It is generally accepted that activated proliferating hepatic stellate cells (HSCs) are responsible for liver fibrosis regardless of the etiology. An exception to this is biliary injury-induced disease in which portal (myo)fibroblasts are the major cells during initial period and are also significantly involved, along with HSCs, at later times of the disease progression (8, 13, 14). Inflammation initiated by the hepatocyte damage plays a critical role both in activation and fibrogenic activity of HSCs. Gut-derived microbial products including Gram-negative bacterial lipopolysaccharide (LPS) enhance inflammation and thus fibrosis during chronic liver injury. Therefore, HSCs have been a topic of intense investigation to discover mechanisms of their responses to inflammatory mediators as well as microbial products. Several lines of enquiry have positively implicated LPS in experimental and human chronic liver disease including non-alcoholic fatty liver disease (NAFLD) (15–18). In contrast, others found inflammatory cytokines, and not serum LPS, to correlate with NAFLD severity (19). However, evidence has emerged showing LPS-induced inhibition of proliferation, reversal of the activated phenotype and mitigation of the fibrogenic activity of HSCs (20–24). This article evaluates such contrasting interactions between LPS and HSCs and discusses the potential of non-inflammatory mimetic(s) of LPS as a therapy for liver fibrosis.

Abbreviations: AP1, Activator protein 1; BAMBI, BMP and activin membrane-bound inhibitor; CCl4, carbon tetrachloride; C/EBP, CCAAT/enhancer-binding protein; ECM, extracellular matrix; ERK, extracellular-signal-regulated kinase; GFAP, glial fibrillary acidic protein; HBV, hepatitis B virus; HCV, hepatitis C virus; HSC, hepatic stellate cell; IFN, interferon; IL, interleukin; IRAK, Interleukin-1 receptor-associated kinase-like; IRF, interferon-regulatory factor; JNK, c-Jun N-terminal kinases; KO, knockout; LBP, lipopolysaccharide-binding protein; LPS, lipopolysaccharide; MAPK, mitogen-activated protein kinase; MMP, matrix metalloproteinase; NADPH, reduced nicotinamide adenine dinucleotide phosphate; NFkB, nuclear factor kappa-light-chain-enhancer of activated B cells; PAMP, pathogen-associated molecular pattern; PDGF, platelet-derived growth factor; P-Mfb, periportal myofibroblasts; PPAR, peroxisome proliferator-activated receptor; PRR, pattern recognition receptor; ROS, reactive oxygen species; SEC, sinusoidal endothelial cell; SMAD, small mother against decapentaplegic; TGF, transforming growth factor; SOCS, suppressor of cytokine signaling; STAT, Signal transducer and activator of transcription; TIMP, tissue inhibitor of metalloproteinases; TIR, Toll/interleukin-1 receptor; TIRAP, TIR domain containing adaptor protein; TLR, toll-like receptor; TNF, tumor necrosis factor; TRAIL, TNF-related apoptosis-inducing ligand; TRAM, TRIF-related adaptor molecule; TRIF, TIR-domain-containing adapter-inducing interferon-β); WT, wild type.

DISRUPTION OF HEPATIC STRUCTURE AND FUNCTION IN CHRONIC LIVER INJURY

The liver receives nearly 70–75% blood from the portal vein and 25–30% from the hepatic artery at the portal triads. The portal veins and hepatic arteries branch after entry into the liver, and eventually the venous and arterial blood mixes up in the capillaries known as "sinusoids." The sinusoids are lined by specialized endothelial cells with no underlying true continuous basement membrane. The sinusoidal endothelial cells (SECs) possess sieve plates that have pores (~100 nm diameter) called "fenestrations." The liver-resident macrophages, Kupffer cells, are found within the sinusoids adhering to the endothelial cells, whereas HSCs reside in the "Disse's space" between the SECs and the parenchymal cells (hepatocytes), the main cells responsible for the liver's metabolic function (25). Highly coordinated interactions between the major cell types of the liver (hepatocytes, stellate cells, SECs, Kupffer cells and biliary epithelial cells) via physical contacts and soluble mediators are critical to the liver's physiological functions and maintenance of homeostasis. This balance is disrupted during injury, and persistent injury leads to chronic fibrotic liver disease and its systemic complications.

LIPOPOLYSACCHARIDE AND LIVER INJURY

Lipopolysaccharide (LPS), a highly inflammatory endotoxin, belongs to the family of gut-derived microbial products known as pathogen-associated molecular patterns (PAMPs). It is a component of the Gram-negative bacterial cell membrane and is composed of three units, O antigen or O polysaccharide, core oligosaccharide and the active constituent lipid A. LPS mediates its cellular effects through toll-like receptor 4 (TLR4), a type I transmembrane protein with an extracellular leucine-rich repeat domain and a cytoplasmic domain homologous to the cytoplasmic domain of the human interleukin (IL)-1 receptor (26). However, association of lipid A with LPS-binding protein (LBP), a soluble protein that increases the affinity and potency of LPS, is required for the subsequent binding to soluble or membrane-bound CD14. CD14 does not have intracellular domain and therefore the LBP-CD14/LPS complex must bind to TLR4. LPS-induced transmembrane signaling also requires TLR4-associated extracellular (MD2) and intracellular (MyD88, TRAM, TRIF, and TIRAP) adapter components (**Figure 1**). LPS instigates several signaling cascades (NFkB, interferon-regulatory factors [IRFs], p38, ERK1/2, and JNK mitogen-activated protein kinases, AP1, etc.) in the immune and inflammatory cells coupled to the expression of cytokines including TNF, IL1α, IL1β, IL6, IL10, and type 1 and type 2 interferons (IFNs), chemokines and several other biologically active mediators (27–31) that are critical to liver injury, repair and fibrogenesis. Interestingly,

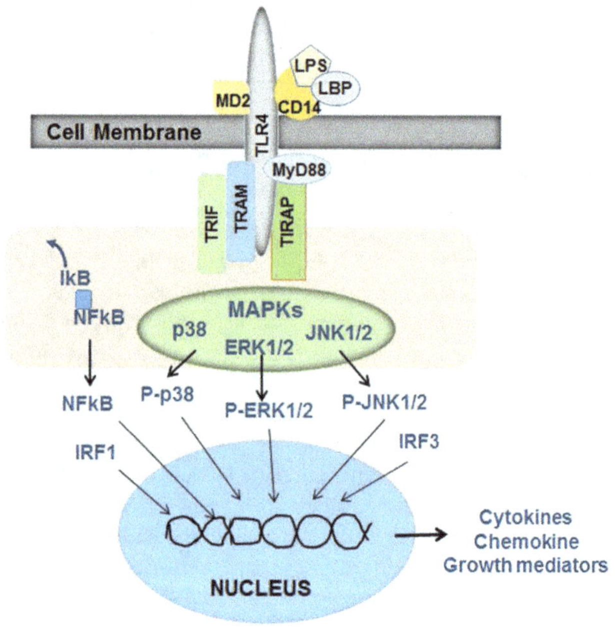

FIGURE 1 | Schematic of LPS-induced signaling in inflammatory cells. LPS in association with LBP (LPS-binding protein) binds to CD14, which then stimulates TLR4 signaling. The adapter proteins MD2 (on the outer side of the cell membrane), and TRIF (TIR-domain-containing adapter-inducing interferon-β), TRAM (TRIF-related adaptor molecule), MyD88 and TIRAP (Toll-Interleukin 1 receptor domain containing adaptor protein) that are associated with the intracellular part of TLR4 are required for LPS-induced and TLR4-stimulated activation of intracellular signaling via NFkB, mitogen activated protein kinases (MAPKs) p38, ERK1/2, and JNK1/2 and well as interferon-regulatory factor (IRF) 1 and 3. Translocation of these activated transcription factors to the nucleus and their subsequent binding to appropriate promoter regions on the DNA instigate transcription of a several cytokines, chemokines and growth mediators specific to a given cell type. The released mediators then act on target cells to promote pathophysiological processes. Adapted from Schwabe et al. (27), Akira et al. (28).

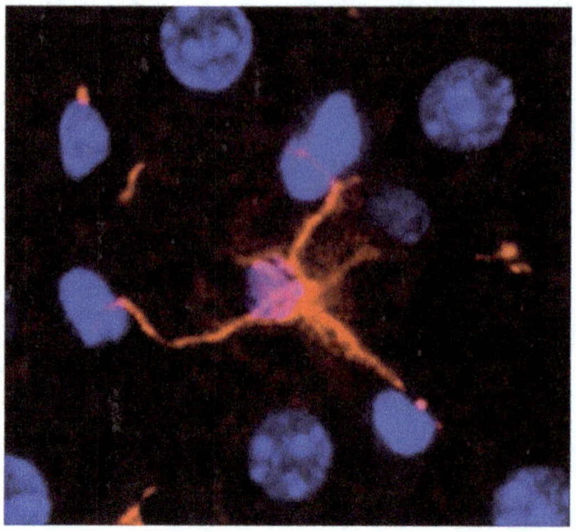

FIGURE 2 | A normal mouse liver section stained for desmin (expressed by hepatic stellate cell, HSC). An HSC can be seen connecting with 4 hepatocytes. Nuclei were stained with DAPI. Adapted from Gandhi (38, 39).

LPS can also elicit cellular response in a MyD88-independent manner (32, 33), and macrophages from Cd14-null mice were shown to produce TNF in response to lipid A (33). Thus, it is important to identify the precise mechanisms of a specific response of a given cell to LPS for better understanding of the pathophysiological processes.

MULTIFUNCTIONAL HEPATIC STELLATE CELLS (HSCs)

HSCs are located in the Disse's space and are the major storage site of vitamin A within their cytoplasmic lipid droplets (34). HSCs can be identified by vitamin A autofluorescence and expression of cytoskeletal intermediate filament desmin and/or glial fibrillary acidic protein (GFAP). However, zonal expression of these markers as well as retinoid-storage by HSCs is variable (35, 36). It is estimated that about 25% of HSCs may not contain vitamin A (34, 37). Although their cell body is small (~10 μm), HSCs demonstrate physical contact with 2–3 adjacent hepatocytes, SECs and even Kupffer cells and other cells in the sinusoidal lumen via long cytoplasmic processes (38, 39) (**Figure 2**). Thus, from their strategic location, HSCs are able to influence the functions of almost all hepatic cell types by juxtacrine (contact) and autocrine/paracrine (via released soluble mediators) mechanisms (38–40).

HSCs produce and react with the potent vasoconstrictor endothelin-1 and vasodilator nitric oxide (41–43), which regulate sinusoidal blood flow by inducing HSC contraction and relaxation, respectively (44–46). LPS stimulates the synthesis of both endothelin-1 and nitric oxide by HSCs, and LPS-induced vascular resistance of the previously normal liver is mitigated by endothelin receptor antagonism (47). HSCs also demonstrate remarkable ability to recruit inflammatory and immune cells, and influence their survival and functions (22, 23, 38–40, 48–54). Furthermore, evidence has emerged showing an important role of HSCs in liver regeneration and hepatocellular carcinoma (55–58). With these powerful characteristics, the strategically located HSCs regulate hepatic vascular tone, liver injury and regeneration, and hepatic immunological tolerance.

ACTIVATION OF HSCs AND LIVER FIBROSIS

Physiologically quiescent HSCs transdifferentiate into highly proliferative, fibrogenic and contractile myofibroblastic activated phenotype (aHSCs) during liver injury (**Figure 3**). Once activated, HSCs produce excessive amounts of extracellular matrix (ECM) components, which include fibrillary collagens and fibronectin (59). The net deposition of the ECM is regulated by matrix metalloproteinases (MMPs) and tissue inhibitors of metalloproteinases (TIMPs). Kupffer cells are a major source of several MMPs whereas HSCs are the major source of TIMPs. HSCs also produce MMPs. During fibrosis development, the predominance of increased expression of TIMPs and down-regulation of the expression of MMPs (collagenases) is

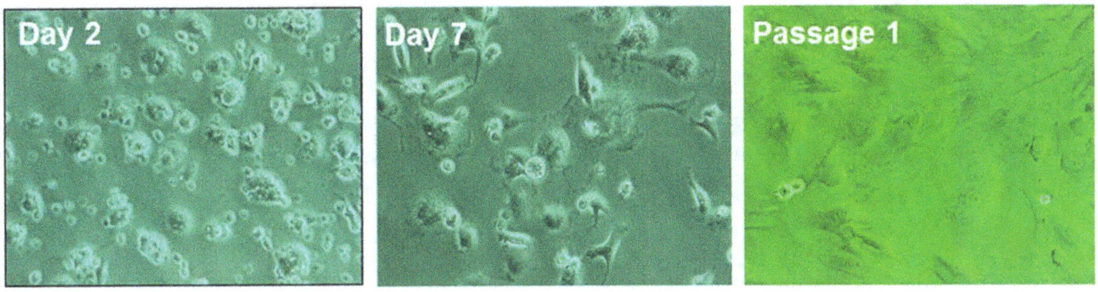

FIGURE 3 | Rat HSCs on day 2, day 7 of culture and in passage 1. On day 2, the cells show typical morphology of quiescent phenotype, and on day 7 of myofibroblast-like phenotype. The passagesd cells are fully activated showing myofibroblastic phenotype. Adapted from Gandhi (38, 39).

a major cause of progressive ECM deposition. This topic is extensively reviewed by Campana and Iredale (60).

The "initiation" phase of HSC activation begins with the loss of retinoid stores and down-regulation of peroxisome proliferator-activated receptor γ (PPARγ), accompanied by the expression of smooth muscle alpha-actin (αSMA) (via up-regulation of its transcription factor c-Myb) and platelet-derived growth factor β receptor (PDGFβR) (8, 9, 59). It is not entirely clear whether the loss of retinoids is a cause or a consequence of HSC activation. For example, supplementation of the culture medium with retinoic acid retards the rate of HSC activation (61), and the expression of lecithin-retinol acyltransferase (LRAT), an enzyme responsible for the accumulation of retinol as its esters, is lost during HSC activation (62). It was shown that the energy required for activation of HSCs is derived from triglycerides stored in the lipid droplets through autophagic/lysosomal degradation (63). However, mice that lack LRAT are devoid of lipid droplets (62, 64), and yet are similarly susceptible to bile duct ligation (BDL)- or CCl4-induced fibrosis as the wild type (WT) mice, and LRAT-deficient HSCs are similarly activated as WT HSCs (62). Since HSCs are the exclusive cell type to express LRAT in the liver, these results suggest that retinoids may not be absolutely essential for HSC quiescence. Further work is necessary to understand the role of retinoids and triglycerides stored in the lipid droplets in HSC activation.

It is generally accepted that in almost all etiologies of fibrosis, factors derived from injured/dying hepatocytes including apoptotic bodies, danger-associated molecular patterns (DAMPs), reactive oxygen species (ROS) and hedgehog ligands are the initial stimuli for HSC activation (8, 65, 66). High mobility group box 1 (HMGB1), a prominent DAMP released by dying/damaged hepatocytes, is shown to induce activation of HSCs, and also to elicit profibrogenic signals in combination with transforming growth factor-beta 1 (TGFβ) (67). Upon phagocytosis of hepatocyte apoptotic bodies and stimulation with DAMPs, Kupffer cells synthesize and release multiple cytokines, ROS and growth factors such as platelet-derived growth factor (PDGF) that promote activation and proliferation of HSCs (8, 68).

The "initiation phase" is followed by the "perpetuation" phase, as the injury stimulus persists. In this, activated Kupffer cells, modified capillarized SECs, and infiltrating neutrophils and lymphocytes cause HSCs to remain activated and/or cause their further activation and proliferation (8, 9). In this phase, TNFα produced by inflammatory macrophages, including Kupffer cells, stimulates survival signals in HSCs, whereas TGFβ1 induces activation as well as fibrogenic signals. Other cytokines prominently involved in HSC activation, proliferation and fibrosis are IL17, IL1α, and IL1β (67). Importantly, aHSCs themselves produce ROS, pro-inflammatory cytokines and chemokines, and express cell adhesion molecules to recruit circulating inflammatory and immune cells, and retain activated phenotype (8, 9, 69–71). Furthermore, highly activated passaged HSCs and human activated HSC cell line (LX1cells) were shown to increase their expression of αSMA, TGFβ1, and collagen 1a1 upon phagocytosis of hepatocyte-derived apoptotic bodies (65).

Elimination of the injury stimulus causes aHSCs to undergo apoptosis (72), senescence (73), or reversal to quiescent or the so-called "inhibited phenotype" (iHSC) leading to regression of fibrosis (8, 13, 74–76). IL10 and IL22 can be critically involved in the fibrosis reversal process as evidenced by IL10-induced inhibition of the expression of the activation markers in aHSCs (77–79), and IL10- and IL22-induced aHSC death by senescence (80, 81). It is important to note that iHSCs can be rapidly re-activated upon return of the injury stimulus causing accelerated development of fibrosis (75).

In the injured liver Kupffer cells as well as aHSCs are the major source of TGFβ, which is considered to be the most potent cytokine to stimulate ECM synthesis in aHSCs. The autocrine and paracrine stimulation of aHSCs by TGFβ activates the transcription factor complex P-SMAD2/3-SMAD4 (SMAD, small mother against decapentaplegic) and reduced nicotinamide adenine dinucleotide phosphate (NADPH) oxidase-mediated activation of p35-CCAAT/enhancer-binding protein beta (p35-C/EBPβ) (9, 81, 82). Other mediators such as angiotensin II, leptin, ethanol (alcohol) metabolite acetaldehyde and ROS are also major contributors of the synthesis and deposition of excessive amounts of ECM components from aHSCs.

Fas/FasL interactions are also critical to liver injury and fibrosis with an important role of Kupffer cells, which increase the expression of FasL upon phagocytosis of apoptotic bodies (68). Resistance of mice lacking Fas (lpr mice) to injury and fibrosis after bile duct ligation (BDL) (83) indicates that injury to hepatocytes and/or biliary epithelial cells is a critical stimulus

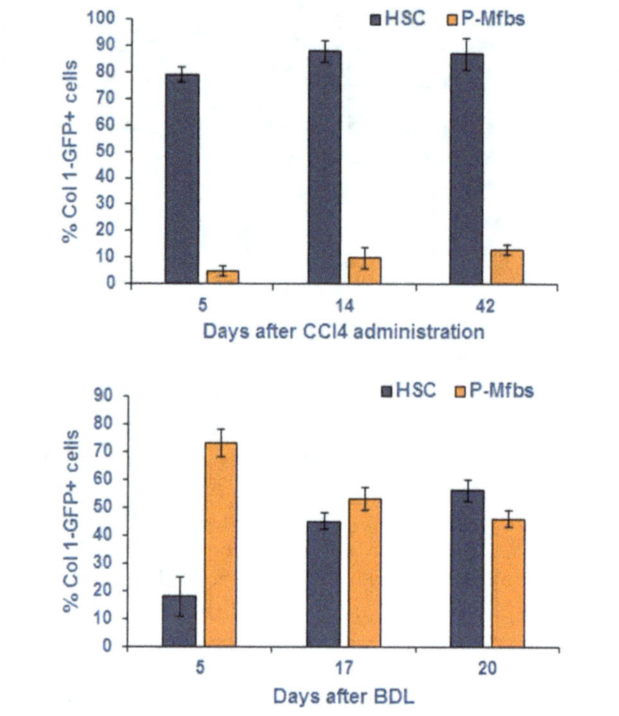

FIGURE 4 | Activated HSCs and P-Mfbs during carbon tetrachloride- or bile duct-ligation-induced liver injury in mice. The cells were identified by flow cytometry using green fluorescence protein (GFP) under collagen 1 promoter. GFP+ and vitamin A+ (HSCs) or GFP+ and vitamin A- cells were separated by flow. Note that HSCs but not P-Mfbs increase in CCl4-induced inflammatory injury and fibrosis, but the number of both cell types increase after BDL. Adapted from Iwaisako et al. (82).

for fibrogenesis. As liver injury and fibrosis progress, Fas/FasL interaction can also be a mechanism of limiting fibrosis through apoptosis of aHSCs (84). In contrast, portal myofibroblasts (P-Mfbs) are resistant to Fas/FasL-induced apoptosis (85), indicating their apparent predominance as the fibrogenic cell in biliary injury. It is shown that 5 and 20 days, respectively, after BDL, ~73 and 43% of the fibrogenic cells were found to be activated P-Mfbs as compared to ~18 and 51% aHSCs (82) (**Figure 4**). In this study, aHSCs and P-Mfbs were distinguished based on the presence (HSC) or absence (P-Mfb) of vitamin A (82), and a significant population of HSCs is devoid of or strongly deficient in vitamin A (34, 35, 37). A comprehensive comparative examination of the mechanisms underlying biliary and other types of liver fibrosis and precise identification of the responsible cells at various stages of its progression will be needed.

CD14/TLR4-INDEPENDENT LPS-INDUCED INFLAMMATORY RESPONSE BY HSCs

Effective clearance of bacterial endotoxins is an important function of the liver, primarily performed by Kupffer cells and hepatocytes (86–88). Plasma concentrations of LPS and other microbial products are very low or undetectable in physiology, but increase during both acute and chronic liver damage because of increased gut permeability and reduced hepatic clearance (15, 89–92). Gut-derived microbial products are critically involved in complications of endotoxemia occurring in acute and chronic liver injury, HCV infection, obstructive jaundice, cholestasis and chronic alcoholic and non-alcoholic hepatitis (93–98). A recent analysis of the association between serum LPS and chronic liver disease in >6,500 subjects found that serum LPS can be predictive of advanced liver disease (17). Because inflammation is critical to activation and fibrogenic activity of HSCs, LPS has gained much attention as a driver of liver injury, inflammation and fibrosis.

The pro-inflammatory LBP/CD14/TLR4-mediated effects of LPS on Kupffer cells, neutrophils and immune cells implicated in liver damage have been well-characterized (99–101). Activation-dependent response of rat HSCs to LPS by releasing MCP-1 (102) provided evidence for their possible role in hepatic inflammation. In these experiments, high (100 ng/ml) concentration of LPS and serum-supplemented medium were used (102). LPS was later found to stimulate the synthesis of nitric oxide, endothelin-1, TNFα and IL6 in both quiescent and activated rat HSCs at concentration as low as 1–10 ng/ml in serum-free condition (20, 21, 43, 103). This indicated that rat HSCs respond to LPS independent of CD14/TLR4 as serum is the source of LBP, which is produced by hepatocytes but not HSCs (21). These findings are of significant importance because LPS causes liver injury in CD14-independent manner (104); LPS-induced production of TNFα and IL6 in wild type (WT), TLR4-knockout (KO) and CD14-KO mice was similar following partial hepatectomy (105); and bile duct ligation or CCl4 administration elicited similar liver injury in WT, TLR4-mutant (C3H/HeJ) or TLR4-KO mice (23, 106). LPS also elicited similar inflammatory response in HSCs from WT and TLR4-KO (23) or CD14-KO mice (107). Interestingly, although quiescent rat and human HSCs possess very low (negligible) expression of TLR4, LPS induced NFkB activation and stimulated the synthesis of inflammatory cytokines in rat (21) but not human (108) quiescent HSCs (qHSCs). Whereas, both rat and human HSCs express TLR4 upon activation (21, 108), mouse qHSCs contain abundant expression of TLR4 (106). These findings indicate species-specific differences in CD14/TLR4-dependence or -independence of LPS effects may have important implications in hepatic pathophysiology.

In addition to the pro-inflammatory cytokines and chemokines, LPS also stimulates secretion of anti-inflammatory cytokines such as IL10 from HSCs (51). Transcriptomic analysis demonstrated that the repertoire of factors expressed by rat aHSCs and modulated by LPS was much extensive and included numerous cytokines/chemokines, cell adhesion molecules, signal transduction factors, as well as growth mediators (22). Obviously, the direct actions of LPS on HSCs are of critical importance in acute and chronic liver injury.

PRO- AND ANTI-FIBROGENIC EFFECTS OF LPS ON HSCs

As described above, inflammation, initiated by apoptotic bodies, DAMPs and cytokines released by injured/dying hepatocytes, plays a critical role in HSC activation and liver fibrosis. With continued presence of the injury stimulus, dying hepatocytes, Kupffer cells, recruited lymphocytes and even HSCs contribute to the persistent inflammatory environment. The role of Kupffer cells in hepatic inflammation and fibrosis has been investigated extensively, and depletion or blockade of Kupffer cells with gadolinium chloride was found to mitigate liver fibrosis in several murine models of liver injury including that by CCl4, dimethylnitrosamine and BDL (109–111). There is also evidence for a crucial role of the recruited blood-derived macrophages in liver fibrosis and their switch to anti-inflammatory (restorative) phenotype during its resolution (112, 113). These restorative macrophages may induce apoptosis of aHSCs or their reversal to either quiescent or inhibited phenotype (75, 114).

Although LPS has been implicated in liver fibrosis through its pro-inflammatory effects, whether its direct actions on HSCs has a role in fibrogenesis has remained relatively unexplored. LPS was found to inhibit DNA synthesis, concentration-dependently, in activated rat HSCs in presence or absence of serum, the source of LBP (20, 21). This observation is intriguing as activation and proliferation of HSCs are essential components of the initiation and progression of fibrosis. Recent work by Sharma and coworkers confirmed that LPS inhibits proliferation of culture-activated aHSCs as determined by Ki67 labeling *in vitro*, and even HSCs isolated from LPS-treated CCl4-induced chronically injured liver showed size reduction and reduced Ki67 labeling as compared to the cells from rats that did not receive LPS (24). This effect of LPS *in vivo* is impressive since hepatic inflammation was augmented, and indicated that LPS may arrest or mitigate HSC proliferation to limit ongoing fibrosis development in the inflammatory environment (i.e., in the presence of injury stimulus). On the other hand, LPS stimulates NFkB activation (a pro-inflammatory and pro-survival pathway) in HSCs (23, 103, 108), importance of which was confirmed by the observation showing reduced hepatic fibrogenesis after NFkB inhibition (114). It is apparent that such contemporaneous stimulation of the opposing signaling pathways can be of significant importance in regulating expansion of HSCs in the fibrotic liver (see **Figure 5** for schematic of opposing effects of LPS on HSC activation and fibrosis).

LPS-induced inhibition of DNA synthesis in qHSCs (21) suggested that it may not have direct effect on their activation. However, LPS-preconditioned qHSCs are activated upon incubation with TGFβ or when co-cultured with Kupffer cells (106), a main source of TGFβ in the liver (110, 115, 116). LPS was found to down-modulate the expression of BMP and activin membrane-bound inhibitor (BAMBI), a pseudoreceptor for TGFβ1, in qHSCs thereby sensitizing them to TGFβ1-induced activation and fibrogenic activity (106). In this regard, Kupffer cells were shown to become more sensitive to the effects of LPS after bile duct ligation and exhibited significant increase in phagocytic activity, oxidative burst, and cytokine production (117). Kupffer cells isolated from LPS-injected mice were reported to show increased expression of TNFα, IL6 and TGFβ (118), and at high concentrations, LPS promotes autophagy/lipophagy, down-regulates BAMBI and enhances TGFβ1 signaling in activated HSCs and HSC cell line (119). However, LPS does not stimulate the synthesis of TGFβ in purified HSCs (22, 23), and LPS administration to naïve mice also does not increase the expression of TGFβ (23). Furthermore, hepatic expression of BAMBI was not altered in mice that received chronic CCl4 treatment or in LPS-challenged culture-activated HSCs, but it was down-regulated in the livers of naïve mice upon acute LPS treatment (23). Because HSCs (and not hepatocytes or Kupffer cells) express BAMBI (106), these data suggest that its down-regulation occurring early during liver injury may not be sustained in the chronic phase. On the contrary, up-regulation of TGFβ-receptors in aHSCs (23, 24) could be a more dominant mechanism of liver fibrosis. TGFβ1 may also self-regulate its effects by modulating BAMBI expression. For example, TGFβ1 causes up-regulation of BAMBI mRNA and protein in HEPG2 cells via the P-SMAD2/3-4 transcriptional pathway (119), and stimulation of WNT/β-catenin signaling increases BAMBI in colorectal tumor cells (120). Since LPS increases nuclear accumulation of β-catenin in human hepatoma cell lines (121), it will be important to determine whether LPS ± TGFβ1 induce SMAD and/or Wnt/β-catenin signaling in qHSCs or aHSCs and regulate BAMBI, TGFβ-R1 and TGFβ-R2 expression both *in vivo* and *in vitro* for better understanding of the pathway: LPS → Kupffer cells/HSCs → BAMBI → TGFβ1 → activation of HSCs/fibrosis.

At 21 days after BDL, hepatic fibrosis was reported to be 30-50% less in CD14-deficient and in LBP-deficient mice than in the WT mice (122). However, there was no difference in lymphocyte and neutrophil infiltration but activation of macrophages was lower in CD14-KO mice as determined by the expression of Cd11b, a component of the C3 complement receptor primarily expressed on myeloid cells (i.e., macrophages and monocytes) (123). Saito and coworkers proposed that depletion of neutrophils does not have significant effect on BDL-induced fibrosis but LPS-stimulated Kupffer cells enhance hepatic fibrogenesis (123). The TLR4 mutant (C3H/HeJ) mice were also found to show much less CCl4- or BDL-induced fibrosis as compared to the WT mice (106). In contrast, C57BL/6J (B6-WT) and B6.B10ScN-Tlr4$^{lps-del}$/JthJ (TLR4-KO) mice demonstrated similar susceptibility to CCl4-induced fibrosis as analyzed by Sirius red staining, collagen I expression and hydroxyproline concentration, although necroinflammation and liver injury were lower in the latter (23). The expression of TNFα and CXCL1 increased similarly in CCl4-treated WT mice and TLR4-KO mice but that of antifibrogenic IFNγ increased only in WT mice (23). Furthermore, the expression of αSMA and the number of desmin-positive cells increased similarly in CCl4-treated WT and TLR4-KO mice suggesting that TLR4 activation is not necessary for activation and proliferation of HSCs. It is apparent that hepatocyte injury-induced activation of Kupffer cells and HSCs and also inflammation are more relevant to HSC activation and fibrosis. While these data demonstrate that LPS/TLR4 interaction may not be critical to fibrosis development in chronic liver disease, activation of TLR4 as well as TLR5, TLR7, and TLR9 was actually found to be beneficial in chronic hepatitis B virus infection by reducing the viral replication (124). Such effects of LPS and other PAMPs on TLRs can be self-limiting mechanisms of chronic liver disease in majority of HBV-infected subjects.

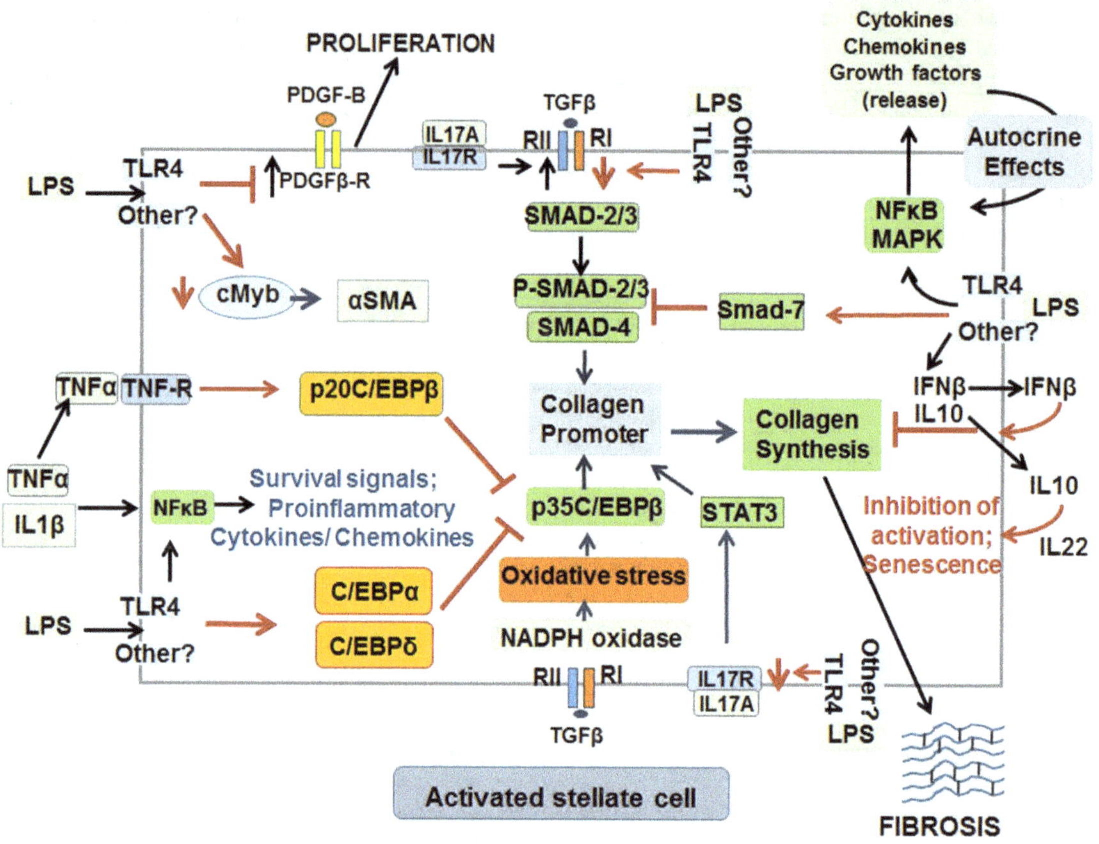

FIGURE 5 | Schematic representation of pro- and anti-fibrogenic effects of LPS on activated HSCs. Although LPS may act through TLR4 on aHSCs, it can also exert effects in a non-TLR4 pathway that has not been identified yet. LPS by stimulating synthesis of several cytokines and chemokines, via stimulation of NFkB and MAPK pathways, promotes survival (TNFα and IL1β) in an autocrine manner. The mediators released thus can also stimulate ECM synthesis, migration and proliferation of aHSCs. LPS down-regulates cMyb transcription factor and thus reduces the expression of α-SMA, a major marker of aHSCs. By down-regulating PDGFβR, LPS mitigates proliferation of aHSCs. LPS inhibits TGFβ-induced ECM synthesis by down-regulating TGFβR1, by increasing expression of SMAD7, C/EBPα, C/EBPδ, and p20C/EBPβ. IL17 can act directly on HSCs to stimulate ECM synthesis and by up-regulating TGFβRII. However, by down-regulating the expression of IL17R, LPS can reduce IL17-induced ECM synthesis by aHSCs. Finally, increased production of IL10 and IFNβ by LPS-stimulated aHSCs can be a mechanism of inhibition of ECM synthesis, activation and promotion of senescence.

In contrast to the down-modulatory effect of LPS on aHSCs (*in vivo* and *in vitro*), augmentation of CCl4-induced liver fibrosis in mice was reported within a very short time of just 4 h following administration of 10 mg/kg LPS (125). LPS administration (0.5 mg/kg; 3 times a week) from the beginning of NASH-inducing choline-deficient L-amino acid-defined (CDAA) diet in mice was also reported to increase inflammation, activation of HSCs and pericellular fibrosis (126). It should be noted that CDAA diet does not cause obesity or insulin resistance in rats, in contrast to mice that develop obesity and insulin resistance and limited fibrosis (127). Nevertheless, LPS effect described above contradict our observations that CCl4-induced hepatic fibrosis is not altered at 24 h after intraperitoneal administration of 5 mg/kg LPS (24). However, αSMA expression was strongly reduced by LPS *in vivo*, and HSCs isolated from LPS-treated CCl4-fibrotic rats showed reduced size, proliferation and expression of Acta 2, cMyb, PDGFβR, TGFβR1, Col1a1, and fibronectin but increased expression of TNFα, IL6, CXCL1 (24). CCl4-induced liver fibrosis was also not affected by a weakly inflammatory lipid A-derivative monophosphoryl lipid A although it caused reduction in αSMA expression in HSCs both *in vivo* and *in vitro* (24). In regard to whether LPS is really critical in promoting or mitigating fibrogenesis, antibiotic treatment of mice was found to reduce BDL- as well as CCl4-induecd fibrosis (106). However, much stronger CCl4-induced fibrosis was observed in germ-free mice as well as Myd88/Trif-deficient mice compared to the WT mice (128). Furthermore, repopulation of Gram-negative microbes (*E. coli*, the source of LPS) following dysbiosis did not affect fibrosis when compared to mice that did not receive *E. coli* (128). A recent investigation also reported that monocytes-derived macrophages stimulated with LPS and monosodium urate increase MMP3 and MMP9 in aHSCs and down-modulate pro-fibrogenic markers (129). These data and the observations showing unique interactions between HSCs and LPS (20–23) suggest that LPS has a dual role as a promoter of liver fibrosis by causing inflammation, and contemporaneously limit fibrosis by its direct effects on aHSCs.

OTHER LPS-STIMULATED PATHWAYS REGULATING LIVER FIBROSIS

The livers of chronically CCl4-treated rats were found to contain several apoptotic aHSCs, which increased further when oxidative stress was induced by administration of tert-butylhydroperoxide (130, 131). *In vitro* experiments confirmed that oxygen-free radicals cause apoptosis of aHSCs (130). Thus, although LPS-stimulated synthesis of free radicals in Kupffer cells (99) and HSCs (103) are generally considered as pro-fibrogenic, the same molecules appear to instigate signaling mechanism of cell death and prevent aHSC proliferation and fibrogenic activity. Along the same line, although autocrine or paracrine actions of TNFα on aHSCs provide NFkB activation-induced cell survival mechanisms, TNFα also stimulates binding of p20C/EBPβ and C/EBPδ to Cola1 promoter and thus represses p35C/EBPβ-induced transcription and fibrosis (132, 133). Interestingly, TGFβ1 has been shown to induce and increase SMAD7 (an inhibitor of pro-fibrogenic P-SMAD2/3) in several cell types including HSCs (134–136). This suggests a feed-back inhibition of pro-fibrogenic action of TGFβ1 in aHSCs. LPS increases SMAD7, and p20C/EBPβ and C/EBPδ (inhibitors of p35C/EBPβ) expression and down-regulates cMyb (a transcription factor for αSMA) expression in aHSCs *in vivo* and *in vitro* (24). Because LPS also strongly stimulates TNFα synthesis by HSCs (20–23, 103), the autocrine loop of its action on inhibitory C/EBP pathway might be a limiting mechanism of fibrogenesis (**Figure 5**).

IL17A promotes not only activation of inflammatory cells, but also stimulates collagen synthesis by HSCs through activation of signal transducer and activator of transcription 3 (STAT3) (137). In contrast, another study reported that IL17 does not directly cause activation of HSCs or induce fibrogenic response, but increases TGFβRII expression in HSCs sensitizing them to TGFβ1/SMAD2/3-induced collagen 1 synthesis (138). LPS down-regulates TGFβR in aHSCs (22, 23), and does not affect IL17A expression although it increases gene transcript of IL17F by more than 10-fold (22). Because IL17A and IL17F share the same receptors (IL17Ra and IL17Rc) (139), a similar fibrogenic effect of IL17F via autocrine pathway in HSCs may not be ruled out. However, microarray analysis showed robust decrease in Il17ra and Il17re in aHSCs stimulated with LPS (22). These findings indicate that LPS-induced down-regulation of both TGFβR and IL17R may limit fibrogenesis during chronic liver injury.

While pro-inflammatory and pro-fibrogenic mediators are produced by various cells during chronic liver injury, there is also abundant evidence for contemporaneous generation of anti-inflammatory and anti-fibrogenic factors such as IL10 and IL13. IL10-KO mice show increased neutrophil infiltration and hepatic fibrosis during repeated CCl4 administration (140). Kupffer cells produce IL13 and not IL10 under basal conditions, and LPS stimulates secretion of IL10 but not of IL13 from them (141–143). HSCs also produce IL10 spontaneously, which is strongly stimulated by LPS (22, 50). Such increased production of IL10 and IL13 can be yet another pathway of limiting liver fibrosis.

IL22 is an interesting cytokine that can be a part of anti-fibrotic mechanisms due to its ability to promote senescence and apoptosis of aHSCs both *in vivo* and *in vitro* (80). These effects of IL22 were found to be mediated via the activation of STAT3 and suppressor of cytokine signaling 3 (SOCS3) (144). However, STAT3 activation was also reported to be a mechanism of IL17-induced collagen synthesis by aHSCs via an IL6-dependent autocrine pathway, and deletion of IL22 exacerbated CCl4- as well as BDL-induced fibrosis (137). Furthermore, leptin-induced JAK2/STAT3 activation increased ECM synthesis and thereby fibrosis, and SOCS-3 activation negatively regulated JAK/STAT signaling (144).

Interferons (IFN) are a family of natural glycoproteins with antiviral activity, and type I IFNs (IFNα and IFNβ) have been widely used for viral eradication in patients with chronic viral hepatitis (145, 146). IFNα treatment was found to resolve liver fibrosis by causing significant reduction in the number of aHSCs (147–151). IFNβ was also shown to exhibit antifibrotic property and has been used to treat chronic HCV infection (150, 151). Recombinant human IFNβ decreased the expression of αSMA, collagen I and III, TGFβ1, PDGF-BB and SMAD4 in culture-activated rat or human HSCs, and increased SMAD7 expression (152). LPS stimulates IFNβ expression in HSCs (22, 49, 52) and it is likely that this can be an autocrine-inhibitory loop to reduce fibrosis. Interestingly, HSC-released IFNβ was found to be a major cytokine to cause autophagy in hepatocytes as a cell survival mechanism (**Figure 5**), but it could also induce acute liver injury through activation of IRF1 signaling in mice upon concanavalin A challenge (49, 50, 52).

PERSPECTIVE

The well-orchestrated communications between the various liver cell types maintain the physiological function of the organ despite exposure to numerous toxic substances, microbial and viral products, food- and environ-derived antigens, and drugs and xenobiotics on a regular basis. During liver injury, this mechanism is disrupted with an immediate repair response that involves activation of HSCs and/or P-Mfbs, resulting in increased production of ECM causing liver fibrosis. This mechanism involves mediators produced by the resident cells (hepatocytes, Kupffer cells, endothelial cells and cholangiocytes) as well as recruited inflammatory and immune cells. Upon termination of the injury stimulus, fibrosis is resolved and the system returns back to the physiologic state. However, persistence of injury stimulus causes progression of fibrosis to cirrhosis and, in some cases, hepatocellular carcinoma. The liver also has a remarkable ability to produce mediators that instigate mechanisms of resistance to fibrosis. Although the levels of a highly pro-inflammatory endotoxin (LPS) are elevated, and it has been implicated in fibrosis progression, evidence also indicates that it can reverse the activated fibrogenic phenotype of HSC to non-fibrogenic phenotype. It is of interest that LPS can exert this effect in absence of CD14/TLR4, which is essential for the generation of pro-inflammatory cytokines and chemokines from cells such as Kupffer cells, monocyte, and neutrophils. Development of LPS mimetics that do not engage CD14/TLR4 but still can act on activated HSCs will be a novel way to reverse these cells to the non-fibrogenic phenotype for treating liver fibrosis.

SYNOPSIS

This article describes the pro-fibrogenic as well as antifibrogenic effects of Gram-negative bacterial endotoxin lipopolysaccharide (LPS). This highly pro-inflammatory mediator is implicated in liver injury, inflammation, and fibrosis of various etiologies. Experiments using animal models of liver fibrosis and isolated cells showed that LPS stimulates synthesis of cytokines including TNFα, IL6, IL1β, and PDGF in Kupffer cells and infiltrating inflammatory and immune cells. These mediators cause activation and proliferation of the fibrogenic hepatic stellate cells (HSCs). In response to mediators such as TGFβ released by Kupffer cells and HSCs themselves, HSCs produce extracellular matrix (ECM) components (collagen I, collagen III, fibronectin) causing fibrosis of the liver. In contrast, LPS acts on activated HSCs directly and reduces the expression of the activation marker α-SMA through down-regulation of its transcription factor for cMyb. LPS also increases expression of SMAD7, p20-C/EBPβ, C/EBPα and C/EBPδ in activated HSCs, which are inhibitors of pro-fibrogenic signaling induced by TGFβ and other pro-fibrogenic mediators. Furthermore, LPS down-regulates TGFβR1 expression in activated HSCs thus mitigating TGFβ-induced fibrogenic activity. LPS stimulates the synthesis of anti-fibrogenic cytokines type 1 interferons and IL10 in HSCs. LPS also stimulates the synthesis of TNFα in HSCs and Kupffer cells. While TNFα is a pro-inflammatory cytokine that promotes survival of HSCs, it also stimulates p20-C/EBPβ and C/EBPδ that block p35C/EBPβ-induced ECM synthesis. The down-modulation of the markers of activation and fibrosis is observed in the HSCs isolated from the fibrotic liver treated *in vivo* with LPS. However, the short-term 24 h treatment with LPS *in vivo* increases inflammation and does not cause reduction in fibrosis. Finally, the antifibrogenic effects of LPS can be mimicked by its weakly inflammatory mimetic monophosphoryl lipid A. Such opposing effects of LPS can be potentially important in limiting liver fibrosis.

AUTHOR CONTRIBUTIONS

CG is responsible for the concept and writing of this manuscript.

REFERENCES

1. Pinzani M, Rosselli M, Zuckermann M. Liver cirrhosis. *Best Pract Res Clin Gastroenterol.* (2011) 25:281–90. doi: 10.1016/j.bpg.2011.02.009
2. Pinzani M. Hepatic fibrosis: a global clinical problem. In: Gandhi CR, Pinzani M, editors. *Stellate Cells in Health and Disease.* London: Elsevier/Academic Press. (2015). p. 29–39. doi: 10.1016/B978-0-12-800134-9.00003-8
3. Kochanek KD, Murphy SL, Xu J, Xu J, Tajada-Vera B. Deaths: final data for 2014. *Natl Vital Stat Rep.* (2016) 65:1–122.
4. European Association for the Study of the Liver. EASL recommendations on treatment of hepatitis C 2018. *J Hepatol.* (2018) 69:461–511. doi: 10.1016/j.jhep.2018.03.026
5. Shah H, Bilodeau M, Burak KW, Cooper C, Klein M, Ramji A, et al. The management of chronic hepatitis C: 2018 guideline update from the Canadian association for the study of the liver. Canadian association for the study of the liver. *CMAJ.* (2018) 190:E677–7. doi: 10.1503/cmaj.170453
6. Mann J, Mann DA. Transcriptional regulation of hepatic stellate cells. *Adv Drug Deliv Rev.* (2009) 61:497–512. doi: 10.1016/j.addr.2009.03.011
7. Page A, Mann DA, Mann J. The mechanisms of HSC activation and epigenetic regulation of HSCs phenotypes. *Curr Pathobiol Rep.* (2014) 2:163–70. doi: 10.1007/s40139-014-0052-0
8. Hasegawa D, Wallace MC, Friedman SL. Stellate cells and hepatic fibrosis. In: Gandhi CR, Pinzani M, editors. *Stellate Cells in Health and Disease.* London: Elsevier/Academic Press (2015). p. 41–62. doi: 10.1016/B978-0-12-800134-9.00004-X
9. Gandhi CR. Hepatic stellate cell activation and pro-fibrogenic signals. *J Hepatol.* (2017) 67:1104–5. doi: 10.1016/j.jhep.2017.06.001
10. Iredale JP. Models of liver fibrosis: exploring the dynamic nature of inflammation and repair in a solid organ. *J Clin Invest.* (2007) 117:539–48. doi: 10.1172/JCI30542
11. Liedtke C, Luedde T, Sauerbruch T, Scholten D, Streetz K, Tacke F, et al. Experimental liver fibrosis research: update on animal models, legal issues and translational aspects. *Fibrogenesis Tissue Repair.* (2013) 6:19. doi: 10.1186/1755-1536-6-19
12. Rombouts K. Hepatic stellate cell culture models. In: Gandhi CR, Pinzani M, editors. *Stellate Cells in Health and Disease.* London: Elsevier/Academic Press (2015). p. 15–27. doi: 10.1016/B978-0-12-800134-9.00002-6
13. Koyama Y, Wang P, Brenner DA, Kisseleva T. Stellate cells, portal myofibroblasts, epithelial-to-mesenchymal transition. In: Gandhi CR, Pinzani M, editors. *Stellate Cells in Health and Disease.* London: Elsevier/Academic Press (2015). p. 87–106. doi: 10.1016/B978-0-12-800134-9.00006-3
14. Mederacke I, Hsu CC, Troeger JS, Huebener P, Mu X, Dapito DH, et al. Fate tracing reveals hepatic stellate cells as dominant contributors to liver fibrosis independent of its aetiology. *Nat Commun.* (2013) 4:2823. doi: 10.1038/ncomms3823
15. Soares JB, Pimentel-Nunes P, Roncon-Albuquerque R, Leite-Moreira A. The role of lipopolysaccharide/toll-like receptor 4 signaling in chronic liver diseases. *Hepatol Int.* (2010) 4:659–72. doi: 10.1007/s12072-010-9219-x
16. Sharifnia T, Antoun J, Verriere TG, Suarez G, Wattacheril J, Wilson KT, et al. Hepatic TLR4 signaling in obese NAFLD. *Am J Physiol Gastrointest Liver Physiol.* (2015) 309:G270–8. doi: 10.1152/ajpgi.00304.2014
17. Männistö V, Färkkilä M, Pussinen P, Jula A, Männistö S, Lundqvist A, et al. Serum lipopolysaccharides predict advanced liver disease in the general population. *J Hep Rep.* (2019) 1:345–52. doi: 10.1016/j.jhepr.2019.09.001
18. Carpino G, del Ben M, Pastori D, Carnevale R, Baratta F, Overi D, et al. Increased liver localization of lipopolysaccharides in human and experimental non-alcoholic fatty liver disease. *Hepatology.* (2019) doi: 10.1002/hep.31056. [Epub ahead of print].
19. du Plessis J, Korf H, van Pelt J, Windmolders P, Vander Elst I, Verrijken A, et al. Pro-inflammatory cytokines but not endotoxin-related parameters associate with disease severity in patients with nafld. *PLoS ONE.* (2016) 11:e0166048. doi: 10.1371/journal.pone.0166048
20. Uemura T, Gandhi CR. Inhibition of DNA synthesis in cultured hepatocytes by endotoxin-conditioned medium of activated stellate cells is transforming growth factor-β- and nitric oxide-independent. *Br J Pharmacol.* (2001) 133:1125–33. doi: 10.1038/sj.bjp.0704151
21. Thirunavukkarasu C, Uemura T, Wang LF, Watkins S, Gandhi CR. Normal rat hepatic stellate cells respond to endotoxin in LBP-independent manner to

produce inhibitor(s) of DNA synthesis in hepatocytes. *J Cell Physiol.* (2005) 204:654–65. doi: 10.1002/jcp.20366

22. Harvey SAK, Dangi A, Tandon A, Gandhi CR. The transcriptomic response of rat hepatic stellate cells to endotoxin: implications for hepatic inflammation and immune regulation. *PLoS ONE.* (2013) 8:e82159. doi: 10.1371/journal.pone.0082159
23. Kumar S, Wang J, Shanmukhappa SK, Gandhi CR. TLR4-independent CCl4-induced fibrosis and lipopolysaccharide-induced acute liver injury in mice: role of hepatic stellate cells. *Am J Pathol.* (2017) 187:1356–67. doi: 10.1016/j.ajpath.2017.01.021
24. Sharma A, Verma AK, Kofron M, Kudira R, Miethke A, Wu T, et al. Lipopolysaccharide reverses hepatic stellate cell activation via modulation of c-Myb, SMADs and C/EBP transcription factors. *Hepatology.* (2020) doi: 10.1002/hep.31188. [Epub ahead of print].
25. Gandhi CR. Cellular anatomy of the liver. In McManus LM, Mitchell RN, editors. *Pathobiology of Human Disease: A Dynamic Encyclopedia of Disease Mechanisms*, Amsterdam: Elsevier Press (2014). p. 1759–69. doi: 10.1016/B978-0-12-386456-7.04201-5
26. Medzhitov R, Preston-Hurlburt P, Janeway CA Jr. A human homologue of the *Drosophila* toll protein signals activation of adaptive immunity. *Nature.* (1997) 388:394–7. doi: 10.1038/41131
27. Schwabe RF, Seki E, Brenner DA. Toll-like receptor signaling in the liver. *Gastroenterology.* (2006) 130:1886–900. doi: 10.1053/j.gastro.2006.01.038
28. Akira S, Uematsu S, Takeuchi O. Pathogen recognition and innate immunity. *Cell.* (2006) 124:783–801. doi: 10.1016/j.cell.2006.02.015
29. Poltorak A, He X, Smirnova I, Liu MY, van Huffel C, Du X, et al. Defective LPS signaling in C3H/HeJ and C57BL/10ScCr mice: mutations in Tlr4 gene. *Science.* (1998) 282:2085–8. doi: 10.1126/science.282.5396.2085
30. Silhavy TJ, Kahne D, Walker S. The bacterial cell envelope. *Cold Spring Harb Perspect Biol.* (2010) 2:a000414. doi: 10.1101/cshperspect.a000414
31. Mahla RS, Reddy MC, Prasad DV, Kumar H. Sweeten PAMPs: role of sugar complexed pamps in innate immunity and vaccine biology. *Front Immunol.* (2013) 4:248. doi: 10.3389/fimmu.2013.00248
32. Jiang Z, Georgel P, Du X, Shamel L, Sovath S, Mudd S, et al. CD14 is required for MyD88-independent LPS signaling. *Nat Immunol.* (2005) 6:565–70. doi: 10.1038/ni1207
33. Kawai T, Adachi O, Ogawa T, Takeda K, Akira S. Unresponsiveness of MyD88-deficient mice to endotoxin. *Immunity.* (1999) 11:115–22. doi: 10.1016/S1074-7613(00)80086-2
34. Wake K. Perisinusoidal stellate cells (fat-storing cells, interstitial cells, lipocytes), their related structure in and around the liver sinusoids, vitamin A-storing cells in extrahepatic organs. *Int Rev Cytol.* (1980) 66:303–53. doi: 10.1016/S0074-7696(08)61977-4
35. Geerts A. History, heterogeneity, developmental biology, functions of quiescent hepatic stellate cells. *Semin Liver Dis.* (2001) 21:311–35. doi: 10.1055/s-2001-17550
36. Pinzani M, Gandhi CR, editiors. Stellate cells: history and early work. *Stellate Cells in Health and Disease.* London: Elsevier/Academic Press (2015). p. 1–13. doi: 10.1016/B978-0-12-800134-9.00001-4
37. Sztark F, Dubroca J, Latry P, Quinton A, Balabaud C, Bioulac-Sage P. Perisinusoidal cells in patients with normal liver histology. a morphometric study. *J Hepatol.* (1986) 2:358–69. doi: 10.1016/S0168-8278(86)80047-2
38. Gandhi CR. Hepatic stellate cells. In: Monga SP, editor. *Molecular Pathology of Liver Diseases.* New York, NY: Springer (2010). p. 53–80. doi: 10.1007/978-1-4419-7107-4_5
39. Gandhi CR. Stellate cells in Hepatic immunological tolerance. In Gandhi CR, Pinzani M, editors. *Stellate Cells in Health and Disease. London, UK: Elsevier/Academic Press.* (2015). p. 227–49. doi: 10.1016/B978-0-12-800134-9.00014-2
40. Gandhi CR. Stellate cells in regulation of hepatocyte survival and function. In Gandhi CR, *Pinzani M,* editors. *Stellate Cells in Health and Disease. London, UK: Elsevier/Academic Press.* (2015). p. 209–25. doi: 10.1016/B978-0-12-800134-9.00013-0
41. Gabriel A, Kuddus R, Rao AS, Watkins WD, Gandhi CR. Superoxide-induced changes in endothelin (ET) receptors and stimulation of ET-1 synthesis in hepatic stellate cells. *J Hepatol.* (1998) 29:614–27. doi: 10.1016/S0168-8278(98)80157-8
42. Gabriel A, Kuddus R, Rao AS, Gandhi CR. Down-regulation of endothelin receptors by transforming growth factor ß1 in hepatic stellate cells. *J Hepatol.* (1999) 30:440–50. doi: 10.1016/S0168-8278(99)80103-2
43. Gandhi CR, Uemura T, Kuddus RH. Endotoxin causes up-regulation of endothelin receptors in cultured hepatic stellate cells via nitric oxide-dependent and -independent mechanisms. *Br J Pharmacol.* (2000) 131:319–27. doi: 10.1038/sj.bjp.0703577
44. Kawada N, Tran-Thi TA, Klein H, Decker K. The contraction of hepatic stellate (Ito) cells stimulated with vasoactive substances. possible involvement of endothelin 1 and nitric oxide in the regulation of the sinusoidal tonus. *Eur J Biochem.* (1993) 213:815–23. doi: 10.1111/j.1432-1033.1993.tb17824.x
45. Rockey DC, Weisiger RA. Endothelin induced contractility of stellate cells from normal and cirrhotic rat liver: implications for regulation of portal pressure and resistance. *Hepatology.* (1996) 24:233–40. doi: 10.1002/hep.510240137
46. Zhang JX, Pegoli W Jr, Clemens MG. Endothelin-1 induces direct constriction of hepatic sinusoids. *Am J Physiol.* (1994) 266:G624–32. doi: 10.1152/ajpgi.1994.266.4.G624
47. Gandhi CR, Kuddus RH, Nemoto EM, Murase N. Endotoxin treatment causes up-regulation of endothelin system in the liver: amelioration of increased portal resistance by endothelin receptor antagonism. *J Gastroenterol Hepatol.* (2001) 6:61–9. doi: 10.1046/j.1440-1746.2001.02419.x
48. Stewart R, Dangi A, Huang C, Murase N, Kimura S, Stolz DB, et al. A novel mouse model of depletion of stellate cells clarifies their role in ischemia/reperfusion- and endotoxin-induced acute liver injury. *J Hepatol.* (2014) 60:298–305. doi: 10.1016/j.jhep.2013.09.013
49. Rani, R, Tandon A, Wang J, Kumar S, Gandhi CR. Stellate cells orchestrate concanavalin A-induced acute liver damage. *Am J Pathol.* (2017) 187:2008–19. doi: 10.1016/j.ajpath.2017.05.015
50. Rani R, Kumar S, Sharma A, Mohanty SK, Donnelly B, Tiao GT, et al. Mechanisms of Concanavalin A-induced cytokine synthesis by hepatic stellate cells: distinct roles of interferon regulatory factor-1 in liver injury. *J Biol Chem.* (2018) 293:18466–76. doi: 10.1074/jbc.RA118.005583
51. Dangi A, Sumpter T, Kimura S, Stolz DB, Murase N, Raimondi G, et al. Selective expansion of allogeneic regulatory T cells by hepatic stellate cells: role of endotoxin and implications for allograft tolerance. *J Immunol.* (2012) 188:3667–77. doi: 10.4049/jimmunol.1102460
52. Dangi A, Huang C, Tandon A, Stolz D, Wu T, Gandhi CR. Endotoxin-stimulated rat hepatic stellate cells induce autophagy in hepatocytes as a survival mechanism. *J Cell Physiol.* (2016) 231:94–105. doi: 10.1002/jcp.25055
53. Sumpter T, Dangi A, Matta B, Huang C, Stolz D, Vodovotz Y, et al. Hepatic stellate cells undermine the allostimulatory function of liver myeloid dendritic cells via STAT3-dependent induction of IDO. *J Immunol.* (2012) 189:3848–58. doi: 10.4049/jimmunol.1200819
54. Kumar S, Wang J, Thomson AW, Gandhi CR. Hepatic stellate cells increase the immunosuppressive function of natural $Foxp3^{+}$ regulatory T cells via IDO-induced AhR activation. *J Leukoc Biol.* (2017) 101:429–38. doi: 10.1189/jlb.2A0516-239R
55. Preziosi ME, Monga SP. Update on the mechanisms of liver regeneration. *Semin Liver Dis.* (2017) 37:141–51. doi: 10.1055/s-0037-1601351
56. Dapito DH, Schwabe RF. Hepatic stellate cells and liver cancer. In Gandhi CR, Pinzani M, editors. *Stellate Cells in Health and Disease.* London: Elsevier/Academic Press (2015). p. 145–162. doi: 10.1016/B978-0-12-800134-9.00 009-9
57. Cook D, Achanta S, Hoek JB, Ogunnaike BA, Vadigepalli R. Cellular network modeling and single cell gene expression analysis reveals novel hepatic stellate cell phenotypes controlling liver regeneration dynamics. *BMC Syst Biol.* (2018) 12:86. doi: 10.1186/s12918-018-0605-7
58. Sircana A, Paschetta E, Saba F, Molinaro F, Musso G. Recent insight into the role of fibrosis in nonalcoholic steatohepatitis-related hepatocellular carcinoma *Int J Mol Sci.* (2019) 20:1745. doi: 10.3390/ijms200 71745
59. Hernandez-Gea V, Friedman SL. Pathogenesis of liver fibrosis. *Annu Rev Pathol.* (2011) 6:425–56. doi: 10.1146/annurev-pathol-011110-130246

60. Campana L, Iredale J. Matrix Metalloproteinases and their inhibitors. In Gandhi CR, Pinzani M, editors. *Stellate Cells in Health and Disease.* London: Elsevier/Academic Press (2015). p. 107–24. doi: 10.1016/B978-0-12-800134-9.00007-5
61. Chi X, Anselmi A, Watkins S, Gandhi, CR. Prevention of cultured stellate cell transformation and endothelin-B receptor up-regulation by retinoic acid. *Br J Pharmacol.* (2003) 139:765–74. doi: 10.1038/sj.bjp.0705303
62. Kluwe J, Wongsiriroj N, Troeger JS, Gwak GY, Dapito DH, Pradere JP, et al. Absence of hepatic stellate cell retinoid lipid droplets does not enhance hepatic fibrosis but decreases hepatic carcinogenesis. *Gut.* (2011) 60:1260–8. doi: 10.1136/gut.2010.209551
63. Hernandez-Gea V, Ghiasi-Nejad Z, Rozenfeld R, Gordon R, Fiel MI, Yue Z, et al. Autophagy releases lipid that promotes fibrogenesis by activated hepatic stellate cells in mice and in human tissues. *Gastroenterology.* (2012) 142:938–46. doi: 10.1053/j.gastro.2011.12.044
64. Blaner WS, O'Byrne SM, Wongsiriroj N, Kluwe J, D'Ambrosio DM, Jiang H, et al. Hepatic stellate cell lipid droplets: a specialized lipid droplet for retinoid storage. *Biochim Biophys Acta.* (2009) 1791:467–73. doi: 10.1016/j.bbalip.2008.11.001
65. Canbay A, Taimr P, Torok, N, Higuchi H, Friedman S, Gores GJ. Apoptotic body engulfment by a human stellate cell line is profibrogenic. *Lab Invest.* (2003) 83:655–63. doi: 10.1097/01.LAB.0000069036.63405.5C
66. Omenetti A, Choi S, Michelotti G, Diehl AM. Hedgehog signaling in the liver. *J Hepatol.* (2011) 54:366–73. doi: 10.1016/j.jhep.2010.10.003
67. Ignat SR, Dinescu S, Hermenean A, Costache, M. Cellular interplay as a consequence of inflammatory signals leading to liver fibrosis development. *Cells.* (2020) 9:E461. doi: 10.3390/cells9020461
68. Canbay A, Feldstein AE, Higuchi H, Werneburg N, Grambihler A, Bronk SF, et al. Kupffer cell engulfment of apoptotic bodies stimulates death ligand and cytokine expression. *Hepatology.* (2003) 38:1188–98. doi: 10.1053/jhep.2003.50472
69. Pinzani M, Marra F. Cytokine receptors and signaling in hepatic stellate cells. *Semin Liver Dis.* (2001) 21:397–416. doi: 10.1055/s-2001-17554
70. Marra F, Caligiuri A. Cytokine production and signaling in stellate cells. In Gandhi CR, Pinzani M. editors. *Stellate Cells in Health and Disease.* London: Elsevier/Academic Press (2015). p. 63–86. doi: 10.1016/B978-0-12-800134-9.00005-1
71. Tacke F, Weiskirchen R. Update on hepatic stellate cells: pathogenic role in liver fibrosis and novel isolation techniques. *Expert Rev Gastroenterol Hepatol.* (2012) 6:67–80. doi: 10.1586/egh.11.92
72. Iredale JP, Benyon RC, Pickering J, McCullen M, Northrop M, Pawley S, et al. Mechanisms of spontaneous resolution of rat liver fibrosis. Hepatic stellate cell apoptosis and reduced hepatic expression of metalloproteinase inhibitors. *J Clin Invest.* (1998) 102:538–49. doi: 10.1172/JCI1018
73. Krizhanovsky V, Yon M, Dickins RA, Hearn S, Simon J, Miething C, et al. Senescence of activated stellate cells limits liver fibrosis. *Cell.* (2008) 134:657–67. doi: 10.1016/j.cell.2008.06.049
74. Issa R, Zhou X, Constandinou CM, Fallowfield J, Millward-Sadler H, Gaca, MD, et al. Spontaneous recovery from micronodular cirrhosis: evidence for incomplete resolution associated with matrix cross-linking. *Gastroenterology.* (2004) 126:1795–808. doi: 10.1053/j.gastro.2004.03.009
75. Kisseleva T, Cong M, Paik Y, Scholten D, Jiang C, Benner C, et al. Myofibroblasts revert to an inactive phenotype during regression of liver fibrosis. *Proc Natl Acad Sci USA.* (2012) 109:9448–53. doi: 10.1073/pnas.1201840109
76. Troeger JS, Mederacke I, Gwak GY, Dapito DH, Mu X, Hsu CC, et al. Deactivation of hepatic stellate cells during liver fibrosis resolution in mice. *Gastroenterology.* (2012) 143:73–83. doi: 10.1053/j.gastro.2012.06.036
77. Huang YH, Shi MN, Zheng WD, Zhang LJ, Chen ZX, Wang XZ. Therapeutic effect of interleukin-10 on CCl4-induced hepatic fibrosis in rats. *World J Gastroenterol.* (2006) 12:1386–91. doi: 10.3748/wjg.v12.i9.1386
78. Huang YH, Chen MH, Guo QL, Chen YX, Zhang LJ, Chen ZX, et al. Interleukin-10 promotes primary rat hepatic stellate cell senescence by upregulating the expression levels of p53 and p21. *Mol Med Rep.* (2018) 17:5700–7. doi: 10.3892/mmr.2018.8592
79. Chen E, Cen Y, Lu D, Luo W, Jiang H. IL-22 inactivates hepatic stellate cells via downregulation of the TGF-1/Notch signaling pathway. *Mol Med Rep.* (2018) 17:5449–5453. doi: 10.3892/mmr.2018.8516
80. Kong X, Feng D, Wang H, Hong F, Bertola A, Wang FS, et al. Interleukin-22 induces hepatic stellate cell senescence and restricts liver fibrosis in mice. *Hepatology.* (2012) 56:1150–9. doi: 10.1002/hep.25744
81. Weng HL, Liu Y, Chen JL, Huang T, Xu LJ, Godoy P, et al. The etiology of liver damage imparts cytokines transforming growth factor beta1 or interleukin-13 as driving forces in fibrogenesis. *Hepatology.* (2009) 50:230–43. doi: 10.1002/hep.22934
82. Iwaisako K, Jiang C, Zhang M, Cong M, Moore-Morris TJ, Park TJ, et al. Origin of myofibroblasts in the fibrotic liver in mice. *Proc Natl Acad Sci USA.* (2014) 111:E3297–305. doi: 10.1073/pnas.1400062111
83. Canbay A, Higuchi H, Bronk SF, Taniai M, Sebo TJ, Gores GJ. Fas enhances fibrogenesis in the bile duct ligated mouse: a link between apoptosis and fibrosis. *Gastroenterology.* (2002) 123:1323–30. doi: 10.1053/gast.2002.35953
84. Saile B, Knittel T, Matthes N, Schott P, Ramadori G. CD95/CD95L-mediated apoptosis of the hepatic stellate cell. A mechanism terminating uncontrolled hepatic stellate cell proliferation during hepatic tissue repair. *Am J Pathol.* (1997) 151:1265–72.
85. Ramadori G, Saile B. Mesenchymal cells in the liver–one cell type or two? *Liver.* (2002) 22:283–94. doi: 10.1034/j.1600-0676.2002.01726.x
86. Nolan JP. Endotoxin, reticuloendothelial function, liver injury. *Hepatology.* (1981) 1:458–65. doi: 10.1002/hep.1840010516
87. van Bossuyt H, de Zanger RB, Wisse E. Cellular and subcellular distribution of injected lipopolysaccharide in rat liver and its inactivation by bile salts. *J Hepatol.* (1988) 7:325–37. doi: 10.1016/S0168-8278(88)80005-9
88. Fox ES, Thomas P, Broitman SA. Clearance of gut-derived endotoxins by the liver. *Gastroenterology.* (1989) 96:456–61. doi: 10.1016/0016-5085(89)91571-0
89. Triger DR, Boyer TD, Levin J. Portal and systemic bacteraemia and endotoxaemia in liver disease. *Gut.* (1978) 19:935–9. doi: 10.1136/gut.19.10.935
90. Lumsden AB, Henderson JM, Kutner MH. Endotoxin levels measured by a chromogenic assay in portal, hepatic and peripheral venous blood in patients with cirrhosis. *Hepatology.* (1988) 8:232–6. doi: 10.1002/hep.1840080207
91. Bomzon A, Blendis LM. The nitric oxide hypothesis and the hyperdynamic circulation in cirrhosis. *Hepatology.* (1994) 20:1343–50. doi: 10.1002/hep.1840200535
92. Caradonna L, Mastronardi ML, Magrone T, Cozzolongo R, Cuppone R, Manghisi OG, et al. Biological and clinical significance of endotoxemia in the course of hepatitis C virus infection. *Curr Pharm Des.* (2002) 8:995–1005. doi: 10.2174/1381612024606983
93. Kocsar LT, Bertok L, Varteresz V. Effect of bile acids on the intestinal absorption of endotoxin in rat. *J Bacteriol.* (1969) 100:220–3. doi: 10.1128/JB.100.1.220-223.1969
94. Adachi Y, Moore LE, Bradford BU, Gao W, Thurman RG. Antibiotics prevent liver injury in rats following long-term exposure to ethanol. *Gastroenterology.* (1995) 108:218–24. doi: 10.1016/0016-5085(95)90027-6
95. Greve JWM, Gouma DJ, Buurman WA. Complications in obstructive jaundice: role of endotoxins. *Scand J Gastroenterol.* (1992) 194 (Suppl. 194):8–12. doi: 10.3109/00365529209096019
96. Sasatomi K, Noguchi K, Sakisaka S, Sata M, Tanikawa, KA. bNormal accumulation of endotoxin in biliary epithelial cells in primary biliary cirrhosis and primary sclerosing cholangitis. *J Hepatol.* (1998) 29:409–16. doi: 10.1016/S0168-8278(98)80058-5
97. Draper LR, Gyure LA, Hall JG, Robertson D. Effect of alcohol on the integrity of the intestinal epithelium. *Gut.* (1983) 24:399–404. doi: 10.1136/gut.24.5.399
98. Parlesak A, Schafer C, Schutz T, Bode JC, Bode C. Increased intestinal permeability to macromolecules and endotoxemia in patients with chronic alcohol abuse in different stages of alcohol-induced liver disease. *J Hepatol.* (2000) 32:742–7. doi: 10.1016/S0168-8278(00)80242-1
99. Su GL. Lipopolysaccharides in liver injury: molecular mechanisms of Kupffer cell activation. *Am J Physiol Gastrointest Liver Physiol.* (2002) 283:G256–65. doi: 10.1152/ajpgi.00550.2001
100. Gandhi CR. Kupffer Cells. In Monga SP, editor. *Molecular Pathology of Liver Diseases.* New York, NY: Springer (2010). p. 81–96. doi: 10.1007/978-1-4419-7107-4_6

101. Sabroe I, Dower SK, Whyte MK. The role of Toll-like receptors in the regulation of neutrophil migration, activation, apoptosis. *Clin Infect Dis.* (2005) 41(Suppl. 7):S421–6. doi: 10.1086/431992
102. Sprenger H, Kaufmann A, Garn H, Lahme B, Gemsa D, Gressner, AM. Differential expression of monocyte chemotactic protein-1 (MCP-1) in transforming rat hepatic stellate cells. *J Hepatol.* (1999) 30:88–94. doi: 10.1016/S0168-8278(99)80011-7
103. Thirunavukkarasu C, Watkins SC, Gandhi CR. Mechanisms of endotoxin-induced NO, IL-6, TNF-alpha production in activated rat hepatic stellate cells: role of p38 MAPK. *Hepatology.* (2006) 44:389–98. doi: 10.1002/hep.21254
104. Haziot A, Lin XY, Zhang F, Goyert SM. The induction of acute phase proteins by lipopolysaccharide uses a novel pathway that is CD14-independent. *J Immunol.* (1998) 160:2570–072.
105. Campbell JS, Riehle KJ, Brooling JT, Bauer RL, Mitchell C, Fausto N. Proinflammatory cytokine production in liver regeneration is Myd88-dependent, but independent of Cd14, Tlr2, Tlr4. *J Immunol.* (2006) 176:2522–8. doi: 10.4049/jimmunol.176.4.2522
106. Seki E, de Minicis S, Osterreicher CH, Kluwe J, Osawa Y, Brenner DA, et al. TLR4 enhances TGF-beta signaling and hepatic fibrosis. *Nat Med.* (2007) 13:1324–32. doi: 10.1038/nm1663
107. Gandhi CR. Hepatic fibrosis is independent of the effects of endotoxin (*Lipopolysaccharide*) on hepatic stellate cells. *FASEB J.* (2017) 31:A328.7
108. Paik YH, Schwabe RF, Bataller R, Russo MP, Jobin C, Brenner DA. Toll-like receptor 4 mediates inflammatory signaling by bacterial lipopolysaccharide in human hepatic stellate cells. *Hepatology.* (2003) 37:1043–55. doi: 10.1053/jhep.2003.50182
109. Muriel P, Escobar Y. Kupffer cells are responsible for liver cirrhosis induced by carbon tetrachloride. *J Appl Toxicol.* (2003) 23:103–8. doi: 10.1002/jat.892
110. Rivera CA, Bradford BU, Hunt KJ, Adachi Y, Schrum LW, Koop DR, et al. Attenuation of CCl4 induced hepatic fibrosis by GdCl3 treatment or dietary glycine. *Am J Physiol Gastrointest Liver Physiol.* (2001) 281:G200–7. doi: 10.1152/ajpgi.2001.281.1.G200
111. Sakaida I, Hironaka K, Terai S, Okita K. Gadolinium chloride reverses dimethylnitrosamine (DMN)-induced rat liver fibrosis with increased matrix metalloproteinases (MMPs) of Kupffer cells. *Life Sci.* (2003) 72:943–59. doi: 10.1016/S0024-3205(02)02342-1
112. Thomas JA, Pope C, Wojtacha D, Robson AJ, Gordon-Walker TT, Hartland S, et al. Macrophage therapy for murine liver fibrosis recruits host effector cells improving fibrosis, regeneration, function. *Hepatology.* (2011) 53:2003–15. doi: 10.1002/hep.24315
113. Ramachandran P, Pellicoro A, Vernon MA, Boulter L, Aucott RL, Ali A, et al. Differential Ly-6C expression identifies the recruited macrophage phenotype, which orchestrates the regression of murine liver fibrosis. *Proc Natl Acad Sci USA.* (2012) 109:E3186–95. doi: 10.1073/pnas.1119964109
114. Oakley F, Meso M, Iredale JP, Green K, Marek CJ, Zhou X, et al. Inhibition of inhibitor of kappaB kinases stimulates hepatic stellate cell apoptosis and accelerated recovery from rat liver fibrosis. *Gastroenterology.* (2005) 128:108–20. doi: 10.1053/j.gastro.2004.10.003
115. Duffield JS, Forbes SJ, Constandinou CM, Clay S, Partolina M, Vuthoori S, et al. Selective depletion of macrophages reveals distinct, opposing roles during liver injury and repair. *J Clin Invest.* (2005) 115:56–65. doi: 10.1172/JCI200522675
116. Friedman SL, Arthur MJ. Activation of cultured rat hepatic lipocytes by Kupffer cell conditioned medium. Direct enhancement of matrix synthesis and stimulation of cell proliferation via induction of platelet-derived growth factor receptors. *J Clin Invest.* (1989) 84:1780–5. doi: 10.1172/JCI114362
117. Minter RM, Fan MH, Sun J, Niederbichler A, Ipaktchi K, Arbabi S, et al. Altered Kupffer cell function in biliary obstruction. *Surgery.* (2005) 138:236–45. doi: 10.1016/j.surg.2005.04.001
118. El Kasmi KC, Anderson AL, Devereaux MW, Fillon SA, Harris JK, Lovell MA, et al. Toll-like receptor 4-dependent Kupffer cell activation and liver injury in a novel mouse model of parenteral nutrition and intestinal injury. *Hepatology.* (2012) 55:1518–28. doi: 10.1002/hep.25500
119. Sekiya T, Oda T, Matsuura K, Akiyama T. Transcriptional regulation of the TGF-beta pseudoreceptor BAMBI by TGF-beta signaling. *Biochem Biophys Res Commun.* (2004) 320:680–4. doi: 10.1016/j.bbrc.2004.06.017
120. Sekiya T, Adachi S, Kohu K, Yamada T, Higuchi O, Furukawa Y, et al. Identification of BMP and activin membrane-bound inhibitor (BAMBI), an inhibitor of transforming growth factor-beta signaling, as a target of the beta-catenin pathway in colorectal tumor cells. *J Biol Chem.* (2004) 279:6840–6. doi: 10.1074/jbc.M310876200
121. Wang LJ, Bai L, Su D, Zhang T, Mao ZY. Proinflammatory conditions promote hepatocellular carcinoma onset and progression via activation of Wnt and EGFR signaling pathways. *Mol Cell Biochem.* (2013) 381:173–81. doi: 10.1007/s11010-013-1700-0
122. Isayama F, Hines IN, Kremer M, Milton RJ, Byrd CL, Perry AW, et al. LPS signaling enhances hepatic fibrogenesis caused by experimental cholestasis in mice. *Am J Physiol Gastrointest Liver Physiol.* (2006) 290:G1318–28. doi: 10.1152/ajpgi.00405.2005
123. Saito JM, Bostick MK, Campe CB, Xu J, Maher JJ. Infiltrating neutrophils in bile duct ligated livers do not promote hepatic fibrosis. *Hepatol Res.* (2003) 25:180–91. doi: 10.1016/S1386-6346(02)00247-4
124. Isogawa M, Robek MD, Furuichi Y, Chisari FV. Toll-like receptor signaling inhibits hepatitis B virus replication *in vivo*. *J Virol.* (2005) 79:7269–72. doi: 10.1128/JVI.79.11.7269-7272.2005
125. Chen M, Liu J, Yang W, Ling W. Lipopolysaccharide mediates hepatic stellate cell activation by regulating autophagy and retinoic acid signaling. *Autophagy.* (2017) 13:1813–27. doi: 10.1080/15548627.2017.1356550
126. Nakanishi K, Kaji K, Kitade M, Kubo T, Furukawa M, Saikawa S, et al. Exogenous administration of low-dose lipopolysaccharide potentiates liver fibrosis in a choline-deficient L-Amino-acid-defined diet-induced murine steatohepatitis model. *Int J Mol Sci.* (2019) 20:2724. doi: 10.3390/ijms20112724
127. Kamada Y, Matsumoto H, Tamura S, Fukushima J, Kiso S, Fukui K, et al. Hypoadiponectinemia accelerates hepatic tumor formation in a nonalcoholic steatohepatitis mouse model. *J Hepatol.* (2007) 47:556–64. doi: 10.1016/j.jhep.2007.03.020
128. Mazagova M, Wang L, Anfora AT, Wissmueller M, Lesley SA, Miyamoto Y, et al. Commensal microbiota is hepatoprotective and prevents liver fibrosis in mice. *FASEB J.* (2015) 29:1043–55. doi: 10.1096/fj.14-259515
129. Robert S, Gicquel T, Bodin A, Fautrel A, Barreto E, Victoni T, et al. Influence of inflammasome pathway activation in macrophages on the matrix metalloproteinase expression of human hepatic stellate cells. *Int Immunopharmacol.* (2019) 72:12–20. doi: 10.1016/j.intimp.2019.03.060
130. Thirunavukkarasu C, Watkins S, Gandhi, CR. Superoxide-induced apoptosis of activated rat hepatic stellate cells. *J Hepatol.* (2004) 41:567–75. doi: 10.1016/j.jhep.2004.06.023
131. Jameel NM, Thirunavukkarasu C, Wu T, Watkins C, Friedman SL, Gandhi CR. p38-MAPK and caspase-3-mediated superoxide-induced apoptosis of rat hepatic stellate cells: reversal by retinoic acid. *J Cell Physiol.* (2009) 218:157–66. doi: 10.1002/jcp.21581
132. Houglum K, Buck M, Kim DJ, Chojkier M. TNF-alpha inhibits liver collagen-alpha 1(I) gene expression through a tissue-specific regulatory region. *Am J Physiol.* (1998) 274:G840–7. doi: 10.1152/ajpgi.1998.274.5.G840
133. Iraburu MJ, Dominguez-Rosales JA, Fontana L, Auster A, García-Trevijano ER, Covarrubias-Pinedo A, et al. Tumor necrosis factor alpha down-regulates expression of the alpha1 (I) collagen gene in rat hepatic stellate cells through a p20C/EBPbeta- and C/EBPdelta-dependent mechanism. *Hepatology.* (2000) 31:1086–93. doi: 10.1053/he.2000.5981
134. Zhao J, Crowe DL, Castillo C, Wuenschell C, Chai Y, Warburton D. Smad7 is a TGF-beta-inducible attenuator of Smad2/3-mediated inhibition of embryonic lung morphogenesis. *Mech Dev.* (2000) 93:71–81. doi: 10.1016/S0925-4773(00)00281-1
135. Tahashi Y, Matsuzaki K, Date M, Yoshida K, Furukawa F, Sugano Y, et al. Differential regulation of TGF-β signal in hepatic stellate cells between acute and chronic rat liver injury. *Hepatology.* (2002) 35:49–61. doi: 10.1053/jhep.2002.30083
136. Quezada M, Wang J, Hoang V, McGee EA. Smad7 is a transforming growth factor-beta-inducible mediator of apoptosis in granulosa cells. *Fertil Steril.* (2012) 97:1452–9.e1-6. doi: 10.1016/j.fertnstert.2012.03.024
137. Meng F, Wang K, Aoyama T, Grivennikov SI, Paik Y, Scholten D, et al. Interleukin-17 signaling in inflammatory, Kupffer cells, hepatic stellate cells exacerbates liver fibrosis in mice. *Gastroenterology.* (2012) 143:765–76.e3 doi: 10.1053/j.gastro.2012.05.049

138. Fabre T, Kared H, Friedman SL, Shoukry NH. IL-17A enhances the expression of profibrotic genes through upregulation of the TGF-β receptor on hepatic stellate cells in a JNK-dependent manner. *J Immunol.* (2014) 193:3925–33. doi: 10.4049/jimmunol.1400861
139. Kolls JK, Lindén A. Interleukin-17 family members and inflammation. *Immunity.* (2004) 21:467–76. doi: 10.1016/j.immuni.2004.08.018
140. Louis H, van Laethem JL, Wu W, Quertinmont E, Degraef C, van den Berg K, et al. Interleukin-10 controls neutrophilic infiltration, hepatocyte proliferation, liver fibrosis induced by carbon tetrachloride in mice. *Hepatology.* (1998) 28:1607–15. doi: 10.1002/hep.510280621
141. Knolle P, Schlaak J, Uhrig A, Kempf P, Meyer zum Büschenfelde KH, Gerken G. Human Kupffer cells secrete IL-10 in response to lipopolysaccharide (LPS) challenge. *J Hepatol.* (1995) 22:226–9. doi: 10.1016/0168-8278(95)80433-1
142. Matsukawa A, Hogaboam CM, Lukacs NW, Lincoln PM, Evanoff HL, Strieter RM, et al. Expression and contribution of endogenous IL-13 in an experimental model of sepsis. *J Immunol.* (2000) 164:2738–44. doi: 10.4049/jimmunol.164.5.2738
143. Valatas V, Kolios G, Manousou P, Xidakis C, Notas G, Ljumovic D, et al. Secretion of inflammatory mediators by isolated rat Kupffer cells: the effect of octreotide. *Regul Pept.* (2004) 120:215–25. doi: 10.1016/j.regpep.2004.03.009
144. Handy JA, Fu PP, Kumar P, Mells JE, Sharma S, Saxena NK, et al. Adiponectin inhibits leptin signalling via multiple mechanisms to exert protective effects against hepatic fibrosis. *Biochem J.* (2011) 440:385–395. doi: 10.1042/BJ20102148
145. Bonkovsky HL. Therapy of hepatitis C: other options. *Hepatology.* (1997) 26:S143–51. doi: 10.1002/hep.510260725
146. Hoofnagle JH, di Bisceglie AM. The treatment of chronic viral hepatitis. *N Engl J Med.* (1997) 336:347–56. doi: 10.1056/NEJM199701303360507
147. Fort J, Pilette Veal CN, Oberti F, Gallois Y, Douay O, et al. Effects of long-term administration of interferon alpha in two models of liver fibrosis in rats. *J Hepatol.* (1998) 29:263–70. doi: 10.1016/S0168-8278(98)80012-3
148. Okanoue T, Itoh Y, Minami M, Sakamoto S, Yasui K, Sakamoto M, et al. Interferon therapy lowers the rate of progression to hepatocellular carcinoma in chronic hepatitis C but not significantly in an advanced stage: a retrospective study in 1148 patients. viral hepatitis therapy study group. *J Hepatol.* (1999) 30:653–9. doi: 10.1016/S0168-8278(99)80196-2
149. Suzuki K, Aoki K, Ohnami S, Yoshida K, Kazui T, Kato N, et al. Adenovirus-mediated gene transfer of interferon alpha improves dimethylnitrosamine-induced liver cirrhosis in rat model. *Gene Ther.* (2003) 10:765–73. doi: 10.1038/sj.gt.3301949
150. Habersetzer F, Boyer N, Marcellin P, Bailly F, Ahmed SN, Alam J, et al. A pilot study of recombinant interferon beta-1a for the treatment of chronic hepatitis C. *Liver.* (2000) 20:437–41. doi: 10.1034/j.1600-0676.2000.020006437.x
151. Shen H, Zhang M, Minuk GY, Gong Y. Different effects of rat interferon alpha, beta and gamma on rat hepatic stellate cell. *BMC Cell Biol.* (2002) 3:9–13. doi: 10.1186/1471-2121-3-9
152. Rao HY, Wei L, Wang JH, Fei R, Jiang D. Inhibitory effect of human interferon-beta-1a on activated rat and human hepatic stellate cells. *J Gastroenterol Hepatol.* (2010) 25:1777–84. doi: 10.1111/j.1440-1746.2010.06264.x

7

Metabolomic Signatures of Autoimmune Hepatitis in the Development of Cirrhosis

Shan-shan Li[1,2], Ming Niu[3], Jing Jing[2], Ying Huang[2], Zi-teng Zhang[2], Shuai-shuai Chen[2], Ge-zi Shi[2], Xian He[1,2], Hai-zhu Zhang[1], Xiao-he Xiao[2], Zheng-sheng Zou[2], Yue-cheng Yu[4]* and Jia-bo Wang[2,5]**

[1] School of Pharmacy and Chemistry, Dali University, Dali, China, [2] Department of Liver Diseases, Fifth Medical Center of Chinese PLA General Hospital, Beijing, China, [3] Department of Poisoning Treatment, Fifth Medical Center of Chinese PLA General Hospital, Beijing, China, [4] Liver Diseases Center of General Hospital of PLA Eastern Theater Command, Bayi Hospital Affiliated to Nanjing University of Chinese Medicine, Nanjing, China, [5] School of Traditional Chinese Medicine, Capital Medical University, Beijing, China

***Correspondence:**
Jia-bo Wang
jiabo_wang@ccmu.edu.cn
Yue-cheng Yu
gslsycy@163.com
Zheng-sheng Zou
zszou302@163.com

Objectives: Autoimmune hepatitis (AIH) can progress into severe outcomes, i.e., decompensated cirrhosis, from remarkable and persistent inflammation in the liver. Considering the energy-expending nature of inflammation, we tried to define the metabolomics signatures of AIH to uncover the underlying mechanisms of cirrhosis development and its metabolic biomarkers.

Methods: Untargeted metabolomics analysis was performed on sera samples from 79 AIH patients at the stages (phenotypes) of non-cirrhosis ($n = 27$), compensated cirrhosis ($n = 22$), and decompensated cirrhosis ($n = 30$). Pattern recognition was used to find unique metabolite fingerprints of cirrhosis with or without decompensation.

Results: Out of the 294 annotated metabolites identified, 2 metabolic fingerprints were found associated with the development of cirrhosis (independent of the decompensated state, 42 metabolites) and the evolution of decompensated cirrhosis (out of 47 metabolites), respectively. The cirrhosis-associated fingerprints (eigenmetabolite) showed better capability to differentiate cirrhosis from non-cirrhosis patients than the aminotransferase-to-platelet ratio index. From the metabolic fingerprints, we found two pairs of metabolites (Mesobilirubinogen/6-Hydroxynicotinic acid and LysoPA(8:0/0:0)/7alpha-Hydroxycholesterol) calculated as ratio of intensities, which revealed robust abilities to identify cirrhosis or predict decompensated patients, respectively. These phenotype-related fingerprint metabolites featured fundamental energy supply disturbance along with the development of AIH cirrhosis and progression to decompensation, which was characterized as increased lipolysis, enhanced proteolysis, and increased glycolysis.

Conclusions: Remodeling of metabolism to meet the liver inflammation-related energy supply is one of the key signatures of AIH in the development of cirrhosis and decompensation. Therefore, drug regulation metabolism has great potential in the treatment of AIH.

Keywords: liver cirrhosis, autoimmune hepatitis, metabolomics, metabolic pathway, biomarkers

INTRODUCTION

Autoimmune hepatitis (AIH) is an inflammatory disease of the liver mediated by an abnormal autoimmune response (1). The pathogenesis of AIH is not fully understood. AIH patients may have long-term asymptomatic tissue inflammation, but they are often not diagnosed, thus losing treatment opportunities. When clinical symptoms appear, the disease may have progressed to a more severe stage, and may even further progress to cirrhosis, decompensation of liver function and eventually liver failure (2, 3). AIH cirrhosis has no specific clinical manifestations in the compensated stage; When the disease progresses to the decompensated stage, liver dysfunction and portal hypertension will appear. Decompensated patients may also experience symptoms such as gastrointestinal bleeding, liver ascites, and coma. Liver transplantation is an effective treatment for decompensated patients (4), but AIH may recur after transplantation. Although AIH is a disease mediated by autoimmune abnormalities and autoantibodies are important for the diagnosis of AIH, serum autoantibodies do not reflect the severity of the disease in AIH patients (5). Looking for biomarkers that can predict the progression of liver cirrhosis and malignancy in AIH patients is of immense significance in the clinical prognosis and understanding of the underlying mechanism of disease progression.

AIH is mainly characterized by liver inflammation, which is essentially a chronic and unresolved liver inflammatory damage (6). Inflammation is an energy-expensive biological process that requires a large amount of energy and intermediary metabolites for the synthesis of inflammatory factors and immune response (7). Continuous hepatic inflammation inevitably causes significant metabolic changes and induces a wide range of catabolic dysfunction, which may be involved in the progression of the disease. The liver is the main metabolic organ, responsible for most of the body's metabolic processes such as synthesis, decomposition, and transformation (8), thus, it is very important to study AIH from the perspective of metabolism.

Metabolomics is a phenotypic method for studying metabolites, small molecule substrates, and intermediary metabolites, which directly reflects potential biochemical activity and state of cells/tissues (9). Furthermore, it is a powerful method to explore specific biomarkers of liver diseases (10). In recent years, non-targeted metabolomics has been applied to the study of AIH-related biomarkers (11–13), but there is no research related to disease progression of AIH.

Here, we report the findings of untargeted and whole spectrum metabolomic study in sera from 79 AIH patients and compare the metabolic markers of liver cirrhosis and decompensation. The aim of this study is to characterize the sera metabolite fingerprints specific to patients with compensated or decompensated AIH cirrhosis, and to identify potential prognostic biomarkers of AIH.

MATERIALS AND METHODS

Study Design

We explored the sera samples of hospitalized AIH patients in the Biobank of Fifth Medical Center of Chinese PLA General Hospital from October 31st, 2015 to May 19th, 2017. Patients diagnosed with AIH and where adequate clinical information was available, were selected for the study. This research scheme was approved by the Ethics Committee of the hospital based on the ethical principles of the Declaration of Helsinki, and written informed consent was obtained from all patients. Their sera had to be deposited within 4 days after diagnosis. Patients with competitive etiologies were excluded. There are 89 AIH patients initially screened, and 10 of them were excluded due to competitive etiologies. Among those 10 excluded patients, 8 had concurrent drug-induced liver injury and 2 had alcoholic liver disease. Finally, 79 patients were enrolled in the study. The enrolled samples were divided into three groups: non-cirrhosis (NC) ($n = 27$), compensated cirrhosis (CC) ($n = 22$), and decompensated cirrhosis (DC) ($n = 30$) groups, according to the international clinical guidelines (14). Based on untargeted metabolomics, we acquired numerous metabolites (metabolome profile) with significant difference ($P < 0.05$ and FC >1.5 or <0.67) by comparing CC and DC with NC and marked them as (CC+DC)/NC. Metabolites identified in metabolome profiles were considered as ones with cirrhosis-associated metabolome features. Similarly, by comparing CC or DC with NC, they were marked as CC/NC and DC/NC, respectively. The excluded part of DC/NC can be considered as decompensation-associated metabolome features. Also, hierarchical clustering was used to screen out the metabolic fingerprints, which consisted of a cluster of metabolites with high area under curve (AUC) of the receiver operating characteristic (ROC) analysis and P-values, in differentiating each group (phenotype). Furthermore, the phenotype-associated fingerprint metabolites were projected to one eigenmetabolite by reducing the dimension, which is defined as the first principal component in unsupervised principal component analysis (PCA) (15). The eigenmetabolite was further investigated to discover relationships with demographics, biochemistry, complications, and clinical evaluation models. Finally, metabolic pathways of phenotype-associated fingerprint metabolites were analyzed to interpret the underlying mechanisms of the metabolic drivers in the evolution of AIH.

Samples Preparation and Chromatographic Conditions

The biobanked serum were processed according to the literature (16). Quality control samples (QC) were prepared by mixing 10 μL from each sample to be analyzed. Chromatographic column: ZORBOX RRHD C18 analytical column (2.1 mm i.d. × 100 mm, 1.8 μm i.d., Agilent Technologies, USA). Column temperature: 30°C. Sample temperature: 4°C. The mobile phase was composed of solvent A: Water with 0.1% formic acid in positive mode of Q-TOF, pure water in negative mode, mobile phase B: Acetonitrile. Flow rate: 0.30 mL/min; Sample injection size: 4 μL. Chromatographic gradient elution conditions: 0–1 min, 100% (A); 1–9 min, 100%-60% (A); 9–19 min, 60–10% (A); 19–21 min, 10–0% (A); 21–25 min, 100% (B).

Mass Spectrum Condition

An Agilent 6550 Q-TOF LC/MS with an electrospray ionization source (ESI) in positive and negative ion modes was used.

TABLE 1 | Clinical information comparison between liver disease patients with NC, CC, and DC.

	Non-cirrhosis (*n* = 27)	Compensated cirrhosis (*n* = 22)	Decompensated cirrhosis (*n* = 30)	P^a	P^b
Age/year	51(42,56)	54(50,63)	57.5(51.0,67.0)	0.224	0.274
Female, *n* (%)	27(100.0)	18(81.8)	28(93.3)	–	–
ALT/U·L^{-1}	30.0(12.0,96.0)	35.5(20.3,145.8)	32.0(22.0,76.8)	0.26	0.663
AST/U·L^{-1}	59.0(26.0,121.0)	75.0(30.8,171.5)	49.5(36.8,117.8)	0.148	0.788
AST/ALT	1.4(1.1,2.2)	1.6(0.9,2.4)	1.8(1.3,2.7)	0.702	0.404
ALP/U·L^{-1}	105.0(79.0,184.0)	135.0(114.8,190.8)	118.5(90.3,224.0)	0.067	0.437
GGT/U·L^{-1}	67.0(15.0,197.0)	94.0(48.3,164.3)	49.5(26.3,181.5)	0.501	0.47
TBil /mg·dl^{-1}	14.2(10.2,22.4)	22.3(13.5,61.4)	26.6(11.8,83.5)	0.03	0.624
DBil/μmo·L^{-1}	5.7(3.3,12.0)	11.6(5.3,47.1)	14.5(5.4,66.5)	0.027	0.657
IgA/g·L^{-1}	2.6(1.9,3.5)	2.9(1. 9,4.6)	3.7(2.4,6.2)	0.488	0.154
IgG/g·L^{-1}	15.0(12.1,21.3)	21.6(15.5,24.0)	20.4(16.2,25.8)	0.062	0.97
IgM/g·L^{-1}	1.2(0.8,1.7)	1.7(0.9,2.9)	1.7(1.1,2.3)	0.093	0.795
CHE/U·L^{-1}	5241.0(4877.0,7125.0)	4192.0(2938.3,6100.5)	2883.0(1984.8,4037.3)	0.011	0.005
INR/IU	1.0(0.9,1.0)	1.1(1.0,1.2)	1.1(1.0,1.3)	0.005	0.194
TC/mmol·L^{-1}	4.2(3.7,5.0)	3.8(2.8,4.7)	3.3(2.7,4.0)	0.151	0.243
TG/mmol·L-1	1.1(0.9,1.5)	1.3(0.8,1.7)	1.0(0.8,1.6)	0.96	0.535
ALB/g·L-1	36.0(34.0,40.0)	33.0(29.5,37.0)	29.5(25.8,33.3)	0.025	0.05
WBC/mm^3	5140.0(4340.0,6800.0)	3825.0(3155.0,4777.5)	3850.0(2852.5,5010.0)	0.005	0.926
PLT/10^9·L^{-1}	195.0(168.0,223.0)	101.0(62.5,158.0)	84.0(53.5,124.5)	<0.01	0.229
TBA/umol·L-1	22.0(7.0,37.0)	35.5(17.3,97.8)	47.0(16.0,108.3)	0.033	0.853
Cr/umol·L-1	59.0(51.0,70.0)	60.0(53.5,65.8)	66.0(60.5,74.3)	0.371	0.081
PT /s	11.2(10.6,11.7)	12.3(11.0,13.7)	12.8(11.2,14.7)	0.008	0.188
ANA	1:100(1:486,1:100)	1:320(1:1,000,1:100)	1:320(1:1000,1:100)	0.102	0.669
γ-globulin/%	24.0(18.0,28.8)	29.4(22.4,33.8)	32.0(25.6,35.0)	0.052	0.4
With ascites (%)	0(0.00)	0(0.00)	26(86.7)	–	–
With HE (%)	0(0.00)	0(0.00)	0(0.00)	–	–
APRI score	31.9(12.8,55.8)	69.9(35.8,185.4)	97.2(38.3,159.9)	0.004	0.697

All clinical information in the table indicates data collected at the time closest to blood collection.
Median and quartile values are provided as Median (upper quartile, lower quartile), unless otherwise noted as n (%). P^a is the significant difference comparison between non-cirrhosis and compensated cirrhosis patients, P^b between compensated and decompensated cirrhosis patients.
ALT, alanine aminotransferase. AST, aspartate transaminase. ALP, alkaline phosphatase. GGT, γ-glutamyl transpeptidase. TBil, total bilirubin. DBil, direct bilirubin. IgA, immunoglobulin A. IgG, immunoglobulin G. IgM, immunoglobulin M. CHE, cholinesterase. INR, international normalized ratio. TC, total cholesterol. TG, triglyceride. ALB, albumin. WBC, white blood cell. PLT, platelet. TBA, total bile acid. Cr, creatinine. PT, prothrombin time. ANA, antinuclear. HE, hepatic encephalopathy. APRI, AST to PLT ratio index.

Non-targeted primary mass spectrometric detection conditions: The mass range of m/z 50–1,200; gas temperature of 225°C in both positive and negative ionization modes; airflow of 13 l/min; the nebulizer of 20 pisg (negative) and 20 pisg (positive); sheath gas temperature of 275°C and sheath gas flow of 12 l/min; electrospray capillary voltage of 3,500 V in negative ionization mode and 4,000 V in positive ionization mode; and nozzle voltage of 2,000 V in the positive and negative ion modes. The acquisition mode was ESI Continuum mode and 14,104 variables were captured in positive ion mode as well as 13,357 variables were captured in negative ion mode.

Statistical Analysis

All variables were normalized in MetaboAnalyst 4.0 (https://www.metaboan-alyst.ca) after being preprocessed in Masshunter Profinder software. Summarized results of the patients' clinical biochemical characteristics for continuous variable are expressed as median (upper quartile, lower quartile), and categorical variables are expressed as numbers and percentage. Comparisons between groups were made with Kruskal-Wallis H test. All statistical analysis was performed using SPSS 21.0 software. The significance level for all statistical tests was set at 0.05. PCA and orthogonal partial least squares discrimination analysis (OPLS-DA) were performed in SIMCA -P 14.1 software. The *P*-values, fold change (FC) and AUC of ROC were obtained from the MetaboAnalyst website. We narrowed down the original variables to fingerprint by *P*-value, FC, and AUC.

RESULTS

Baseline Demographic and Clinical Characteristics of the Study Cohort

The baseline demography and clinical characteristics among NC, CC, and DC groups are described in **Table 1**. There was no difference in the mean ages among the three groups. Except for 6 male patients, female patients accounted for an overwhelming proportion of AIH patients (n = 73, 92.41%). Between NC and CC groups, the levels of TBA, PT, and INR in CC were much higher than those in NC, and the levels of CHE, ALB, PLT, and WBC in CC were significantly lower than those in NC. Significantly lower levels of ALB and CHE were found in DC groups as compared to the CC group. With respect to complications, 86.67% of patients in the DC group had ascites. Besides, there was no hepatic encephalopathy in AIH patients. Aminotransferase-to-platelet ratio index (APRI) score showed an increasing trend along with the development of cirrhosis from NC to CC and DC.

Patients With Cirrhosis Exhibited Different Anabolism and Metabolism Characteristics

Compared to non-cirrhotic AIH patients, those that developed into the cirrhosis stage (CC or DC) showed different characteristics, including sera enzymes, liver-synthesizing proteins, liver-metabolizing metabolites, and coagulation function (**Table 1**). When cirrhosis developed, significant decrease in albumin and white blood cell counts were observed. The coagulation function indices (prothrombin time and international normalized ratio) increased significantly, but were not significant between CC and DC groups. Bilirubin (TBiL and DBiL) increased significantly in the CC group compared to the NC group, indicating potential liver dysfunction of detoxication. Along with the evolving disease stages, cholinesterase decreased significantly. Together, these results indicated a gradual disturbance of liver functions such as anabolism and metabolism in the evolution of AIH.

Liver Cirrhosis and Decompensation Stages Associated With Different Sera Metabolites

We observed significant alterations in the metabolomic profiles from either positive or negative modes of mass spectrometry, in different stages of AIH (**Figures 1A–D**). This indicates that the progression from NC to CC and DC was a major contributor for the alteration of the sera metabolome. To explore the underlying relationship between the evolving stages of AIH and the patterns of sera metabolite levels, we firstly obtained metabolic entities with significant difference ($P < 0.05$) between NC and CC, as well as CC vs. DC. The Venn diagram of these metabolic entities showed over 1,200 metabolites (including both positive and negative modes) that were associated with cirrhosis [(CC+DC) vs. NC]; while over 1,600 metabolites were solely associated with decompensation (DC vs. CC) (**Figures 1E,F**). We then identified 124 and 170 metabolites in these two sets of variables, respectively. Based on these metabolites, we found that the PCA plot of 124 cirrhosis-related metabolites showed an obvious separation of NC from either CC or DC, while CC and DC overlapped (**Figure 1G**). The PCA plot of the 170 decompensation-related metabolites revealed an evident separation of DC from either CC or NC, while CC and NC were located in the same zone (**Figure 1H**). These results indicate two distinct metabolic features associated with cirrhosis or decompensation stages. The fold changes of these annotated metabolites between the study groups are showed in **Supplementary Figure 1**.

Cirrhosis-Associated Sera Metabolites Composed of a Fingerprint for AIH-Related Liver Cirrhosis

To reduce the dimension of the data set and find a unique metabolomic fingerprint of AIH-related liver cirrhosis, we computed the AUC and *P*-values of each of the 124 cirrhosis-related metabolites in differentiating cirrhosis (either CC or DC) from non-cirrhosis (NC). The resulting AUCs and associated *P*-values were used for a hierarchical cluster analysis and shown in a heat-map, indicating the highest relevant cluster (including 42 metabolites) with a highly significant association with cirrhosis [**Supplementary Figure 2 (I)**]. The AUC values in this cluster for cirrhosis ranged from 0.6786 to 0.7835 with significant *P*-values (**Supplementary Tables 1, 3**). Interestingly, the 42-metabolite cluster identified in **Supplementary Figure 2 (I)**, the high AUC values observed in cirrhosis (either CC or DC) were maintained when patients were separated into CC or DC groups [**Supplementary Figure 2(II,III)**]. These results indicate a unique metabolome fingerprint (42 metabolites) among patients with cirrhosis.

To further display the metabolome fingerprint trend in AIH development, we computed an eigenmetabolite (15) using PCA as a representative variable of the aforementioned 42-metabolite cluster. The eigenmetabolite showed progressively decreasing trend across the different stages of AIH and reached a minimum in DC (**Figure 2A**). Interestingly, there was a significant decrease of the eigenmetabolite in CC compared to NC, but no significance was observed between CC and DC. This trend supports the result that the 42 metabolites represented a metabolic fingerprint for AIH-related liver cirrhosis.

Cirrhosis-Associated Metabolic Fingerprint Showed Better Diagnostic Performance in Discerning AIH Cirrhosis Than That of APRI

We found that the cirrhosis-associated metabolic fingerprint (eigenmetabolite) had better capability of identifying cirrhotic from non-cirrhotic patients than APRI (AUC values 0.874 vs. 0.763, **Figures 2B,C**). Collectively, these findings indicate that the 42-metabolite cluster can serve as a fingerprint of sera metabolites, which characteristically differentiated cirrhosis from non-cirrhosis.

Decompensation-Associated Sera Metabolites Composed a Fingerprint for Differentiating Decompensation Stage

Similarly, for each of the 170 metabolites in decompensation-associated metabolome feature, we computed the AUC assessing the differentiation accuracy of each metabolite in decompensated cirrhosis from the compensation stage. The resulting AUCs and associated *P*-values were used for a hierarchical cluster analysis, which identified the highest relevant cluster including 47 metabolites with a highly significant association with cirrhosis (AUC for cirrhosis and significant *P* shown in

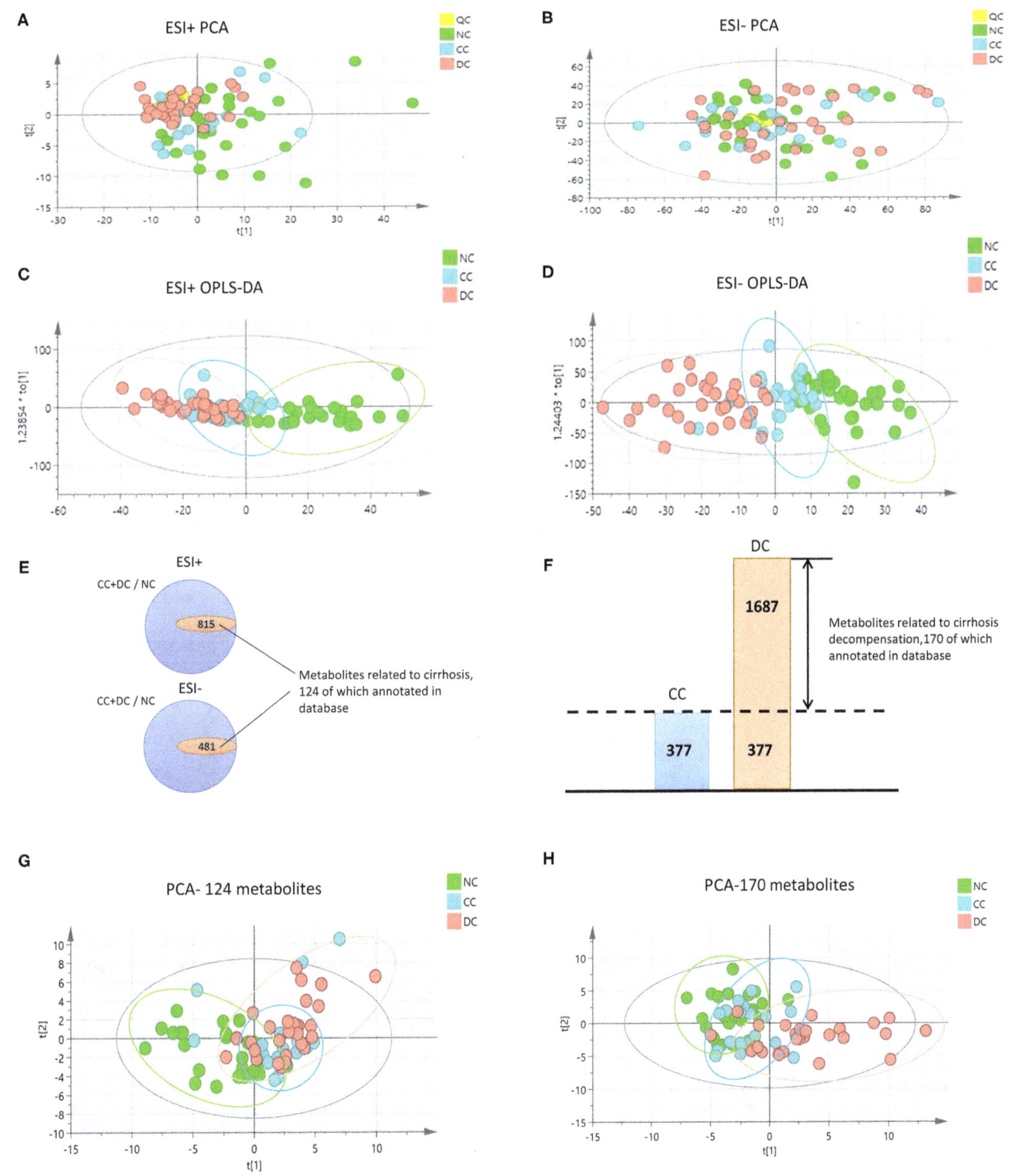

FIGURE 1 | Metabolome profile for cirrhosis at different period. **(A–D)** are PCA and OPLS-DA with whole variables among NC, CC, and DC under positive and negative model. The great difference among NC, CC, and DC under OPLS-DA demonstrated the difference among groups. **(E,F)** Venn diagram. **(E)** The inner parts means the set of variables related to progression of cirrhosis, 124 of which annotated in database was metabolome feature for cirrhosis. **(F)** The part of DC was the set of variables related to decompensation, 170 of which annotated in database was metabolome feature for decompensation. **(G,H)** are PCA among NC, CC, and DC with metabolome feature for cirrhosis and decompensation. They showed that great discrimination of NC and DC respectively.

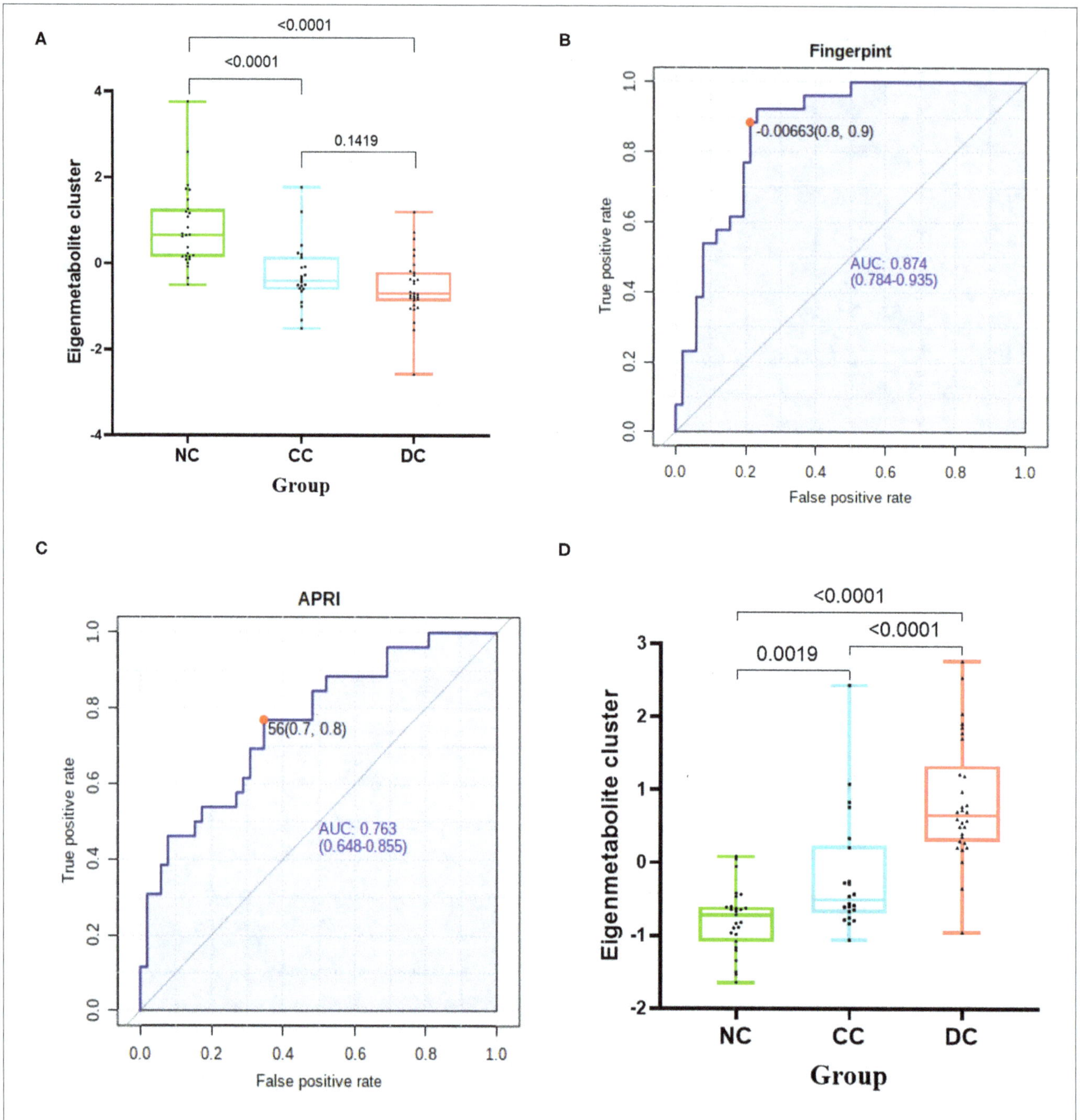

FIGURE 2 | Identification of cirrhosis-related metabolome fingerprint. **(A)** Showed the decreasing trend of eigenmetabolite of metabolome fingerprint along with the progression of cirrhosis. **(B)** Demonstrated the cirrhosis-associated metabolic fingerprint (eigenmetabolite) revealed better capability to identify cirrhotic patients from non-cirrhotic ones(AUC:0.874). **(C)** The ROC curve of APRI in discriminating cirrhosis from non-cirrhotic AIH patients(AUC:0.763). **(D)** Showed that the increasing trend of eigenmetabolite of metabolome fingerprint from NC to CC and DC.

[**Supplementary Figure 3**, **Supplementary Table 2**]). We then computed an eigenmetabolite by PCA, which is representative of the 47-metabolite cluster and correlated the eigenmetabolite with the progression of AIH, from NC to CC and DC (**Figure 2D**). The eigenmetabolite showed an increasing trend and significant differences (all $P < 0.05$) among NC, CC, and DC.

Metabolic Fingerprints Indicating Loss of Liver Anabolic Functions

We further compared trends of the two metabolic fingerprints separately using clinically important indices (14, 17, 18). Cirrhosis-associated eigenmetabolite were significantly higher in NC and CC patients with high-albumin (**Figure 3A**), which

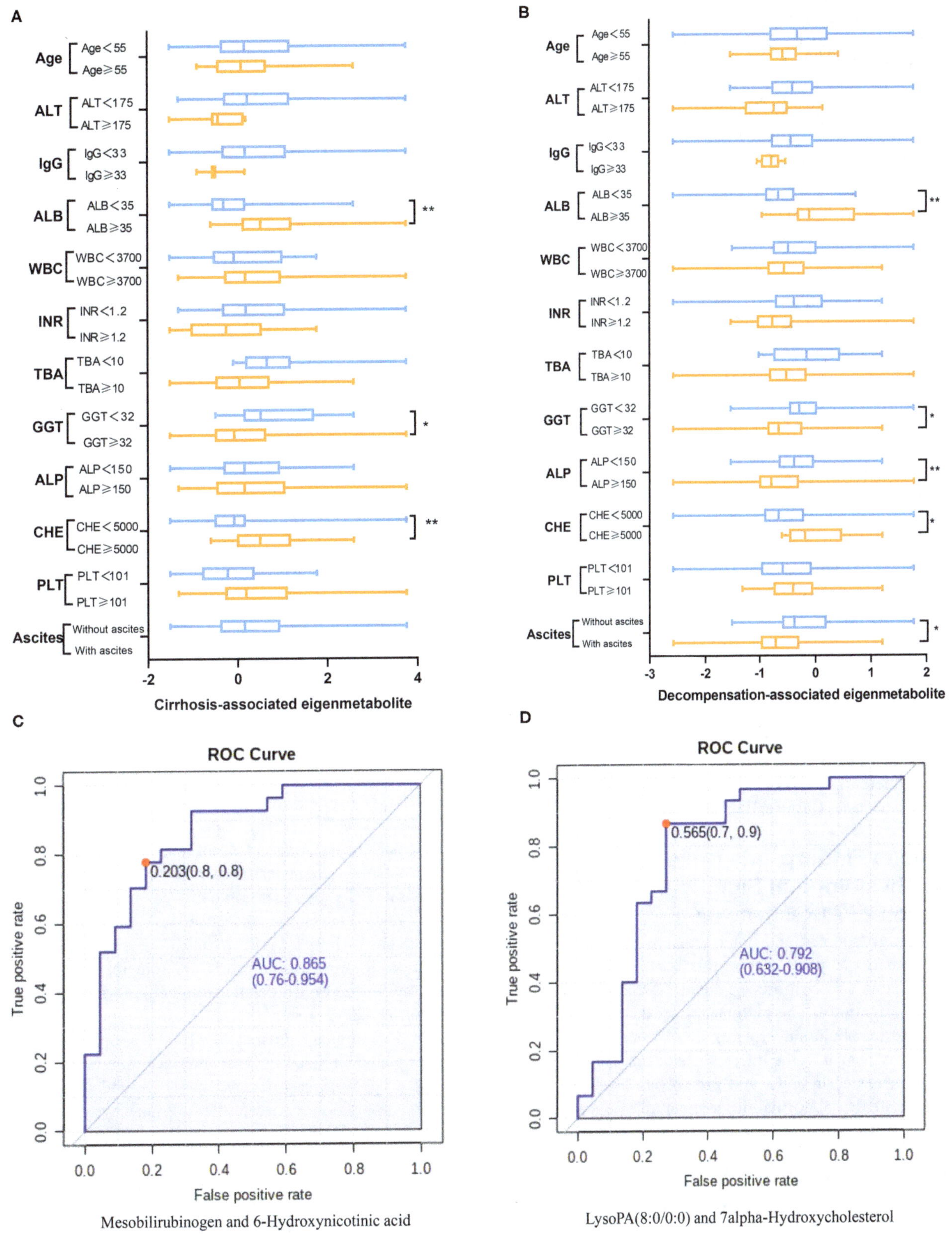

FIGURE 3 | Clinical associations of the two metabolic fingerprints and the diagnostic ability of paired metabolites. **(A)** Comparison between clinical indices and the cirrhosis-associated fingerprint (eigenmetabolite) in NC and CC patients. **(B)** Comparison between clinical indices and the decompensation-associated fingerprint (eigenmetabolite) in CC and DC patients. **(C)** The diagnosis ability of intensity ratio between Mesobilirubinogen and 6-Hydroxynicotinic acid to differentiate NC and CC. **(D)** The diagnosis ability of intensity ratio between LysoPA(8:0/0:0) and 7alpha-Hydroxycholesterol to differentiate CC and DC(The units of each index are indicated in **Table 1**).

indicates the loss of liver anabolic function in cirrhotic AIH patients. Albumin-associated scores may be useful to evaluate long-term prognosis in patients with autoimmune-related hepatic cirrhosis (19). Similarly, high level of eigenmetabolite was observed in patients with high cholinesterase. In some clinical indices, decompensation-associated metabolic fingerprint in CC and DC patients had significant alterations in their subgroups (**Figure 3B**). Notably, significant *P*-value also existed between patients with low-albumin and high-albumin indicating further loss of liver anabolic functions in decompensated cirrhotic patients. In addition, high level of alkaline phosphatase corelated with low level of decompensation-associated eigenmetabolite, indicating low anabolic liver function (20, 21). Besides, low levels of eigenmetabolite were observed in patients with high γ-glutamyl transpeptidase in cirrhosis and decompensated patients. Gamma-glutamyl transpeptidase and albumin were independent predictors of significant fibrosis (22, 23). In cirrhotic patients with ascites, low level of decompensation-associated eigenmetabolite was observed compared to non-ascites patients.

Paired Metabolites Reveal Diagnostic and Prognostic Capability for AIH

From the cirrhosis-associated fingerprint, a metabolites pair—Mesobilirubinogen and 6-Hydroxynicotinic acid—was further screened out to construct a novel diagnostic parameter to identify AIH-related cirrhosis patients (**Figure 3C**). The diagnostic ability of such paired metabolites is based on the intensity ratio, which was 0.865 of AUC. The intensity ratio of paired metabolites can eliminate the differences between instruments and provide better methodology and good applicability for clinical use. Similarly, another metabolites pair—LysoPA(8:0/0:0) and 7alpha-Hydroxycholesterol—was screened out from the decompensation-associated fingerprint and achieved 0.792 of AUC in differentiating decompensated cirrhosis from non-decompensated ones (**Figure 3D**).

Metabolic Fingerprints Have Potential Pathophysiological Significance in the Evolution of AIH Cirrhosis

Several energy sources and intermediary metabolites in the plasma of patients with liver cirrhosis changed significantly compared to non-cirrhosis patients, which indicates a particularly significant energy metabolism disorder. We found that the two metabolic fingerprints are obviously related to the energy supply related to the interference of metabolic pathways, especially increased lipolysis and proteolysis (**Figure 4**). These results indicate that abnormalities in metabolic fingerprints may be involved in the progression of the disease.

AIH Cirrhosis Associates With Increased Lipolysis

In the two metabolic fingerprints for different stages of AIH, a typical feature is that a series of metabolites related to long-chain fatty acids (e.g.,12,13-DHOME, trans-2-Enoyl-OPC4-CoA, Docosadienoyl-CoA, Tetrac-osatetraenoyl-CoA and (S)-3-Hydroxydodecanoyl-CoA, etc.) are significantly reduced (**Supplementary Tables 1, 2**). Increased lipolysis and suppressed lipogenesis strikingly promote the energy supplying flux by fatty acids.

AIH Cirrhosis Associates With Increased Proteolysis

Due to a large amount of energy expenditure, a key feature of decompensated liver cirrhosis was observed to be used as energy supply by proteolysis (**Figure 4**). Several proteolysis markers Glutaminylphenylalanine, Hydroxyprolyl-Tyrosine, and Glutaminyltryptophan, and incomplete breakdown products of protein catabolism, increased significantly in DC group compared to the NC or CC groups (**Supplementary Table 3**).

DISCUSSION

This paper is the first study utilizing untargeted and whole-spectrum metabolomics approach in sera samples of AIH patients without cirrhosis or with cirrhosis at either compensation or decompensation stages. We identified two metabolic fingerprints for different stages of AIH. The fingerprint of metabolites related to liver cirrhosis includes 42 metabolites, reflecting the characteristic metabolic changes in the process of AIH progression to liver cirrhosis, without distinguishing between compensatory and decompensated states. Compared to non-invasive liver cirrhosis evaluation index APRI, liver cirrhosis-related metabolite fingerprints have a better diagnostic ability to distinguish between non-cirrhosis and liver cirrhosis. The metabolic fingerprint related to decompensation includes 47 metabolites, reflecting the characteristic metabolic changes from cirrhosis to the decompensated stage. These metabolic characteristics provide a new perspective to understand the underlying mechanism of AIH disease progression. Specifically, the analysis of pathway enrichment by combining two metabolic fingerprints indicates that AIH progresses to liver cirrhosis and decompensated stage, which is manifested by obvious disturbances in metabolic processes related to energy supply, and nutrient metabolism is the basic characteristic of decomposition and consumption. These metabolic characteristics are further strengthened from compensated cirrhosis to decompensated cirrhosis.

AIH-related immune response may be caused by the autoantigens of initial CD4+ T cells (24), which further forms continuous immune response and inflammatory reaction. There are many studies on the relationship between immunology and metabolism (25–27), but little is known about the metabolic adaptation and characteristics of AIH disease progression. AIH is mainly characterized by liver interface inflammation. As the disease progresses, it produces energy dependence, leading to energy competition between the immune system and other programs in the body. At the same time, the energy supply in the body is obviously disordered, and nutrients (such as lipids and proteins) are consumed in large quantities (7),which manifests as increased lipolysis and proteolysis. In this study, we found that a group of pathways involved in energy metabolism constituting the metabonomic characteristics of AIH. L-kynurenine and its further breakdown products carry out diverse biological functions, including dilating blood vessels during inflammation and regulating the immune response (28, 29). The elevation of

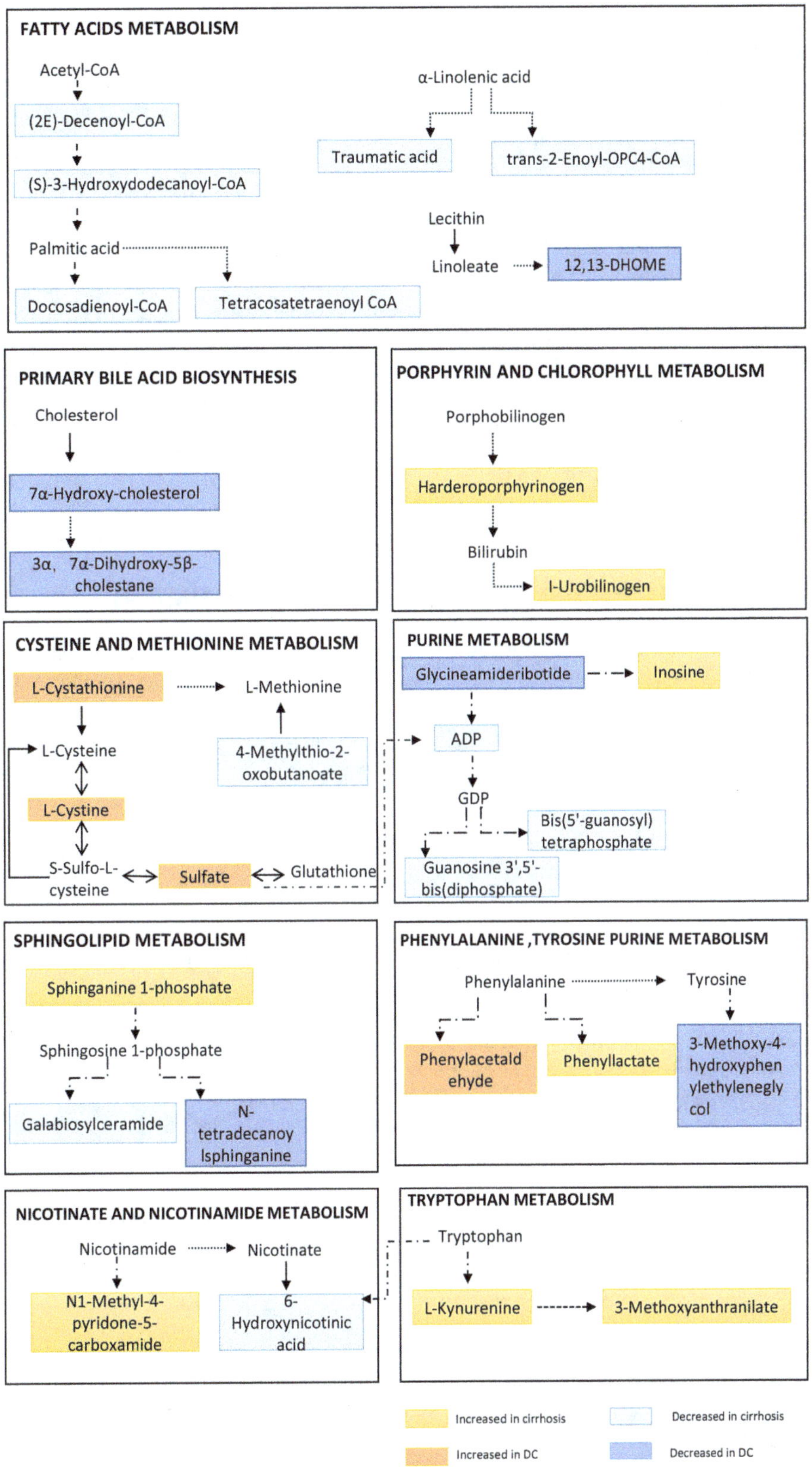

FIGURE 4 | Pathway enrichment of metabolites in metabolome fingerprint. A typical feature is that a series of metabolites related to long-chain fatty acids (e.g., 12,13-DHOME, trans-2-Enoyl-OPC4-CoA and Docosadienoyl-CoA, etc.) are significantly reduced. And, a key feature of decompensated liver cirrhosis was observed to be used as energy supply by proteolysis (incomplete breakdown products of protein catabolism increased significantly in DC group).

L-kynurenine is associated with the presence of inflammation and energy expenditure (7).

We also observed significant decrease of 7alpha-hydroxycholesterol (the catalyzing product of Cyp7a1) in decompensated autoimmune hepatic cirrhosis (30). Previous studies have shown that Cyp7a1 is positively associated with liver inflammation (31, 32). Cyp7a1 is the rate-limiting enzyme in the "classic pathway" of bile acids synthesis. The reduction of bile acid synthesis will inevitably cause the dynamic balance of enterohepatic circulation, which will lead to persistent inflammation in the liver (33). In addition, bile acids can help emulsify fat, enhance lipolysis, and improve the solubility of lipids by forming mixed micelles, promote the absorption of lipids in the intestine, and improve lipolysis. And, the interaction between bile acids and intestinal microbiota is not unidirectional. It is necessary to study the intestinal bacteria of AIH patients to elucidate the potential impact of gut microbial on bile acids metabolism and its further effects on liver immune and metabolic microenvironments. Interestingly, the metabolites related to long-chain fatty acids in the metabolic fingerprint of cirrhosis are all reduced, which indicate that β-oxidation of fatty acids is enhanced, and the body needs to consume a lot of energy for immune response and immune cell activation and proliferation (34). There are many proteins with incomplete catabolism in the fingerprint of decompensated metabolism. These findings imply that proteolysis may increase due to energy requirements. In previous reports, the skeletal muscles of rats have a significant accumulation of sphinganine and sphingosine after exercise, which may be related to the increase in energy requirements. Furthermore, ceramide promotes apoptosis whereas sphingosine-1-phosphate can inhibit apoptosis and induce cell growth. So, the reaction will tend to transform to sphingosine. Therefore, Galabiosyl ceramide and N-tetradecanoyl sphinganine will decrease (35).

Based on the favorable aspects of metabolic reprogramming mechanisms of AIH, we can explore the utility of characteristic metabolites to facilitate diagnosis or monitoring of disease progression. We therefore found that the intensity ratio of a pair of metabolites [Mesobilirubinogen and 6-Hydroxynicotinic acid] can be applied to recognizing cirrhosis in AIH patients; furthermore, the paired metabolites [LysoPA(8:0/0:0) and 7alpha-Hydroxycholesterol] can predict the development of decompensated cirrhosis for AIH. Since the intensity ratio of paired metabolites can eliminate the system bias of instruments in different laboratories, these metabolite pairs can be much easier to be applied in clinical settings. Compared with targeted quantitation of metabolites by mass spectrometry, the intensity ratio of paired metabolites is much cheaper and simpler (36).

In summary, liver metabolic dysfunction featuring enhanced lipolysis and increased proteolysis, may play an important role in the pathogenesis and progression of liver cirrhosis in AIH patients. The established metabolic fingerprint profile related to liver cirrhosis and decompensation can be used as a resource for metabolic adaptation and metabolic reprogramming of AIH, and provide guidance for future clinical prognosis, mechanisms, and new treatment research. Furthermore, this finding suggests that metabolic reprogramming may be a new direction in treating AIH.

ETHICS STATEMENT

The studies involving human participants were reviewed and approved by Medical Ethics Committee of Fifth Medical Center of Chinese PLA General Hospital. The patients/participants provided their written informed consent to participate in this study.

AUTHOR CONTRIBUTIONS

J-bW, Y-cY, and Z-sZ were responsible for the study concept and design. S-sL, JJ, S-sC, YH, ZS, G-zS, and XH performed sample collection, conducted LC-MS data analysis, and manuscript preparation. S-sL and J-bW drafted the manuscript. Z-tZ, H-zZ, Z-sZ, and Y-cY reviewed and modified the manuscript. MN helped with data analysis. All authors contributed to the article and approved the submitted version.

REFERENCES

1. Giorgina MV, Diego V, Albert JC, Michael PM, Edward LK, John MV. Autoimmune hepatitis. *Nat Rev Dis Primers.* (2018) 4:18018. doi: 10.1038/nrdp.2018.18
2. Mieli-Vergani G, Vergani D, Czaja AJ, Manns MP, Krawitt EL, Vierling JM, et al. Autoimmune hepatitis. *Nat Rev Dis Primers.* (2018) 4:18017. doi: 10.1038/nrdp.2018.17
3. Pape S, Schramm C, Gevers TJ. Clinical management of autoimmune hepatitis. *United European Gastroenterol J.* (2019) 7:1156–63. doi: 10.1177/2050640619872408
4. Liberal R, Grant CR. Cirrhosis and autoimmune liver disease: current understanding. *World J Hepatol.* (2016) 8:1157–68. doi: 10.4254/wjh.v8.i28.1157
5. Czaja AJ. Diagnosis and management of autoimmune hepatitis: current status and future directions. *Gut Liver.* (2016) 10:177. doi: 10.5009/gnl15352
6. Sucher E, Sucher R, Gradistanac T, Brandacher G, Schneeberger S, Berg T. Autoimmune hepatitis-immunologically triggered liver pathogenesis-diagnostic and therapeutic strategies. *J Immunol Res.* (2019) 2019:9437043. doi: 10.1155/2019/9437043
7. Clària J, Moreau R, Fenaille F, Amorós A, Junot C, Gronbaek H, et al. Orchestration of tryptophan-kynurenine pathway, acute decompensation, and acute-on-chronic liver failure in cirrhosis. *Hepatology.* (2019) 69:1686–701. doi: 10.1002/hep.30363
8. Trefts E, Gannon M, Wasserman DH. The liver. *Curr Biol.* (2017) 27: R1147–51. doi: 10.1016/j.cub.2017.09.019
9. Bujak R, Struck-Lewicka W, Markuszewski MJ, Kaliszan R. Metabolomics for laboratory diagnostics. *J Pharm Biomed Anal.* (2015) 113:108–20. doi: 10.1016/j.jpba.2014.12.017
10. Yu M, Zhu Y, Cong Q, Wu C. Metabonomics research progress on liver diseases. *Can J Gastroenterol Hepatol.* (2017) 2017:8467192. doi: 10.1155/2017/8467192

11. Zhou C, Jia HM, Liu YT, Yu M, Chang X, Ba YM, et al. Metabolism of glycerophospholipid, bile acid and retinol is correlated with the early outcomes of autoimmune hepatitis. *Mol bioSyst.* (2016) 12:1574–85. doi: 10.1039/C6MB00092D
12. Wang JB, Pu SB, Sun Y, Li ZF, Niu M, Yan XZ, et al. Metabolomic profiling of autoimmune hepatitis: the diagnostic utility of nuclear magnetic resonance spectroscopy. *J Proteome Res.* (2014) 13:3792–801. doi: 10.1021/pr500462f
13. Lytton SD, Osiecki M, MałgorzataWozniak, Cukrowska B, Wierzbicka A, Goliszek M, Socha P, et al. Tryptophan-kynurenine profile in pediatric autoimmune hepatitis. *Immunol Res.* (2019) 67:39–47. doi: 10.1007/s12026-019-9068-1
14. EASL Clinical Practice Guidelines: autoimmune hepatitis. *J Hepatol.* (2015) 63:971–1004. doi: 10.1016/j.jhep.2015.06.030
15. Moreau R, Clària J, Aguilar F, Fenaille F, Lozano JJ, Junot C, et al. Blood metabolomics uncovers inflammation-associated mitochondrial dysfunction as a potential mechanism underlying ACLF. *J Hepatol.* (2020) 72:688–701. doi: 10.1016/j.jhep.2019.11.009
16. Zhang L, Niu M, Wei AW, Tang JF, Tu C, Bai ZF, et al. Risk profiling using metabolomic characteristics for susceptible individuals of drug-induced liver injury caused by Polygonum multiflorum. *Arch Toxicol.* (2020) 94:245–56. doi: 10.1007/s00204-019-02595-3
17. Czaja AJ. Diagnosis and management of autoimmune hepatitis. *Clin Liver Dis.* (2015) 19:57–79. doi: 10.1016/j.cld.2014.09.004
18. Mack CL, Adams D, Assis DN, Kerkar N, Manns MP, Mayo MJ, et al. Diagnosis and management of autoimmune hepatitis in adults and children: 2019 practice guidance and guidelines from the American Association for the study of liver diseases. *Hepatology.* (2020) 72:671–722. doi: 10.1002/hep.31065
19. Song Y, Yang H, Lin L, Jiang K, Liu WT, Wang BM, et al. [Albumin-to-bilirubin scores for assessing the prognosis in autoimmune hepatitis-related cirrhosis]. *Zhonghua Gan Zang Bing Za Zhi.* (2019) 27:772–6. doi: 10.3760/cma.j.issn.1007-3418.2019.10.007
20. Lynch KD, Chapman RW, Keshav S, Montano-Loza AJ, Mason AL, Kremer AE, et al. Effects of vedolizumab in patients with primary sclerosing cholangitis and inflammatory bowel diseases. *Clin Gastroenterol Hepatol.* (2020) 18:179–87.e6. doi: 10.1016/j.cgh.2019.05.013
21. Trauner M, Gulamhusein A, Hameed B, Caldwell S, Shiffman ML, Landis C, et al. The nonsteroidal farnesoid X receptor agonist cilofexor (GS-9674) improves markers of cholestasis and liver injury in patients with primary sclerosing cholangitis. *Hepatology.* (2019) 70:788–801. doi: 10.1002/hep.30509
22. Li Q, Lu C, Li W, Huang Y, Chen L. The gamma-glutamyl transpeptidase-to-albumin ratio predicts significant fibrosis and cirrhosis in chronic hepatitis B patients. *J Viral Hepat.* (2017) 24:1143–50. doi: 10.1111/jvh.12751
23. Liu L, Lan Q, Lin L, Lu J, Ye C, Tao Q, et al. Gamma-glutamyl transpeptidase-to-platelet ratio predicts the prognosis in HBV-associated acute-on-chronic liver failure. *Clin Chim Acta.* (2018) 476:92–7. doi: 10.1016/j.cca.2017.11.017
24. Brahim I, Brahim I, Hazime R, Admou B. [Autoimmune hepatitis: immunological diagnosis]. *Presse Med.* (2017) 46:1008–19. doi: 10.1016/j.lpm.2017.08.012
25. Gatza E, Wahl DR, Opipari AW, Sundberg TB, Reddy P, Liu C, et al. Manipulating the bioenergetics of alloreactive T cells causes their selective apoptosis and arrests graft-versus-host disease. *Sci Transl Med.* (2011) 3:67ra8. doi: 10.1126/scitranslmed.3001975
26. Ito K, Ito K. Metabolism and the control of cell fate decisions and stem cell renewal. *Annu Rev Cell Dev Biol.* (2016) 32:399–409. doi: 10.1146/annurev-cellbio-111315-125134
27. Vander Heiden MG, DeBerardinis RJ. Understanding the intersections between metabolism and cancer biology. *Cell.* (2017) 168:657–69. doi: 10.1016/j.cell.2016.12.039
28. Cervenka I, Agudelo LZ, Ruas JL. Kynurenines: tryptophan's metabolites in exercise, inflammation, and mental health. *Science.* (2017) 357:eaaf9794. doi: 10.1126/science.aaf9794
29. Yin J, Ren W, Yang G, Duan J, Huang X, Fang R, et al. L-Cysteine metabolism and its nutritional implications. *Mol Nutr Food Res.* (2016) 60:134–46. doi: 10.1002/mnfr.201500031
30. Liu H, Pathak P, Boehme S, Chiang JY. Cholesterol 7α-hydroxylase protects the liver from inflammation and fibrosis by maintaining cholesterol homeostasis. *J Lipid Res.* (2016) 57:1831–44. doi: 10.1194/jlr.M069807
31. Chambers KF, Day PE, Aboufarrag HT, Kroon PA. Polyphenol effects on cholesterol metabolism via bile acid biosynthesis, CYP7A1: a review. *Nutrients.* (2019) 11:2588. doi: 10.3390/nu11112588
32. Ferrell JM, Pathak P, Boehme S, Gilliland T, Chiang JYL. Deficiency of both farnesoid X Receptor and Takeda G protein-coupled receptor 5 exacerbated liver fibrosis in mice. *Hepatology.* (2019) 70:955–70. doi: 10.1002/hep.30513
33. Hartmann P, Chu H, Duan Y, Schnabl B. Gut microbiota in liver disease: too much is harmful, nothing at all is not helpful either. *Am J Physiol Gastrointest Liver Physiol.* (2019) 316:G563–G573. doi: 10.1152/ajpgi.00370.2018
34. Baranowski M, Błachnio-Zabielska AU, Charmas M, Helge JW, Dela F, Ksiazek M, et al. Exercise increases sphingoid base-1-phosphate levels in human blood and skeletal muscle in a time- and intensity-dependent manner. *Eur J Appl Physiol.* (2015) 115:993–1003. doi: 10.1007/s00421-014-3080-x
35. Nguyen P, Leray V, Diez M, Serisier S, Le Bloc'h J, Siliart B, et al. Liver lipid metabolism. *J Anim Physiol Anim Nutr (Berl).* (2008) 92:272–83. doi: 10.1111/j.1439-0396.2007.00752.x
36. Ribbenstedt A, Ziarrusta H, Benskin JP. Development, characterization and comparisons of targeted and non-targeted metabolomics methods. *PLoS ONE.* (2018) 13:e0207082. doi: 10.1371/journal.pone.0207082

8

Novel Anti-inflammatory Treatments in Cirrhosis: A Literature-Based Study

Thit Mynster Kronborg[1], Henriette Ytting[1], Lise Hobolth[1], Søren Møller[2,3] and Nina Kimer[1,4]*

[1] Gastro Unit, Medical Division, Amager-Hvidovre University Hospital, Hvidovre, Denmark, [2] Department of Clinical Physiology and Nuclear Medicine 260, Center for Functional and Diagnostic Imaging and Research, Amager-Hvidovre Hospital, Hvidovre, Denmark, [3] Department of Clinical Medicine, Faculty of Health Sciences, University of Copenhagen, Copenhagen, Denmark, [4] Novo Nordisk Foundation Centre for Basic Metabolic Research, Faculty of Health Sciences, University of Copenhagen, Copenhagen, Denmark

Correspondence:
Thit Mynster Kronborg
thit.mynster.kronborg@regionh.dk

Liver cirrhosis is a disease characterised by multiple complications and a poor prognosis. The prevalence is increasing worldwide. Chronic inflammation is ongoing in liver cirrhosis. No cure for the inflammation is available, and the current treatment of liver cirrhosis is only symptomatic. However, several different medical agents have been suggested as potential healing drugs. The majority are tested in rodents, but few human trials are effectuated. This review focuses on medical agents described in the literature with supposed alleviating and curing effects on liver cirrhosis. Twelve anti-inflammatory, five antioxidative, and three drugs with effects on gut microflora and the LPS pathway were found. Two drugs not categorised by the three former categories were found in addition. In total, 42 rodent studies and seven human trials were found. Promising effects of celecoxib, aspirin, curcumin, kahweol, pentoxifylline, diosmin, statins, emricasan, and silymarin were found in cirrhotic rodent models. Few indices of effects of etanercept, glycyrrhizin arginine salt, and mitoquinone were found. Faecal microbiota transplantation is in increasing searchlight with a supposed potential to alleviate cirrhosis. However, human trials are in demand to verify the findings in this review.

Keywords: liver cirrhosis, inflammation, treatment, cytokines, anti-oxidation, cirrhosis models

INTRODUCTION

Liver cirrhosis is a chronic disease with increasing prevalence. Its most common aetiologies are alcohol consumption, viral hepatitis, obesity, diabetes mellitus, and metabolic syndrome leading to non-alcoholic steatohepatitis as a part of non-alcoholic fatty liver disease (1). In general, liver cirrhosis results from ongoing fibrosis formation, and further progression leads to portal hypertension, hepatic encephalopathy, and an increased risk of organ failure and hepatocellular carcinoma (HCC), which is associated with high mortality (2).

Chronic inflammation in alcoholic liver disease is mediated by a direct response to alcohol and an indirect inflammatory response to gut microbiota-derived lipopolysaccharide (LPS), leading to a stronger oxidative-inflammatory response (3). With ongoing systemic inflammation, endothelial dysfunction, and fibrogenesis (4) evolve in the liver and are associated with elevated inflammatory cytokines and immune cell activation (5). The inflammation may be caused by translocation over the bowel wall of pathogens or derived pathogen-associated molecular patterns (PAMPs) and damage-associated molecular patterns (DAMPs). These are products of microbial origin produced by pathogens and not by the host. Products from apoptotic cells (6) translocate into the portal and systemic circulation via an impaired intestinal barrier. With a continuous injury, the PAMPs and DAMPs can activate hepatic stellate cells (HSC's) with unwanted adverse effects (6). The HSC's are a source of myofibroblasts and portal fibroblasts, which drive the fibrogenic process (2). When quiescent, HSC's mainly act as vitamin A reserves, but they can abundantly secrete extracellular matrix proteins and different proteinases that elicit unwanted liver architecture remodelling when activated.

Currently, there is no cure for this chronic inflammation in cirrhosis, and treatment mainly focuses on symptomatic relief. When ascites develops in the decompensated stage, diuretics, and albumin infusion improve fluid retention and circulatory function after paracentesis. Non-selective beta-blockers (NSBB's) decreases portal hypertension and are used for long-term treatment as primary and secondary prophylaxis of bleeding from oesophageal varices (7, 8). Hepatic encephalopathy can be reversed using antibiotics and lactulose, as the encephalopathy is often triggered by infections and constipation (9).

There is a reduced incidence of HCC in patients treated with NSBB's (10). The underlying mechanism might be a reduction in bacterial translocation from the gut, which may diminish the portal load of PAMP's and thus the hepatic inflammation.

As hepatic inflammation and neo-angiogenesis are critical drivers in the pathogenesis of HCC, the beta-adrenergic blockade may impede angiogenesis through inhibition of vascular endothelial growth factor production and prevent HCC (11). The preliminary studies need further scientific explorations to support this hypothesis.

Diuretics are the first choice treatment of ascites in decompensated cirrhosis (8, 12). However, side effects of diuretics include fluid- and electrolyte disturbances, dehydration, and renal impairment. Albumin infusion is used to prevent the development of hepatorenal syndrome (HRS) and relieve circulatory disturbances in decompensated cirrhosis (13, 14).

In addition to its osmotic effects, albumin has an immunomodulatory effect (14–16) that is measurable by significantly reduced interleukine-6 (IL-6) response in high dose albumin treatment (14). Thus, albumin may improve survival and prevent complications in decompensated cirrhosis, and its immunomodulatory effects require further exploration as they relate to the prevention of acute-on-chronic liver failure (ACLF).

Both inflammation and oxidative stress are considered key elements in the pathology of cirrhosis. When the liver is injured, it may increase reactive oxygen and nitrogen species (ROS, RNS). These intermediates can induce pro-fibrogenic mechanisms. The oxidative stress causes injury by an alteration of DNA, proteins and lipids, resulting in activation of the hepatic stellate cells; hence one of the triggers of fibrogenesis also elicited by inflammatory pathways. Oxidative stress and inflammation are tightly related and can create a vicious cycle to aggravate liver injuries (17).

Multiple pathways are relevant and interesting when seeking to treat liver cirrhosis. In particular, the chronic and systemic inflammatory and oxidative mechanisms that mediate several complications in cirrhosis suggest that inflammatory cascades are possible targets for the treatment of cirrhosis. The available therapy is inadequate in treating fibrogenesis and liver tissue inflammation, and novel targets and therapies are wanted.

The present review aims to evaluate possible anti-inflammatory agents as potential drug candidates that may alleviate, cure or increase survival among patients with liver cirrhosis.

METHODS

A search of the literature published during the last 10 years was conducted in PubMed and Medline. Titles and abstracts were searched for the following key terms in different combinations: "cirrhosis," "liver cirrhosis," "cohort," "inflammation," "anti-inflammatory," "chronic liver disease," "drugs," "targets," "cure." The complete search strategy is described in **Supplementary Table 1**. Following agreement among the authors, specific searches were then carried out that include the following terms combined with "liver cirrhosis":

"silymarin," "anti-TNF-α," "curcumin," "faecal microbiota transplantation," "enoxaparin," "etanercept," "artesunate," "celecoxib," "aspirin," "kahweol," "mitoquinone," "glycyrrhizin arginine salt," "pentoxifylline," "statin," "emricasan," "lanifibranor," "formyl peptide receptor 2 (WKYMVm)," "tanshinone."

Inclusion criteria for the studies were their full text being in English, and their design being clinical trials, clinical studies, comparative studies, multi-centre studies, case reports, and observational studies. Interventional studies were considered regardless of whether they had a control group or were blinded. In addition, studies evaluating the safety, efficacy, and therapeutic mechanisms of pharmacological agents with anti-inflammatory effects in humans were included, and studies evaluating

Abbreviations: ACLF, acute on chronic liver failure; α-SMA, α-smooth muscle actin; ALT, alanine aminotransferase; ALP, alkaline phosphatase; AMP, antimicrobial peptide; AST, aspartate aminotransferase; BDL, bile duct ligation; CCl_4, carbon tetrachloride; cCK18, cleaved cytokeratine-18; COX, cyclooxygenase; CTGF, connective tissue growth factor; eNOS, endothelial nitric oxide synthase; flCK18, full-length cytokeratine 18; FMT, faecal microbiota transplantation; GPx, glutathione peroxidase; GR, glutathione reductase; GSH, glutathione reductase/reduced glutathione; GST, glutathione-S-transferase; HBV, Hepatitis B virus; HCC, hepatocellular carcinoma; HCV, Hepatitis C virus; HE, hepatic encephalopathy; HRS, hepatorenal syndrome; HSC, hepatic stellate cells; HVPG, hepatic venous pressure gradient; HYP, hydroxyproline; ICAM-1, intercellular adhesion molecule 1; IL-6, interleukine-6; Keap-1, Kelch-like ECH-associated protein 1; KLF2, Krüppel-like factor 2; LDL, low density lipoprotein; LFA-1, lymphocyte function-associated antigen 1; LPS, lipopolysaccharide; MDA, malondialdehyde, measure of lipid peroxidation; MSCs, mesenchymal stem cells; NADPH, nicotinamide adenine dinucleotide phosphate; NFkB, nuclear factor-kB; NO, nitrogen oxide; NOS, nitrogen oxygen synthase; Nrf2, Nuclear factor erythroid 2-realted factor 2; PARs, protease activated receptors; PDGF, platelet derived growth factor; PPARα, peroxisome proliferator-activated receptor-α; RCT, randomised controlled trial; ROS, reactive oxygen species; SBP, spontaneous bacterial peritonitis; SOD, superoxide dismutase; STAT3, signal transducer and activator 3; Supp., supplementary; TAA, thioacetamide; TBARS, thiobarbituric acid reactive substances; TGF-β, transforming growth factor-β; TNF-α, tumour necrosis factor-α; VEGF, vascular endothelial growth factor; WKYMVm, a hexapeptide.

inflammatory mechanisms in rodent models were also assessed to support our understanding of immunological mechanisms.

Selected studies using rodent models were considered for inclusion, as the differentiation between fibrosis and cirrhosis differs markedly from that in humans. Hence, mentioning cirrhosis was a criterion in rodent studies. Cell model studies were considered relevant only when combined with human- or rodent studies fulfilling all other search criteria.

Studies with an exclusive focus on fibrosis, steatosis, steatohepatitis, and viral hepatitis without cirrhosis were excluded.

RESULTS

Literature searches were conducted between the 6th of March and the 16th of May 2021. The initial search strategy resulted in 57,853 general hits, which were subsequently reduced to 1,337 drug search-related hits.

After excluding duplicates and irrelevant papers and following the above-stated in- and exclusion criteria, the abstracts of 351 publications were identified and screened for studies evaluating pharmacological agents' safety, efficacy, and therapeutic mechanisms with anti-inflammatory effects in cirrhosis.

Another 16 papers were found during a manual search of reference lists and bibliographies (**Figure 1**, Trial flow chart). The remaining 275 papers were excluded due to their primary focus on fibrosis, with no mentioning of cirrhosis or because of a lack of investigations into inflammatory or antioxidative pathways. Seventy-six publications were considered relevant to the research question as evaluated by the authors (SM, NK, and TMK). Of these, 27 studies explored the clinical effects of the included anti-inflammatory drugs in human studies without a particular focus on the anti-inflammatory markers, and these were excluded (see **Supplementary Table 2**).

Forty-two studies explored potential anti-inflammatory mechanisms of drugs in animal models, and seven studies explored these same drug mechanisms in humans.

Tables 1A,B lists the included studies.

Agents were assessed according to their pathway mechanisms.

Anti-inflammatory Mediators

Twelve different anti-inflammatory mediators acting on several pathways were evaluated in 30 animal studies and five human studies. Cytokines were most often used as a marker for inflammation. Cytokines are regulatory peptides released by activated cells and act as crucial mediators in immune and inflammatory disorders. Increasing evidence support a major role for several cytokines in liver diseases (**Figure 2**) (66).

The following agents are reported to interfere with the immune system, with potential beneficial effects:

Celecoxib (25–29, 67), *aspirin* (30, 31), *etanercept* (32), *curcumin* (33–39), *kahweol* (40, 41), *pentoxifylline* (42, 68), *diosmin* (42–44), *glycyrrhizin arginine salt* (45), *statins* (18, 19, 46–50), *emricasan* (20–22, 51, 69) *and lanifibranor* (52) *and formayl receptor 2 agonist—WKYMVm* (53).

In addition, 27 human studies with various methodologies investigated the mechanisms but did not report anti-inflammatory endpoints. These are listed in **Supplementary Table 2**.

Celecoxib

Celecoxib is a cyclooxygenase-2 (COX-2) inhibitor used in the treatment of arthritis (70, 71). COX-2, an enzyme expressed due to inflammation, is increased in inflammatory, vascular endothelial lining, and expressed by Kupffer cells in the cirrhotic liver (72, 73). Celecoxib has anti-inflammatory effects to relieve cirrhosis complications and reduce portal hypertension in several rat studies (25–29, 67) (**Supplementary Table 3a**). Celecoxib was administered to prevent cirrhosis in experimental animal models where cirrhosis was induced by peritoneal injections of thioacetamide (TAA). However, no human studies with anti-inflammatory endpoints have been carried out with celecoxib.

Aspirin

Aspirin is a COX-inhibitor that acts on the nuclear factor kappa B (NFkB), which transcript adhesion molecules in endothelial cells and vascular smooth muscle cells, which affect macrophage and T lymphocyte adherence (30). In addition, aspirin may enhance interferon-α-induced growth inhibition and apoptosis in HCC (74), but few studies have investigated aspirin as a single treatment for cirrhosis.

In rats with TAA-induced cirrhosis, aspirin markedly reduces fibrogenesis with a macroscopic and histologic improvement of the liver tissue compared to controls (30, 31).

While biomarkers of inflammation were not assessed in these studies (30), serum bilirubin levels were significantly lower in the aspirin-treated cirrhotic rats than in the untreated cirrhotic rats (31).

So far, no human studies of aspirin as a treatment of inflammation have investigated specific molecular or anti-inflammatory biomarkers or inflammation cascades. Clinical endpoints investigated are listed in **Supplementary Table 2** (75–77).

Etanercept

TNF-α is a cytokine produced in immune cells, and it is shown that hepatic signalling through the TNF-R1-receptor is essential for liver regeneration (78). TNF-α activates the NFkB-pathway, which mediates protective and anti-apoptotic effects but also initiates transcription of inflammatory mediator genes (79). However, TNF-α is also a proinflammatory mediator capable of inducing apoptosis and liver destruction (79). Etanercept is a TNF-α antagonist and an approved drug for autoimmune diseases, e.g., inflammatory bowel disease and rheumatoid arthritis. A single rat study (32) found that TNF-α levels were neutralised combined with a significantly lower expression of TNF-R1 by etanercept exposure. Surprisingly, a retrospective study of patients with various immune-related diseases receiving TNF-α-inhibitors found an increased hazard ratio for developing cirrhosis. Immunological pathways were not further assessed, and its endpoints are listed in **Supplementary Table 2** (80).

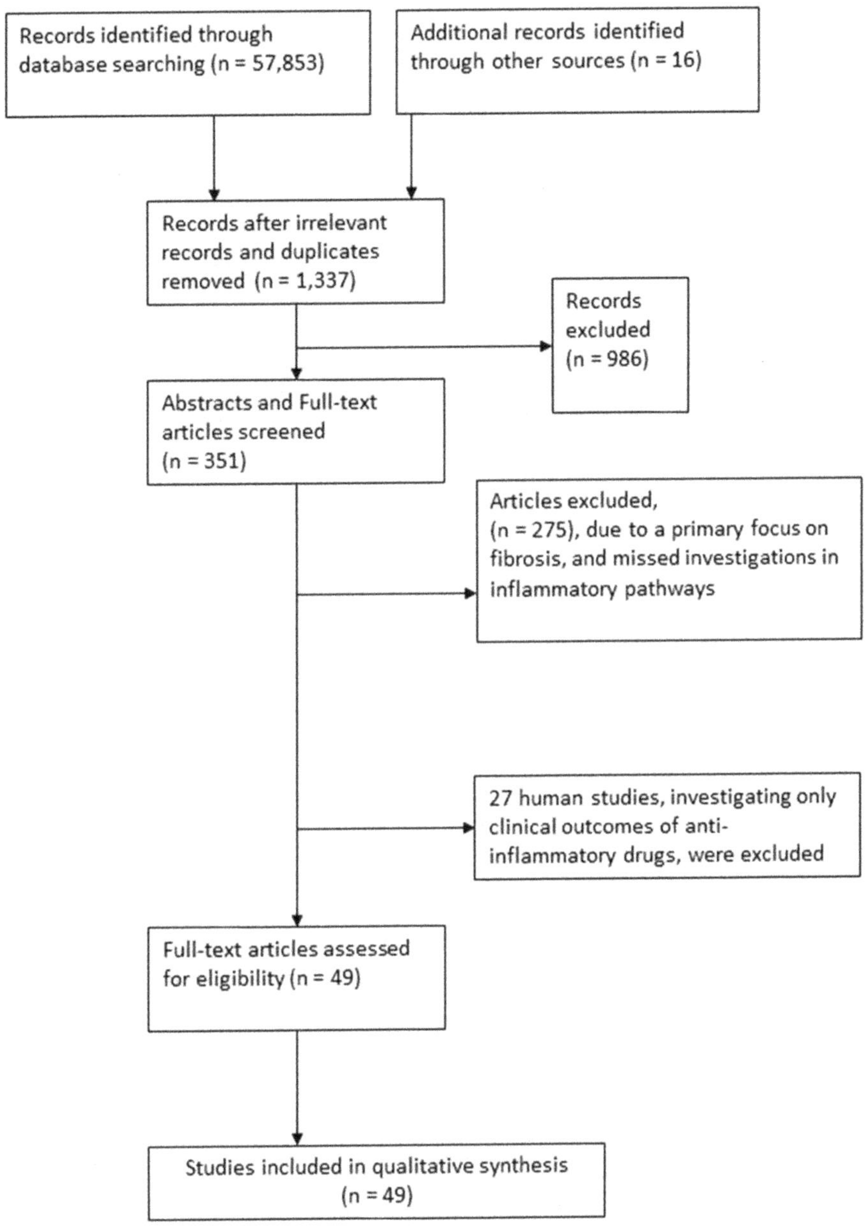

FIGURE 1 | Trial flow chart.

Curcumin

Curcumin is a derivative of turmeric, which appears to have anti-inflammatory, antioxidant, plus anticarcinogenic effects (81).

Curcumin has an increasing effect on the signalling molecules nuclear factor erythroid 2-related factor 2 (Nrf-2), Nrf2-NFkB (measured as mRNA) and protein expression (34), and a decrease in the cytokines TGF-1β and TNF-α and in IL-10 (33). In addition, curcumin reduces alanine aminotransferase (ALT) levels in hamsters and rats with CCl_4-induced cirrhosis (33, 35).

Curcumin may also reduce the expression of α-smooth muscle actin (α-SMA), a phenotypic marker of HSC-activation, and COX-2 combined with lactulose (35). In addition curcumin increases SIRT3, a sirtuin with a pivotal role in fatty acid oxidation and reduction of cellular reactive oxygen species (ROS) in the liver, which is decreased in cirrhotic rats (36). Furthermore, mRNA expression of the signalling molecules AMPK, CPT-1A, IDH2, and MnSOD was increased by curcumin, indicating reduced oxidative stress.

Curcumin was found to reduce protein expressions of eNOS, COX-2, VEGF, p-VEGFR2, and p-Erk in cirrhotic rats (37). The impact of curcumin on inflammatory markers was investigated by Cai et al. (38) and by Hernández-Aquino et al. (39)

(**Supplementary Table 3b**). Curcumin appeared to decrease the levels of LPS-TLR4-related downstream inflammatory cytokines in the liver, specifically, TNF-α, IL-1β, IL-6, and CINC-1/IL-8. The decreases were mediated by decreased LPS levels and innate inflammation in the curcumin-treated group, not due to decreased LPS absorption but enhanced LPS clearance and detoxification in the liver (38). In addition, restoration of MMP-9, MMP-2, MMP-13m NFkB, IL-1, IL-10, TGF-β, connective tissue growth factor (CTGF), collagen, α-SMA, and Smad3+7 was also induced by curcumin as well as a decrement in activated hepatic stellate cells (39).

Overall, curcumin seems to decrease inflammatory responses, ameliorate fibrosis and portal hypertension, and attenuate splanchnic hyperdynamic circulation at least partly by inducing vasoconstriction through inhibition of eNOS and decreasing mesenteric angiogenesis via VEGF blockade.

In humans, a recent double-blind placebo-controlled trial demonstrated the effects of curcumin vs. placebo on disease severity in cirrhosis. However, specific anti-inflammatory effects have not been addressed in humans, see **Supplementary Table 2** (82).

Kahweol

The LPS-induced inflammatory response is a crucial driver in systemic inflammation, most likely caused by bacterial translocation of PAMPs and DAMPs from the gut into blood circulation (6). The LPS signal transducer activates NFkB. Signal transducer and activator 3 (STAT3) is another transcriptional factor involved in the NFkB-pathway. Inhibition of these two factors could reduce the inflammatory responses (83).

Kahweol is a coffee-specific compound of coffee beans that exhibits anticarcinogenic, anti-tumour progressive, and anti-inflammatory properties (84), probably via affection of the NFkB and STAT3 signalling.

Seo et al. investigated kahweol's antifibrotic and anti-inflammatory effect on mouse liver Kupffer cells and hepatocytes

TABLE 1A | Human studies (*N* = 7).

Study ID	Species	Intervention	Methods	Aim	Results
Zafra et al. (18)	Humans	Statins (Simvastatin 40 mg, once 12 h before and once 1 h before the study)	Randomised, double-blind, placebo-controlled trial. 30 patients with liver cirrhosis	Impact on hepatic nitric oxide release and hepatic resistance	Increased hepatosplanchnic output of nitric oxide products. Decreased hepatic resistance
Kaplan et al. (19)	Humans	Statins (Simvastatin 40 mg/day for up to 24 months)	Prospective, multi-centre, double-blind, randomised clinical trial	To investigate the potential reduction of incident hepatic decompensation events among patients at high risk for hepatic decompensation	Not yet available
Frenette et al. (20)	Humans	Emricasan (25 mg twice daily for 3 months, and afterwards 25 mg daily open label)	Multi-centre study, randomised placebo-controlled trial of 86 patients	To investigate the effect of Emricasan on liver function in cirrhosis	Decrease of full-length CK-18 and caspase 3/7. No decrease in cleaved CK-18. Improvement of MELD and Child-Pugh score after 3 months due to improvement in INR and bilirubin
Garcia-Tsao et al. (21)	Humans	Emricasan (25 mg twice daily for 28 days)	Multi-centre, open-label clinical study of 23 patients	Impact on portal hypertension	No significant change in HVPG overall, but sig. decrease in severe PH, AST, ALT, cCK18, and caspase-3/7.
Garcia-Tsao et al. (22)	Humans	Emricasan (5, 25, and 50 mg twice daily for up to 48 weeks)	Multi-centre, double-blinded, randomised clinical study of 263 patients	Testing earlier results of Emricasan decreasing portal hypertension in NASH-related cirrhosis	No significant difference in HVPG for any emricasan dose vs. placebo. Sig. decrease of biomarkers (including Caspase 3/7, cCK18, and flCK18) at week 24, returned to baseline by week 48
Bajaj et al. (23)	Humans	FMT (15 capsules)	Randomised, single-blind, placebo-controlled clinical trial. 20 patients with cirrhosis and recurrent HE	Safety, tolerability, and impact on mucosal/stool microbiota and brain function	Similar episodes of infections and HE in both groups. Reduced LBP in FMT-group. Reduced IL-6 expression post-FMT
Bajaj et al. (24)	Humans	FMT (15 capsules)	Randomised, single-blind, placebo-controlled trial of 20 patients with cirrhosis and recurrent HE	Effect of FMT on the gut-brain axis, inflammation (IL-6 and LPS-binding protein)	Reduced HE-occurrence. Reduced serum IL-6 and LBP

TABLE 1B | Rodent studies ($N = 42$).

ID	Species	Drug	Methods	Aim	Results
Gao et al. (25)	Rats	Celecoxib (20 mg/kg/day)	TAA-induced cirrhosis for 16 weeks during celecoxib administration	Inhibition of COX-2 by celecoxib, reduction of intestinal inflammatory transport	Improvement of intestinal epithelial barrier integrity, blocked inflammatory transport, and diminished progression of cirrhosis
Gao et al. (26)	Rats	Celecoxib (20 mg/kg/day)	TAA-induced cirrhosis for 16 weeks during celecoxib administration	Effect of celecoxib on portal hypertension and the mechanisms behind it.	Dual effects on intrahepatic fibrosis and angiogenesis, Modulation of VEGF/VEGFR-2
Wen et al. (27)	Rats	Celecoxib (20 mg/kg/day)	TAA-induced cirrhosis for 16 weeks during celecoxib administration	Effect on the epithelial-mesenchymal transition of hepatocytes	Amelioration of fibrosis and cirrhosis through suppression of mesenchymal biomarkers. Reduction of intrahepatic inflammation and inhibition of TGF-β1/Smad pathway.
Gao et al. (2)	Rats	Celecoxib (20 mg/kg/day)	TAA-induced cirrhosis for 16 weeks during celecoxib and octreotide administration	Anti-angiogenesis effect of octreotide and celecoxib on cirrhotic portal hypertension	Celecoxib and octreotide relieved fibrogenesis, micro-hepatic arterioportal fistulas, and intrahepatic angiogenesis.
Su et al. (28)	Rats	Celecoxib (20 mg/kg/day)	TAA-induced cirrhosis for 16 weeks during celecoxib administration	To investigate whether celecoxib alleviates liver fibrosis by inhibiting hepatocyte apoptosis via the ER stress response	Celecoxib reduces hepatic apoptosis in TAA-induced cirrhotic rats.
Tang et al. (29)	Rats	Celecoxib (20 mg/kg/day)	TAA-induced cirrhosis for 8 weeks before concomitant continued induction with celecoxib	To examine the impacts of splenomegaly on the development of cirrhosis and assessment of the effects of celecoxib on the splenomegaly and cirrhotic liver.	Celecoxib ameliorates cirrhosis via reducing inflammatory cytokines and immune cells derived from the spleen and suppressing oxidative stress.
Li et al. (30)	Rats	Aspirin (low dose aspirin: 30 mg/kg/day, high dose aspirin: 300 mg/kg/day) and enoxaparin (2 mg/kg/day)	TAA-induced cirrhosis for 4 weeks during aspirin and/or enoxaparin administration	To examine effects of aspirin and enoxaparin in liver function, coagulation index, and histopathology in a rat model of liver fibrosis	Sign. improvement in fibrosis grade in low-dose aspirin, high-dose aspirin, and enoxaparin treated rats.
Assy et al. (31)	Rats	Aspirin (300 mg/kg daily) and enoxaparin (2 mg/kg/day) for 5 weeks	TAA-induced cirrhosis	To examine the effect of aspirin and enoxaparin on fibrosis progression and regenerative activity in a rat model of liver cirrhosis and to determine if the drugs are beneficial in animals with advanced fibrosis or cirrhosis undergoing partial hepatectomy	Sig. improvement in fibrosis grade in both aspirin and enoxaparin group. Improvement of hepatic regenerative activity sig. improved in the aspirin group, unchanged in the enoxaparin group
Abdul-Hamid et al. (32)	Rats	Etanercept (2 mg/kg subcutaneous twice a week for 5 months)	TAA-induced cirrhosis during treatment with etanercept	To clarify the effect of etanercept on the development of cirrhosis and hemosiderosis in rats, highlighting the implication and distribution pattern of hepatic TNF-R1	Diminished expression of hepatic TNF-R1, attenuation of collagen and hemosiderin accumulation, and preservation of hepatic histoarchitecture
Abo-Zaid et al. (33)	Rats	Curcumin (150, 200 or 250 mg/kg/day for 6 weeks)	CCl_4-induced cirrhosis during curcumin injections	To evaluate the immune regulatory effect of curcumin in hepatic cirrhotic rats	IL-10 sig. increased in curcumin groups, TNF-α and TGF-1β decreased. Curcumin tended to retain the normal structure of liver tissues.
Macías-Pérez et al. (34)	Hamsters	Curcumin (30 mg/kg/day for 4 weeks)	CCl_4-induced cirrhosis before Curcumin administration	To evaluate reversal of cirrhosis by doxazosin, carvedilol, and curcumin and studying possible modulation of Nrf-2 and NF-kB	a/b adrenergic blockers with curcumin reverse hepatic damage, possibly as a result of adrenergic antagonism on HSC and conceivably by the increase of Nrf-2/NF-kB mRNA ratio

(Continued)

TABLE 1B | Continued

ID	Species	Drug	Methods	Aim	Results
Kyuong et al. (35)	Rats	Curcumin (10 mg/mL orally for 4 weeks)	DMN induced cirrhosis	To investigate the hepatoprotective effect of curcumin. Comparison of curcumin and lactulose treatment in cirrhotic rats	Increased electrical conductivity when treated with curcumin or lactulose compared to the cirrhotic model, sig. levels of attenuated fibrosis and decreased inflammatory response after curcumin and lactulose.
Chenari et al. (36)	Rats	Curcumin (100 mg/kg/day for 4 weeks)	BDL-induced cirrhosis	To explore the hepatoprotective activity of curcumin via measuring expression of SIRT3, AMPK, CPT-1A, IDH2, and MnSOD and lipid profile	Increase of SIRT3, AMPK, CPT-1A, IDH2, and MnSOD and improvement of lipid profile when fed curcumin
Hsu et al. (37)	Rats	Curcumin (600 mg/kg/day for 2 weeks)	CBDL-induced cirrhosis	To evaluate the effects of curcumin as an antiproliferative, anti-inflammatory, and anti-angiogenic agent	Decrease of flow in the superior mesenteric artery and increased resistance. Sig. reduction of eNOS, COX2, VEGF, and pErk. Decrease of portosystemic shunting, induction of vasoconstriction. Amelioration of portal hypertension.
Cai et al. (38)	Rats	Curcumin (200 mg/kg/day for 12 weeks)	CCl_4-induced cirrhosis	To test the anti-endotoxemia effect of curcumin on induced cirrhosis in rats, elucidate the underlying molecular mechanism.	Improvement of physiological condition, amelioration of liver injury, reduction of inflammatory cytokines in serum and liver tissue, a decrease of LPS in a peripheral vein
Hernández-Aquino et al. (39)	Rats	Curcumin (100 mg/kg twice a day for 3 weeks)	CCl_4-induced cirrhosis partly before Curcumin administration	To investigate fibrosis reduction in cirrhotic rats and to determine the canonical/non-canonical Smad3 pathways and HSC activation/deactivation induced by curcumin	Reduced liver damage, restoration of levels of MMP-9, MMP-2, Nf-kB, IL-1, IL-10, TGF-β, CTGF, Col-1, MMP-13, Smad-7, α-SMA, and Smad-3. Decrement in hepatic stellate cells
Seo et al. (40)	Mouse liver cell model	Kahweol (doses not specified)	Addition of kahweol in LPS-Kupffer cells and hepatocytes	Effect of kahweol on liver inflammation	Decrease of LPS-induced production of IL-1a, IL-1b, IL-6, and TNF-α. Downregulation of phosphor-NF-kB and—signal transducer and activator of transcription 3 expression.
Arauz et al. (41)	Mice	Kahweol (200 mg/kg twice a day caffeinated or decaffeinated for 8 weeks)	TAA-induced cirrhosis during coffee administration.	Antifibrotic properties of coffee	Blockade of TGF-1β and connective tissue growth factor.
Ali et al. (42)	Rats	Pentoxifylline (100 mg/kg/day) and/or diosmin (50 mg/kg/day) for 28 days	BDL-cirrhotic rats	Effects on inflammatory response oxidative balance, cytoglobin	Downregulation of Keap-1/Nrf-2/GSH and NF-kB-p65/p38-MAPK pathways
Ali et al. (43)	Rats	Diosmin (100 mg/kg/day) and sildenafil (10 mg/kg twice daily) for 4 weeks	BDL-induced cirrhosis	Effects of diosmin on fibrotic markers, oxidation levels, and diverse oxidative markers	Downregulation of NF-kB-p65, P38-MAPK, Keap-1, and iNos.
Tahir et al. (44)	Rats	Diosmin (10 mg/kg or 20 mg/kg for 4 weeks)	Ethanol-induced cirrhosis, diosmin before ethanol (increasing dose of ethanol for 28 days).	Efficacy of diosmin on hepatotoxicity, free radicals, oxidative status, transcription factors, and inflammatory markers.	Diosmin normalised CYP 450 2E1 and alcohol dehydrogenase, attenuated oxidative stress, and alleviated ethanol-induced NF-kB activation as well as TNF-α, COX-2, and iNos.

(Continued)

TABLE 1B | Continued

ID	Species	Drug	Methods	Aim	Results
Zhang et al. (45)	Rats	Glycyrrhizin arginine salt (75 or 150 mg/kg for 2 weeks)	BDL-induced cirrhosis	Effect of glycyrrhizin arginine salt on cirrhosis	Decrease of serum bilirubin, AST, 8-isoprostane and malondialdehyde, Slower fibrogenesis. Reduction of bile salt pool, hydroxyproline, TGF-β1, α -SMA, TNF-α, MMP-2, and MMP-9.
Tripathi et al. (46)	Rats	Statin, 25 mg/kg/day for CCl_4- and TAA induced cirrhosis, 5 mg/kg/day for BDL cirrhosis (simvastatin for 3 days)	CCl_4-, BDL, and TAA induced cirrhosis	Effect on ACLF	Prevention of ACLF-complications and improved survival. Reduction of inflammation and oxidation markers
Meireles et al. (47)	Rats	Statin (simvastatin 5 mg/kg/day for 3 days)	BDL induced cirrhosis	Impact of cirrhotic microcirculation and hepatoprotection	Aggravation of microvascular dysfunction and upregulation of inflammatory pathways; prevention of endothelial dysfunction
Uschner et al. (48)	Rats	Statin (atorvastatin 15 mg/kg for 7 days)	BDL + CCl_4-induced cirrhosis	Investigation of angiogenesis and the hedgehog pathway.	Inhibition of the non-canonical Hh-pathway and angiogenesis.
Shirin et al. (49)	Rats	Statin (atorvastatin 1, 10 or 20 mg/kg/day, rosuvastatin 2.5, 5, 10, or 20 mg/kg/day for 12 weeks)	TAA-induced cirrhosis concomitantly with atorvastatin/rosuvastatin/saline.	Prevention of cirrhosis	No inhibition of cirrhosis or oxidative stress
Jang et al. (50)	Rats	Statin and MSCs (1 × 10^6 MSC's two times during 12 weeks, and/or 10 mg/kg/day of simvastatin for 5 weeks)	TAA-induced cirrhosis	Synergistic effect of simvastatin and MSCs on fibrosis	Decreased collagen distribution, lowered hydroxyproline content
Gracia-Sancho et al. (51)	Rats	Emricasan (10 mg/kg/day for 7 days)	CCl_4-induced cirrhosis. *In vitro* experiment on hepatocyte expressions	Effects on haemodynamics, hepatic cells phenotype	Lowered portal pressure, reduced hepatic inflammation, and reduced fibrosis. *In vitro* experiment improved hepatocyte expression
Boyer-Diaz et al. (52)	Rats and human samples	Lanifibranor (100 mg/kg/day for 2 weeks)	TAA-induced cirrhosis for 12 weeks and BDL induced secondary biliary cirrhosis in two separate rat groups. Human samples from liver resections	Therapeutic potential of pan-PPAR activation for the treatment of advanced cirrhosis	For the rats with TAA-cirrhosis: Sig. decrease in portal pressure, reduction of ascites, and cirrhosis regression. Attenuation of the hepatic proinflammatory environment through cytokine expression pattern shift. For human hepatocytes: improvement and amelioration of HSC phenotype and reduction in contraction capacity
Jun et al. (53)	Rats	WKYMVm (2.5 mg/kg twice pr. week for 22 weeks)	BDL-induced cirrhosis	Effects on hepatic regeneration via vascular remodelling, resulting from its pro-angiogenic properties	Improvement of vascular remodelling, inhibition of fibrosis, and enhanced hepatic function
Vilaseca et al. (54)	Rats and human liver cells	Mitoquinone (5 mg/kg/day for 14 days)	HSCs exposed to mitoquinone. CCl_4- and TAA-induced cirrhosis.	Effects of mitoquinone on hepatic oxidative stress, HSC phenotype, inflammation markers, and liver fibrosis	Decrease of proliferation in both HSCs and rats. Decrease in hepatic oxidative stress and diminished fibrosis
Turkseven et al. (55)	Rats	Mitoquinone (10 mg/kg/day for 25 days)	BDL-induced cirrhosis	Effect on oxidative stress, inflammation markers, fibrosis, and mitophagy.	Prevention of inflammation, hepatocyte necrosis, and fibrosis by mitoquinone. Decrease of TNF- α, TGF-1β, collagen, IL-6, IL-1β, and metalloproteinases. Attenuation of apoptosis by reduced expression of cleaved caspase-3.

(Continued)

TABLE 1B | Continued

ID	Species	Drug	Methods	Aim	Results
Zaidi et al. (56)	Rats	Silymarin vs. saline (200 mg/kg twice a week for 8 weeks)	TAA-induced cirrhosis	Effects of silymarin on liver enzymes, antioxidant enzymes, glutathione reductase, and MDA	Restoration of antioxidant enzymes (SOD and GSH), MDA, and catalase activity
Pour et al. (57)	Rats	Silymarin (50 mg/kg/day) and/or lactulose (2 g/kg/day) for 8 weeks	TAA-induced cirrhosis	Possible synergic and healing effects	Decrease in liver enzymes and malondialdehyde levels
Ali et al. (58)	Rats	Curcumin (400 mg/kg), silybin-phytosome (400 mg/kg), alpha-R-lipoic acid (200 mg/kg/day), or saline. For 7 weeks.	TAA-induced cirrhosis	Protective effects	Blockade of malondialdehyde (MDA) and protein carbonyls. Decrease of GSH-depletion, collagen deposition, MMp-2activity, TGF-1β levels, a-SMA, and HSP-47 expression
Abdel-Moneim et al. (59)	Rats	Silymarin (100 mg/kg five times a week for 4 weeks), taurine (100 mg/kg five times a week for 4 weeks), or both, or olive oil	CCl_4-induced cirrhosis	Hepatoprotective effect	Alleviation of thiobarbituric acid reactive substances, reduction of NO levels, and NOS activity. Increase of superoxide dismutase, glutathione peroxidase, and glutathione reductase. Reduction of TGF-1β, IL-6, and TNF-α. Combination therapy decreased adiponectin levels and normalised FFA
Aithal et al. (60)	Rats	Silymarin (100 mg/kg) and/or bone-marrow-derived stromal cells (5.8 mill. cells in 0.5 mL) for 3 weeks	CCl_4-induced cirrhosis	Efficiency and hepatic differentiation potential of BM-MSCs in combination with silymarin	Ameliorated liver tissue damage through immunoregulatory activities. Decrease in liver enzymes and diminished fibrosis. Combination treatment was most efficient compared with individual treatments
Yang et al. (61)	Rats	Tanshinone (10, 20, or 40 mg/kg for 1 week)	CCl_4- and concomitant alcohol-induced cirrhosis	Investigate therapeutic effects of tanshinone by promoting proliferation and differentiation of stem cells.	Improvement of histology, liver markers, and promotion of proliferation and differentiation of endogenous liver stem cells.
Liu et al. (62)	Germ-free Mice	FMT (0.2 mL daily gavage for 3 days)	CCl_4-induced cirrhosis in conventional and germ-free mice.	Effect of colonisation using human donors on cortical and liver inflammation markers	Reduced neuroinflammation, and microglial activation and dysbiosis. Liver inflammation was unaffected.
Chen et al. (63)	Rats	Artesunate (25 mg/kg/day for 8 weeks)	CCl_4-injection and ethanol-induced cirrhosis. Concomitant artesunate or oil solution	Effect of artesunate on bacterial translocation and gut microbiota	Decrease of IL-6 and TNF-α levels. Positive effect on dysbiosis and reduction of bacterial translocation.
Fortea et al. (64)	Rats	Enoxaparin (40 IU/kg/day or 180 IU/kg/day) vs. saline for 12 weeks	CCl_4-induced cirrhosis, BDL induced cirrhosis.	Effects on advanced cirrhosis	No effect on fibrosis, profibrogenic gene expression, or infection. No amelioration of IL-6 levels. Hepatic arterial dysfunction was corrected.
Cerini et al. (65)	Rats	Enoxaparin (1.8 mg/kg subcutaneously) for 24 and 1 h or daily for 1 week or daily for 3 weeks	CCl_4-induced cirrhosis, TAA-induced cirrhosis, concomitant Enoxaparin.	Effects on hepatic and systemic haemodynamics, fibrosis, and nitric oxide availability	Decreased portal pressure. Reductions in fibrosis, fibrin deposition, HSC-activation (α-SMA, pro-collagen), and desmin expression

in vitro (40). Kahweol was found to limit the production of IL-1α, IL-1β, IL-6, and TNF-α were reduced. Furthermore, this inhibitory effect was associated with the downregulation of LPS-stimulated phosphor-NFkB and STAT3.

Arauz et al. (41) investigated the effects of coffee in rats with TAA-induced cirrhosis. Coffee prevented a weight loss and limited the increase of ALT, alkaline phosphatase (ALP), and gamma-glutamyl transpeptidase observed in cirrhotic controls.

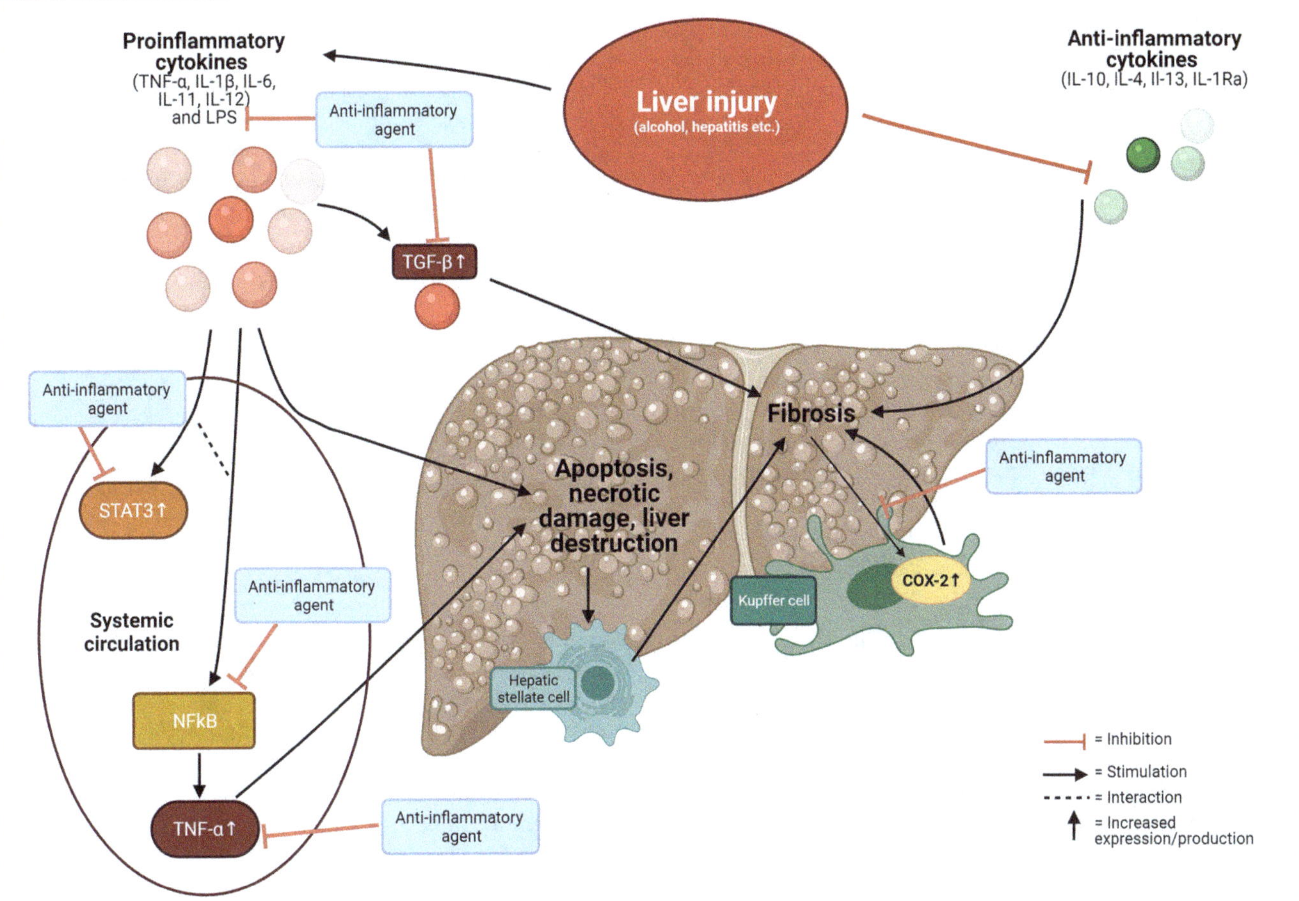

FIGURE 2 | Cytokines in liver disease. Inflammatory responses on various liver injuries and potential targets for anti-inflammatory agents. COX-2, cyclooxygenase–2; IL, interleukin; LPS, lipopolysaccharide; NFkB, nuclear factor-kB; STAT3, signal transducer and activator 3; TGF, transforming growth factor; TNF, tumour necrosis factor.

In addition, significant amelioration of the cytokines TGF-β, CTGF, IL-10, and MMP-13 and α-SMA spikes evolved when coffee was administered to the rats. Thus, the action mechanisms are probably associated with antioxidant properties, mainly with coffee's ability to block the elevation of the profibrogenic cytokine (TGF-β) and the downstream effector CTGF.

No intervention studies in humans have yet explored the anti-inflammatory effects of coffee derivatives in patients with cirrhosis. However, one epidemiologic study is listed in **Supplementary Table 2**.

Pentoxifylline and Diosmin

Pentoxifylline is a non-selective phosphodiesterase inhibitor, which exhibits vasodilator activity on peripheral hepatic blood vessels (85). In addition, it exerts an anti-inflammatory regulation by affecting TGF-β- and tissue inhibitor metalloproteinase-1 (TIMP-1) expressions. Beneficial effects in humans with advanced liver disease have been described (68), and regulating effects of the hepatic stellate cell activity, is suggested to be related to the Hedgehog signalling pathway (86).

Diosmin is a natural flavone reported to prevent hepatic injury through inhibition of NFkB activation (42, 87). In bile duct ligated(BDL)-induced cirrhotic rats, pentoxifylline and diosmin have increased survival (42). A healing effect on the fibrotic markers HYP and TGF-β, and the oxidative markers malondialdehyde (MDA), SOD (superoxide dismutase), glutathione reductase (GSH), and nicotinamide adenine dinucleotide phosphate (NADPH) oxidase activity favoured both diosmin and pentoxifylline; see **Supplementary Table 3c**.

Diosmin has been investigated as a single treatment and in combination with sildenafil (43). Findings about its anti-inflammatory and antioxidant effects are described in **Supplementary Table 3c**. A rodent study (44) confirmed findings of regulation of TNF-α and NFkB activation in rats treated with ethanol and diosmin concomitant for 4 weeks. TNF-α was significantly elevated by ethanol and remitted by the concomitant addition of diosmin. NFkB was investigated by immunohistochemical staining, and the expression was markedly suppressed in diosmin-treated rat groups.

In a clinical trial, 329 patients with cirrhosis were randomised to treatment with pentoxifylline or placebo for 6 months (68).

Pentoxifylline lowered complication rates of bacterial infections, renal insufficiency, hepatic encephalopathy, and gastrointestinal bleeding. Higher TNF-α baseline levels were associated with the development of complications in the absence of pentoxifylline.

Glycyrrhizin Arginine Salt

Glycyrrhizin is the primary active constituent of liquorice root. Liquorice has anti-inflammatory, spasmolytic, laxative, anti-depressive, anti-ulcer, and anti-diabetic effects (88). The statement is supported by a rodent study in which glycyrrhizin combined with arginine seems to protect against hyperammonaemia and hepatic encephalopathy (45).

The therapeutic effects of glycyrrhizin and arginine also change cytokine levels (TGF-β1 and TNF-α), antibodies against matrix metalloproteinases, and biochemical markers of liver function. In this study, significant changes were found to recommend glycyrrhizin arginine salt treatment. Results for its anti-inflammatory effects are listed in **Supplementary Table 3d**.

Statins

Statins have proved antioxidative, antiproliferative, and anti-inflammatory properties and a capacity to improve endothelial function and stimulate neoangiogenesis (89, 90). Statins decrease leukocyte adhesion to endothelial and epithelial cells by inhibiting expression and binding of the integrin LFA-1 and the intercellular adhesion molecule 1 (ICAM-1). Statins also decrease NFkB production, and hence the release of proinflammatory cytokines such as TNF-α and IL-6. This chain of action blocks critical proteins required to form lipid rafts and immune cell activation and growth. They also reduce the levels of oxidative stress (91).

Studies in rats with experimental-induced cirrhosis have shown that statins may prevent LPS-induced ACLF-derived complications and prolong survival. Moreover, statins increase the hepatic sinusoidal function, protect against endothelial dysfunction and the harmful effects of hypovolemic insults. Finally, statins normalise inflammatory markers during critical events such as ACLF and hypovolemia (46, 47) (see **Supplementary Table 3e**). A significant effect of simvastatin, when combined with bone-marrow-derived mesenchymal stem cells, has been demonstrated with amelioration of fibrosis (50) (see **Supplementary Table 3e**). Atorvastatin also reduces portal pressure in CCl_4-cirrhotic rats (48). In human cirrhotic liver samples, Sonic hedgehog (Shh) and Glioma-associated oncogene family zinc finger-2 (Gli-2) mRNA levels, as well as protein expressions, increases (48). Atorvastatin treatment significantly downregulated the hedgehog components Shh and Gli-2 in the BDL and CCl_4-cirrhotic models. Likewise, mRNA levels of α-SMA, collagen-1, and vimentin decreased after atorvastatin treatment.

In contrast, one rat study did not find a significant amelioration of cirrhosis on treatment with atorvastatin or rosuvastatin (49).

Simvastatin may increase the hepato-splanchnic output of nitric oxide products in patients with cirrhosis, thereby improving portal hypertension (18).

Randomised clinical trials have investigated beneficial effects on clinical outcomes such as liver function, rebleeding from oesophageal varices, and survival (92–94), and one ongoing multi-centre trial is also prospectively investigating the potential reduction of hepatic decompensation (19). However, no human studies have explored anti-inflammatory mechanisms in detail; hence, the therapeutic effects of statins are not yet completely understood [for clinical endpoints in human studies (90, 92–104) see **Supplementary Table 2**].

Emricasan

Emricasan is an oral pan-caspase inhibitor with alleviating impact on apoptosis, inflammation, and fibrosis in animal models of liver injury.

Studies have demonstrated how emricasan can inhibit hepatic cell death with reductions in caspase-3-activity in CCl_4-cirrhotic rats, while reducing portal hypertension and hepatic microvascular dysfunction in rats with advanced cirrhosis is also described (51). In addition, three human studies have explored the clinical effects of emricasan (20–22).

Frenette et al. (20) administered emricasan 25 mg in a randomised, double-blinded, placebo-controlled trial. Emricasan reduced cleaved keratin-18 (a marker of apoptosis) relative to placebo, although insignificant, but caspase 3/7 and flCK-18 levels reduced significantly. Garcia-Tsao et al. (21) likewise found reductions in cleaved cytokeratin 18 and caspase-3/7 after 28 days of treatment with emricasan in 22 cirrhotic patients. **Supplementary Table 3** lists anti-inflammatory marker results for the rodent studies.

A recent clinical trial concerning NASH-related cirrhosis by the same authors (22) showed the same biomarker patterns described above. However, the clinical effects on liver biochemistry and portal hypertension were not observed in patients with decompensated NASH-related cirrhosis (69) (see **Supplementary Table 2**).

Lanifibranor

Peroxisome proliferator-activated receptors (PPARs) are present in mammals in three isoforms, and all isoforms have a role in maintaining liver function (105). The pan-PPAR agonist lanifibranor has shown potential to alleviate models of mild liver injury and non-alcoholic fatty liver disease. We found one study of the effects of lanifibranor on cirrhotic rats and on cirrhotic human hepatic cells *in vitro*. Lanifibranor ameliorated fibrosis and portal hypertension in the rats in addition to significant anti-inflammatory effects (**Supplementary Table 3f**) and showed promising results in human hepatic cells. However, no human clinical trials were found.

Formyl Peptide Receptor 2 Agonist—(WKYMVm)

Hexapeptide WKYMVm (Trp-Lys-Tyr-Met-Val-D-Met) is a ligand of the formyl peptide receptor 2. It exhibits anti-inflammatory and angiogenic properties in multiple disease models. The WKYMVm peptide improves vascular remodelling and inhibits fibrosis in a rat model of hepatic failure (53) (See **Supplementary Table 3g**). Furthermore, WKYMVm enhances hepatic function by upregulating the expression of hepatic function markers. These data suggest that the WKYMVm peptide modulates liver function and vascular regeneration in rodent hepatic failure. No human trials are described.

Antioxidants

Seventeen animal studies investigated the effects of five different antioxidant mediators, three of which were investigated in human studies with clinical endpoints): *Curcumin* (33–38), *pentoxifylline* (42, 68), and *diosmin* (42–44) *are described above. Mitoquinone* (54, 55) and *silymarin* (56–60, 106) are described below.

Antioxidant agents seem to attenuate hepatic fibrosis in rodent models (107). The mechanism is partly due to the influence on the activation of hepatic stellate cells, which induce extracellular matrix deposition (**Figure 3**). Several agents have supposed antioxidant effects demonstrated by measurements of reactants as MDA, NADPH oxidase, Nrf2, Keap 1, NFkB, and IkB. NADPH oxidase is highly expressed by Kupffer cells and generates high amounts of ROS during early liver injury. In addition, hepatic stellate cells also seem to express NADPH—generating ROS, which mediates fibrogenic factors (107).

Mitoquinone

Mitochondrial dysfunction appears to play a crucial role in the development and progression of liver cirrhosis. Cirrhotic livers exhibit increased ROS produced by mitochondria. Mitoquinone is a mitochondria-targeted antioxidant, which might relieve the damaging effects of ROS within cirrhotic livers (54, 55). Two rat studies have assessed the effects of treatment with mitoquinone. Thus, Vilaseca et al. (54) found a relieving effect on portal hypertension in rats, as well as on fibrosis and oxidative markers.

Mitochondrial superoxide content was significantly higher in hepatic stellate cells and hepatocytes from cirrhotic rats but not in sinusoidal- or Kupffer cells compared to non-cirrhotic rats, and this effect appeared to be dose-dependent. Similar effects on HSC activity were found in human liver cells exposed to mitoquinone.

Mitoquinone also reduced oxidative stress and reduced portal pressure and intrahepatic vascular resistance in rats with CCl_4-induced cirrhosis. Mitoquinone resulted in a significant reduction in hepatic fibrosis, which points to a potential clinical value of this drug. The activity of the hepatic stellate cells was assessed by the expression of profibrogenic genes and α-SMA, and both markers reduced significantly in cirrhotic rats.

Finally, inflammatory markers in *in vivo* models were measured, and iNOS, IL-6, and IL-1β were all reduced significantly.

In another study of BDL rats, Turkseven et al. (55) also investigated the effects of mitoquinone. Treatment with mitoquinone prevented inflammation, hepatocyte necrosis, and progression of fibrosis. Initially, bile-duct ligation of the rats led to increased gene expression (Qr-PCR) of inflammatory and oxidant markers, and these responses were reduced by mitoquinone. Collagen type col1α1, TGF-β, TNF-α, IL-6, IL-1β, and levels of circulatory TNF-α were all reduced. Furthermore, mitoquinone reduced the protein carbonylation, an indicator of irreversible oxidative protein modification, in cirrhotic rats. Mitoquinone normalised the gene expression of the mitochondrial antioxidant Mn-SOD, Cu/ZnSOD, and catalase impaired by cirrhosis.

Parkin protein expression in mitochondria is an indicator of the removal of dysfunctional mitochondria by autophagy. Parkin protein expression decreases in cirrhosis but increases in rats treated with mitoquinone (55).

Mitoquinone seems to possess both anti-inflammatory and antioxidant effects in human cells and rodent models, but no human studies have yet verified these effects.

Silymarin

Silymarin is an extract of the plant *Silybum marianum* (milk thistle), the main compound being silybin. Silymarin has a low bioavailability and lack solubility in water. Silybin acts by turning off proinflammatory signals derived from NFkB-activation (which is involved in the induction of TNF-α, IL-1, IL-6, and GM-CSF) and induces apoptosis. Silymarin's antioxidant activity is related to its free radical-scavenging and lipid peroxidation inhibition, as demonstrated *in vivo* and *in vitro* (108).

We identified five rodent studies that have assessed the effects of silymarin in cirrhosis models.

Ali et al. (58) investigated the modulatory effects of curcumin, silybin-phytosome, and alpha-R-lipoic acid in rats with TAA-induced cirrhosis. TAA was given at the same time as the intervention. Glutathione depletion, collagen deposition, matrix metalloproteinase-2 activity, TGF-β1 levels and heat shock protein-47 gene expressions- all factors believed to be involved in the development of cirrhosis-, were partially blocked by the combination therapy with curcumin, silybin-phytosome, and alpha-R-lipoic acid. Thus, therapy increased ROS generation and inhibited the activation of hepatic stellate cells, thereby preventing liver cirrhosis.

Zaidi et al. (56) also evaluated the effects of silymarin on rats with TAA-induced cirrhosis. Antioxidant activity was reduced as superoxide dismutase (SOD) and GSH were low, and MDA (measure of lipid peroxidation) and catalase were increased before treatment was initiated. Conversely, silymarin restored SOD and GSH, MDA, and catalase activity.

A possible synergistic effect between silymarin and lactulose has been investigated in a cirrhotic rat model (57) with no significant difference found between treatment groups according to their necro-inflammatory scores.

A combination of silymarin and the amino acid taurine was assessed in a study on CCl_4-induced cirrhosis (59). Silymarin alone and silymarin with taurine restored the TBARS (thiobarbituric acid reactive substances) levels, and the combination treatment significantly reduced NO levels and NOS activity. However, activities of SOD, glutathione peroxidase (GPx), and glutathione reductase (GR) increased significantly in all treatment groups. In addition, glutathione-S-transferase (GST) and reduced glutathione (GSH) increased in rats treated with silymarin alone or the combination treatment.

The cytokines TNF-α, TGF-β1, IL-6, and the proteins leptin and resistin elevated in the cirrhotic model, while adiponectin reduced. All three treatments reduced TGF-β1, IL-6, and leptin,

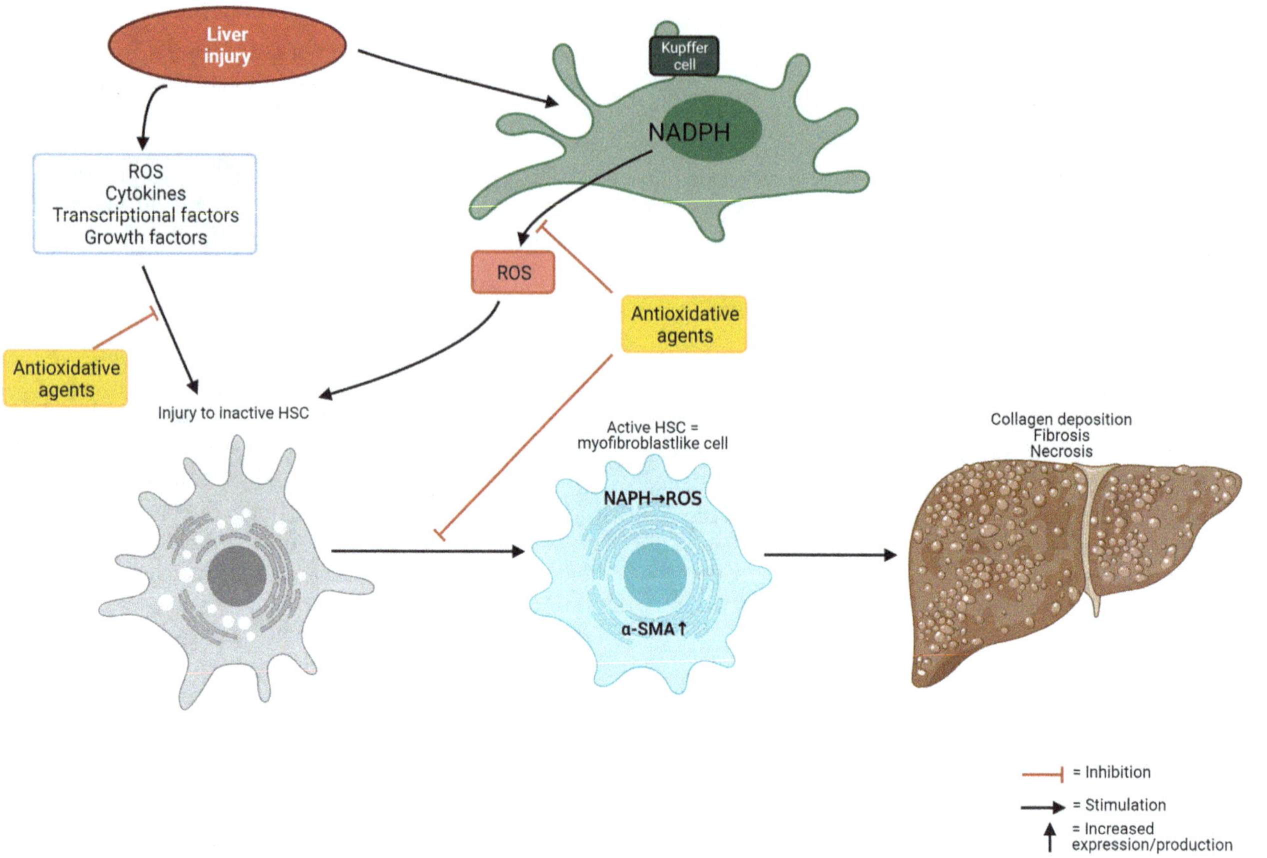

FIGURE 3 | Antioxidative mechanisms. Simplified illustration of oxidative and antioxidative mechanisms affecting liver cells. α-SMA, α-smooth muscle actin; HSC, hepatic stellate cell; NADPH, nicotinamide adenine dinucleotide phosphate; ROS, reactive oxygen species.

but only taurine and the combination taurine and silymarin reduced TNF-α and resistin.

Finally, a combination of bone-marrow-derived stromal cells and silymarin ameliorated liver tissue damage in a CCl_4-cirrhotic rat model through immunoregulatory activities. However, antioxidative markers were not investigated in this study (60).

Only a single cohort study of silymarin has been carried out in humans. Fathalah et al. (106) investigated the effects of high-dose silymarin in decompensated chronic hepatitis C virus (HCV)-cirrhotic patients. The main results improved biochemical liver parameters and Child-Pugh score; however, no oxidative markers were investigated (see **Supplementary Table 2**).

Gut Microflora and the LPS Pathway

Gut dysbiosis with translocation of bacteria and the bacterial product might play a role in the development of complications of cirrhosis. Alleviation of the dysbiosis in the gut flora of patients with cirrhosis, and the effects on LPS, supports that counteracting anti-inflammatory mechanisms are beneficial in cirrhosis.

Our search resulted in four animal studies, two human studies reporting effects on inflammatory markers, and two human studies where only clinical endpoints were considered. Thus, we found three different gut microbial modulation therapies, namely *Faecal microbiota transplantation* (23, 24, 62, 109)*, kahweol* (40, 41) *as described earlier, and artesunate* (63).

Faecal Microbiota Transplantation (FMT)

Among pertinent mechanisms, an increase in LPS leads to hepatocyte damage, which stimulates hepatic macrophages and increases the release of IL-1, IL-6, and TNF-α. Several pathways are involved in the promotion or counteraction of chronic inflammation (40). For example, kahweol affects the LPS pathway in the gut resulting in anti-inflammatory effects (described above). Liu et al. explored the effects faecal microbiota transplantation (FMT) from humans to germ-free and conventional mice (62). They found reduced neuroinflammation and microglial activation and dysbiosis 15 days after FMT exposure, whereas liver inflammation was unaffected. Higher degrees of neuroinflammation in mice regardless of their cirrhosis state was found with faecal microbial colonisation from humans with cirrhosis as compared with mice exposed to colonisation from healthy humans. Bajaj et al. investigated the safety of FMT capsules in patients with cirrhosis and recurrent HE in a Phase 1 randomised, placebo-controlled trial (23). FMT improved duodenal mucosal diversity, dysbiosis, and expression of duodenal antimicrobial peptide (AMP) and reduced lipopolysaccharide-binding protein (LBP). Subsequently, a trial was constructed based on the same cohorts elucidating the effects on inflammatory markers: IL-6 and LPS-binding protein, and bile acids in serum (24). Four weeks of FMT decreased levels of serum IL-6 and LBP compared to the placebo group. In the FMT group, greater deconjugation and secondary bile acid formation were found. In an ongoing study, Woodhouse et al. (109) currently assess if FMT in patients with advanced cirrhosis is effective, feasible, and safe.

Artesunate

Artesunate is an extract of the Chinese herb "Artemisia annua," which has historically been used as an antimalarial drug. It is assumed to affect the pathological bacterial translocation (63), which is thought to be the key driver of spontaneous infection in patients with cirrhosis (110). For example, prophylactic antibacterial treatment is often indicated in patients with ascites and risk of spontaneous bacterial peritonitis. A single study assessed the effects of artesunate in rats with CCl_4-induced cirrhosis (63). Thus, artesunate decreased IL-6 and TNF-α in the cirrhotic liver at week 4, 6, and 8, indicating an effect on inflammatory responses. Microbial diversity in the artesunate group, as compared to controls was increased at week 4 and reduced at weeks 6 and 8. Bacterial genomic DNA products reappeared in rats treated with artesunate after 4 weeks, unlike in the cirrhotic rats not treated with artesunate. No bacteria were detected in the blood in either group. Thus, artesunate decreased the occurrence of bacterial translocation significantly.

No human studies have yet been conducted, but the primary impression of the effects of artesunate is promising according to alleviating the inflammatory factors and the dysbiosis of gut microbiota in cirrhosis.

Deactivation of Hepatic Stellate Cells

Several of the therapeutic agents described are hypothesised to have multiple impacts on different homeostatic and pathophysiological pathways. For example, enoxaparin (30, 31, 64, 65, 111) and tanshinone (61) may have effects that have not yet been classified as direct antifibrotic mechanisms and do not fit into a concrete anti-inflammatory or antioxidative mode of action.

Enoxaparin

Enoxaparin has both anticoagulant and antithrombotic effects (112). A rat experimental study observed a reduction of proliferation and activation of hepatic stellate cells (30). In addition, it has been demonstrated that patients with cirrhosis more frequently exhibit a prothrombotic state than a hypocoagulative state (113, 114).

Enoxaparin has been proven to reduce portal pressure in cirrhotic rats, implying effects beyond the anti-thrombotic (65). Short-term treatment of cirrhotic rats with enoxaparin showed a significant reduction of superoxide content, α-SMA, and mRNA of pro-collagen I and liver fibrosis. In addition, the oxidative stress levels were lower, and fibrosis reduced by 25% after enoxaparin treatment.

However, Fortea et al. (64) did not find an amelioration of fibrosis, biochemical parameters, hepatic endothelial dysfunction, or portal hypertension after enoxaparin treatment of cirrhotic rats. On the contrary, the therapeutic dose of enoxaparin did decrease survival in rats with CCl_4-induced cirrhosis. Enoxaparin as a preventive therapy for portal venous thrombosis in patients with Child-Pugh B-C cirrhosis has been suggested by the authors of one study (111), favouring enoxaparin compared to no treatment. It was found safe and preventive for thrombosis for 34 patients treated for 48 weeks. In addition, the frequency of decompensation reduced, and survival increased in the enoxaparin group.

Tanshinone

Salvia miltiorrhiza (S. miltiorrhiza) is a Chinese herb comprising multiple compounds. Tanshinone is extracted from S. miltiorrhiza and is described as a natural antioxidant with hepatoprotective, antifibrotic, and anticancerogenic effects. In addition, it is supposed to induce stem cell proliferation and differentiation (115). A single rat study investigated the effects in a cirrhotic model (61), where tanshinone improved the histological injury, serological tests, and increased expression of markers indicating newly proliferated stem cells. These effects appeared to be caused by promoting proliferation and differentiation of endogenous liver stem cells. No human trials were found.

DISCUSSION

In the present review, we have identified and explored possible anti-inflammatory and antioxidant agents as potential drug candidates to interfere with the fibrogenesis processes and thereby alleviate the development and perpetuation of complications of cirrhosis. In cirrhotic rodent models we have found promising indices of beneficial anti-inflammatory and antioxidative effects of the COX-2 inhibitor celecoxib, aspirin, curcumin, kahweol, pentoxifylline, diosmin, statins, emricasan, and silymarin. Few indices of effects of etanercept, glycyrrhizin arginine salt, and mitoquinone were found. In addition, FMT is a growing field with the potential to alleviate cirrhosis by a beneficial regulation of the gut flora.

The main limitation of the present review is the lack of human studies assessing anti-inflammatory agents in cirrhosis. The lack makes it difficult to assess the clinical efficacy of the agents discussed and to compare the effects between different studies. The literature offers many experimental studies in rodents where multiple beneficial effects on cirrhosis regarding fibrosis are reported (see **Supplementary Table 3**). However, extrapolating experimental animal studies into a clinically relevant setting is problematic. Nevertheless, several different agents were identified, and many of these showed potential curing or relieving mechanisms and effects in the applied models. However, most of the rodent studies are not comparable since especially the method of inducing cirrhosis differs. The procedures, the duration, and the timing of adding the experimental agents differ vividly.

There are important conflicting results for enoxaparin, statins, and etanercept. In particular, one human study investigating etanercept found significant harmful effects (80). One rat study of statins (49) and enoxaparin (64) showed no intervention effects. Curcumin seems promising in both rodent and human clinical trials. Anti-inflammatory and antifibrotic effects, as well as a positive impact on portal pressure and hemodynamic in rodents combined with favourable clinical outcome in cirrhotic patients, indicates a convincing potential (33–38, 82). Curcumin also has potential effects on quality of life (116). Silymarin is also studied in a different setting and shows potential anti-inflammatory and antioxidative effects in rodents and clinical improvement in patients. Emricasan showed promising alleviating effects in both rodent and human studies on several parameters. Promising clinical effects (20–22) are shown, but only caspase and flCK-18 are measured as anti-inflammatory markers. Hence, the mechanisms are still largely unexplored, and future studies with inflammatory and clinical endpoints are warranted.

Several retrospective studies have suggested that statins can improve mortality in cirrhosis (90, 95, 103). Clinical studies of the anti-portal hypertensive effects of statins have provided encouraging results in recently published trials (93, 97, 102, 117), while other studies have reported a reduced risk of decompensation and death (89, 90, 92, 94), and that statins might reduce the risk of infections in patients with cirrhosis (96). One study also described improved survival during infections among cirrhotic patients undergoing continuing treatment with statins (104). Human studies exploring anti-inflammatory mechanisms in cirrhosis should be highly encouraged.

The anti-inflammatory effects of statins seem to be steps ahead of other agents concerning testing in human trials, mainly due to the similar effect of statins on portal hypertension (93, 97, 102, 117). Novel research implies the anti-inflammatory effects of statins as key drives in lowering the portal pressure, but the immunological impact needs further exploration in humans (89, 91).

Dysbiosis in the gut flora is suspected as a precipitating factor in cirrhotic patients with infections who need antibiotic treatment. FMT could prove to be a valuable "post-treatment" after antibiotic exposure, restoring the potentially harmful effect antibiotics have on microbial diversity and function (118). Initial studies have focused on safety and organ function outcomes in cirrhosis (23), relevant in a complex disease entity. Studies on FMT without prior antibiotics are needed to assess the impact of gut dysbiosis and the inhibition or alleviation of inflammation in decompensated cirrhosis. Future studies are awaited (109) in the search for preventive and treating agents in cirrhosis.

Very few side effects are reported for the main part of the described agents, and safety deserves a primary focus in future investigations of anti-inflammatory agents. Only two safety studies regarding celecoxib are conducted (119, 120).

Real-life clinical trials exploring anti-inflammatory interventions and their safety in patients with liver cirrhosis are notably missing in the literature. Furthermore, data on the combination of anti-inflammatory or antioxidative markers and clinical outcomes are scarce. Human randomised clinical trials, preferably placebo-controlled, are the next step toward clinical application of anti-inflammatory agents. As most inflammation markers are easy to sample by blood tests, this should be possible and feasible to add to clinical protocols.

Autologous macrophage therapy is another promising treatment that seems safe (121); the effects of which are yet to be fully investigated. This is also the case for other autologous cell transplantation, such as mesenchymal stromal cell therapy (122).

In conclusion, we recommend further study of the inflammatory, oxidative, microbiological, and immunological mechanisms and pathways responsible for disease progression in cirrhosis. Known and novel compounds with potential healing effects in cirrhosis are identified and require further exploration. In general, the literature encloses very few human clinical trials on the aspects, and the need for studies is growing. Future studies should include anti-inflammatory biomarkers and clinical endpoints in combination to assess potential immunological agents in the treatment of cirrhosis.

AUTHOR CONTRIBUTIONS

TK, NK, and SM contributed to conception and design of the review. TK performed the literature searches and wrote the first draught of the manuscript. NK and TK assessed the literature searches. All authors critically revised the litterature and contributed to manuscript revision, read, and approved the submitted version.

REFERENCES

1. Smith A, Baumgartner K, Bositis C. Cirrhosis: diagnosis and management. *Am Fam Physician.* (2019) 100:759–70.
2. Zhang CY, Yuan WG, He P, Lei JH, Wang CX. Liver fibrosis and hepatic stellate cells: etiology, pathological hallmarks and therapeutic targets. *World J Gastroenterol.* (2016) 22:10512–22. doi: 10.3748/wjg.v22.i48.10512
3. Park BJ, Lee YJ, Lee HR. Chronic liver inflammation: clinical implications beyond alcoholic liver disease. *World J Gastroenterol.* (2014) 20:2168–75. doi: 10.3748/wjg.v20.i9.2168
4. Albillos A, Lario M, Álvarez-Mon M. Cirrhosis-associated immune dysfunction: distinctive features and clinical relevance. *J Hepatol.* (2014) 61:1385–96. doi: 10.1016/j.jhep.2014.08.010
5. Koyama Y, Brenner DA. Liver inflammation and fibrosis. *J Clin Invest.* (2017) 127:55–64. doi: 10.1172/JCI88881

6. Simbrunner B, Mandorfer M, Trauner M, Reiberger T. Gut-liver axis signaling in portal hypertension. *World J Gastroenterol.* (2019) 25:5897–917. doi: 10.3748/wjg.v25.i39.5897
7. Reiberger T, Mandorfer M. Beta adrenergic blockade and decompensated cirrhosis. *J Hepatol.* (2017) 66:849–59. doi: 10.1016/j.jhep.2016.11.001
8. Kockerling D, Nathwani R, Forlano R, Manousou P, Mullish BH, Dhar A. Current and future pharmacological therapies for managing cirrhosis and its complications. *World J Gastroenterol.* (2019) 25:888–908. doi: 10.3748/wjg.v25.i8.888
9. Angeli P, Bernardi M, Villanueva C, Francoz C, Mookerjee RP, Trebicka J, et al. EASL clinical practice guidelines for the management of patients with decompensated cirrhosis. *J Hepatol.* (2018) 69:406–60. doi: 10.1016/j.jhep.2018.03.024
10. Thiele M, Albillos A, Abazi R, Wiest R, Gluud LL, Krag A. Non-selective beta-blockers may reduce risk of hepatocellular carcinoma: a meta-analysis of randomized trials. *Liver Int.* (2015) 35:2009–16. doi: 10.1111/liv.12782
11. Thiele M, Wiest R, Gluud LL, Albillos A, Krag A. Can non-selective beta-blockers prevent hepatocellular carcinoma in patients with cirrhosis? *Med Hypotheses.* (2013) 81:871–4. doi: 10.1016/j.mehy.2013.08.026
12. Pose E, Cardenas A. Translating our current understanding of ascites management into new therapies for patients with cirrhosis and fluid retention. *Dig Dis.* (2017) 35:402–10. doi: 10.1159/000456595
13. Caraceni P, Riggio O, Angeli P, Alessandria C, Neri S, Foschi FG, et al. Long-term albumin administration in decompensated cirrhosis (ANSWER): an open-label randomised trial. *Lancet.* (2018) 391:2417–29. doi: 10.1016/S0140-6736(18)30840-7
14. Fernández J, Clària J, Amorós A, Aguilar F, Castro M, Casulleras M, et al. Effects of albumin treatment on systemic and portal hemodynamics and systemic inflammation in patients with decompensated cirrhosis. *Gastroenterology.* (2019) 157:149–62. doi: 10.1053/j.gastro.2019.03.021
15. Wilde B, Katsounas A. Immune dysfunction and albumin-related immunity in liver cirrhosis. *Mediators Inflamm.* (2019) 2019:7537649. doi: 10.1155/2019/7537649
16. Bernardi M, Angeli P, Claria J, Moreau R, Gines P, Jalan R, et al. Albumin in decompensated cirrhosis: new concepts and perspectives. *Gut.* (2020) 69:1127–38. doi: 10.1136/gutjnl-2019-318843
17. Li S, Hong M, Tan HY, Wang N, Feng Y. Insights into the role and interdependence of oxidative stress and inflammation in liver diseases. *Oxid Med Cell Longev.* (2016) 2016:4234061. doi: 10.1155/2016/4234061
18. Zafra C, Abraldes JG, Turnes J, Berzigotti A, Fernández M, García-Pagán JC, et al. Simvastatin enhances hepatic nitric oxide production and decreases the hepatic vascular tone in patients with cirrhosis. *Gastroenterology.* (2004) 126:749–55. doi: 10.1053/j.gastro.2003.12.007
19. Kaplan DE, Mehta R, Garcia-Tsao G, Albrecht J, Aytaman A, Baffy G, et al. SACRED: Effect of simvastatin on hepatic decompensation and death in subjects with high-risk compensated cirrhosis: statins and cirrhosis: reducing events of decompensation. *Contemp Clin Trials.* (2021) 104:106367. doi: 10.1016/j.cct.2021.106367
20. Frenette CT, Morelli G, Shiffman ML, Frederick RT, Rubin RA, Fallon MB, et al. Emricasan improves liver function in patients with cirrhosis and high model for end-stage liver disease scores compared with placebo. *Clin Gastroenterol Hepatol.* (2019) 17:774–83.e4. doi: 10.1016/j.cgh.2018.06.012
21. Garcia-Tsao G, Fuchs M, Shiffman M, Borg BB, Pyrsopoulos N, Shetty K, et al. Emricasan (IDN-6556) lowers portal pressure in patients with compensated cirrhosis and severe portal hypertension. *Hepatology.* (2019) 69:717–28. doi: 10.1002/hep.30199
22. Garcia-Tsao G, Bosch J, Kayali Z, Harrison SA, Abdelmalek MF, Lawitz E, et al. Randomized placebo-controlled trial of emricasan for non-alcoholic steatohepatitis-related cirrhosis with severe portal hypertension. *J Hepatol.* (2020) 72:885–95. doi: 10.1016/j.jhep.2019.12.010
23. Bajaj JS, Salzman NH, Acharya C, Sterling RK, White MB, Gavis EA, et al. Fecal microbial transplant capsules are safe in hepatic encephalopathy: a phase 1, randomized, placebo-controlled trial. *Hepatology.* (2019) 70:1690–703. doi: 10.1002/hep.30690
24. Bajaj JS, Salzman N, Acharya C, Takei H, Kakiyama G, Fagan A, et al. Microbial functional change is linked with clinical outcomes after capsular fecal transplant in cirrhosis. *JCI Insight.* (2019) 4:e133410. doi: 10.1172/jci.insight.133410
25. Gao JH, Wen SL, Tong H, Wang CH, Yang WJ, Tang SH, et al. Inhibition of cyclooxygenase-2 alleviates liver cirrhosis via improvement of the dysfunctional gut-liver axis in rats. *Am J Physiol - Gastrointest Liver Physiol.* (2016) 310:G962–72. doi: 10.1152/ajpgi.00428.2015
26. Gao JH, Wen SL, Yang WJ, Lu YY, Tong H, Huang ZY, et al. Celecoxib ameliorates portal hypertension of the cirrhotic rats through the dual inhibitory effects on the intrahepatic fibrosis and angiogenesis. *PLoS ONE.* (2013) 8:e0146617. doi: 10.1371/journal.pone.0069309
27. Wen SL, Gao JH, Yang WJ, Lu YY, Tong H, Huang ZY, et al. Celecoxib attenuates hepatic cirrhosis through inhibition of epithelial-to-mesenchymal transition of hepatocytes. *J Gastroenterol Hepatol.* (2014) 29:1932–42. doi: 10.1111/jgh.12641
28. Su W, Tai Y, Tang SH, Ye YT, Zhao C, Gao JH, et al. Celecoxib attenuates hepatocyte apoptosis by inhibiting endoplasmic reticulum stress in thioacetamide-induced cirrhotic rats. *World J Gastroenterol.* (2020) 26:4094–107. doi: 10.3748/wjg.v26.i28.4094
29. Tang S, Huang Z, Jiang J, Gao J, Zhao C, Tai Y, et al. Celecoxib ameliorates liver cirrhosis via reducing inflammation and oxidative stress along spleen-liver axis in rats. *Life Sci.* (2021) 272:119203. doi: 10.1016/j.lfs.2021.119203
30. Li CJ, Yang ZH, Shi XL, Liu DL. Effects of aspirin and enoxaparin in a rat model of liver fibrosis. *World J Gastroenterol.* (2017) 23:6412–9. doi: 10.3748/wjg.v23.i35.6412
31. Assy N, Hussein O, Khalil A, Luder A, Szvalb S, Paizi M, et al. The beneficial effect of aspirin and enoxaparin on fibrosis progression and regenerative activity in a rat model of cirrhosis. *Dig Dis Sci.* (2007) 52:1187–93. doi: 10.1007/s10620-006-9595-1
32. Abdul-Hamid M, Ahmed RR, Moustafa N, Nady R. The antifibrogenic effect of etanercept on development of liver cirrhosis induced by thioacetamide in rats. *Ultrastruct Pathol.* (2017) 41:23–35. doi: 10.1080/01913123.2016.1256361
33. Abo-Zaid MA, Shaheen ES, Ismail AH. Immunomodulatory effect of curcumin on hepatic cirrhosis in experimental rats. *J Food Biochem.* (2020) 44:e13219. doi: 10.1111/jfbc.13219
34. Macías-Pérez JR, Vázquez-López BJ, Muñoz-Ortega MH, Aldaba-Muruato LR, Martínez-Hernández SL, Sánchez-Alemán E, et al. Curcumin and α/β-Adrenergic antagonists cotreatment reverse liver cirrhosis in hamsters: Participation of Nrf-2 and NF-κB. *J Immunol Res.* (2019) 2019:3019794. doi: 10.1155/2019/3019794
35. Kyung EJ, Kim HB, Hwang ES, Lee S, Choi BK, Kim JW, et al. Evaluation of hepatoprotective effect of curcumin on liver cirrhosis using a combination of biochemical analysis and magnetic resonance-based electrical conductivity imaging. *Mediators Inflamm.* (2018) 2018:5491797. doi: 10.1155/2018/5491797
36. Chenari S, Safari F, Moradi A. Curcumin enhances liver SIRT3 expression in the rat model of cirrhosis. *Iran J Basic Med Sci.* (2017) 20:1306–11. doi: 10.22038/IJBMS.2017.9609
37. Hsu SJ, Lee JY, Lin TY, Hsieh YH, Huang HC, Lee FY, et al. The beneficial effects of curcumin in cirrhotic rats with portal hypertension. *Biosci Rep.* (2017) 37:BSR20171015. doi: 10.1042/BSR20171015
38. Cai Y, Lu D, Zou Y, Zhou C, Liu H, Tu C, et al. Curcumin protects against intestinal origin endotoxemia in rat liver cirrhosis by targeting PCSK9. *J Food Sci.* (2017) 82:772–80. doi: 10.1111/1750-3841.13647
39. Hernández-Aquino E, Quezada-Ramírez MA, Silva-Olivares A, Ramos-Tovar E, Flores-Beltrán RE, Segovia J, et al. Curcumin downregulates Smad pathways and reduces hepatic stellate cells activation in experimental fibrosis. *Ann Hepatol.* (2020) 19:497–506. doi: 10.1016/j.aohep.2020.05.006
40. Seo HY, Kim MK, Lee SH, Hwang JS, Park KG, Jang BK. Kahweol ameliorates the liver inflammation through the inhibition of NF-κB and STAT3 activation in primary kupffer cells and primary hepatocytes. *Nutrients.* (2018) 10:863. doi: 10.3390/nu10070863
41. Arauz J, Moreno MG, Cortés-Reynosa P, Salazar EP, Muriel P. Coffee attenuates fibrosis by decreasing the expression of TGF-β and CTGF in a murine model of liver damage. *J Appl Toxicol.* (2013) 33:970–9. doi: 10.1002/jat.2788
42. Ali FEM, Bakr AG, Abo-youssef AM, Azouz AA, Hemeida RAM. Targeting Keap-1/Nrf-2 pathway and cytoglobin as a potential protective mechanism of diosmin and pentoxifylline against cholestatic liver cirrhosis. *Life Sci.* (2018) 207:50–60. doi: 10.1016/j.lfs.2018.05.048

43. Ali FEM, Azouz AA, Bakr AG, Abo-youssef AM, Hemeida RAM. Hepatoprotective effects of diosmin and/or sildenafil against cholestatic liver cirrhosis: the role of Keap-1/Nrf-2 and P38-MAPK/NF-κB/iNOS signaling pathway. *Food Chem Toxicol.* (2018) 120:294–304. doi: 10.1016/j.fct.2018.07.027
44. Tahir M, Rehman MU, Lateef A, Khan R, Khan AQ, Qamar W, et al. Diosmin protects against ethanol-induced hepatic injury via alleviation of inflammation and regulation of TNF-α and NF-κB activation. *Alcohol.* (2013) 47:131–9. doi: 10.1016/j.alcohol.2012.12.010
45. Zhang H, Lin Y, Zhen Y, Hu G, Meng X, Li X, et al. Therapeutic effect of glycyrrhizin arginine salt on rat cholestatic cirrhosis and its mechanism. *Am J Chin Med.* (2018) 46:1111–27. doi: 10.1142/S0192415X18500581
46. Tripathi DM, Vilaseca M, Lafoz E, Garcia-Calderó H, Viegas Haute G, Fernández-Iglesias A, et al. Simvastatin prevents progression of acute on chronic liver failure in rats with cirrhosis and portal hypertension. *Gastroenterology.* (2018) 155:1564–77. doi: 10.1053/j.gastro.2018.07.022
47. Meireles CZ, Pasarin M, Lozano JJ, García-Calderó H, Gracia-Sancho J, García-Pagán JC, et al. Simvastatin attenuates liver injury in rodents with biliary cirrhosis submitted to hemorrhage/resuscitation. *Shock.* (2017) 47:370–7. doi: 10.1097/SHK.0000000000000734
48. Uschner FE, Ranabhat G, Choi SS, Granzow M, Klein S, Schierwagen R, et al. Statins activate the canonical hedgehog-signaling and aggravate non-cirrhotic portal hypertension, but inhibit the non-canonical hedgehog signaling and cirrhotic portal hypertension. *Sci Rep.* (2015) 5:14573. doi: 10.1038/srep14573
49. Shirin H, Sharvit E, Aeed H, Gavish D, Bruck R. Atorvastatin and rosuvastatin do not prevent thioacetamide induced liver cirrhosis in rats. *World J Gastroenterol.* (2013) 19:241–8. doi: 10.3748/wjg.v19.i2.241
50. Jang YO, Kim SH, Cho MY, Kim KS, Park KS, Cha SK, et al. Synergistic effects of simvastatin and bone marrow-derived mesenchymal stem cells on hepatic fibrosis. *Biochem Biophys Res Commun.* (2018) 497:264–71. doi: 10.1016/j.bbrc.2018.02.067
51. Gracia-Sancho J, Manicardi N, Ortega-Ribera M, Maeso-Díaz R, Guixé-Muntet S, Fernández-Iglesias A, et al. Emricasan ameliorates portal hypertension and liver fibrosis in cirrhotic rats through a hepatocyte-mediated paracrine mechanism. *Hepatol Commun.* (2019) 3:987–1000. doi: 10.1002/hep4.1360
52. Boyer-Diaz Z, Aristu-Zabalza P, Andrés-Rozas M, Robert C, Ortega-Ribera M, Fernández-Iglesias A, et al. Pan-PPAR agonist lanifibranor improves portal hypertension and hepatic fibrosis in experimental advanced chronic liver disease. *J Hepatol.* (2021) 74:1188–99. doi: 10.1016/j.jhep.2020.11.045
53. Jun JH, Park SY, Park S, Park HJ, Kim JY, Park GT, et al. Formyl peptide receptor 2 alleviates hepatic fibrosis in liver cirrhosis by vascular remodeling. *Int J Mol Sci.* (2021) 22:1–4. doi: 10.3390/ijms22042107
54. Vilaseca M, García-Calderó H, Lafoz E, Ruart M, López-Sanjurjo CI, Murphy MP, et al. Mitochondria-targeted antioxidant mitoquinone deactivates human and rat hepatic stellate cells and reduces portal hypertension in cirrhotic rats. *Liver Int.* (2017) 37:1002–12. doi: 10.1111/liv.13436
55. Turkseven S, Bolognesi M, Brocca A, Pesce P, Angeli P, Di Pascoli M. Mitochondria-targeted antioxidant mitoquinone attenuates liver inflammation and fibrosis in cirrhotic rats. *Am J Physiol - Gastrointest Liver Physiol.* (2020) 318:G298–304. doi: 10.1152/ajpgi.00135.2019
56. Zaidi SNF, Mahboob T. Prevention of liver cirrhosis by Silymarin. *Pak J Pharm Sci.* (2017) 30:1203–11.
57. Ghobadi Pour M, Mirazi N, Alaei H, Moradkhani S, Rajaei Z, Monsef Esfahani A. Effects of lactulose and silymarin on liver enzymes in cirrhotic rats. *Can J Physiol Pharmacol.* (2017) 95:522–9. doi: 10.1139/cjpp-2016-0454
58. Ali SO, Darwish HAEM, Ismail NAEF. Modulatory effects of curcumin, silybin-phytosome and alpha-R-lipoic acid against thioacetamide-induced liver cirrhosis in rats. *Chem Biol Interact.* (2014) 216:26–33. doi: 10.1016/j.cbi.2014.03.009
59. Abdel-Moneim AM, Al-Kahtani MA, El-Kersh MA, Al-Omair MA. Free radical-scavenging, anti-inflammatory/anti-fibrotic and hepatoprotective actions of taurine and silymarin against CCl4 induced rat liver damage. *PLoS ONE.* (2015) 10:e0144509. doi: 10.1371/journal.pone.0144509
60. Aithal AP, Bairy LK, Seetharam RN, Kumar N. Hepatoprotective effect of bone marrow-derived mesenchymal stromal cells in CCl4-induced liver cirrhosis. *3 Biotech.* (2021) 11:107. doi: 10.1007/s13205-021-02640-y
61. Yang N, Chen H, Gao Y, Zhang S, Lin Q, Ji X, et al. Tanshinone IIA exerts therapeutic effects by acting on endogenous stem cells in rats with liver cirrhosis. *Biomed Pharmacother.* (2020) 132:110815. doi: 10.1016/j.biopha.2020.110815
62. Liu R, Kang JD, Sartor RB, Sikaroodi M, Fagan A, Gavis EA, et al. Neuroinflammation in murine cirrhosis is dependent on the gut microbiome and is attenuated by fecal transplant. *Hepatology.* (2020) 71:611–26. doi: 10.1002/hep.30827
63. Chen YX, Lai LN, Zhang HY, Bi YH, Meng L, Li XJ, et al. Effect of artesunate supplementation on bacterial translocation and dysbiosis of gut microbiota in rats with liver cirrhosis. *World J Gastroenterol.* (2016) 22:2949–59. doi: 10.3748/wjg.v22.i10.2949
64. Fortea JI, Zipprich A, Fernandez-Mena C, Puerto M, Bosoi CR, Almagro J, et al. Enoxaparin does not ameliorate liver fibrosis or portal hypertension in rats with advanced cirrhosis. *Liver Int.* (2018) 38:102–12. doi: 10.1111/liv.13510
65. Cerini F, Vilaseca M, Lafoz E, García-Irigoyen O, García-Calderó H, Tripathi DM, et al. Enoxaparin reduces hepatic vascular resistance and portal pressure in cirrhotic rats. *J Hepatol.* (2016) 64:834–42. doi: 10.1016/j.jhep.2015.12.003
66. Tilg H. Cytokines and liver diseases. *Can J Gastroenterol.* (2001) 15:661–8. doi: 10.1155/2001/746736
67. Gao JH, Wen SL, Feng S, Yang WJ, Lu YY, Tong H, et al. Celecoxib and octreotide synergistically ameliorate portal hypertension via inhibition of angiogenesis in cirrhotic rats. *Angiogenesis.* (2016) 19:501–11. doi: 10.1007/s10456-016-9522-9
68. Lebrec D, Thabut D, Oberti F, Perarnau JM, Condat B, Barraud H, et al. Pentoxifylline does not decrease short-term mortality but does reduce complications in patients with advanced cirrhosis. *Gastroenterology.* (2010) 138:1755–62. doi: 10.1053/j.gastro.2010.01.040
69. Frenette C, Kayali Z, Mena E, Mantry PS, Lucas KJ, Neff G, et al. Emricasan to prevent new decompensation in patients with NASH-related decompensated cirrhosis. *J Hepatol.* (2021) 74:274–82. doi: 10.1016/j.jhep.2020.09.029
70. Krasselt M, Baerwald C. Celecoxib for the treatment of musculoskeletal arthritis. *Expert Opin Pharmacother.* (2019) 20:1689–702. doi: 10.1080/14656566.2019.1645123
71. Puljak L, Marin A, Vrdoljak D, Markotic F, Utrobicic A, Tugwell P. Celecoxib for osteoarthritis. *Cochrane Database Syst Rev.* (2017) 2017:CD009865. doi: 10.1002/14651858.CD009865.pub2
72. Mohammed NA, El-Aleem SA, El-Hafiz HA, McMahon RFT. Distribution of constitutive (COX-1) and inducible (COX-2) cyclooxygenase in postviral human liver cirrhosis: a possible role for COX-2 in the pathogenesis of liver cirrhosis. *J Clin Pathol.* (2004) 57:350–4. doi: 10.1136/jcp.2003.012120
73. El-Bassiouny A, Zoheiry MMK, Nosseir MMF, El-Ahwany EG, Ibrahim RA, El-Bassiouni NEI. Expression of cyclooxygenase-2 and transforming growth factor-beta 1 in HCV-induced chronic liver disease and hepatocellular carcinoma. *MedGenMed.* (2007) 9:45.
74. Li T, Dong ZR, Guo ZY, Wang CH, Tang ZY, Qu SF, et al. Aspirin enhances IFN-α-induced growth inhibition and apoptosis of hepatocellular carcinoma via JAK1/STAT1 pathway. *Cancer Gene Ther.* (2013) 20:366–74. doi: 10.1038/cgt.2013.29
75. Jiang ZG, Feldbrügge L, Tapper EB, Popov Y, Ghaziani T, Afdhal N, et al. Aspirin use is associated with lower indices of liver fibrosis among adults in the United States. *Aliment Pharmacol Ther.* (2016) 43:734–43. doi: 10.1111/apt.13515
76. Shin S, Lee SH, Lee M, Kim JH, Lee W, Lee HW, et al. Aspirin and the risk of hepatocellular carcinoma development in patients with alcoholic cirrhosis. *Medicine.* (2020) 99:e19008. doi: 10.1097/MD.0000000000019008
77. Lee TY, Hsu YC, Tseng HC, Yu SH, Lin JT, Wu MS, et al. Association of daily aspirin therapy with risk of hepatocellular carcinoma in patients with chronic hepatitis B. *JAMA Intern Med.* (2019) 179:633–40. doi: 10.1001/jamainternmed.2018.8342
78. Böhm F, Köhler UA, Speicher T, Werner S. Regulation of liver regeneration by growth factors and cytokines. *EMBO Mol Med.* (2010) 2:294–305. doi: 10.1002/emmm.201000085
79. Baeck C, Tacke F. Balance of inflammatory pathways and interplay of immune cells in the liver during homeostasis and injury. *EXCLI J.* (2014) 13:67–81.

80. Tang KT, Dufour JF, Chen PH, Hernaez R, Hutfless S. Antitumour necrosis factor-α agents and development of new-onset cirrhosis or non-alcoholic fatty liver disease: a retrospective cohort. *BMJ Open Gastroenterol.* (2020) 7:e000349. doi: 10.1136/bmjgast-2019-000349
81. Qiu P, Sun J, Man S, Yang H, Ma L, Yu P, et al. Curcumin attenuates N-Nitrosodiethylamine-induced liver injury in mice by utilizing the method of metabonomics. *J Agric Food Chem.* (2017) 65:2000-7. doi: 10.1021/acs.jafc.6b04797
82. Nouri-Vaskeh M, Malek Mahdavi A, Afshan H, Alizadeh L, Zarei M. Effect of curcumin supplementation on disease severity in patients with liver cirrhosis: a randomized controlled trial. *Phyther Res.* (2020) 34:1446-54. doi: 10.1002/ptr.6620
83. He G, Karin M. NF-κB and STAT3- key players in liver inflammation and cancer. *Cell Res.* (2011) 21:159-68. doi: 10.1038/cr.2010.183
84. Cárdenas C, Quesada AR, Medina MA. Anti-angiogenic and anti-inflammatory properties of kahweol, a coffee diterpene. *PLoS ONE.* (2011) 6:e23407. doi: 10.1371/annotation/38262cc6-07cc-4074-8ce7-2181d4d0fbdc
85. Bektas S, Karakaya K, Can M, Bahadir B, Guven B, Erdogan N, et al. The effects of tadalafil and pentoxifylline on apoptosis and nitric oxide synthase in liver ischemia/reperfusion injury. *Kaohsiung J Med Sci.* (2016) 32:339-47. doi: 10.1016/j.kjms.2016.05.005
86. Li H, Hua J, Guo CX, Wang WX, Wang BJ, Yang DL, et al. Pentoxifylline inhibits liver fibrosis via hedgehog signaling pathway. *J Huazhong Univ Sci Technol - Med Sci.* (2016) 36:372-6. doi: 10.1007/s11596-016-1594-7
87. Zheng Y, Zhang R, Shi W, Li L, Liu H, Chen Z, et al. Metabolism and pharmacological activities of the natural health-benefiting compound diosmin. *Food Funct.* (2020) 11:8472-92. doi: 10.1039/D0FO01598A
88. Dastagir G, Rizvi MA. Review *Glycyrrhiza glabra L.* (Liquorice). *Pak J Pharm Sci.* (2016) 29:1727-33.
89. Tsochatzis EA, Bosch J. Statins in cirrhosis—ready for prime time. *Hepatology.* (2017) 66:697-9. doi: 10.1002/hep.29277
90. Bang UC, Benfield T, Bendtsen F. Reduced risk of decompensation and death associated with use of statins in patients with alcoholic cirrhosis. a nationwide case-cohort study. *Aliment Pharmacol Ther.* (2017) 46:673-80. doi: 10.1111/apt.14243
91. Pose E, Trebicka J, Mookerjee RP, Angeli P, Ginès P. Statins: old drugs as new therapy for liver diseases? *J Hepatol.* (2019) 70:194-202. doi: 10.1016/j.jhep.2018.07.019
92. Pollo-Flores P, Soldan M, Santos UC, Kunz DG, Mattos DE, da Silva AC, et al. Three months of simvastatin therapy vs. placebo for severe portal hypertension in cirrhosis: a randomized controlled trial. *Dig Liver Dis.* (2015) 47:957-63. doi: 10.1016/j.dld.2015.07.156
93. Abraldes JG, Villanueva C, Aracil C, Turnes J, Hernandez-Guerra M, Genesca J, et al. Addition of simvastatin to standard therapy for the prevention of variceal rebleeding does not reduce rebleeding but increases survival in patients with cirrhosis. *Gastroenterology.* (2016) 150:1160-70.e3. doi: 10.1053/j.gastro.2016.01.004
94. Abraldes JG, Albillos A, Bañares R, Turnes J, González R, García-Pagán JC, et al. Simvastatin lowers portal pressure in patients with cirrhosis and portal hypertension: a randomized controlled trial. *Gastroenterology.* (2009) 136:1651-8. doi: 10.1053/j.gastro.2009.01.043
95. Huang YW, Lee CL, Yang SS, Fu SC, Chen YY, Wang TC, et al. Statins reduce the risk of cirrhosis and its decompensation in chronic hepatitis b patients: a nationwide cohort study. *Am J Gastroenterol.* (2016) 111:976-85. doi: 10.1038/ajg.2016.179
96. Motzkus-Feagans C, Pakyz AL, Ratliff SM, Bajaj JS, Lapane KL. Statin use and infections in veterans with cirrhosis. *Aliment Pharmacol Ther.* (2013) 38:611-8. doi: 10.1111/apt.12430
97. Bishnu S, Ahammed SKM, Sarkar A, Hembram J, Chatterjee S, Das K, et al. Effects of atorvastatin on portal hemodynamics and clinical outcomes in patients with cirrhosis with portal hypertension: a proof-of-concept study. *Eur J Gastroenterol Hepatol.* (2018) 30:54-9. doi: 10.1097/MEG.0000000000001006
98. Kumar S, Grace ND, Qamar AA. Statin use in patients with cirrhosis: a retrospective cohort study. *Dig Dis Sci.* (2014) 59:1958-65. doi: 10.1007/s10620-014-3179-2
99. Simon TG, Bonilla H, Yan P, Chung RT, Butt AA. Atorvastatin and fluvastatin are associated with dose-dependent reductions in cirrhosis and hepatocellular carcinoma, among patients with hepatitis C virus: results from ERCHIVES. *Hepatology.* (2016) 64:47-57. doi: 10.1002/hep.28506
100. Mohanty A, Tate JP, Garcia-Tsao G. Statins are associated with a decreased risk of decompensation and death in veterans with hepatitis c-related compensated cirrhosis. *Gastroenterology.* (2016) 150:430-40.e1. doi: 10.1053/j.gastro.2015.10.007
101. Chang FM, Wang YP, Lang HC, Tsai CF, Hou MC, Lee FY, et al. Statins decrease the risk of decompensation in hepatitis B virus- and hepatitis C virus-related cirrhosis: a population-based study. *Hepatology.* (2017) 66:896-907. doi: 10.1002/hep.29172
102. Abd-Elsalam S, Elwan N, Salah R, Hamisa M, Shady E, Hawash N. Evaluation of portal pressure by doppler ultrasound in patients with cirrhosis before and after simvastatin administration - a randomized controlled trial. *F1000Research.* (2018) 7:256. doi: 10.12688/f1000research.13915.1
103. Kaplan DE, Serper MA, Mehta R, Fox R, John B, Aytaman A, et al. Effects of hypercholesterolemia and statin exposure on survival in a large national cohort of patients with cirrhosis. *Gastroenterology.* (2019) 156:1693-706.e12. doi: 10.1053/j.gastro.2019.01.026
104. Hung TH, Tsai CC, Lee HF. Statin use in cirrhotic patients with infectious diseases: a population-based study. *PLoS ONE.* (2019) 14:e0215839. doi: 10.1371/journal.pone.0215839
105. Liss KHH, Finck BN. PPARs and nonalcoholic fatty liver disease. *Biochimie.* (2017) 136:65-74. doi: 10.1016/j.biochi.2016.11.009
106. Fathalah WF, Aziz MAA, Soud NHA El, Raziky MES El. High dose of silymarin in patients with decompensated liver disease: a randomized controlled trial. *J Interf Cytokine Res.* (2017) 37:480-7. doi: 10.1089/jir.2017.0051
107. Bataller R, Schwabe RF, Choi YH, Yang L, Paik YH, Lindquist J, et al. NADPH oxidase signal transduces angiotensin II in hepatic stellate cells and is critical in hepatic fibrosis. *J Clin Invest.* (2003) 112:1383-94. doi: 10.1172/JCI18212
108. Federico A, Dallio M, Loguercio C. Silymarin/Silybin and chronic liver disease: a marriage of many years. *Molecules.* (2017) 22:191. doi: 10.3390/molecules22020191
109. Woodhouse CA, Patel VC, Goldenberg S, Sanchez-Fueyo A, China L, O'Brien A, et al. PROFIT, a PROspective, randomised placebo controlled feasibility trial of faecal microbiota transplantation in cirrhosis: study protocol for a single-blinded trial. *BMJ Open.* (2019) 9:e023518. doi: 10.1136/bmjopen-2018-023518
110. Cirera I, Martin Bauer T, Miguel N, Vila J, Grande L, Taurá P, et al. Bacterial translocation of enteric organisms in patients with cirrhosis. *J Hepatol.* (2001) 34:32-7. doi: 10.1016/S0168-8278(00)00013-1
111. Villa E, Cammà C, Marietta M, Luongo M, Critelli R, Colopi S, et al. Enoxaparin prevents portal vein thrombosis and liver decompensation in patients with advanced cirrhosis. *Gastroenterology.* (2012) 143:1253-60.e4. doi: 10.1053/j.gastro.2012.07.018
112. Frizelle S, Schwarz J, Huber SA, Leslie K. Evaluation of the effects of low molecular weight heparin on inflammation and collagen deposition in chronic coxsackievirus B3-induced myocarditis in A/J mice. *Am J Pathol.* (1992) 141:203-9
113. Tripodi A, Primignani M, Chantarangkul V, Dell'Era A, Clerici M, de Franchis R, et al. An imbalance of pro- vs anti-coagulation factors in plasma from patients with cirrhosis. *Gastroenterology.* (2009) 137:2105-11. doi: 10.1053/j.gastro.2009.08.045
114. Lisman T, Leebeek FWG. Hemostatic alterations in liver disease: a review on pathophysiology, clinical consequences, and treatment. *Dig Surg.* (2007) 24:250-8. doi: 10.1159/000103655
115. Shi MJ, Dong BS, Yang WN, Su SB, Zhang H. Preventive and therapeutic role of Tanshinone IIA in hepatology. *Biomed Pharmacother.* (2019) 112:108676. doi: 10.1016/j.biopha.2019.108676
116. Nouri-Vaskeh M, Afshan H, Malek Mahdavi A, Alizadeh L, Fan X, Zarei M. Curcumin ameliorates health-related quality of life in patients with liver cirrhosis: a randomized, double-blind placebo-controlled trial. *Complement Ther Med.* (2020) 49:102351. doi: 10.1016/j.ctim.2020.102351
117. Pose E, Napoleone L, Amin A, Campion D, Jimenez C, Piano S, et al. Safety of two different doses of simvastatin plus rifaximin in decompensated cirrhosis (LIVERHOPE-SAFETY): a randomised, double-blind, placebo-controlled, phase 2 trial. *Lancet Gastroenterol Hepatol.* (2020) 5:31-41. doi: 10.1016/S2468-1253(19)30320-6

118. Bajaj JS, Kakiyama G, Savidge T, Takei H, Kassam ZA, Fagan A, et al. Antibiotic-associated disruption of microbiota composition and function in cirrhosis is restored by fecal transplant. *Hepatology.* (2018) 68:1549–58. doi: 10.1002/hep.30037
119. Clària J, Kent JD, López-Parra M, Escolar G, Ruiz-del-Arbol L, Ginès P, et al. Effects of celecoxib and naproxen on renal function in nonazotemic patients with cirrhosis and ascites. *Hepatology.* (2005) 41:579–87. doi: 10.1002/hep.20595
120. Guevara M, Abecasis R, Terg R. Effect of celecoxib on renal function in cirrhotic patients with ascites. a pilot study. *Scand J Gastroenterol.* (2004) 39:385–6. doi: 10.1080/00365520310008205
121. Moroni F, Dwyer BJ, Graham C, Pass C, Bailey L, Ritchie L, et al. Safety profile of autologous macrophage therapy for liver cirrhosis. *Nat Med.* (2019) 25:1560–5. doi: 10.1038/s41591-019-0599-8
122. Takeuchi S, Tsuchiya A, Iwasawa T, Nojiri S, Watanabe T, Ogawa M, et al. Small extracellular vesicles derived from interferon-γ pre-conditioned mesenchymal stromal cells effectively treat liver fibrosis. *npj Regen Med.* (2021) 6:19. doi: 10.1038/s41536-021-00132-4

9

The Emerging Role of Macrophages in Chronic Cholangiopathies Featuring Biliary Fibrosis: An Attractive Therapeutic Target for Orphan Diseases

*Massimiliano Cadamuro[1], Noemi Girardi[1], Gregory J. Gores[2], Mario Strazzabosco[3] and Luca Fabris[1,3]**

[1] Department of Molecular Medicine, University of Padua, Padua, Italy, [2] Division of Gastroenterology and Hepatology and the Mayo Clinic Center for Cell Signaling in Gastroenterology, Mayo Clinic, Rochester, NY, United States, [3] Liver Center, Department of Medicine, Yale University, New Haven, CT, United States

***Correspondence:**
Luca Fabris
luca.fabris@unipd.it

Cholangiopathies are a heterogeneous group of chronic liver diseases caused by different types of injury targeting the biliary epithelium, such as genetic defects and immune-mediated attacks. Notably, most cholangiopathies are orphan, thereby representing one of the major gaps in knowledge of the modern hepatology. A typical hallmark of disease progression in cholangiopathies is portal scarring, and thus development of effective therapeutic approaches would aim to hinder cellular and molecular mechanisms underpinning biliary fibrogenesis. Recent lines of evidence indicate that macrophages, rather than more conventional cell effectors of liver fibrosis such as hepatic stellate cells and portal fibroblasts, are actively involved in the earliest stages of biliary fibrogenesis by exchanging a multitude of cues with cholangiocytes, which promote their recruitment from the circulating compartment owing to a senescent or an immature epithelial phenotype. Two cholangiopathies, namely primary sclerosing cholangitis and congenital hepatic fibrosis, are paradigmatic of this mechanism. This review summarizes current understandings of the cytokine and extracellular vesicles-mediated communications between cholangiocytes and macrophages typically occurring in the two cholangiopathies to unveil potential novel targets for the treatment of biliary fibrosis.

Keywords: primary sclerosing cholangitis, congenital hepatic fibrosis, monocyte, cholangiocyte, biliary repair

INTRODUCTION

Cholangiopathies are a heterogeneous group of liver diseases targeting the biliary epithelium of different etiologies including genetic defects (causing Alagille syndrome, cystic fibrosis-related cholangiopathy, and polycystic and fibropolycystic liver diseases) and immune-mediated attacks (causing primary biliary cholangitis and primary sclerosing cholangitis) (1–3). Their clinical evolution is generally much slower than liver diseases aimed at the hepatocytes, spanning over years or decades, and depends on the balance between the manifestations related to the bile duct injury such as cholestasis, ductopenia (or conversely, exuberant bile duct expansion), and portal/biliary fibrosis (4). Whereas, cholestasis related to the impaired ability of the biliary epithelium to alkalinize or fluidify the primary bile produced by the hepatocytes is a common manifestation observed in most of them, biliary fibrosis is a variable occurrence (5). However, if present, biliary fibrosis is a major determinant of disease progression as it is responsible for the disease's most feared complications such as portal hypertension and biliary cirrhosis, and it bears an increased risk of malignant transformation into cholangiocarcinoma (6, 7). Clinically, management of cholangiopathies still represents one of the major gaps in modern hepatology knowledge in terms of both early detection and effective treatment (3). To date, only a few pharmacological therapies have been proven to be effective and only in limited pathology conditions (urosodeoxycholic acid, obeticholic acid, and bezafibrate in primary biliary cholangitis), while the vast majority of cholangiopathies are still orphan. Liver transplantation remains the only option when the disease is advanced (8–10). Major efforts for developing effective therapeutic strategies in cholangiopathies should be devoted to halt biliary fibrogenesis (4, 11). For many years, understanding of the mechanisms of biliary fibrosis has relied on studies performed in animal models where biliary fibrosis develops in a rapid manner not consistent with what is observed in humans (such as the bile duct ligation in rodents), or in animal models where the primary dysfunction affects the hepatocyte rather than the cholangiocyte [such as the *multidrug resistance* (*mdr*)*2*-KO mouse] (12–14). These studies have lent support to the notion that biliary fibrogenesis is an intricate process where multiple cell types are actively involved. Following biliary injury, cholangiocytes lining the finest ramifications of the biliary tree, abutting the canals of Hering, become activated in a so-called "ductular reaction" (2, 15–17). They start to secrete a huge variety of mediators like cytokines, chemokines, and growth factors, and to express a rich repertoire of receptors that enable them to communicate extensively with portal fibroblasts and hepatic stellate cells, the ultimate effectors of the deposition of new extracellular matrix (ECM) components (2, 18). Cell interactions between the epithelial and the mesenchymal compartments are molded by the further involvement of inflammatory cell types recruited from the blood such as neutrophils, macrophages, and lymphocytes (19, 20). Among them, macrophages behave as emerging players in biliary fibrogenesis since the initial phase, and deciphering their involvement has provided insights with translational significance (19, 21, 22). Therefore, the aim of the present review is to draw attention to some recent observations highlighting the role played by macrophages in biliary fibrosis, derived from experimental models of bile duct injury with progressive portal scarring, which recapitulates the phenotype of primary sclerosing cholangitis (PSC) and congenital hepatic fibrosis (CHF), as they may shed light on novel therapeutic approaches.

GENERAL CONCEPTS ON THE INVOLVEMENT OF MACROPHAGES IN FIBROSIS

Macrophages are a cellular population extensively represented in the liver that display a wide heterogeneity dependent upon their developmental origin (resident or infiltrating macrophages) and their polarization (inflammatory or anti-inflammatory) regulated by microenvironmental cues, such as danger signals, and cellular debris taken up by phagocytosis. In normal conditions, liver-resident macrophages, or Kupffer cells (KC), are mainly localized in the perisinusoidal space to ensure tissue homeostasis, antimicrobial defense, and proper metabolism (23, 24). In disease conditions, macrophages play a central role in host defense against infections as well as in tissue repair (25). In these cases, infiltrating macrophages can be recruited following mobilization of circulating monocytes from bone marrow and the spleen. In mouse, the tissue origin of infiltrating macrophages can be assessed by a distinct phenotype. In fact, bone marrow-derived monocytes are Ly-6C high (Ly-6C^{hi}) and express several receptors such as C-C chemokine receptor type 2 (CCR2) and receptors for pathogen and damage associated molecular patterns (PAMPs and DAMPs, respectively), while the spleen-derived macrophages are Ly-6C low (Ly-6C^{lo}) and are less equipped with the receptor machinery (26). Moreover, macrophages possess a high level of cell plasticity, enabling them to respond to a huge variety of both endogenous and exogenous stimuli, interact with multiple cell types, and direct mechanisms underlying tissue repair and regeneration. Following ligand interaction with its receptor(s), macrophages activate a number of cellular responses including phagocytosis, endocytosis, and secretion of soluble mediators like cytokines, chemokines, and growth factors (27, 28). Thanks to these properties, once stimulated, macrophages may exert a range of functions including cell adhesion and migration, antigen presentation, and effector functions in the immune response. Exogenous ligands are bound by receptors involved in the recognition of opsonins, mainly antibodies produced by the complement activation, or through the direct recognition of carbohydrates, proteins, lipids and nucleic acids. In particular, stimulation of different Toll-like receptors (TLR) and lectins expressed by macrophages converge toward the transcription factor NF-kB, whose activation regulates production of proinflammatory and profibrotic mediators (29). Macrophages can also express the receptor for advanced glycation end products (RAGE), a multi-ligand receptor that can bind, among others, the alarmin high-mobility group box-1 (HMGB1), belonging to the DAMP group, and S100 (30). Similar to TLR, RAGE interaction with HMGB1 kindles the pro-inflammatory cascade regulated by NF-kB, with a partial overlap between RAGE and TLRs, since RAGE-deficient macrophages showed a decrease cytokine response following HMGB1 stimulation (29). In response to signals released in an "inflamed" environment, macrophage activation displays marked functional changes that can be roughly divided into M1 (classically activated) or M2 (alternatively activated) phenotypes as the edges of a continuum without a clear demarcation, dependent on the phase and the degree of tissue injury (31). Macrophages undergo M1 activation in the presence of Th1 lymphocytes or upon the effect of multiple pro-inflammatory cytokines, thus increasing their ability to kill intracellular pathogens and contributing to the progression of the inflammatory process. In particular, M1 macrophage differentiation is induced in response to interferon-γ, exposure to microorganisms or microbial products such as lipopolysaccharides (LPS), and cytokines such as tumor necrosis factor-α (TNF-α) (32). M1 macrophages secrete low levels of interleukin (IL)-10 and high levels of IL-1β, IL-6, IL-12, IL-23, and the TNF-α itself, resulting in further activation of Th1 effector cells, thus sustaining a feed-forward loop (33, 34). Beside the secretory profile, the M1 polarization can be identified also by a variety of functional and biochemical phenotypic markers including the overexpression of surface markers, in particular MHC class II and CD86, and the enhanced competence for antigen presentation and microbicide activity (35). Pathogen elimination is indeed facilitated by an increased production of reactive oxygen species (ROS) and nitric oxide (NO), due to the activation of the inducible nitric oxide synthase (iNOS) (36, 37). On the other side of the spectrum, exposure to anti-inflammatory cytokines induces macrophages toward an alternatively activated or M2 phenotype, with increased expression of Ly-6C (Ly-6C^{hi}) and of specific markers such as CD206, Arginase-1, and early growth response gene-2 (Egr2) (38, 39). M2 macrophages do not possess antimicrobial activity due to their inability to produce NO and ROS, and despite the fact that they may express MHC class II proteins, they are inefficient as antigen-presenting cells. Rather, they mostly inhibit the proliferation of T cells, and cooperate with the humoral immune response by regulating the Th2 effectors and stimulating the secretion of immunoglobulins by B cells. Classical inducers of M2 polarization are IL-4 or IL-13, featuring the Th2 response (32, 37). In particular, IL-4 activates the Janus kinase/signal transducer and activator of transcription protein 6 (JAK/STAT6) pathway, which leads to the transcription of several genes, among them *Arachidonate 15-Lipoxygenase, C-C Motif Chemokine Ligand (CCL)22, CCL26, CD23a, Fibronectin 1*, and *suppressor of cytokine signal*, regulating inflammatory cell recruitment and activation and ECM deposition (40, 41). Furthermore, IL-4-stimulated macrophages showed an increased production of anti-inflammatory cytokines (IL-10 and IL-1R antagonist) in conjunction with a reduced expression of proinflammatory/M1-like cytokines (IL-1, TNFα, IL-6, IL-12, and MIP1α), an essential step to dampen inflammation. Furthermore, in animal models of both acute (42, 43) and chronic liver diseases (44), the ability of M2 macrophages to blunt inflammation also relies on the stimulation of apoptosis in M1 macrophages via a IL-10-mediated mechanism, which affects the balance between the anti- and pro-apoptotic proteins Bax and Bcl-2. In addition to the immunomodulatory functions, M2 macrophages are pivotal players in tissue regeneration and repair given their contribution to angiogenesis and ECM remodeling (45). M2 macrophages may stimulate angiogenesis as they secrete high levels of vascular endothelial growth factor (VEGF)-A (45). Furthermore, M2 macrophages can also produce major components of the "scarring" ECM, including fibronectin and collagen, as shown by up-regulation of *Col1a2* and *Col3a1* genes (46). On the other hand, the constitutive activation of arginase in M2 macrophages leads to *de novo* biosynthesis of polyamine and proline, which promotes cell growth and further deposition of collagen in an autocrine loop (47). Moreover, M2 macrophages are responsible for the degradation of the native constituents of ECM by secreting matrix metalloproteinase −9, −12, and −13. While the role of macrophages in liver fibrosis developing in the setting of a parenchymal damage has been extensively studied and has been the subject of recent reviews (21), evidence on their significant contribution to biliary fibrosis have only recently been emerging. Accumulation of macrophages is a distinctive trait of biliary fibrosis, in particular when it is particularly prominent (PSC, CHF). Of note, these conditions share some relevant clinical aspects, as both disorders may develop portal hypertension without progression to full-blown biliary cirrhosis and bear an increased risk of malignant progression toward cholangiocarcinoma.

THE FIBROGENIC ROLE OF MACROPHAGES IN PSC

Among chronic liver diseases, PSC is paradigmatic of the pathophysiological relevance of progressive fibrogenesis, which generates a tight and stiff sheath around the ductal epithelium whereby necroinflammation is less pronounced compared with other inflammatory cholangiopathies. The hallmark of the disease is in fact the development of concentric periductal fibrosis, leading to the narrowing and eventual obliteration of both small and large bile ducts, which at the radiological level results in the formation of diffuse multifocal biliary strictures recognizable as a "beaded" configuration (48). The pathogenesis of PSC is largely unknown but immune-mediated mechanisms are likely involved, although the nature of the triggering factors remains elusive. The frequent association with inflammatory bowel disease, mainly chronic ulcerative colitis, suggests that bacterial components enriched in endotoxins like LPS and delivered to the liver parenchyma through the portal circulation may also be relevant in the pathogenesis of PSC (49). Interesting insights into the mechanisms responsible for biliary fibrosis can derive from a deep phenotyping of the portal cell infiltrate. Using a high-throughput sequencing approach, Govaere et al. found that in PSC, the peribiliary milieu was extensively populated by CCL28$^+$ macrophages already in the early stage of the disease before developing advanced fibrosis in contrast to HCV chronic hepatitis, which instead showed an enrichment in T and B cells in the areas of hepatocellular injury and regeneration (50). Macrophage recruitment to the biliary microenvironment has been confirmed in murine models of PSC (*Mdr2*$^{-/-}$ mouse), where they promote injury and cholestasis (51). Of note, the immunophenotype of macrophages accumulating in the periportal areas of liver sections obtained from PSC patients and *Mdr2*$^{-/-}$ mice, is consistent with an origin from circulating monocytes rather than from the resident KCs (CD68$^+$/CCR2$^+$ in human, CD45$^+$/F4/80$^+$/CD11b^{hi} in mice). In PSC, following the initial pro-inflammatory reaction, the macrophage infiltration of the peribiliary area increased as the fibrotic stage of the disease progressed, encompassing both pro-inflammatory iNOS$^+$ M1 and anti-inflammatory CD206$^+$ M2 phenotypes, with a predominance of M1 in advanced stages (51).

Cell Senescence and Extracellular Vesicle Release Are Distinctive Epithelial Traits Promoting Macrophage Recruitment

In PSC, a distinctive feature of cholangiocytes is cell senescence, an irreversible condition of cell cycle arrest. Senescence is induced by the activation of the N-Ras pathway upon persistence of cellular injury (52), where alterations in cell morphology, increased lysosomal activities, and enhanced DNA damage responses are associated with exuberant pro-inflammatory secretory functions, which involve IL-6, IL-8, CCL2, and plasminogen activator inhibitor 1, and collectively result in the senescence-associated secretory phenotype (SASP). Interestingly, SASP activation in PSC is closely associated with macrophage recruitment. *In vitro* models of cellular senescence, generated by treating normal human cholangiocytes with the inhibitor of apoptosis antagonist BV6 or with LPS, and cholangiocytes isolated from PSC livers, released monocyte chemotactic factors including CCL2/monocyte chemoattractant protein (MCP)-1 and IL-8, regulated by the transcription factor NF-kB, that promoted monocyte migration (51). In particular, strategies aimed at blocking CCR2, the cognate receptor of CCL2/MCP-1, by pharmacological treatment with cenicriviroc (dual antagonist of CCR2/5) or by genetic ablation led to a significant therapeutic gain in mouse models of PSC *in vivo*. In these conditions, the reduction in peribiliary infiltration of monocyte-derived macrophages was paralleled by a stark improvement of fibrosis as well as of cholestatic indexes (53). These findings were reproduced in an experimental model of acute sclerosing cholangitis generated by biliary instillation of BV6, where targeting CCR2-dependent monocyte recruitment significantly attenuated both the inflammatory and fibrotic responses, thus highlighting the concept that macrophage accumulation within the periductal space is a key event since the initial stages of biliary injury (51). Recent data showed that in addition to soluble factors, cholangiocytes can activate macrophages originating from the bone marrow by releasing membrane-derived nanometer-sized (from 40 to 200) extracellular vesicles (EVs) (54). EVs are functionally active, bilayer-delimited particles including miRNA and DAMPs which bear several small biomolecules mediating cell-to-cell communication as a sort of "secret messengers" (55). Apoptotic bodies from dying cells are usually larger than 500 nm, thus EV-mediated DAMP cargo is of particular interest in conditions with negligible cell death by necrosis, as occurred in PSC. Among DAMP, S100A11 is contained in EVs released by primary cholangiocytes derived from *Mdr2*$^{-/-}$ mouse and grown in 3D-structures as cholangioids (54). Of note, S100A1 is a potent agonist of RAGE (56) and highly expressed by macrophages. Upon binding to S100A1, bone marrow-derived macrophages turned to a proinflammatory phenotype involving secretion of TNF-α, IL-1β, and IL-6 associated with M1 polarization, through an NF-kB-dependent mechanism (54). Expression of these proinflammatory cytokines by bone marrow-derived macrophages was suppressed by RAGE manipulation through genetic deletion or selective inhibition by TTP448 or by NF-kB inhibition by TPCA-1. Altogether, these data identify RAGE as an actionable target to hamper macrophage polarization promoted by cholangiocyte-derived EVs (54). The key role played by macrophages in biliary fibrosis featuring PSC, driven by chemokines and EVs originating from senescent cholangiocytes is illustrated in **Figure 1**.

Relationship of Macrophage Activation With Biliary Repair

In PSC, effects of M1-polarized macrophages have also been reported on the level of biliary repair involving hepatic progenitor cells (HPC) (57), whose activation leading to ductular reaction is instrumental in biliary fibrogenesis (4, 16, 58). In cell co-culture studies, bone marrow-derived M1 macrophages promoted a self-renewing phenotype of HPC via activation of the Notch signaling pathway (57). It is important to note that Notch activation in HPC by Jagged1 expressed by myofibroblasts was previously described as a critical pathway promoting HPC differentiation toward the biliary lineage (59). Monocyte/infiltrating macrophage and Notch signaling gene signatures were enriched in PSC liver samples and among core enrichment genes associated with HPC marker Hes Family BHLH Transcription Factor 1 (HES1) (57). Effects of macrophage depletion induced by

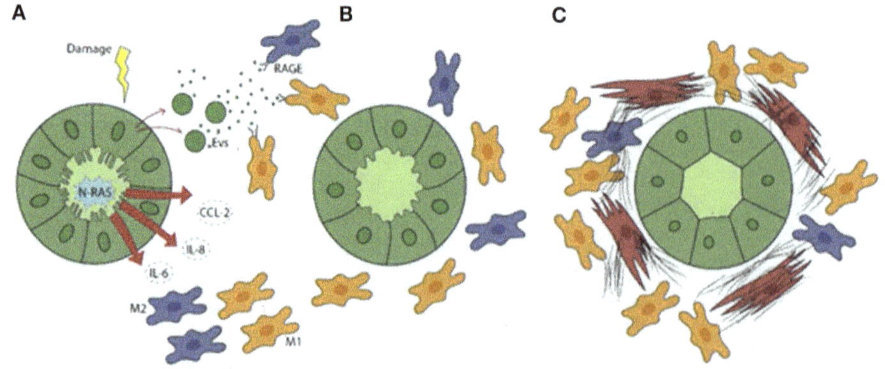

FIGURE 1 | In PSC **(A)**, senescent cholangiocytes harbor activation of N-Ras signaling, resulting in the secretion of the pro-inflammatory mediators IL-6, IL-8, and CCL2, which drive the peribiliary accumulation of both M1 (yellow) and M2 (blue) macrophages. Extracellular vesicles (EVs) containing damage-associated molecular patterns (DAMPs) are also released by senescent cholangiocytes. **(B)** By binding the RAGE receptor expressed by macrophages, EVs further elicit macrophage activation and infiltration. **(C)** M1 macrophages become preponderant in a later phase, when the generation of a dense fibrotic tissue is further enhanced by the accumulation of portal myofibroblasts (brown).

liposome encapsulated clodronate (a bisphosphonate which inhibits the monocyte-macrophage transdifferentiation) have been extensively investigated in another animal model of PSC, generated by mouse feeding with 3,5-diethoxycarbonyl-1,4-dihydrocollidine (DDC). The DDC-fed mouse is characterized by cholangitis and intense biliary fibrosis associated with macrophage recruitment, activation of portal myofibroblasts, and a prominent ductular reaction (60). In DDC-fed mice, macrophage depletion blunted deposition of laminin, a major component of the basement membrane surrounding the bile ducts. When laminin is defective, reactive ductules were confined within the portal area and did not progress to "atypical" ductules (61), which extend beyond the portal tract boundaries into the parenchyma and represent a feature of a more fibrogenic biliary injury. Moreover, macrophage depletion was accompanied by a significant reduction in the proliferative status of cholangiocytes (61), consistent with previous observations identifying the TNF family member TNF-like weak inducer of apoptosis (TWEAK) as the signal emitted by macrophages that is responsible for expansion of HPC by interacting with its receptor Fn14 and stimulation of ductular reactions by activating NFκB signaling (62, 63). However, macrophage depletion induced by liposomal clodronate involves not only bone marrow-derived macrophages, but also liver-resident macrophages (KCs). A study focusing on the role of F4/80$^+$ KCs in the same clodronate-treated DDC model showed that KC depletion was beneficial only in the early phase of biliary injury, while it was detrimental in the regression phase with worsening effects on portal inflammation and fibrosis (64). These data conceivably suggest that KC may play a dual role in sclerosing cholangiopathy in keeping with their marked cell plasticity. Therefore, therapeutic interventions targeting macrophages in sclerosing cholangitis must pay attention to the remarkable heterogeneity of this cell type that cannot be too simplified by the conventional distinction between infiltrating and liver-resident macrophages, and between M1 and M2 phenotypes.

THE FIBROGENIC ROLE OF MACROPHAGES IN CHF

Fibropolycystic liver diseases, which encompass a number of genetic conditions with biliary dysgenesis such as autosomal recessive polycystic kidney disease (ARPKD), CHF, and Caroli's disease (CD), are caused by mutations in the polycystic kidney and hepatic disease 1 (*PKHD1*), the gene encoding for fibrocystin/polyductin (FPC) (65, 66). FPC is a large protein expressed by ductal epithelial cells, such as cholangiocytes, in several cellular compartments including cilia, centromeres, basal bodies, and tight and adherence junctions (65, 66). Although FPC function is unknown, it is likely involved in cell proliferation, cell-cell and cell-matrix interactions, cell differentiation, secretion, and planar cell polarity (67). A common trait of these diseases is the cyst-like enlargement of the intrahepatic bile duct epithelium accompanied by a progressive deposition of fibrotic tissue in the peribiliary region. In the dysgenetic ducts, cholangiocytes present cilium defects and retain features of immaturity reminiscent of a fetal-like behavior (2–4, 19). Worsening fibrosis leads to portal hypertension and related complications, such as variceal bleeding and ascites, and young patients are generally disposed to develop chronic cholangitis (2, 68, 69). Since effective pharmacological treatments are currently lacking, the only curative approaches are based on surgical interventions such as liver resection (in CD) or liver transplantation when portal hypertension or recurrent acute cholangitis lead to life-threatening complications (70).

Epithelial Immaturity of Dysgenetic Ducts Is Characterized by an Overactivation of the β-Catenin Signaling to Stimulate Macrophage Recruitment

Recent findings suggest that in CHF, biliary fibrosis is the result of a chronic, low-grade inflammatory response sustained by macrophages and originating from FPC-defective cholangiocytes akin to "parainflammation," a process of adaptation to an unrestrained cell dysfunction. When cell dysfunction is persistent, the inflammatory response, unable to restore the normal tissue homeostasis, becomes pathologic and can ultimately lead to scarring (71). Interestingly, in a murine model of CHF, the *Pkhd1*$^{del4/del4}$ mouse, macrophages featuring the inflammatory reaction showed a switch of polarization over the disease progression. In fact, macrophages dominating the peribiliary infiltrate in the early stages showed a preponderance of proinflammatory iNOS$^+$ M1 macrophages recruited from the circulating precursors that gradually shift to a profibrotic CD206$^+$ M2 phenotype as the fibrosis progressed (72). Notably, macrophage infiltration was driven by the hectic secretory functions displayed by FPC-defective cholangiocytes dependent upon an over-activation of the β-catenin signaling (72). This perturbation resulted in an exuberant production of several chemokines, in particular of chemokine (C-X-C motif) ligand 1 (CXCL1), CXCL10, and CXCL12, directing the progressive accumulation of macrophages in the pericystic area. Macrophages in turn released TNF-α when M1-preponderant, coupled with transforming growth factor (TGF) β while enriching in M2, which further stimulated the *de novo* expression of integrin αVβ6 by FPC-defective cholangiocytes. Upregulation of integrin αVβ6, the local activator of latent TGFβ (73), is a crucial mechanism in the peribiliary fibrosis that finally leads to the recruitment of portal myofibroblasts and is actively involved in the generation of the several components of the fibrotic ECM, in particular fibronectin and collagen type I. Thus, in *Pkhd1*$^{del4/del4}$ mice, biliary fibrosis is initially promoted by macrophages and involvement of portal myofibroblasts occurs only in a later stage, when fibrosis worsens and associates with the development of portal hypertension (72). The translational significance of macrophage targeting in biliary fibrosis even when related to CHF was confirmed by treating *Pkhd1*$^{del4/del4}$ mice with clodronate *in vivo*. Macrophage depletion was paralleled by a significant reduction in portal fibrosis, which prevented the establishment of portal hypertension (72). Of note, this finding was reproduced in the *cpk/cpk* mice, another model of ARPKD, where macrophage reduction was accompanied by a decreased size of the epithelial cysts not only in the liver, but also in the kidney (74). Besides β-catenin, other signaling anomalies contribute to the pro-inflammatory phenotype activated by FPC deficiency. In fact, the epithelial secretion of CXCL10 is further sustained through an autocrine loop in which the NLRP3 inflammasome complex, once activated, allows the secretion of IL-1β that in turn stimulates CXCL10 secretion through the phosphorylation and activation of the JAK/STAT3 signaling (2, 75). Again, this mechanism is amenable to therapeutic intervention since the *in vivo* treatment of $Pkhd1^{del4/del4}$ mice with AMG-487, an antagonist of CXCR3, the cognate receptor for CXCL10, significantly reduced the extent of M2 infiltrating macrophages together with a significant decrease in the fibrotic and cyst areas (75). **Figure 2** summarizes the sequence of events unleashed by FPC inactivation in cholangiocytes, which results in the progressive peribiliary accumulation of macrophages.

CCL2/MCP-1 Signaling Also Mediates Macrophage Infiltration in Ciliary Dysfunctions

As mentioned, cilium dysfunction represents a defining feature of ductal epithelial cells in these conditions (thereby also termed as "ciliopathies") (76, 77). A crucial protein essential for cilia formation is the intraflagellar transport 88 (IFT88) (78). Inactivation of the *Ift88* gene in mouse ($IFT88^{Orpk}$ mouse) leads to liver cyst expansion associated with deposition of fibrosis, which reproduces the liver phenotype of human ARPKD/CHF, similarly to the $Pkhd1^{del4/del4}$ mouse. This model is also characterized by a massive accumulation of Ly-6C^{hi} infiltrating macrophages near the dysgenetic ducts, which preceded the cyst growth and the onset of biliary fibrosis. Macrophage recruitment was mediated by CCL2/MCP-1 expressed by cholangiocytes harboring cilia dysfunction. Phenotyping of peribiliary macrophages showed enhanced gene expression of profibrotic and proinflammatory mediators including IL-6, VEGF-A, TGFβ, and PDGF-B, which in turn directed accumulation and activation of portal fibroblasts in a later stage that promoted fibrosis progression (79). Notably, in this model the genetic manipulation of CCL2 signaling obtained by generating double KO $IFT88^{Orpk}/FBVCCR2^{-/-}$ mice caused a significant reduction in Ly-6C^{hi} macrophages and in the pericystic fibrosis, but did not affect liver cyst expansion (79). The relevance of CCL2 signaling was confirmed further in the PCK rat, another well-established rodent model ortholog to the human fibropolycystic liver and kidney diseases. Upon treatment with bindarit, a small molecule that inhibits CCL2 expression and activity, the PCK rat reported a reduction in macrophage accumulation accompanied by an amelioration of renal function, but without significant effects on both liver and kidney cyst growth (80). These data are partially in contrast with results obtained treating inducible $Pkd1^{fl/fl}$;*Pax8-rtTA;TetO-Cre* mice with INCB3344, a specific CCR2 antagonist, which showed a reduction of renal cyst enlargement (81).

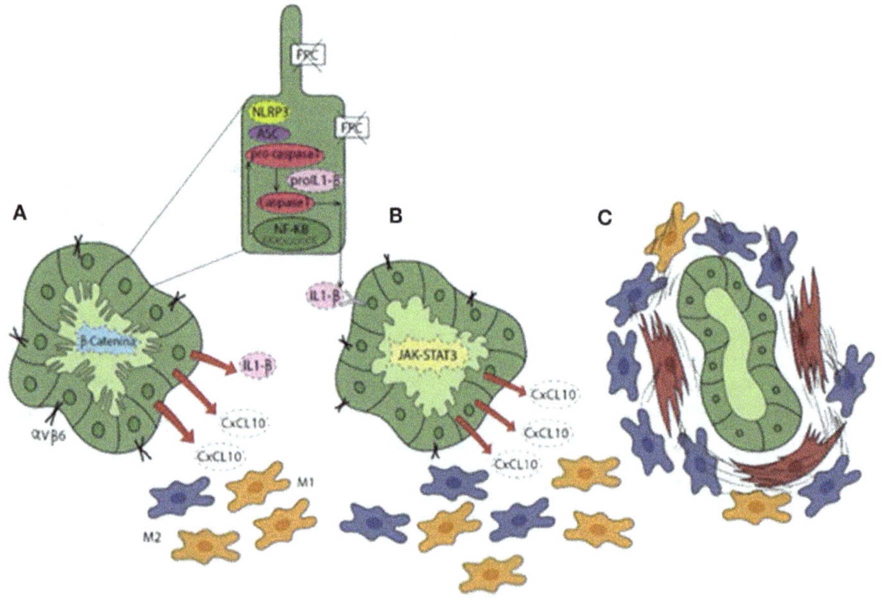

FIGURE 2 | In CHF **(A),** fibrocystin (FPC)-defective cholangiocytes gain an immature (fetal-like) phenotype characterized by an over-activation of the β-catenin signaling. This enables cholangiocytes to secrete a range of pro-inflammatory chemokines (CXCL1, CXCL10, and CXCL12) and to express integrin αVβ6, the local activator of latent TGFβ, a major driver of liver fibrogenesis. In particular, secretion of CXCL10 is sustained by an autocrine/paracrine loop where the activation of the NLRP3 inflammasome stimulates the secretion of IL-1β via the JAK/STAT3 pathway (pale green cholangiocyte) that, in turn, enhances the production of CXCL10. **(A,B)** The exuberant chemokine secretion by cholangiocytes orchestrates the peribiliary accumulation of macrophages, which are initially molded into the M1 phenotype (yellow) prevailing on the M2 (blue). **(C)** At a later stage, increase in M2 macrophages associates with the recruitment of myofibroblasts (brown), which result in the progressive accumulation of peribiliary fibrotic tissue and in the progression of the disease.

TABLE 1 | Anti-macrophage strategies used for *in vivo* treatments.

Drug	Experimental model	Mechanism of action	Readouts and therapeutic effects
Cenicriviroc	C57BL/6. *Mdr2*$^{-/-}$ mice	CCR2 antagonist	Reduction in peribiliary infiltration of monocyte-derived macrophages. Improvement of fibrosis and cholestasis.
Clodronate	DDC fed mice, *Pkhd1*$^{del4/del4}$ mice and *cpk/cpk* mice	Inhibitor of monocyte-macrophage transdifferentiation	Reduction of tissue accumulation of M2 macrophages. Significant decrease in fibrosis; reduction in epithelial cyst size in liver and kidney.
AMG-487	*Pkhd1*$^{del4/del4}$ mice	CXCR3 antagonist (CXCL10 receptor)	Reduction of the extent of CD45^{+} leucocytes (mainly M2 macrophages and CD4^{+} T cells). Decrease of the fibrotic area extent and of the cyst size.
Genetic inhibition of CCL2 signaling	Double KO *IFT88Orpk/FBVCCR2*$^{-/-}$ mice	CCL2 signaling inhibitor	Significant reduction of Ly6c^{hi} macrophages. Improvement of fibrosis.
Bindarit	PCK rat	Inhibitor of CCL2 expression/activity	Significant reduction of macrophage accumulation. Amelioration of renal function.
INCB3344	Inducible *Pkd1fl/fl; Pax8-rtTA; TetO-Cre* mice	CCR2 antagonist	Reduction of renal cyst enlargement.

Collectively, these findings suggest that different mechanisms likely underpin epithelial cyst expansion and biliary fibrosis, and confirm that monocyte-derived macrophages are key drivers of fibrogenesis.

CONCLUSIONS

Mouse models of biliary fibrosis developing in the context of chronic cholangiopathies such as PSC and CHF have revealed that macrophages, in particular the Ly-6C^{hi} population originating from the circulating compartment, hold a crucial role, especially in the initial phase of fibrogenesis. In fact, following an initial bile duct injury, macrophage infiltration of the peribiliary area is an early event preceding the accumulation of the more conventional fibrogenic cell type in the liver, i.e., the portal myofibroblast, ultimately responsible for the deposition of scarring ECM components in the portal area. Interestingly, macrophages are instructed by pro-inflammatory mediators (CCL2, IL-8, CXCL1, CXCL10, CXCL12) or EV-mediated DAMP released by cholangiocytes owing to the gain of a senescent phenotype (as in PSC) or the persistence of an immature, fetal-like ciliary defective phenotype (as in CHF). It would be tempting to speculate on the deep phenotypic similarities that senescence and immaturity, as maturation stages at the opposite ends of the cell life, share at the cholangiocyte level. On the other hand, macrophages populating the peribiliary area show different patterns of polarization over time in the two cholangiopathies. Whilst in PSC, M1 macrophages become preponderant as the disease progresses, in CHF the M1 phenotype dominates the early infiltrate, and is then equated by M2 in a later stage. Nonetheless, macrophages represent ideal targets for drug delivery given their phagocytic functions, and experimental evidence is mounting that their therapeutic targeting provides an attractive strategy to ameliorate biliary fibrosis (21). Of note, this concept is even more relevant in PSC and CHF, which are still orphan diseases and are thus eagerly awaiting novel treatments among cholangiopathies. The relevant therapeutic effects obtained by targeting macrophages in animal models of PSC and CHF are summarized in **Table 1**. Although these observations may serve as a promising starting point for future therapeutic directions, a number of challenges deserve consideration in future studies. First, it will be important to have a deeper understanding of the variable role of macrophages during disease progression, in particular as it relates to the polarization switch, in order to devise more specific macrophage-targeted interventions. Second, it must be underlined that most data herein discussed have been obtained in rodent models, and thus they need translation to human settings. This is of utmost importance as the heterogeneity of liver macrophages in humans is much less investigated compared to mice. Generation of biliary organoids from patient-derived liver biopsy or bile sample may offer a significant asset to tackle this challenge (82). Finally, additional pathogenetic factors such as microbiota and infections, which are particularly relevant in both PSC and CHF, heavily influence macrophage functions, and thus major efforts will be devoted to address this area.

AUTHOR CONTRIBUTIONS

MC designed the study and wrote the first draft. NG wrote the first draft. GG and MS critically reviewed the draft and finalized the manuscript. LF designed the study, critically reviewed the draft and finalized the manuscript.

ACKNOWLEDGMENTS

We thank Arianna Camellato, Department of Architecture, University of Florence, for her valuable support in graphic design.

REFERENCES

1. Strazzabosco M, Fabris L, Spirli C. Pathophysiology of cholangiopathies. *J Clin Gastroenterol.* (2005) 39:S90–102. doi: 10.1097/01.mcg.0000155549.29643.ad
2. Fabris L, Fiorotto R, Spirli C, Cadamuro M, Mariotti V, Perugorria MJ, et al. Pathobiology of inherited biliary diseases: a roadmap to understand acquired liver diseases. *Nat Rev Gastroenterol Hepatol.* (2019) 16:497–511. doi: 10.1038/s41575-019-0156-4
3. Banales JM, Huebert RC, Karlsen T, Strazzabosco M, LaRusso NF, Gores GJ. Cholangiocyte pathobiology. *Nat Rev Gastroenterol Hepatol.* (2019) 16:269–81. doi: 10.1038/s41575-019-0125-y
4. Fabris L, Spirli C, Cadamuro M, Fiorotto R, Strazzabosco M. Emerging concepts in biliary repair and fibrosis. *Am J Physiol Gastrointest Liver Physiol.* (2017) 313:G102–16. doi: 10.1152/ajpgi.00452.2016
5. Tam PKH, Yiu RS, Lendahl U, Andersson ER. Cholangiopathies - Towards a molecular understanding. *EBioMedicine.* (2018) 35:381–93. doi: 10.1016/j.ebiom.2018.08.024
6. Chung BK, Karlsen TH, Folseraas T. Cholangiocytes in the pathogenesis of primary sclerosing cholangitis and development of cholangiocarcinoma. *Biochim Biophys Acta Mol Basis Dis.* (2018) 1864:1390–400. doi: 10.1016/j.bbadis.2017.08.020
7. Cannito S, Milani C, Cappon A, Parola M, Strazzabosco M, Cadamuro M. Fibroinflammatory liver injuries as preneoplastic condition in cholangiopathies. *Int J Mol Sci.* (2018) 19:3875. doi: 10.3390/ijms19123875
8. Nayagam JS, Pereira SP, Devlin J, Harrison PM, Joshi D. Controversies in the management of primary sclerosing cholangitis. *World J Hepatol.* (2016) 8:265–72. doi: 10.4254/wjh.v8.i5.265
9. Terziroli Beretta-Piccoli B, Mieli-Vergani G, Vergani D, Vierling JM, Adams D, Alpini G, et al. The challenges of primary biliary cholangitis: What is new and what needs to be done. *J Autoimmun.* (2019) 105:102328. doi: 10.1016/j.jaut.2019.102328
10. Gerussi A, D'Amato D, Cristoferi L, O'Donnell SE, Carbone M, Invernizzi P. Multiple therapeutic targets in rare cholestatic liver diseases: time to redefine treatment strategies. *Ann Hepatol.* (2020) 19:5–16. doi: 10.1016/j.aohep.2019.09.009
11. Rajapaksha IG, Angus PW, Herath CB. Current therapies and novel approaches for biliary diseases. *World J Gastrointest Pathophysiol.* (2019) 10:1–10. doi: 10.4291/wjgp.v10.i1.1
12. Katzenellenbogen M, Pappo O, Barash H, Klopstock N, Mizrahi L, Olam D, et al. Multiple adaptive mechanisms to chronic liver disease revealed at early stages of liver carcinogenesis in the Mdr2-knockout mice. *Cancer Res.* (2006) 66:4001–10. doi: 10.1158/0008-5472.CAN-05-2937
13. Katzenellenbogen M, Mizrahi L, Pappo O, Klopstock N, Olam D, Jacob-Hirsch J, et al. Molecular mechanisms of liver carcinogenesis in the mdr2-knockout mice. *Mol Cancer Res.* (2007) 5:1159–70. doi: 10.1158/1541-7786.MCR-07-0172
14. Mariotti V, Cadamuro M, Spirli C, Fiorotto R, Strazzabosco M, Fabris L. Animal models of cholestasis: an update on inflammatory cholangiopathies. *Biochim Biophys Acta Mol Basis Dis.* (2019) 1865:954–64. doi: 10.1016/j.bbadis.2018.07.025
15. Roskams TA, Theise ND, Balabaud C, Bhagat G, Bhathal PS, Bioulac-Sage P, et al. Nomenclature of the finer branches of the biliary tree: canals, ductules, and ductular reactions in human livers. *Hepatology.* (2004) 39:1739–45. doi: 10.1002/hep.20130
16. Desmet VJ. Ductal plates in hepatic ductular reactions. Hypothesis and implications. III. Implications for liver pathology. *Virchows Arch.* (2011) 458:271–9. doi: 10.1007/s00428-011-1050-9
17. Strazzabosco M, Fabris L. Development of the bile ducts: essentials for the clinical hepatologist. *J Hepatol.* (2012) 56:1159–70. doi: 10.1016/j.jhep.2011.09.022
18. Sato K, Meng F, Giang T, Glaser S, Alpini G. Mechanisms of cholangiocyte responses to injury. *Biochim Biophys Acta Mol Basis Dis.* (2018) 1864:1262–9. doi: 10.1016/j.bbadis.2017.06.017
19. Fabris L, Strazzabosco M. Epithelial-mesenchymal interactions in biliary diseases. *Semin Liver Dis.* (2011) 31:11–32. doi: 10.1055/s-0031-1272832
20. Sheppard D. Epithelial-mesenchymal interactions in fibrosis and repair. Transforming growth factor-β activation by epithelial cells and fibroblasts. *Ann Am Thorac Soc.* (2015) 12:S21–3. doi: 10.1513/AnnalsATS.201406-245MG
21. Tacke F. Targeting hepatic macrophages to treat liver diseases. *J Hepatol.* (2017) 66:1300–12. doi: 10.1016/j.jhep.2017.02.026
22. Guillot A, Tacke F. Liver macrophages: old dogmas and new insights. *Hepatol Commun.* (2019) 3:730–43. doi: 10.1002/hep4.1356
23. Motta PM. The three-dimensional microanatomy of the liver. *Arch Histol Jpn.* (1984) 47:1–30. doi: 10.1679/aohc.47.1
24. Sung JY, Costerton JW, Shaffer EA. Defense system in the biliary tract against bacterial infection. *Dig Dis Sci.* (1992) 37:689–96. doi: 10.1007/bf01296423
25. Liaskou E, Wilson DV, Oo YH. Innate immune cells in liver inflammation. *Mediators Inflamm.* (2012) 2012:949157. doi: 10.1155/2012/949157
26. Song P, Zhang J, Zhang Y, Shu Z, Xu P, He L, et al. Hepatic recruitment of CD11b+Ly6C+ inflammatory monocytes promotes hepatic ischemia/reperfusion injury. *Int J Mol Med.* (2018) 41:935–45. doi: 10.3892/ijmm.2017.3315
27. Sica A, Invernizzi P, Mantovani A. Macrophage plasticity and polarization in liver homeostasis and pathology. *Hepatology.* (2014) 59:2034–42. doi: 10.1002/hep.26754
28. Ritz T, Krenkel O, Tacke F. Dynamic plasticity of macrophage functions in diseased liver. *Cell Immunol.* (2018) 330:175–82. doi: 10.1016/j.cellimm.2017.12.007
29. Kokkola R, Andersson A, Mullins G, Ostberg T, Treutiger CJ, Arnold B, et al. RAGE is the major receptor for the proinflammatory activity of HMGB1 in rodent macrophages. *Scand J Immunol.* (2005) 61:1–9. doi: 10.1111/j.0300-9475.2005.01534.x
30. Brett J, Schmidt AM, Yan SD, Zou YS, Weidman E, Pinsky D, et al. Survey of the distribution of a newly characterized receptor for advanced glycation end products in tissues. *Am J Pathol.* (1993) 143:1699–712.
31. Mosser DM, Edwards JP. Exploring the full spectrum of macrophage activation. *Nat Rev Immunol.* (2008) 8:958–69. doi: 10.1038/nri2448
32. Sica A, Mantovani A. Macrophage plasticity and polarization: *in vivo* veritas. *J Clin Invest.* (2012) 122:787–95. doi: 10.1172/JCI59643
33. Benoit M, Desnues B, Mege JL. Macrophage polarization in bacterial infections. *J Immunol.* (2008) 181:3733–9. doi: 10.4049/jimmunol.181.6.3733
34. Arango Duque G, Descoteaux A. Macrophage cytokines: involvement in immunity and infectious diseases. *Front Immunol.* (2014) 5:491. doi: 10.3389/fimmu.2014.00491
35. Murray PJ. Macrophage polarization. *Annu Rev Physiol.* (2017) 79:541–66. doi: 10.1146/annurev-physiol-022516-034339
36. Mills CD. Molecular basis of "suppressor" macrophages. *J Immunol.* (1991) 146:2719–23.
37. Mills CD. Anatomy of a discovery: m1 and m2 macrophages. *Front Immunol.* (2015) 6:212. doi: 10.3389/fimmu.2015.00212
38. Jablonski KA, Amici SA, Webb LM, Ruiz-Rosado Jde D, Popovich PG, Partida-Sanchez S, et al. Novel markers to delineate murine M1 and M2 macrophages. *PLoS ONE.* (2015) 10:e0145342. doi: 10.1371/journal.pone.0145342
39. Veremeyko T, Yung AWY, Anthony DC, Strekalova T, Ponomarev ED. Early growth response gene-2 is essential for M1 and M2 macrophage activation and plasticity by modulation of the transcription factor CEBPβ. *Front Immunol.* (2018) 9:2515. doi: 10.3389/fimmu.2018.02515
40. Gordon S, Martinez FO. Alternative activation of macrophages: mechanism and functions. *Immunity.* (2010) 32:593–604. doi: 10.1016/j.immuni.2010.05.007
41. Bao L, Zhang H, Chan LS. The involvement of the JAK-STAT signaling pathway in chronic inflammatory skin disease atopic dermatitis. *JAKSTAT.* (2013) 2:e24137. doi: 10.4161/jkst.24137
42. Bai L, Liu X, Zheng Q, Kong M, Zhang X, Hu R, et al. M2-like macrophages in the fibrotic liver protect mice against lethal insults through conferring apoptosis resistance to hepatocytes. *Sci Rep.* (2017) 7:10518. doi: 10.1038/s41598-017-11303-z

43. Bai L, Fu L, Li L, Ren F, Zheng Q, Liu S, et al. Cellular Mechanisms of Hepatoprotection Mediated by M2-Like Macrophages. *Med Sci Monit.* (2018) 24:2675–82. doi: 10.12659/MSM.907222
44. Wan J, Benkdane M, Teixeira-Clerc F, Bonnafous S, Louvet A, Lafdil F, et al. M2 Kupffer cells promote M1 Kupffer cell apoptosis: a protective mechanism against alcoholic and nonalcoholic fatty liver disease. *Hepatology.* (2014) 59:130–42. doi: 10.1002/hep.26607
45. Corliss BA, Azimi MS, Munson JM, Peirce SM, Murfee WL. Macrophages: an inflammatory link between angiogenesis and lymphangiogenesis. *Microcirculation.* (2016) 23:95–121. doi: 10.1111/micc.12259
46. Ramachandran P, Pellicoro A, Vernon MA, Boulter L, Aucott RL, Ali A, et al. Differential Ly-6C expression identifies the recruited macrophage phenotype, which orchestrates the regression of murine liver fibrosis. *Proc Natl Acad Sci USA.* (2012) 109:E3186–95. doi: 10.1073/pnas.11199 64109
47. Rath M, Müller I, Kropf P, Closs EI, Munder M. Metabolism via arginase or nitric oxide synthase: two competing arginine pathways in macrophages. *Front Immunol.* (2014) 5:532. doi: 10.3389/fimmu.201 4.00532
48. Seo N, Kim SY, Lee SS, Byun JH, Kim JH, Kim HJ, et al. Sclerosing cholangitis: clinicopathologic features, imaging spectrum, and systemic approach to differential diagnosis. *Korean J Radiol.* (2016) 17:25–38. doi: 10.3348/kjr.2016.17.1.25
49. Núñez FP, Quera PR, Gomollón F. Primary sclerosing cholangitis and inflammatory bowel disease: intestine-liver interrelation. Colangitis esclerosante primaria y enfermedad inflamatoria intestinal: interrelación intestino-hígado. *Gastroenterol Hepatol.* (2019) 42:316–25. doi: 10.1016/j.gastrohep.2019.02.004
50. Govaere O, Cockell S, Van Haele M, Wouters J, Van Delm W, Van den Eynde K, et al. High-throughput sequencing identifies aetiology-dependent differences in ductular reaction in human chronic liver disease. *J Pathol.* (2019) 248:66–76. doi: 10.1002/path.5228
51. Guicciardi ME, Trussoni CE, Krishnan A, Bronk SF, Lorenzo Pisarello MJ, et al. Macrophages contribute to the pathogenesis of sclerosing cholangitis in mice. *J Hepatol.* (2018) 69:676–86. doi: 10.1016/j.jhep.2018.05.018
52. Tabibian JH, O'Hara SP, Splinter PL, Trussoni CE, LaRusso NF. Cholangiocyte senescence by way of N-ras activation is a characteristic of primary sclerosing cholangitis. *Hepatology.* (2014) 59:2263–75. doi: 10.1002/hep.26993
53. Puengel T, Krenkel O, Kohlhepp M, Lefebvre E, Luedde T, Trautwein C, et al. Differential impact of the dual CCR2/CCR5 inhibitor cenicriviroc on migration of monocyte and lymphocyte subsets in acute liver injury. *PLoS ONE.* (2017) 12:e0184694. doi: 10.1371/journal.pone.0184694
54. Katsumi T, Guicciardi ME, Azad A, Bronk SF, Krishnan A, Gores GJ. Activated cholangiocytes release macrophage-polarizing extracellular vesicles bearing the DAMP S100A11. *Am J Physiol Cell Physiol.* (2019) 317:C788–99. doi: 10.1152/ajpcell.00250.2019
55. Pegtel DM, Peferoen L, Amor S. Extracellular vesicles as modulators of cell-to-cell communication in the healthy and diseased brain. *Philos Trans R Soc Lond B Biol Sci.* (2014) 369:20130516. doi: 10.1098/rstb.2013.0516
56. Xia C, Braunstein Z, Toomey AC, Zhong J, Rao X. S100 Proteins As an Important Regulator of Macrophage Inflammation. *Front Immunol.* (2018) 8:1908. doi: 10.3389/fimmu.2017.01908
57. Li H, Sun S, Lei Q, Lei P, Cai X, Wan C, et al. M1-Polarized macrophages promote self-renewing phenotype of hepatic progenitor cells with Jagged1-Notch signalling involved: relevance in primary sclerosing cholangitis. *J Immunol Res.* (2018) 2018:4807145. doi: 10.1155/2018/4807145
58. Sato K, Marzioni M, Meng F, Francis H, Glaser S, Alpini G. Ductular reaction in liver diseases: pathological mechanisms and translational significances. *Hepatology.* (2019) 69:420–30. doi: 10.1002/hep.30150
59. Boulter L, Govaere O, Bird TG, Radulescu S, Ramachandran P, Pellicoro A, et al. Macrophage-derived Wnt opposes Notch signaling to specify hepatic progenitor cell fate in chronic liver disease. *Nat Med.* (2012) 18:572–9. doi: 10.1038/nm.2667
60. Fickert P, Stöger U, Fuchsbichler A, Moustafa T, Marschall HU, Weiglein AH, et al. A new xenobiotic-induced mouse model of sclerosing cholangitis and biliary fibrosis. *Am J Pathol.* (2007) 171:525–36. doi: 10.2353/ajpath.2007.061133
61. Best J, Verhulst S, Syn WK, Lagaisse K, van Hul N, Heindryckx F, et al. Macrophage depletion attenuates extracellular matrix deposition and ductular reaction in a mouse model of chronic cholangiopathies. *PLoS ONE.* (2016) 11:e0162286. doi: 10.1371/journal.pone.0162286
62. Yanai M, Tatsumi N, Hasunuma N, Katsu K, Endo F, Yokouchi Y. FGF signaling segregates biliary cell-lineage from chick hepatoblasts cooperatively with BMP4 and ECM components *in vitro. Dev Dyn.* (2008) 237:1268–83. doi: 10.1002/dvdy.21520
63. Bird TG, Lu WY, Boulter L, Gordon-Keylock S, Ridgway RA, Williams MJ, et al. Bone marrow injection stimulates hepatic ductular reactions in the absence of injury via macrophage-mediated TWEAK signaling. *Proc Natl Acad Sci USA.* (2013) 110:6542–7. doi: 10.1073/pnas.13021 68110
64. Jemail L, Miyao M, Kotani H, Kawai C, Minami H, Abiru H, et al. Pivotal roles of Kupffer cells in the progression and regression of DDC-induced chronic cholangiopathy. *Sci Rep.* (2018) 8:6415. doi: 10.1038/s41598-018-24825-x
65. Ward CJ, Hogan MC, Rossetti S, Walker D, Sneddon T, Wang X, et al. The gene mutated in autosomal recessive polycystic kidney disease encodes a large, receptor-like protein. *Nat Genet.* (2002) 30:259–69. doi: 10.10 38/ng833
66. Ward CJ, Yuan D, Masyuk TV, Wang X, Punyashthiti R, Whelan S, et al. Cellular and subcellular localization of the ARPKD protein; fibrocystin is expressed on primary cilia. *Hum Mol Genet.* (2003) 12:2703–10. doi: 10.1093/hmg/ddg274
67. Harris PC, Torres VE. Polycystic kidney disease. *Annu Rev Med.* (2009) 60:321–37. doi: 10.1146/annurev.med.60.101707.125712
68. Turkbey B, Ocak I, Daryanani K, Font-Montgomery E, Lukose L, Bryant J, et al. Autosomal recessive polycystic kidney disease and congenital hepatic fibrosis (ARPKD/CHF). *Pediatr Radiol.* (2009) 39:100–11. doi: 10.1007/s00247-008-1064-x
69. Hoyer PF. Clinical manifestations of autosomal recessive polycystic kidney disease. *Curr Opin Pediatr.* (2015) 27:186–92. doi: 10.1097/MOP.0000000000000196
70. Yonem O, Bayraktar Y. Clinical characteristics of Caroli's disease. *World J Gastroenterol.* (2007) 13:1930–3. doi: 10.3748/wjg.v13.i13.1930
71. Medzhitov R. Origin and physiological roles of inflammation. *Nature.* (2008) 454:428–35. doi: 10.1038/nature07201
72. Locatelli L, Cadamuro M, Spirlì C, Fiorotto R, Lecchi S, Morell CM, et al. Macrophage recruitment by fibrocystin-defective biliary epithelial cells promotes portal fibrosis in congenital hepatic fibrosis. *Hepatology.* (2016) 63:965–82. doi: 10.1002/he p.28382
73. Munger JS, Huang X, Kawakatsu H, Griffiths MJ, Dalton SL, Wu J, et al. The integrin aVb6 binds and activates latent TGFb1: a mechanism for regulating pulmonary inflammation and fibrosis. *Cell.* (1999) 96:319–28.
74. Swenson-Fields KI, Vivian CJ, Salah SM, Peda JD, Davis BM, van Rooijen N, et al. Macrophages promote polycystic kidney disease progression. *Kidney Int.* (2013) 83:855–64. doi: 10.1038/ki.2012.446
75. Kaffe E, Fiorotto R, Pellegrino F, Mariotti V, Amenduni M, Cadamuro M, et al. β-Catenin and interleukin-1β-dependent chemokine (C-X-C motif) ligand 10 production drives progression of disease in a mouse model of congenital hepatic fibrosis. *Hepatology.* (2018) 67:1903–19. doi: 10.1002/he p.29652
76. Gunay-Aygun M. Liver and kidney disease in ciliopathies. *Am J Med Genet C Semin Med Genet.* (2009) 151C:296–306. doi: 10.1002/ajmg.c.30225
77. Reiter JF, Leroux MR. Genes and molecular pathways underpinning ciliopathies. *Nat Rev Mol Cell Biol.* (2017) 18:533–47. doi: 10.1038/nrm.2017.60
78. Qin H, Rosenbaum JL, Barr MM. An autosomal recessive polycystic kidney disease gene homolog is involved in intraflagellar transport in C. elegans ciliated sensory neurons. *Curr Biol.* (2001) 11:457–61. doi: 10.1016/s0960-9822(01)00122-1
79. Zimmerman KA, Song CJ, Gonzalez-Mize N, Li Z, Yoder BK. Primary cilia disruption differentially affects the infiltrating and resident macrophage compartment in the liver. *Am J Physiol Gastrointest Liver Physiol.* (2018) 314:G677–89. doi: 10.1152/ajpgi.00381.2017

80. Zoja C, Corna D, Locatelli M, Rottoli D, Pezzotta A, Morigi M, et al. Effects of MCP-1 inhibition by bindarit therapy in a rat model of polycystic kidney disease. *Nephron*. (2015) 129:52–61. doi: 10.1159/000369149
81. Cassini MF, Kakade VR, Kurtz E, Sulkowski P, Glazer P, Torres R, et al. Mcp1 promotes macrophage-dependent cyst expansion in autosomal dominant polycystic kidney disease. *J Am Soc Nephrol*. (2018) 29:2471–81. doi: 10.1681/ASN.2018050518
82. Fiorotto R, Amenduni M, Mariotti V, Fabris L, Spirli C, Strazzabosco M. Liver diseases in the dish: iPSC and organoids as a new approach to modeling liver diseases. *Biochim Biophys Acta Mol Basis Dis*. (2019) 1865:920–8. doi: 10.1016/j.bbadis.2018.08.038

10

Metabolomics Profiling and Diagnosis Biomarkers Searching for Drug-Induced Liver Injury Implicated to *Polygonum multiflorum*

Ying Huang[1,2], Xu Zhao[2], Zi-teng Zhang[2], Shuai-shuai Chen[2], Shan-shan Li[2], Zhuo Shi[2], Jing Jing[2], Ang Huang[3], Yu-ming Guo[2], Zhao-fang Bai[2], Zheng-sheng Zou[3], Xiao-he Xiao[2], Jia-bo Wang[2]* and Ming Niu[2,4]**

[1] College of Pharmacy, Hunan University of Chinese Medicine, Changsha, China, [2] China Military Institute of Chinese Medicine, Fifth Medical Center of Chinese PLA General Hospital, Beijing, China, [3] Center for Non-Infectious Liver Disease, Fifth Medical Center of Chinese PLA General Hospital, Beijing, China, [4] Department of Poisoning Treatment, Fifth Medical Center of Chinese PLA General Hospital, Beijing, China

***Correspondence:**
Ming Niu
nmbright@163.com
Jia-bo Wang
pharm_sci@126.com
Xiao-he Xiao
pharmacy302xxh@126.com

Aim: The diagnosis of drug-induced liver injury (DILI) remains a challenge and the cases of *Polygonum multiflorum* Thunb. (PM) induced DILI (PM-DILI) have received much attention This study aimed to identify a simple and high-efficiency approach to PM-DILI diagnosis via metabolomics analysis.

Methods: Plasma metabolites in 13 PM-DILI patients were profiled by liquid chromatography along with high-resolution mass spectrometry. Meanwhile, the metabolic characteristics of the PM-DILI were compared with that of autoimmune hepatitis (AIH), hepatitis B (HBV), and healthy volunteers.

Results: Twenty-four metabolites were identified to present significantly different levels in PM-DILI patients compared with HBV and AIH groups. These metabolites were enriched into glucose, amino acids, and sphingolipids metabolisms. Among these essential metabolites, the ratios of P-cresol sulfate vs. phenylalanine and inosine vs. bilirubin were further selected using a stepwise decision tree to construct a classification model in order to differentiate PM-DILI from HBV and AIH. The model was highly effective with sensitivity of 92.3% and specificity of 88.9%.

Conclusions: This study presents an integrated view of the metabolic features of PM-DILI induced by herbal medicine, and the four-metabolite decision tree technique imparts a potent tool in clinical diagnosis.

Keywords: drug-induced liver injury, metabolomics, autoimmune hepatitis, hepatitis B, *Polygonum multiflorum* Thunb 3

INTRODUCTION

Drug-induced liver injury (DILI) includes an assorted array of symptoms caused by exposure to synthetic or natural drugs, and the incidence rate is 1–10 in 100,000, approximately. DILI is one of the major reasons for the effects of withdrawal of drugs (1). A sustained growth in the number of patients with DILIs has been recorded in recent years, particularly due to the rapid expansion of the use of natural herbal medicines, including traditional Chinese medicines (TCM) and herbal healthcare products (2–4). DILI patients can deteriorate due to acute liver failure (ALF), and more than half of ALF patients have been reported to be attributed to DILI (5). The early diagnosis of DILI is crucial to ameliorate the therapeutic outcome.

However, the diagnosis of DILI is quite challenging due to the lack of specific and reliable biomarkers (6), and largely depending on excluding diagnosis. Moreover, the diagnostic approach is complex and time-consuming (7). Recently, *Tomoyoshi* et al. reported that γ-Glu-citrulline and ALT have the potential to differentiate DILI from other liver diseases, including hepatitis B (HBV), and hepatitis C (HCV) (8). Furthermore, in our previous study, nine biomarkers obtained by means of ^{1}H NMR were employed in the differential diagnosis of AIH from other diseases that are commonly confused with AIH, including DILI (9). However, the efficiency of these biomarkers in the differentiation of DILI and viral hepatitis (VH) is unclear. Therefore, we need to focus on identifying more specific biomarkers of DILI.

Metabolomics focuses on the global metabolic changes that occur in response to disturbances in living systems, and has emerged as a powerful tool for disease diagnosis and pathogenic investigations (10). In the present study, the metabolites DILI patients were examined by metabolomics involving the use of liquid chromatography mass spectrometry (LC/MS). Due to the rise in number of cases of *Polygonum multiflorum* Thunb. (PM) induced DILI (PM-DILI) which has received much attention in Asian countries (e.g., China, Japan, and Korea), as well as European and North American countries (11, 12). PM-DILI was explored in this study. We identified a highly specific set of metabolites (i.e., P-cresol sulfate, phenylalanine, inosine, and bilirubin) that were able to effectively differentiate PM-DILI patients from patients with other applicable diseases and healthy controls.

MATERIALS AND METHODS

Patients

A total of 58 plasma samples were obtained from patients in the fifth Medical center of Chinese PLA general hospital. Thirteen PM-DILI patients, 12 AIH patients, 24 HBV patients, and 9 healthy controls were recruited after they provided informed consent; the study protocol was approved by the Medical Ethics Committee of the Fifth Medical Center of Chinese PLA General Hospital. The diagnoses of all patients were made according to international codified criteria (7, 13, 14). The plasma samples of AIH and HBV patients were collected during acute exacerbation while hospitalized. The clinical baseline characteristics, including gender, age, and the main parameters of the liver markers, are summarized in **Table 1**.

TABLE 1 | Clinical baseline characteristics of all participants[a].

Variable (Mean ± SD)	AIH	CON	DILI	HBV
Gender (F/M)[b]	9/3	2/7	6/7	2/22
Age (y)	52.8 ± 11.5	51 ± 16	45.8 ± 13	45.0 ± 9.6
IgG (g/L)	35.3 ± 3.7	9.7 ± 2.2	32.2 ± 5.4	29.5 ± 4.5
IgM (g/L)	33.6 ± 5.4	1.8 ± 1.2	28.8 ± 17.1	30.1 ± 10.7
Bilirubin (μmol/L)	26.5 ± 17.2	12 ± 7	85.8 ± 90.5	252.0 ± 127.5
ALT (U/L)	55.8 ± 24.4	31 ± 11	372.2 ± 424.5	76.6 ± 55.3
AST (U/L)	62.9 ± 26.9	27 ± 10	210.2 ± 202.3	111.0 ± 69.1
ALP (U/L)	183.1 ± 94.7	77 ± 40	127.9 ± 48.7	134.6 ± 35.7

[a]*SD, standard deviation; AIH, autoimmune hepatitis; CON, health controls; DILI, Drug-induced liver injuries; HBV, hepatitis; IgG, immunoglobulin G; IgM, immunoglobulin M; ALT, alanine aminotransferase; AST, aspartate aminotransferase; ALP, alkaline phosphatase.*
[b]*F for female and M for male.*

Sample Preparation

Pre-prandial venous blood samples were collected in the morning using lithium heparin tubes (BD Vacutainer; 6 mL; Becton, Dickinson and Company, Franklin Lakes, NJ, USA), and the plasma was collected by centrifugation at 1,000 g at 4°C for 15 min. The plasma samples were immediately stored at −80°C until they were used for the metabolomics analysis. Prior to the LC/MS analysis, 600 μl of acetonitrile was added to 200 μl of plasma, which was thawed at room temperature, for sample purification. The samples were then centrifuged at 10,000 g for 10 min at 4°C. Subsequently, the supernatants were transferred into sample vials.

UHPLC/MS-QTOF Measurement

Four-microliter samples were injected and separated using an Infinity 1290 UHPLC system (Agilent Technologies, SA, USA), ZORBAX SB 300 C18 column (100 × 2.1 mm with a 1.8-μm particle size, Agilent Technologies, SA, USA). The column temperature was maintained at 35°C. The system was operated at a flow rate of 0.3 mL/min with solvent A (water) and solvent B (acetonitrile), and 0.1% of formic acid was also added for the positive mode. The gradient elution program was as follows: 5.00% B for min 0–1; 5%–40% B for min 1–9; 40–90% B for min 9–19; 90–100% B for min 19–21; and 100% A for min 21–25. The total run time was 30 min for each analysis. The mass data were acquired with an Agilent 6550A Q-TOF mass spectrometer (Agilent Technologies, SA, USA) in the full scan mode (80–1,200 m/z) in both the positive and negative ion modes using an Agilent Jet Stream ESI source. In the positive mode, the capillary voltage was set to 4,000 V with a nozzle voltage of 500 V. In the negative mode, the capillary voltage was set to −3,000 V with a nozzle voltage of −500 V. The other source parameters were as follows: the nebulizer was set to 45 psig; the drying gas temperature was maintained at 225°C; the flow rate was 11 L/min; and the voltages of the fragmentor, skimmer 1, and octupole RF peak were 230, 0, and 750 V, respectively. During the analysis, two groups of reference masses of 121.0509 m/z (purine; [$C_5H_4N_4$

+ H]+) and 922.0098 m/z (HP-0921; $[C_{18}H_{18}O_6N_3P_3F_{24} + H]^+$) in positive mode and 112.9885 m/z (ammonium trifluoroacetate $[C_2H_4O_2NF_3 - NH_4]^-$) and 1,033.9881 m/z (HP-0921 + ammonium trifluoroacetate $[C_{20}H_{22}O_8N_4P_3F_{27} - NH_4]^-$) in negative mode, were continuously injected to obtain high-accuracy mass correction. To ensure the stability and repeatability of the LC-MS systems, the QC sample was obtained from 10 μl of each sample and then analyzed together with the other samples. Five replicates of the QC sample were performed on the system before the sample sequence. The QC samples were also inserted, and every five samples were analyzed.

Data Processing and Statistical Analysis

The peak alignment and data filtering were processed using Mass Profinder (version B.06.00, Agilent Technologies, SA, USA). For the molecular feature extraction, up to 2,000 compounds with peak height above 300 counts were extracted. GeneSpring (version 13.1.1, Agilent Technologies, SA, USA) was used for the normalization and statistical analysis. Only variables that were present in 70% of at least one group were included in the analysis, to reduce noise. The normalized data was analyzed using the Wilcoxon Mann-Whitney Test with $p < 0.05$ and a fold change > 2 set as the level of statistical significance. SIMCA 13.0 (Umetrics, Umeå, Sweden) was used for the multivariate analysis, principal component analysis (PCA) and orthogonal projection to latent structures discriminate analysis (OPLS-DA) were applied with Pareto scaling. Finally, the metabolites with greater variable importance in the projection value (VIP > 1) and correlation coefficient value (|Pcorr| > 0.5) in the OPLS-DA analysis were considered statistically significant.

Biomarker Identification

The compounds that exhibited significant changes were selected as the candidate biomarkers and identified using the METLIN database (http://metlin.scripps.edu/). The pathway analysis of the potential biomarkers was carried out with MetaboAnalyst

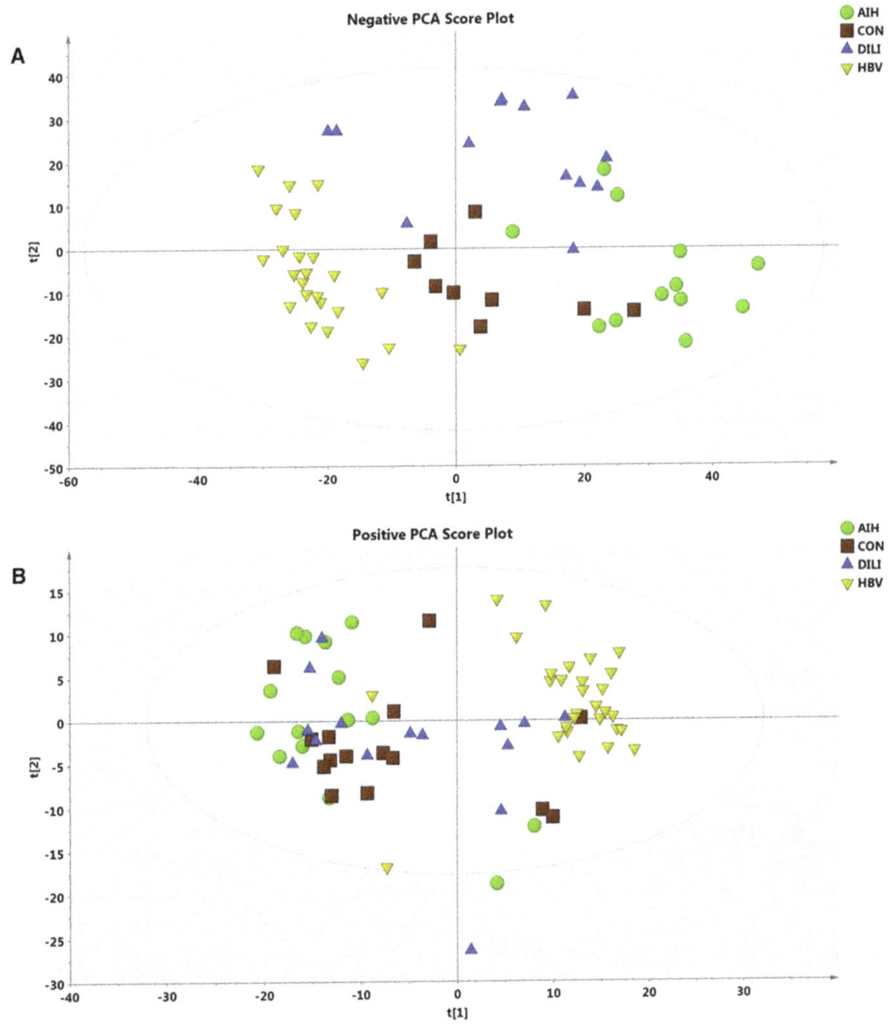

FIGURE 1 | Score plot of PCA model for AIH, CON, DILI, and HBV with the first two principal components. **(A)** The PCA1 and PCA2 explained 27% variation under ESI- mode. **(B)** The PCA1 and PCA2 explained 35% variation under ESI+ mode.

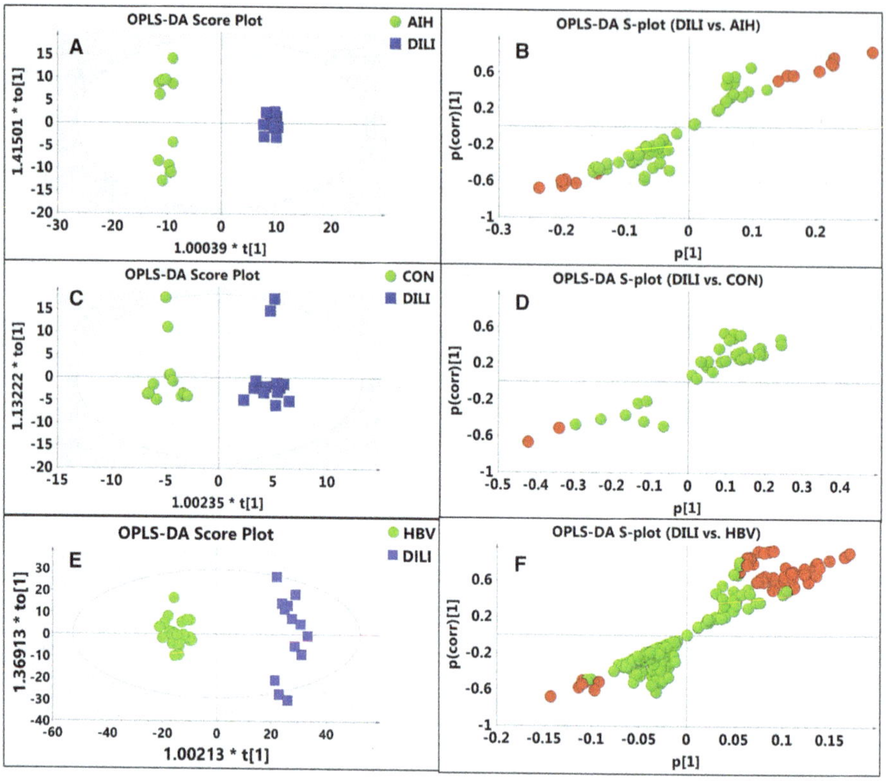

FIGURE 2 | Discrimination of DILI patients from AIH, HBV, and healthy controls according to orthogonal projection to latent structures discriminate analysis (OPLS-DA) model in the ESI- mode. The points in red indicate the identified biomarkers. **(A)** Score plot of the OPLS-DA model for the pair-wise comparisons between the AIH and DILI; **(B)** S-plot of the OPLS-DA model for the AIH and DILI; **(C)** Score plot of the OPLS-DA model for the CON and DILI; **(D)** S-plot of the OPLS-DA model for the CON and DILI; **(E)** Score plot of the OPLS-DA model for the HBV and DILI; **(F)** S-plot of the OPLS-DA model for the HBV and DILI.

3.0 (http://www.metaboanalyst.ca/) based on the Kyoto Encyclopedia of Genes and Genomes (KEGG) pathways library for humans (http://www.genome.jp/kegg/). The differences were considered significant when the test p value was below 0.05.

Decision Tree Learning for the PM-DILI Diagnosis

The classification and regression tree analysis (CRT) was calculated with IBM SPSS 22.0 for Windows, and the Gini algorithm together with a 10-fold cross-validation was used to determine the best split for each node. Receiver operating characteristic (ROC) testing was performed to further evaluate the performances of the established models in the diagnoses of the different patients. The diagnostic values were assessed using the sensitivity, specificity, and area under the curve (AUC).

RESULTS

Plasma Metabolomic Study of the Patients

The representative UHPLC-MS base peak ion (BPI) current chromatograms in the positive and negative ion modes for the human sera from each group, were visually compared. Using the optimized analysis protocol, such as peak alignment and normalization, we obtained 3,995 molecular features.

Pattern Recognition Analysis and Biomarker Screening

After data normalization, log transformation, and Pareto scaling, 850 metabolites were identified to be significantly different between the PM-DILI and other groups by multivariate analysis. PCA was used as an unsupervised method to examine the overall differences among groups and revealed that the metabolites in PM-DILI were vastly different from the other groups (**Figure 1**). OPLS-DA (**Figures 2, 3**) was then used as a supervised method capable of performing classification and discrimination analysis to comprehensively examine the metabolites and revealed significant differences in the paired groups. Based on the criteria of VIP > 1 and a |P(corr)| > 0.5, the 217 molecular-feature ions from the ESI+ and ESI− mode analyses were combined to further identify the molecular formulas. The accurate mass charge ratios of these ions were tentatively identified against the online METLIN database. Finally, a total of 24 potential biomarkers, including 9 metabolites in ESI+ mode and 15 metabolites in ESI− mode, were identified and listed in **Table 2**.

The average normalized quantities of the identified metabolites were orderly clustered and plotted on a heat map based on their Pearson correlation coefficients. The metabolic differences between the PM-DILI and other groups are mapped in **Figure 4** according to the KEGG pathways

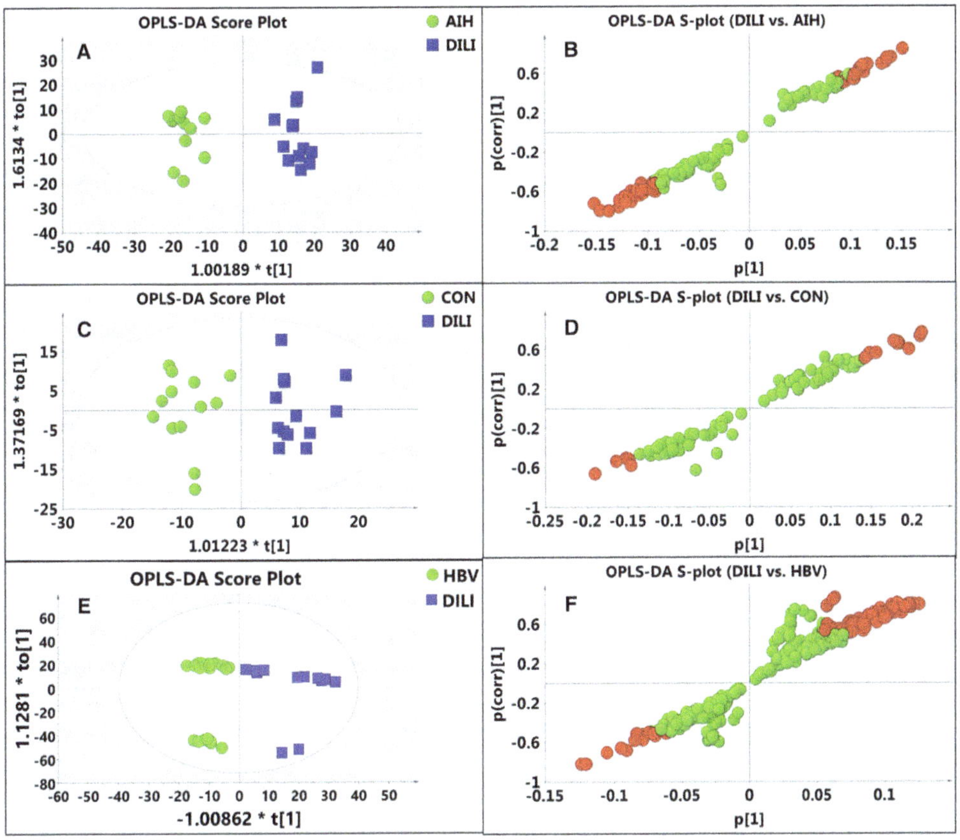

FIGURE 3 | Discrimination of DILI patients from AIH, HBV, and healthy controls according to orthogonal projection to latent structures discriminate analysis (OPLS-DA) model in the ESI+ mode. The points in red indicate the identified biomarkers. **(A)** Score plot of the OPLS-DA model for the pair-wise comparisons between the AIH and DILI; **(B)** S-plot of the OPLS-DA model for the AIH and DILI; **(C)** Score plot of the OPLS-DA model for the CON and DILI; **(D)** S-plot of the OPLS-DA model for the CON and DILI; **(E)** Score plot of the OPLS-DA model for the HBV and DILI; **(F)** S-plot of the OPLS-DA model for the HBV and DILI.

database. We found that the disturbances of some metabolic pathways, such as the metabolisms of three essential amino acids (i.e., tryptophan, valine, phenylalanine), glycerophospholipid metabolism, primary bile acid biosynthesis, and sphingolipid metabolism may specifically contribute to PM-DILI but not to other diseases.

Decision Tree Learning for PM-DILI Diagnosis

The 276 randomly combined pairs of 24 identified metabolites were employed to create a decision tree model for the differential diagnosis of the PM-DILI from other diseases using SPSS software. Ultimately, the best two pairs, the ratios of P-cresol sulfate vs. phenylalanine and inosine vs. bilirubin, were selected. Along with a 10-fold cross-validation, the decision tree for PM-DILI prediction achieved sensitivity (positive predictive values) of 92.3%, specificity (negative predictive values) of 88.9%, accuracy of 89.8%, and an error risk of 0.205 $\pm$ 0.061. The ROC curve for this decision tree is plotted in **Figure 5**, and it yielded an AUC of 0.931.

DISCUSSION

DILI has always been an important cause of ALF, and the diagnosis of DILI remains a challenge. In the present study, plasma metabolomics were employed to investigate the metabolic differences between PM-DILI, HBV, AIH patients, and healthy individuals, to identify a simple and high probability method of diagnosis of PM-DILI.

Different Metabolic Features of PM-DILI and Relevant Diseases

Based on the results of the current analysis, we found that a few essential amino acids and glucose metabolites play important roles in the differentiation of PM-DILI from other symptomatically similar diseases and healthy states. The consumption of glucose leads to increased glucuronic acid volume through the pentose and glucuronate interconversion pathway in HBV and increased 2-Deoxy-D-ribose-5P (dR5P) volume through the pentose phosphate pathway in AIH. It is well known that glucuronic acid conjugates with xenobiotics, such as drugs and bilirubin, with a high probability of making them more water-soluble and eliminating them from the body through

TABLE 2 | Identification of significantly changed metabolites.

Metabolites name	RT (min)	Formula	Mass[a] (m/z)
Data from the ESI− mode			
4-Cresol	1.20	C7H8O	107.0503
Phenylalanine	1.06	C9H11NO2	164.0729
P-cresol sulfate	1.34	C7H8O4S	187.0042
Oxalosuccinic acid	1.33	C6H6O7	189.0027
D-Glucuronic acid	0.90	C6H10O7	193.0388
Deoxyribose 5-phosphate	3.31	C5H11O7P	213.0217
Melatonin	3.97	C13H16N2O2	231.1098
Inosine	12.66	C10H12N4O5	267.0696
PA(17:2(9Z,12Z)/0:0)[a]	18.70	C20H37O7P	419.2069
(25S)-5β-cholestane-3α,7α,12α,26-tetrol	23.11	C27H48O4	435.3601
Glycochenodeoxycholate	4.33	C26H43NO5	448.2976
LysoPE (0:0/22:6(4Z,7Z,10Z,13Z,16Z,19Z))[b]	13.94	C27H44NO7P	524.2746
Taurocholate	15.00	C26H45NO8S	530.2818
PA(14:1(9Z)/13:0)[c]	19.20	C30H57O8P	575.3758
PG(14:1(9Z)/18:3(6Z,9Z,12Z))[d]	6.53	C38H67O10P	713.4488
CoA	15.02	C21H36N7O16P3S	766.1094
Data from the ESI+ mode			
Valine	1.02	C5H11NO2	118.0875
Methionine	1.05	C5H11NO2S	150.0585
Phenylalanine	1.06	C9H11NO2	166.0875
Coniferyl aldehyde	18.76	C10H10O3	179.0719
Tyrosine	1.05	C9H11NO3	182.0776
Phytosphingosine	11.75	C18H39NO3	318.3045
PE (17:2(9Z,12Z)/0:0)[e]	10.42	C22H42NO7P	464.2905
Bilirubin	19.93	C33H36N4O6	585.2639
DG(17:2(9Z,12Z)/20:0/0:0)[f]	19.93	C40H74O5	635.5741

[a] *$[M-H]^-$ for the ESI− mode and $[M+H]^+$ for the ESI+ mode.*
[b] *Compound in the pathway is LPA.*
[c] *Compound in the pathway is L-2-LPE.*
[d] *Compound in the pathway is PA.*
[e] *Compound in the pathway is PG.*
[f] *Compound in the pathway is L-1-LPE.*
[g] *Compound in the pathway is DG.*

the urine or bile (15). In the present study, the significantly elevated levels of D-glucuronic acid observed in the HBV patients might induce impairment in liver detoxification. The pentose phosphate pathway is the primary pathway for the generation of nicotinamide adenine dinucleotide phosphate (NADPH), which is beneficial in the prevention of oxidative stress (16–18). It can be deduced that AIH patients endure more oxidative stress than PM-DILI patients. Considering that the metabolites of the TCA cycle and LysoPE were elevated in PM-DILI and AIH patients, glycerophospholipid metabolism might have been accelerated by the degradation of phosphoethanolamine (PE) to provide adequate energy in these patients.

In addition to glucose metabolism, changes in plasma AA concentrations may also have influenced various biological functions by impairing hepatic function and subsequently caused hyperinsulinemia and hyperglucagonemia (19). For example, methionine (Met) was upregulated in HBV and decreased in AIH and PM-DILI, and the change of Met is frequently associated with the change of related metabolites, such as taurine and cysteine (20). Taurocholic acid is a conjugate of taurine and cholic acid and was observed in our study, which contrasts with the changes in Met. Furthermore, a stepwise increase in the plasma levels of valine was observed from AIH to PM-DILI to HBV. Valine is one of the branched-chain amino acids that have a stimulatory effect on glutamine synthesis and is a major source of nitrogen (21–23). Given that the liver plays a role in the regulation of the glutamine synthesis (24), plasma levels of valine may reflect changes in hepatic function. Additionally, γ- glutamyl dipeptides, the biomarkers for many liver diseases (8), are also synthesized from glutamate, which suggests that valine has the potential to discriminate PM-DILI from other liver diseases.

Furthermore, a few metabolites of amino acids observed in this study were also able to differentiate PM-DILI from other diseases. For example, melatonin is an indolamine product of tryptophan and is involved in the regulation of circadian rhythms. Melatonin also possesses an ability to modulate numerous molecular pathways, including those related to cellular injury (25), oxidative stress (26–28), and inflammation (29–32). The plasma melatonin is altered in different diseases and pathological states; i.e., decreased levels are associated with the hyperactivation of the immune system (33), and elevated levels are correlated with the severity of cirrhosis and hepatic encephalopathy (34). In our study, melatonin were reduced in AIH group and elevated in HBV group compared to the PM-DILI and healthy group. It can be concluded that the levels of melatonin in AIH may be downregulated by abnormal autoimmune reactions against hepatocytes and the liver injuries of HBV patients could be more serious than those of the PM-DILI patients.

Moreover, sphingolipid metabolism was abnormal in the AIH and HBV patients compared to the PM-DILI patients. Sphingolipids have been reported to play important roles in mediating many biological functions, such as cell growth, apoptosis, senescence, and differentiation (35–38). Phytosphingosine is structurally similar to sphingosine and is a precursor of ceramide, which is also regarded as an important cellular signal for inducing apoptosis. Phytosphingosine was downregulated in the HBV patients and upregulated in the AIH patients, but no significant difference was observed between the PM-DILI patients and healthy controls. Thus, it could be inferred that apoptosis was not obvious in PM-DILI patients.

Diagnostic Potentials of the Differential Metabolites

The underlying mechanisms of DILI induced by distinctive drugs may also be different. However, the changes in some metabolites in the plasma might be similar among the DILI samples (8). In this study, all the metabolites with significant changes were regarded as candidate biomarkers, whose diagnostic potentials need to be investigated. In order to precisely differentiate DILI (PM-DILI) cases from cases with other liver diseases, a decision tree analysis that can be used in clinical settings was implemented. Considering the error of each detection, we performed the decision tree analysis with the ratios of identified

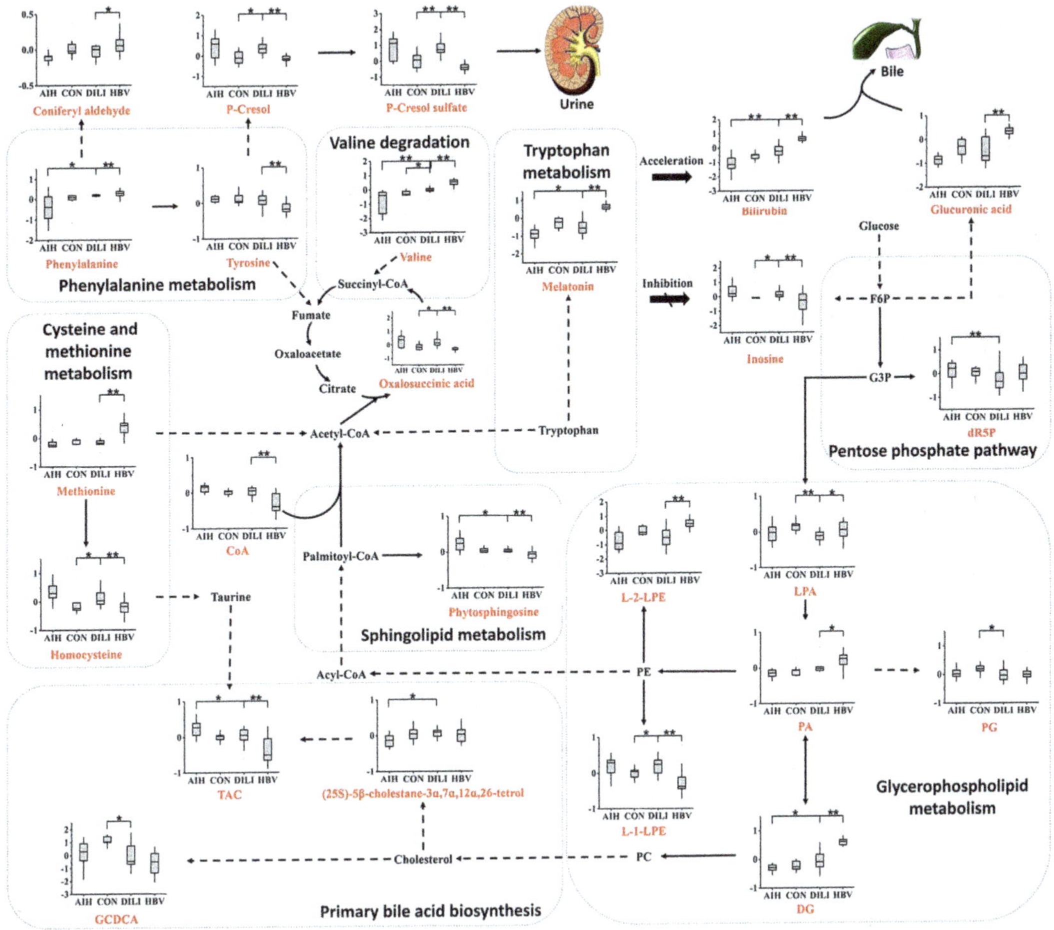

FIGURE 4 | Metabolic network of the significantly changed metabolites. The significantly changed metabolites are shown under the normalized contents. All the *P* values were calculated using Mann-Whitney Test, * and ** represent $p < 0.05$ and $p < 0.01$ compared with the DILI group, respectively. DG, 1,2-diacylglycerol; dR5P, deoxyribose 5-phosphate; PA, phosphatidic acid; PC, phosphatidylcholine; PE, phosphoethanolamine; PG, phosphatidylglycerol; L-1-LPE, L-1-lysophosphoethanolamine; L-2-LPE, L-2-lysophosphoethanolamine; LPA, lysophosphatidic acid; TCA, taurocholic acid; GCDCA, glycochenodeoxycholic acid; F6P, fructose-6-phosphate; G6P, glucose-6-phosphate.

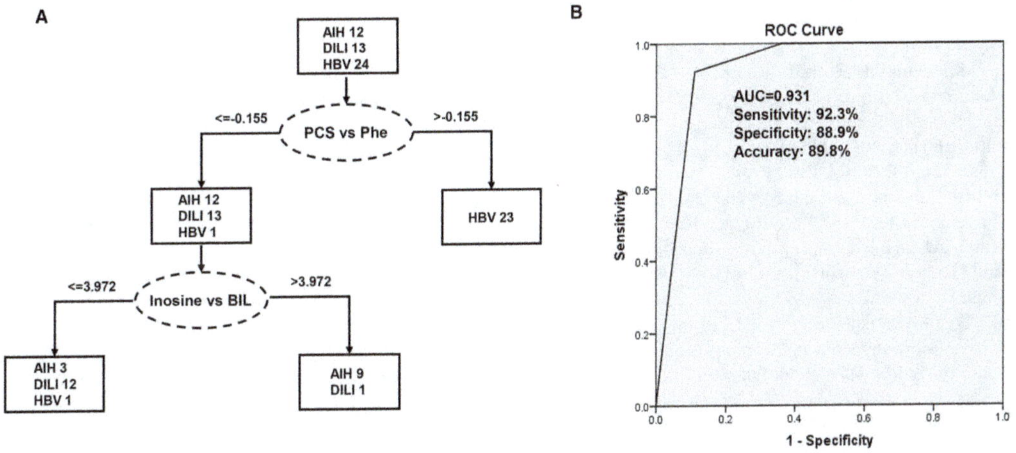

FIGURE 5 | Decision tree classification model for the differential diagnosis of DILI. PCS, P-cresol sulfate; Phe, phenylalanine; BIL, bilirubin. **(A)** Flowchart of the discriminating DILI based on the two ratios of four marker metabolites; **(B)** Results of the ROC tests that correspond to flowchart A.

metabolites. The results indicated that the ratios of P-cresol sulfate vs. phenylalanine and inosine vs. bilirubin need to be investigated for their potential utility in the differential diagnosis of DILI.

CONCLUSION

In summary, our LC–HRMS-based metabolic profiling analysis of plasma samples provides an integrated view of the metabolic features of PM induced DILI. The differential metabolites between DILI and relevant liver diseases were screened and identified, and the results indicated that the metabolic alterations in DILI were mainly related to amino acid and sphingolipid metabolisms. These findings can potentially provide valuable information for the diagnoses of DILI. The diagnostic potentials of the differential metabolites found in the plasma samples revealed that the ratios of P-cresol sulfate vs. phenylalanine and inosine vs. bilirubin exhibited good sensitivity and specificity in differentiating DILI from AIH and HBV. Hence, these factors have great potential as biomarkers of DILI in clinical diagnosis.

ETHICS STATEMENT

The studies involving human participants were reviewed and approved by Medical Ethics Committee of Fifth Medical Center of Chinese PLA General Hospital. The patients/participants provided their written informed consent to participate in this study. Written informed consent was obtained from the individual(s) for the publication of any potentially identifiable images or data included in this article.

AUTHOR CONTRIBUTIONS

YH and MN: LC-MS data analysis and manuscript preparation. YH: sample collection and preparation. MN, J-bW, and X-hX: experimental design. XZ, Z-tZ, S-sC, S-sL, ZS, JJ, AH, Y-mG, Z-fB, and Z-sZ: helped in execution of research. All authors contributed to the article and approved the submitted version.

REFERENCES

1. DeSanty KP, Amabile CM. Antidepressant-induced liver injury. *Annal Pharmacother.* (2007) 41:1201–11. doi: 10.1345/aph.1K114
2. Navarro VJ. Herbal and dietary supplement hepatotoxicity. *Semin Liver Dis.* (2009) 29:373–82. doi: 10.1055/s-0029-1240006
3. Navarro VJ, Barnhart H, Bonkovsky HL, Davern T, Fontana RJ, Grant L, et al. Liver injury from herbals and dietary supplements in the U.S. Drug-induced liver injury network. *Hepatology.* (2014) 60:1399–408. doi: 10.1002/hep.27317
4. Teschke R, Wolff A, Frenzel C, Schulze J, Eickhoff A. Herbal hepatotoxicity: a tabular compilation of reported cases. *Liver Int.* (2012) 32:1543–56. doi: 10.1111/j.1478-3231.2012.02864.x
5. Lee WM. Acute liver failure in the United States. *Semin Liver Dis.* (2003) 23:217–26. doi: 10.1055/s-2003-42641
6. Lewis JH. The art and science of diagnosing and managing drug-induced liver injury in 2015 and beyond. *Clin Gastroenterol Hepatol.* (2015) 13:2173–89.e2178. doi: 10.1016/j.cgh.2015.06.017
7. Chalasani NP, Hayashi PH, Bonkovsky HL, Navarro VJ, Lee WM, Fontana RJ. ACG clinical guideline: the diagnosis and management of idiosyncratic drug-induced liver injury. *Am J Gastroenterol.* (2014) 109:950–66. doi: 10.1038/ajg.2014.131
8. Soga T, Sugimoto M, Honma M, Mori M, Igarashi K, Kashikura K, et al. Serum metabolomics reveals gamma-glutamyl dipeptides as biomarkers for discrimination among different forms of liver disease. *J Hepatol.* (2011) 55:896–905. doi: 10.1016/j.jhep.2011.01.031
9. Wang JB, Pu SB, Sun Y, Li ZF, Niu M, Yan XZ, et al. Metabolomic profiling of autoimmune hepatitis: the diagnostic utility of nuclear magnetic resonance spectroscopy. *J Proteome Res.* (2014) 13:3792–801. doi: 10.1021/pr500462f
10. Nicholson JK, Wilson ID. Opinion: understanding 'global' systems biology: metabonomics and the continuum of metabolism. *Nat Rev Drug Discov.* (2003) 2:668–76. doi: 10.1038/nrd1157
11. Park GJ, Mann SP, Ngu MC. Acute hepatitis induced by Shou-Wu-Pian, a herbal product derived from *Polygonum multiflorum. J Gastroenterol Hepatol.* (2001) 16:115–7. doi: 10.1046/j.1440-1746.2001.02309.x
12. Lei X, Chen J, Ren J, Li Y, Zhai J, Mu W, et al. Liver damage associated with *Polygonum multiflorum* thunb.: a systematic review of case reports and case series. *Evid Based Complement Alternat Med.* (2015) 2015:459749. doi: 10.1155/2015/459749
13. Hennes EM, Zeniya M, Czaja AJ, Parés A, Dalekos GN, Krawitt EL, et al. Simplified criteria for the diagnosis of autoimmune hepatitis. *Hepatology.* (2008) 48:169–76. doi: 10.1002/hep.22322
14. European Association for the Study of the Liver. EASL 2017 clinical practice guidelines on the management of hepatitis B virus infection. *J Hepatol.* (2017) 67:370–98. doi: 10.1016/j.jhep.2017.03.021
15. Beyoglu D, Smith RL, Idle JR. Dog bites man or man bites dog? The enigma of the amino acid conjugations. *Biochem Pharmacol.* (2012) 83:1331–9. doi: 10.1016/j.bcp.2011.12.031
16. Horecker BL. The pentose phosphate pathway. *J Biol Chem.* (2002) 277:47965–71. doi: 10.1074/jbc.X200007200
17. Patra KC, Hay N. The pentose phosphate pathway and cancer. *Trends Biochem Sci.* (2014) 39:347–54. doi: 10.1016/j.tibs.2014.06.005
18. Spaans SK, Weusthuis RA, van der Oost J, Kengen SW. NADPH-generating systems in bacteria and archaea. *Front Microbiol.* (2015) 6:742. doi: 10.3389/fmicb.2015.00742
19. Morgan MY, Marshall AW, Milsom JP, Sherlock S. Plasma amino-acid patterns in liver disease. *Gut.* (1982) 23:362–70. doi: 10.1136/gut.23.5.362
20. Holecek M. Three targets of branched-chain amino acid supplementation in the treatment of liver disease. *Nutrition.* (2010) 26:482–90. doi: 10.1016/j.nut.2009.06.027
21. Dam G, Keiding S, Munk OL, Ott P, Buhl M, Vilstrup H, et al. Branched-chain amino acids increase arterial blood ammonia in spite of enhanced intrinsic muscle ammonia metabolism in patients with cirrhosis and healthy subjects. *Am J Physiol Gastrointest Liver Physiol.* (2011) 301:G269–77. doi: 10.1152/ajpgi.00062.2011
22. Ruderman NB, Berger M. The formation of glutamine and alanine in skeletal muscle. *J Biol Chem.* (1974) 249:5500–6.
23. Odessey R, Khairallah EA, Goldberg AL. Origin and possible significance of alanine production by skeletal muscle. *J Biol Chem.* (1974) 249:7623–9.
24. Brosnan JT. Interorgan amino acid transport and its regulation. *J Nutr.* (2003) 133 (6 Suppl. 1):2068s–72s. doi: 10.1093/jn/133.6.2068S
25. Wang X. The antiapoptotic activity of melatonin in neurodegenerative diseases. *CNS Neurosci Ther.* (2009) 15:345–57. doi: 10.1111/j.1755-5949.2009.00105.x
26. Zhang HM, Zhang Y. Melatonin: a well-documented antioxidant with conditional pro-oxidant actions. *J Pineal Res.* (2014) 57:131–46. doi: 10.1111/jpi.12162
27. Manchester LC, Coto-Montes A, Boga JA, Andersen LP, Zhou Z, Galano A, et al. Melatonin: an ancient molecule that makes oxygen metabolically tolerable. *J Pineal Res.* (2015) 59:403–19. doi: 10.1111/jpi.12267
28. Garcia JJ, Lopez-Pingarron L, Almeida-Souza P, Tres A, Escudero P, García-Gil FA, et al. Protective effects of melatonin in reducing oxidative stress and in preserving the fluidity of biological membranes: a review. *J Pineal Res.* (2014) 56:225–37. doi: 10.1111/jpi.12120

29. Jin H, Wang Y, Zhou L, Liu L, Zhang P, Deng W, et al. Melatonin attenuates hypoxic pulmonary hypertension by inhibiting the inflammation and the proliferation of pulmonary arterial smooth muscle cells. *J Pineal Res.* (2014) 57:442–50. doi: 10.1111/jpi.12184
30. Chen J, Chen G, Li J, Qian C, Mo H, Gu C, et al. Melatonin attenuates inflammatory response-induced brain edema in early brain injury following a subarachnoid hemorrhage: a possible role for the regulation of pro-inflammatory cytokines. *J Pineal Res.* (2014) 57:340–7. doi: 10.1111/jpi.12173
31. Borges Lda S, Dermargos A, da Silva Junior EP, Weimann E, Lambertucci RH, Hatanaka E. Melatonin decreases muscular oxidative stress and inflammation induced by strenuous exercise and stimulates growth factor synthesis. *J Pineal Res.* (2015) 58:166–72. doi: 10.1111/jpi.12202
32. Cano Barquilla P, Pagano ES, Jimenez-Ortega V, Fernandez-Mateos P, Esquifino AI, Cardinali DP. Melatonin normalizes clinical and biochemical parameters of mild inflammation in diet-induced metabolic syndrome in rats. *J Pineal Res.* (2014) 57:280–90. doi: 10.1111/jpi.12168
33. Marseglia L, D'Angelo G, Manti S, Salpietro C, Arrigo T, Barberi I, et al. Melatonin and atopy: role in atopic dermatitis and asthma. *Int J Mol Sci.* (2014) 15:13482–93. doi: 10.3390/ijms150813482
34. Chojnacki C, Wachowska-Kelly P, Blasiak J, Reiter RJ, Chojnacki J. Melatonin secretion and metabolism in patients with hepatic encephalopathy. *J Gastroenterol Hepatol.* (2013) 28:342–7. doi: 10.1111/jgh.12055
35. Bourbon NA, Sandirasegarane L, Kester M. Ceramide-induced inhibition of Akt is mediated through protein kinase Czeta: implications for growth arrest. *J Biol Chem.* (2002) 277:3286–92. doi: 10.1074/jbc.M110541200
36. Hu W, Xu R, Zhang G, Jin J, Szulc ZM, Bielawski J, et al. Golgi fragmentation is associated with ceramide-induced cellular effects. *Mol Biol Cell.* (2005) 16:1555–67. doi: 10.1091/mbc.e04-07-0594
37. Stover T, Kester M. Liposomal delivery enhances short-chain ceramide-induced apoptosis of breast cancer cells. *J Pharmacol Exp Ther.* (2003) 307:468–75. doi: 10.1124/jpet.103.054056
38. Birbes H, El Bawab S, Obeid LM, Hannun YA. Mitochondria and ceramide: intertwined roles in regulation of apoptosis. *Adv Enzyme Regul.* (2002) 42:113–29. doi: 10.1016/S0065-2571(01)00026-7

11

Bile Acid Receptor Therapeutics Effects on Chronic Liver Diseases

*Vik Meadows[1,2], Lindsey Kennedy[3], Debjyoti Kundu[2], Gianfranco Alpini[1,3] and Heather Francis[1,3]**

[1] Richard L. Roudebush VA Medical Center, Indiana University School of Medicine, Indianapolis, IN, United States, [2] Department of Biochemistry and Molecular Biology, Indiana University School of Medicine, Indianapolis, IN, United States, [3] Division of Gastroenterology and Hepatology, Department of Medicine, Indiana University School of Medicine, Indianapolis, IN, United States

***Correspondence:**
Heather Francis
heafranc@iu.edu

In the past ten years, our understanding of the importance of bile acids has expanded from fat absorption and glucose/lipid/energy homeostasis into potential therapeutic targets for amelioration of chronic cholestatic liver diseases. The discovery of important bile acid signaling mechanisms, as well as their role in metabolism, has increased the interest in bile acid/bile acid receptor research development. Bile acid levels and speciation are dysregulated during liver injury/damage resulting in cytotoxicity, inflammation, and fibrosis. An increasing focus to target bile acid receptors, responsible for bile acid synthesis and circulation, such as Farnesoid X receptor and apical sodium-dependent bile acid transporter to reduce bile acid synthesis have resulted in clinical trials for treatment of previously untreatable chronic liver diseases such as non-alcoholic steatohepatitis and primary sclerosing cholangitis. This review focuses on current bile acid receptor mediators and their effects on parenchymal and non-parenchymal cells. Attention will also be brought to the gut/liver axis during chronic liver damage and its treatment with bile acid receptor modulators. Overall, these studies lend evidence to the importance of bile acids and their receptors on liver disease establishment and progression.

Keywords: bile acid, chronic liver disease, obeticholic acid, ursodeoxycholic acid, bile acid receptor

INTRODUCTION

Focal studies of hepatic secretion led to the critical analysis and understanding of bile and its circulation connecting the liver and intestine (1). Bile acids (BAs) are heterogenous compounds whose chemical and amphipathic properties result from the enzymatic breakdown of insoluble cholesterol (2). Since their isolation from bile, the field of BA chemistry has provided intensive study of their complex chemical nature and the physiological effects of their dynamic composition in circulating bile (2–5).

Hepatic BA build up leads to inflammation, necrosis, and apoptosis of various liver cells which then affects BA synthesis and transport perpetuating BA-induced damage (2, 3). Due to the extensive knowledge and research concerning hepatic BA formation and secretion, it is natural to assume BAs contribute to chronic liver damage. The increased synthesis of BAs in combination with interrupted BA signaling can lead to adverse effects in patients of chronic liver diseases. It is estimated that 1.5 billion people worldwide suffer from chronic liver diseases whose complications, cirrhosis and liver cancer, result in 2 million deaths globally (6). Chronic liver diseases have an increased burden in the health care system due to the frequent hospital readmissions, accompanying hepatic decompensation, and risk for infection as liver damage progresses (6). Many chronic liver diseases, such as primary sclerosing cholangitis (PSC) and non-alcoholic fatty liver disease (NAFLD), have minimal treatment options requiring liver transplantation as the only permanent remedy (6, 7).

Various therapeutics have been FDA-approved for clinical trials aiming to improve liver function and relieve adverse effects of disrupted BA signaling. This article serves as a brief review of BA signaling and function in various chronic liver diseases and their regulation of the gut microbiome.

CIRCULATION, MODIFICATION, AND FUNCTION OF BILE ACIDS

Bile Acid Synthesis and Transport

The catabolism of cholesterol into BAs in the parenchyma is tightly regulated by over 17 enzymes, preferentially expressed in the liver, that are involved in the synthesis and alteration of BAs into bile salts (8, 9). Impairment of these mechanisms can result in cholestasis, liver damage, impaired lipid metabolism, and other maladies (3, 5, 8). Modifications and conjugations of BAs affect their solubility, hydrophobicity, and receptor binding affinity (8, 10). BA synthesis and conjugations are summarized in **Figure 1** (reprinted with permission from Molinaro et al. Trends Endocrinol Metab).

Bile acids are secreted into the bile canaliculi by hepatocytes, draining to the bile ducts located in the portal triad. Cholangiocytes are the epithelial cells lining the bile ducts and assist in BA modification and circulation by cholehepatic shunting, the process in which BAs are reabsorbed from the bile and returned to hepatocytes (11–14). The intrahepatic bile duct system allows BAs to flow into the intestinal lumen through the common hepatic duct in response to food ingestion to assist in emulsification, metabolism and absorption of dietary lipids and fat-soluble vitamins (A, D, E, and K). Alternatively, BAs are deposited in the gallbladder for storage and prevention of cholesterol-crystallization and gallstone formation (10, 15). Approximately 95% of BAs are reabsorbed in the distal ileum by the apical sodium-dependent bile acid transporter (ASBT; alternatively known as ileal bile acid transporter, IBAT) and delivered to the liver through the portal system via enterohepatic or portal circulation (16–18). The gut microbiome is capable of deconjugating primary bile acids and converting them to secondary bile acids prior to absorption or fecal excretion which affects gut microbiome community, BA pool, and liver health (8, 19, 20).

Aside from their important roles in digestion, BAs can behave as signaling molecules in carbohydrate and lipid metabolism, energy expenditure, and hepatic disease (20–22). BAs and activation of their downstream targets including G-protein-coupled bile acid receptor (TGR5), transforming growth factor-α (TGF-α) and sphingosine-1-phosphate receptor-2 (S1PR2) stimulate cholangiocyte proliferation and contribute to the progression of cholangiocarcinoma [CCA, *in vivo* and *in vitro* (21–25)]. Alternatively, Farnesoid X Receptor (FXR) is down regulated in hepatocellular carcinoma (HCC) (26). It has been shown that FXR via increased CYP450 epoxygenase activity suppress NF-κB signaling thereby reducing hepatic inflammation (27, 28). Further exploration into the anti-inflammatory role of FXR and assessment of BA direct or indirect targets may provide understanding of chronic cholestatic disease establishment and progression.

Intrahepatic and Extrahepatic Bile Acid Modification

The catabolism of cholesterol results in the formation of the primary BAs, cholic acid (CA) or chenodeoxycholic acid (CDCA), through the major (classical) pathway or the minor (alternative/acidic) pathway, respectively (29). Cholehepatic shunting alters the BA pool via biliary ASBT transport, multidrug resistance cassette 3 (MDR3, human; multidrug resistance cassette 2, mice), and organic solute transporter α-β (OSTα-β) BA secretion into the peribiliary plexus prior to reaching the hepatic sinusoids (30). Ileal bile acid binding protein (IBABP) is expressed in large cholangiocytes to sequester BAs preventing biliary cytotoxicity (30, 31). CA and CDCA/Ursodeoxycholic acid (UDCA) are converted to deoxycholic acid (DCA) and lithocholic acid (LCA), respectively, via 7α/β-dihydroxylation by various species of the commensal gut microbiota in the gastrointestinal tract (32). Human secondary BAs (DCA and LCA) are capable of being circulated back to the liver via enterohepatic circulation leading to an increased hepatic levels of damaging hydrophobic BAs (32).

DYSREGULATION OF BILE ACIDS IN CHRONIC LIVER DISEASES

PSC and PBC

PSC and Primary Biliary Cholangitis (PBC) are rare cholestatic liver diseases that affect the biliary system. PSC is an idiopathic disease with cholestasis, inflammation and eventual fibrosis resulting from strictures of intra- and extrahepatic bile ducts (33). PSC is one of the most common causes for liver transplantation (LT) (33). Due to its heterogenous and spontaneous progression, effective medical therapies have not yet been developed (33). Fat-soluble vitamin deficiency can occur in PSC patients as a result of decreased bile flow and secretion. It has also been shown that PSC has a positive correlation with ulcerative colitis (UC), a form of inflammatory bowel disease (IBD). PSC/IBD patients display

Abbreviations: ALKP/ALP, Alkaline phosphatase; ASBT, apical sodium bile acid transporter; AST, aspartate aminotransferase; Bas, bile acids; FXR, Farnesoid X receptor; CA, cholic acid; CCA, cholangiocarcinoma; CDCA, chenodeoxycholic acid; DCA, deoxycholic acid; HCC, hepatocellular carcinoma; IBABP, ileal bile acid binding protein; IBD, irritable bowel disease; IBAT, ileal bile acid transporter; LCA, lithocholic acid; LDL, low density lipoprotein; MDR2, multidrug resistance cassette 2; MDR3, multidrug resistance cassette 3; NAFLD, non-alcoholic fatty liver disease; NASH, non-alcoholic steatohepatitis; OCA, Obeticholic acid; OSTα-β, organic solute transporter α-β; PBC, primary biliary cholangitis; PSC, primary sclerosing cholangitis; TBA, total bile acid; TGR5, Takeda G protein coupled receptor 5; UDCA, Ursodeoxycholic acid.

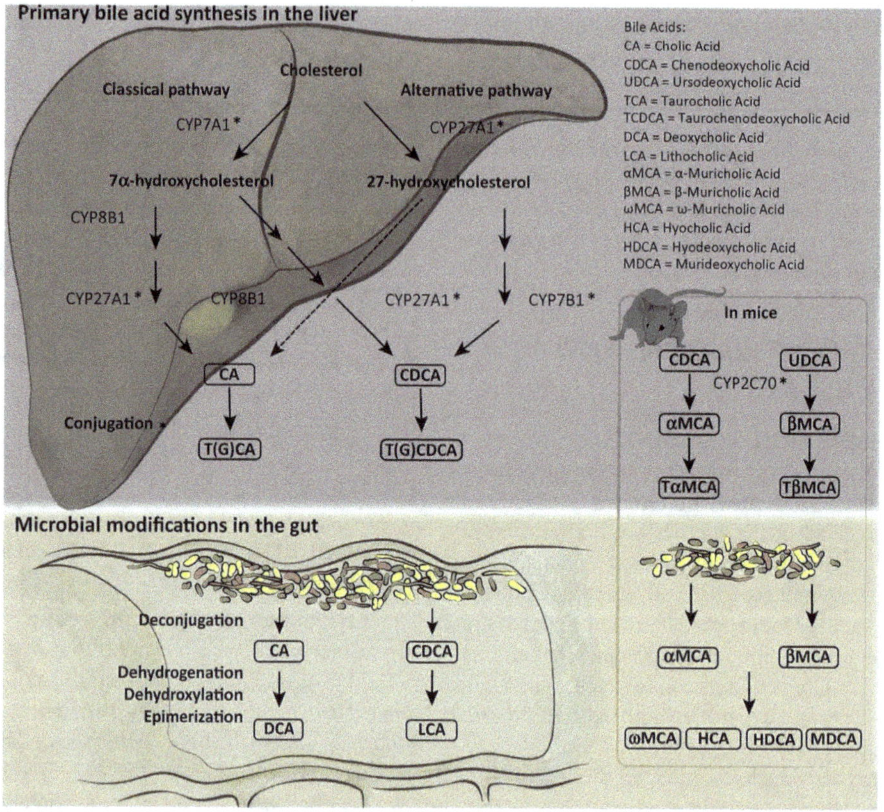

FIGURE 1 | Human and mouse bile acid synthesis and conjugation. Cholesterol catabolism results in the creation of primary bile acids (BAs) through either the classical pathway, accomplished by Cytochrome P450 7A1 (CYP7A1), or the alternative/acidic pathway, conducted by Cytochrome P450 27A1 (CYP27A1). Alteration by various cytochrome P450 family of enzymes allows for the creation of cholic acid (CA) and chenodeoxycholic acid (CDCA). Primary BAs can become conjugated to glycine or taurine prior to secretion to the biliary ductules. Deconjugation and reconjugation occurs in the distal ileum through bacterial intervention creating secondary BAs: lithocholic acid (LCA) or deoxycholic acid (DCA). Mice have additional primary BAs: Ursodeoxycholic acid (UDCA) and α- and β-muricholic acid. The murine specific primary BAs created by cytochrome P450 2C70 (CYP2C70) can also be conjugated to glycine or taurine prior to secretion into bile duct and alteration by gut microbiota into secondary BAs. Figure reprinted with permission from Molinaro et al. Trends Endocrinol Metab.

altered BA fecal excretion and decreased gut microbiome diversity compared to healthy or IBD patient controls (34). Patients with PSC have decreased expression of hepatic FXR, TGR5, and S1PR2 (35). The multidrug resistance cassette 2 knock-out mouse (MDR2$^{-/-}$) is a mouse model utilized to mimic the PSC phenotype including increased cholestasis, intrahepatic bile duct mass and hepatic inflammation due to hepatic BA build up (36, 37). This murine model has been useful for identifying effects of potential therapeutics, such as UDCA. Meng et al. reported that UDCA treatment in Mdr2$^{-/-}$ mice reduced serum TBA, elevated hepatic expression of BA transporters, and reduced hepatic inflammation and collagen deposition (36).

PBC is a chronic auto-immune disease, predominantly affecting middle-aged women, that results in biliary ductopenia and cholestasis. Li et al. reported elevated serum levels of total BAs (TBA) and FGF19 in cirrhotic PBC patients compared to healthy controls and non-cirrhotic PBC patients (38). Similarly, Trottier et al. demonstrated elevated BAs in serum samples from both PBC and PSC compared to healthy controls (39). Ursodeoxycholic acid (UDCA), an epimer of CDCA, was the first FDA-approved treatment for PBC. Despite increased bile flow, lower liver enzyme levels, and decreased serum BA levels, one in three PBC patients will have a limited or no response to treatment, strengthening the need for effective therapeutic intervention of PBC progression (33, 40–45).

NAFLD

NAFL and non-alcoholic steatohepatitis (NASH) are two of the most common hepatic diseases worldwide due to an increase of sedentary lifestyle and consumption of a high-fat/high-cholesterol diet (46, 47). Its prevalence has demonstrated positive correlation with an increasing number of obese and type II diabetic patients (46). Currently, there are no approved therapies for the treatment of NAFL and NASH aside from a change of diet and exercise for gradual weight loss.

BA signaling is disrupted in NAFL and NASH patients yielding great interest in the search for exogenous methods of BA regulation (48, 49). Mouzaki et al. uncovered greater fecal BA secretion and increased primary to secondary BA ratio in NASH patients compared to healthy controls (49). Ferslew et al. found elevated serum BAs in NASH patients, compared to healthy controls, with an increase of taurine- and glycine-conjugated BAs (48). Benedict and Zhang proposed that FXR suppression of hepatic inflammation may ameliorate NAFLD progression (50).

HCC and CCA

HCC is currently the third leading cause of cancer deaths worldwide. HCC affects parenchymal cells in the liver, which make up to 70% of the liver tissue. HCC develops in chronic liver disease or cirrhotic liver patients and is usually detected through various imaging methods prior to diagnosis. Patients with HCC can be asymptomatic or present with a range of symptoms including cirrhosis-related pain. The underlying chronic liver injury, and difficulty in diagnosis, both contribute to HCCs high mortality. CCA is a rare but devastating cancer with poor prognosis. Patients present with jaundice, pruritus (intense itch) and acholic (pale) stool due to reduced bile and bilirubin excretion. Due to the intimate relationship between hepatocytes, cholangiocytes and BAs it is important to investigate BA signaling in the establishment and progression of HCC and CCA.

Demonstrating a shift in the BA pool during cancer development, Changbumrung et al. reported elevated ratios for trihydroxy to dihydroxy BAs and for glycine-conjugated to taurine-conjugated BAs in patients with HCC and CCA compared to healthy patients (51). Luo et al. demonstrated a similar trend with elevated glycine-conjugated BAs in hepatic injury patients, ranging from hepatitis B viral infection to cirrhosis, compared to healthy controls suggesting taurine-conjugated BAs as a potential sensitive biomarker for liver injury (52). This increase in BA pool size is due to reduced inhibition of BA synthesis. FXR activation has been indicated to have anti-cancer properties, with decreased expression in progressing human HCC lesions, since its downstream effects include inhibition of BA synthesis and cell proliferation (26, 53). Guo et al. reported decreased FXR expression in HCC tumor lesions, indicating a hindering role in HCC development and progression (26). Wolfe et al. found a decrease of FXR expression in HCC tumor lesions, compared to normal liver tissue, with increasing tumor development stage (53). Similarly, Liu et al. reported decreased small heterodimer partner (SHP) and FXR expression in human HCC compared to paired healthy control (54). Erice et al. demonstrated FXR expression in CCA samples negatively correlates with advanced cancer progression and lymph node invasion. In contrast to FXR, TGR5 expression is elevated in CCA tumors compared to controls (25). This discovery is likely due to cholangiocyte requirement of TGR5 for BA-induced proliferation and anti-apoptosis signaling (55, 56). Additional BA receptors, such as S1PR2, have been found to have elevated expression in human CCA tumors, as shown by Liu et al. (57). Taken together these studies indicate that altered BAs may serve to enhance HCC and CCA progression during disease development.

CURRENT BILE ACID-RELATED THERAPIES OF CHRONIC LIVER DISEASES

Bile Acid Therapies

The use of synthetic or naturally occurring BAs to reduce gallstone formation, aid in lipid absorption following gastric surgeries, and assist in reduction of cholestasis has increased in recent years. UDCA is a hydrophilic BA conjugated to undergo enterohepatic circulation or deconjugated and converted into LCA by the gut microbiome and excreted into feces. UDCA was the first FDA-approved therapy for PBC patients exhibiting altered serum liver enzyme levels (41). UDCA has been a staple therapy due to its ability to prevent gallstone formation, increasing bicarbonate secretion to prevent acidification of bile, and positive side effect profile as compared to treatment with CDCA (18, 41, 58). In many PBC patients, long-term UDCA treatment when administered at early stage of disease increases survival rate, lowers liver enzyme serum levels, and improves liver histology (41, 43, 59, 60). Regardless of its beneficial effects, 30–40% of PBC patients do not respond to UDCA treatment.

UDCA treatment can improve liver histology and serum ALT/ASP levels in PSC patients, however, data supporting any long-term efficacy or long-term survival are lacking (61). Moreover, UDCA prescribed at high doses increased medical complications and mortality in PSC patients (61–64). PSC patients treated with norUDCA, a side chain shortened homolog of UDCA, exhibited reduced ALP serum levels compared to placebo in a dose-dependent manner, however norUDCA's effects on PSC progression, long-term survival, and mortality have not been investigated (65).

Bile Acid Receptor/Transporter Agonists and Antagonists

Obeticholic acid (OCA, Ocaliva) is an FDA-approved, synthetic derivative of CDCA and is a high affinity ligand for the nuclear bile acid receptor, FXR (40). FXR is a nuclear BA receptor that when expressed is capable of reducing BA synthesis, increasing expression of BA transporters and modulating lipoprotein metabolism (66). OCA has been studied as a potential therapeutic drug in the treatment of various chronic liver diseases (40, 44). Following Phase II and Phase III clinical trials, it has been suggested that OCA treatment can be delivered in conjunction with UDCA in PBC, or as a monotherapy in patients who do not tolerate UDCA, respectively (67, 68). Adverse events including pruritus occurred in nearly all patients and was observed to occur in a dose dependent manner (67, 68). The beneficial effects of OCA as a monotherapy are currently being investigated in various clinical trials (7, 67, 69). The use of OCA has promising effects on improving liver enzyme levels, lowering plasma bilirubin and IgM levels, and has recently been shown to improve or stabilize liver fibrosis and biliary injury in PBC patients with cirrhosis (68, 69). Despite promising outcomes in

PBC patients, long-term effects of OCA on disease progression and patient survival are still being investigated.

In the Farnesoid X Receptor Ligand Obeticholic Acid in NASH Treatment (FLINT) clinical trial, NASH patients treated with OCA presented with improved fibrosis scores, elevated low-density lipoprotein (LDL) and increased average weight loss compared to placebo control (46, 70). NASH patients treated with OCA also had increased ALP levels compared to placebo control (46). The effects of OCA on insulin resistance and the observed improvement of lipid absorption were not sustained following termination of OCA treatment (46). Further investigation into the short-term and long-term effects of OCA on liver function and injury are warranted and are actively being explored in the Randomized Global Phase III Study to Evaluate the Impact on NASH with Fibrosis of Obeticholic Acid Treatment (REGENERATE) clinical trial assessing FXR activation in the treatment of NASH (71). Translational Research and Evolving Alcoholic hepatitis Treatment (TREAT) consortium conducted phase II clinical trial utilizing OCA on patients with moderately severe alcoholic hepatitis (AH) that was completed in 2018, however currently no data is available on this study (72). The Phase 3 Study of Obeticholic Acid in Patients with Primary Biliary Cirrhosis (POISE) double-blind, placebo controlled clinical trial has been one of the few to publish results demonstrating OCA's long-term safety and effectiveness (69). POISE study data showed that three-year OCA treatment reduced or stabilized hepatic collagen deposition and ductular injury in PBC patients with cirrhosis (69). The Combination OCA and Statins for Monitoring of Lipids (CONTROL) clinical trial study found increased LDL in NASH patients treated with OCA (5, 10, or 25 mg) indicating altered lipid metabolism (73). The observed increase in LDL cholesterol was reduced in NASH patients concurrently treated with OCA and atorvastatin, a statin utilized to reduce endogenous cholesterol production (73). The authors noted that these two drugs were well-tolerated when utilized together, addressing the observed increase in LDL cholesterol following OCA treatment in NASH patients, but remained inconclusive with respect to the combinatorial effect on hepatic injury (70, 73). Eaton et al. observed that decompensated patients with cirrhotic PSC and PBC, OCA treatment led to the development of jaundice and elevated liver enzyme levels (74). While the long-term benefits of OCA are still being evaluated in various liver diseases, it is still being explored as a potential.

During normal enterohepatic circulation, IBAT/ASBT is responsible for the reabsorption of BAs in the intestinal tract prior to secretion into the portal blood system (75). Additionally, ASBT is responsible for cholehepatic shunting of BAs between cholangiocytes and hepatocytes, which ultimately increases hepatic BA pool. A common symptom of chronic cholestatic liver disease is pruritus, intense itching of the dermis due

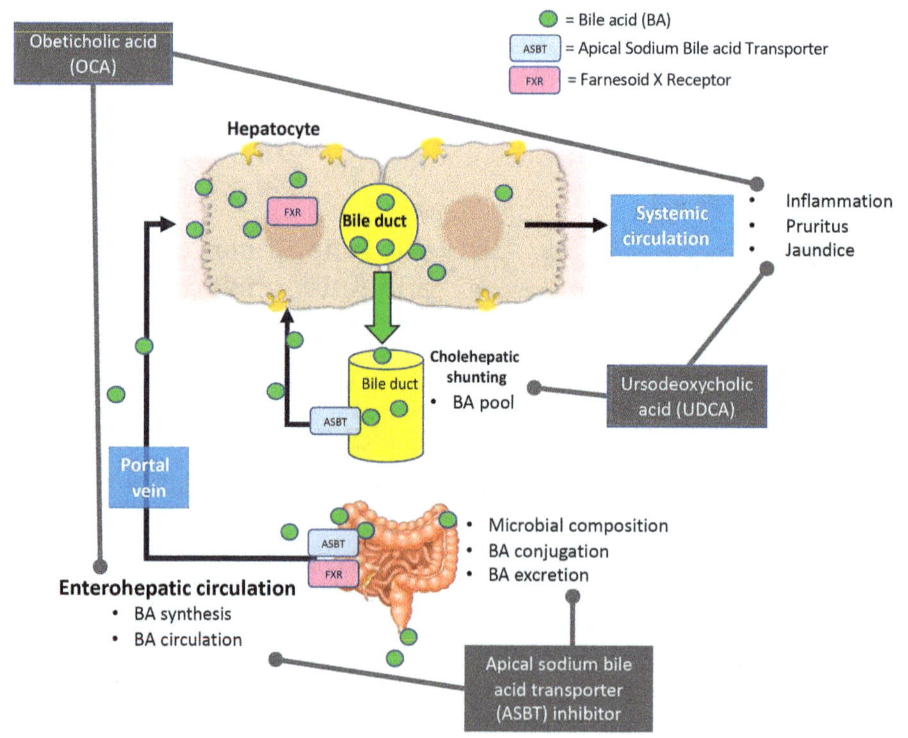

FIGURE 2 | Current bile acid receptor therapeutics and their effects in bile acid signaling. Briefly, Obeticholic acid (OCA) reduces bile acid (BA) synthesis, circulating BA levels, and hepatic inflammation. This treatment may cause adverse effects such as pruritus and jaundice (in decompensated PBC patients). Ursodeoxycholic acid (UDCA) alters BA pool and reduced hepatic inflammation and damage. In some cases, UDCA treatment has led to development of pruritus. Apical sodium bile acid transporter (ASBT) inhibitors affect bile acid synthesis, circulation, secretion, and microbial composition in the intestine.

to increased BA deposition (75). IBAT/ASBT inhibitors are potential therapeutic candidates for this detrimental symptom (76). Pilot studies conducted with various synthetic IBAT/ASBT inhibitors have demonstrated variable results. The Al-Dury et al. study reported patients who continued through A4250 (synthetic IBAT/ASBT inhibitor) received relief from itching, but pruritus returned during wash-out and BA sequestrant treatment. Despite improvement of pruritus and lowered serum BAs, many patients in the A4250 study dropped out early due to abdominal pain and diarrhea (76). Similar benefits were identified in the pilot study of GSK2330672 (synthetic IBAT/ASBT inhibitor), PBC patients resulted with lowered serum BAs and increased serum FGF19. The most common adverse events in this treatment cohort were headaches and diarrhea, which provides reason to limit the treatment length in patients with pruritus (77).

BA RECEPTOR AGONIST EFFECTS ON THE GUT/LIVER AXIS DURING LIVER DISEASE

BA species affect and regulate gut microbial species composition (32). BA species and concentrations in different portions of the gastrointestinal tract can result in increased side effects including increased intestinal permeability and BA-induced diarrhea (78). Elevated hydrophobic BAs in the colon are capable of inducing inflammation which is reduced following CDCA treatment alleviating the increased toxicity from insoluble BA concentrations and mast cell secretory factors (i.e., histamine or nerve growth factor NGF) (78, 79).

A small cohort of PBC patients exhibited altered gut microbiome composition, compared to healthy controls, which was partially reversed following 6-month UDCA treatment (80). This study found eight-PBC associated genera and a reduction in normal gut microbiome associated microbial members including *Faecalibacterium*, *Bacteroides*, *Sutterella*, and *Oscillospira* spp. A study from Selmi et al. implicated increased *N. aromaticivorans* population is responsible for the induction of PBC (81). Tang et al. reported increased epithelial infiltration of *Enterobacteriaceae* in PBC patients indicating increased permeability and decreased gastrointestinal immune response in diseased patients (80).

The gastrointestinal epithelial barrier plays an important role in maintaining BA enterohepatic circulation homeostasis and reduced inflammation from lipopolysaccharide (LPS) leakage. BA circulation is necessary to avoid damaging increases in colonic BAs that result in inflammation and intestinal damage (78). Song et al. found that CDCA was capable of reducing paracellular permeability and increased cell-to-cell tight junctions via FXR activation in mice (82). Removal of commensal gut microbiota in Mdr2$^{-/-}$ mice resulted in increased serum liver enzyme levels, cholangiocyte senescence, and circulating primary BAs (37). Alternatively, Li et al. discovered a depletion of BA induced damage to the colon and reduced mast cell activation and degranulation in FXR$^{-/-}$ mice or *Z*-guggulsterone treated mast cells (79).

The role of the gut microbiome in BA homeostasis is still being investigated. The disruption of the gut-liver axis can allow infiltration of microbes, or their metabolic products, into the enterohepatic circulation to prolong disease (83). Chronic liver disease patients all maintain their own gut microbiome signature that inherently play a role in disease development. Future studies of BA-associated therapeutics should consider effects on the gut microbiome and their metabolites in relation to changing BA pool/circulation and chronic liver disease.

CONCLUSION

BA signaling, and therapeutics that alter them, have effects on the gut microbiome and organs outside of the liver. The use of BA receptor agonists and antagonists and their indirect effects (BA pool, synthesis, circulation, and the gut microbiome composition) is summarized in **Figure 2**. The human and mouse gut microbiome fluctuates with the increase or decrease of BAs, which can lead to increased inflammation and intestinal malabsorption (19, 37, 80, 84–86). In depth exploration of BA signaling and circulation during chronic liver diseases may provide insight to disease amelioration or treatment strategies. Understanding the role of the gut microbiome on BA modification and circulation may allow for innovative concurrent treatment for the reductions of inopportune side effects of the currently investigated treatments, OCA and UDCA.

AUTHOR CONTRIBUTIONS

VM and HF drafted manuscript. VM, LK, DK, GA, and HF edited and approved final version of manuscript. VM and HF arranged figures.

REFERENCES

1. Reuben A. The biliary cycle of Moritz Schiff. *Hepatology.* (2005) 42:500–5. doi: 10.1002/hep.20823
2. Hofmann AF, Hagey LR. Bile acids: chemistry, pathochemistry, biology, pathobiology, and therapeutics. *Cell Mol Life Sci.* (2008) 65:2461–83. doi: 10.1007/s00018-008-7568-6
3. Chiang JY. Bile acids: regulation of synthesis. *J Lipid Res.* (2009) 50:1955–66. doi: 10.1194/jlr.R900010-JLR200
4. Chiang JY. Bile acid metabolism and signaling. *Compr Physiol.* (2013) 3:1191–212. doi: 10.1002/cphy.c120023
5. Hofmann AF, Hagey LR. Key discoveries in bile acid chemistry and biology and their clinical applications: history of the last eight decades. *J Lipid Res.* (2014) 55:1553–95. doi: 10.1194/jlr.R049437
6. Moon AM, Singal AG, Tapper EB. Contemporary epidemiology of chronic liver disease and cirrhosis. *Clin Gastroenterol Hepatol.* (2019). doi: 10.1016/j.cgh.2019.07.060. [Epub ahead of print].
7. Jhaveri MA, Kowdley KV. New developments in the treatment of primary biliary cholangitis - role of obeticholic acid. *Ther Clin Risk Manag.* (2017) 13:1053–60. doi: 10.2147/TCRM.S113052

8. Russell DW. The enzymes, regulation, and genetics of bile acid synthesis. *Annu Rev Biochem.* (2003) 72:137–74. doi: 10.1146/annurev.biochem.72.121801.161712
9. Liu Y, Rong Z, Xiang D, Zhang C, Liu D. Detection technologies and metabolic profiling of bile acids: a comprehensive review. *Lipids Health Dis.* (2018) 17:121. doi: 10.1186/s12944-018-0774-9
10. de Aguiar Vallim TQ, Tarling EJ, Edwards PA. Pleiotropic roles of bile acids in metabolism. *Cell Metab.* (2013) 17:657–69. doi: 10.1016/j.cmet.2013.03.013
11. Hofmann AF. Current concepts of biliary secretion. *Dig Dis Sci.* (1989) 34: 16S–20. doi: 10.1007/BF01536657
12. Glaser SS, Alpini G. Activation of the cholehepatic shunt as a potential therapy for primary sclerosing cholangitis. *Hepatology.* (2009) 49:1795–7. doi: 10.1002/hep.22969
13. Hofmann AF, Zakko SF, Lira M, Clerici C, Hagey LR, Lambert KK, et al. Novel biotransformation and physiological properties of norursodeoxycholic acid in humans. *Hepatology.* (2005) 42:1391–8. doi: 10.1002/hep.20943
14. Alpini G, Glaser S, Baiocchi L, Francis H, Xia X, Lesage G. Secretin activation of the apical Na+-dependent bile acid transporter is associated with cholehepatic shunting in rats. *Hepatology.* (2005) 41:1037–45. doi: 10.1002/hep.20653
15. Cai JS, Chen JH. The mechanism of enterohepatic circulation in the formation of gallstone disease. *J Membr Biol.* (2014) 247:1067–82. doi: 10.1007/s00232-014-9715-3
16. Chiang JY. Recent advances in understanding bile acid homeostasis. *F1000Res.* (2017) 6:2029. doi: 10.12688/f1000research.12449.1
17. Chiang JY. Regulation of bile acid synthesis: pathways, nuclear receptors, and mechanisms. *J Hepatol.* (2004) 40:539–51. doi: 10.1016/j.jhep.2003.11.006
18. Tonin F, Arends I. Latest development in the synthesis of ursodeoxycholic acid (UDCA): a critical review. *Beilstein J Org Chem.* (2018) 14:470–83. doi: 10.3762/bjoc.14.33
19. Kang JD, Myers CJ, Harris SC, Kakiyama G, Lee IK, Yun BS, et al. Bile acid 7α-dehydroxylating gut bacteria secrete antibiotics that inhibit clostridium difficile: role of secondary bile acids. *Cell Chem Biol.* (2019) 26:27–34 e4. doi: 10.1016/j.chembiol.2018.10.003
20. Jia ET, Liu ZY, Pan M, Lu JF, Ge QY. Regulation of bile acid metabolism-related signaling pathways by gut microbiota in diseases. *J Zhejiang Univ Sci B.* (2019) 20:781–92. doi: 10.1631/jzus.B1900073
21. Zhou H, Hylemon PB. Bile acids are nutrient signaling hormones. *Steroids.* (2014) 86:62–8. doi: 10.1016/j.steroids.2014.04.016
22. Dawson PA. Roles of Ileal ASBT and OSTalpha-OSTbeta in regulating bile acid signaling. *Dig Dis.* (2017) 35:261–6. doi: 10.1159/000450987
23. Werneburg NW, Yoon JH, Higuchi H, Gores GJ. Bile acids activate EGF receptor via a TGF-alpha-dependent mechanism in human cholangiocyte cell lines. *Am J Physiol Gastrointest Liver Physiol.* (2003) 285:G31–6. doi: 10.1152/ajpgi.00536.2002
24. Deutschmann K, Reich M, Klindt C, Droge C, Spomer L, Haussinger D, et al. Bile acid receptors in the biliary tree: TGR5 in physiology and disease. *Biochim Biophys Acta Mol Basis Dis.* (2018) 1864:1319–25. doi: 10.1016/j.bbadis.2017.08.021
25. Erice O, Labiano I, Arbelaiz A, Santos-Laso A, Munoz-Garrido P, Jimenez-Aguero R, et al. Differential effects of FXR or TGR5 activation in cholangiocarcinoma progression. *Biochim Biophys Acta Mol Basis Dis.* (2018) 1864:1335–44. doi: 10.1016/j.bbadis.2017.08.016
26. Guo F, Xu Z, Zhang Y, Jiang P, Huang G, Chen S, et al. FXR induces SOCS3 and suppresses hepatocellular carcinoma. *Oncotarget.* (2015) 6:34606–16. doi: 10.18632/oncotarget.5314
27. Wang YD, Chen WD, Wang M, Yu D, Forman BM, Huang W. Farnesoid X receptor antagonizes nuclear factor kappaB in hepatic inflammatory response. *Hepatology.* (2008) 48:1632–43. doi: 10.1002/hep.22519
28. Gai Z, Visentin M, Gui T, Zhao L, Thasler WE, Hausler S, et al. Effects of farnesoid X receptor activation on arachidonic acid metabolism, NF-kB signaling, and hepatic inflammation. *Mol Pharmacol.* (2018) 94:802–11. doi: 10.1124/mol.117.111047
29. Molinaro A, Wahlstrom A, Marschall HU. Role of bile acids in metabolic control. *Trends Endocrinol Metab.* (2018) 29:31–41. doi: 10.1016/j.tem.2017.11.002
30. Xia X, Francis H, Glaser S, Alpini G, LeSage G. Bile acid interactions with cholangiocytes. *World J Gastroenterol.* (2006) 12:3553–63. doi: 10.3748/wjg.v12.i22.3553
31. Luo ZL, Cheng L, Wang T, Tang LJ, Tian FZ, Xiang K, et al. Bile acid transporters are expressed and heterogeneously distributed in rat bile ducts. *Gut Liver.* (2019) 13:569–75. doi: 10.5009/gnl18265
32. Ridlon JM, Kang DJ, Hylemon PB, Bajaj JS. Bile acids and the gut microbiome. *Curr Opin Gastroenterol.* (2014) 30:332–8. doi: 10.1097/MOG.0000000000000057
33. Tabibian JH, Bowlus CL. Primary sclerosing cholangitis: a review and update. *Liver Res.* (2017) 1:221–30. doi: 10.1016/j.livres.2017.12.002
34. Vaughn BP, Kaiser T, Staley C, Hamilton MJ, Reich J, Graiziger C, et al. A pilot study of fecal bile acid and microbiota profiles in inflammatory bowel disease and primary sclerosing cholangitis. *Clin Exp Gastroenterol.* (2019) 12:9–19. doi: 10.2147/CEG.S186097
35. Song WS, Park HM, Ha JM, Shin SG, Park HG, Kim J, et al. Discovery of glycocholic acid and taurochenodeoxycholic acid as phenotypic biomarkers in cholangiocarcinoma. *Sci Rep.* (2018) 8:11088. doi: 10.1038/s41598-018-29445-z
36. Meng F, Kennedy L, Hargrove L, Demieville J, Jones H, Madeka T, et al. Ursodeoxycholate inhibits mast cell activation and reverses biliary injury and fibrosis in Mdr2(-/-) mice and human primary sclerosing cholangitis. *Lab Invest.* (2018) 98:1465–77. doi: 10.1038/s41374-018-0101-0
37. Tabibian JH, O'Hara SP, Trussoni CE, Tietz PS, Splinter PL, Mounajjed T, et al. Absence of the intestinal microbiota exacerbates hepatobiliary disease in a murine model of primary sclerosing cholangitis. *Hepatology.* (2016) 63:185–96. doi: 10.1002/hep.27927
38. Li Z, Lin B, Lin G, Wu Y, Jie Y, Li X, et al. Circulating FGF19 closely correlates with bile acid synthesis and cholestasis in patients with primary biliary cirrhosis. *PLoS ONE.* (2017) 12:e0178580. doi: 10.1371/journal.pone.0178580
39. Trottier J, Bialek A, Caron P, Straka RJ, Heathcote J, Milkiewicz P, et al. Metabolomic profiling of 17 bile acids in serum from patients with primary biliary cirrhosis and primary sclerosing cholangitis: a pilot study. *Dig Liver Dis.* (2012) 44:303–10. doi: 10.1016/j.dld.2011.10.025
40. Bowlus CL. Obeticholic acid for the treatment of primary biliary cholangitis in adult patients: clinical utility and patient selection. *Hepat Med.* (2016) 8:89–95. doi: 10.2147/HMER.S91709
41. Floreani A, Mangini C. Primary biliary cholangitis: old and novel therapy. *Eur J Intern Med.* (2018) 47:1–5. doi: 10.1016/j.ejim.2017.06.020
42. P.Jansen LM. New therapies target the toxic consequences of cholestatic liver disease. *Expert Rev Gastroenterol Hepatol.* (2018) 12:277–85. doi: 10.1080/17474124.2018.1424538
43. ter Borg PC, Schalm SW, Hansen BE, van Buuren HR, Dutch PBC Study Group. Prognosis of ursodeoxycholic acid-treated patients with primary biliary cirrhosis. results of a 10-yr cohort study involving 297 patients. *Am J Gastroenterol.* (2006) 101:2044–50. doi: 10.1111/j.1572-0241.2006.00699.x
44. Trivedi PJ, Hirschfield GM, Gershwin ME. Obeticholic acid for the treatment of primary biliary cirrhosis. *Expert Rev Clin Pharmacol.* (2016) 9:13–26. doi: 10.1586/17512433.2015.1092381
45. Zhang Y, Jiang R, Zheng X, Lei S, Huang F, Xie G, et al. Ursodeoxycholic acid accelerates bile acid enterohepatic circulation. *Br J Pharmacol.* (2019) 176:2848–63. doi: 10.1111/bph.14705
46. Makri E, Cholongitas E, Tziomalos K. Emerging role of obeticholic acid in the management of nonalcoholic fatty liver disease. *World J Gastroenterol.* (2016) 22:9039–43. doi: 10.3748/wjg.v22.i41.9039
47. Benedict M, Zhang X. Non-alcoholic fatty liver disease: an expanded review. *World J Hepatol.* (2017) 9:715–32. doi: 10.4254/wjh.v9.i16.715
48. Ferslew BC, Xie G, Johnston CK, Su M, Stewart PW, Jia W, et al. Altered bile acid metabolome in patients with nonalcoholic steatohepatitis. *Dig Dis Sci.* (2015) 60:3318–28. doi: 10.1007/s10620-015-3776-8
49. Mouzaki M, Wang AY, Bandsma R, Comelli EM, Arendt BM, Zhang L, et al. Bile acids and dysbiosis in non-alcoholic fatty liver disease. *PLoS ONE.* (2016) 11:e0151829. doi: 10.1371/journal.pone.0151829
50. Armstrong LE, Guo GL. Role of FXR in liver inflammation during nonalcoholic steatohepatitis. *Curr Pharmacol Rep.* (2017) 3:92–100. doi: 10.1007/s40495-017-0085-2
51. Changbumrung S, Tungtrongchitr R, Migasena P, Chamroenngan S. Serum unconjugated primary and secondary bile acids in patients with cholangiocarcinoma and hepatocellular carcinoma. *J Med Assoc Thai.* (1990) 73:81–90.

52. Luo L, Aubrecht J, Li D, Warner RL, Johnson KJ, Kenny J, et al. Assessment of serum bile acid profiles as biomarkers of liver injury and liver disease in humans. *PLoS ONE.* (2018) 13:e0193824. doi: 10.1371/journal.pone.0193824
53. Wolfe A, Thomas A, Edwards G, Jaseja R, Guo GL, Apte U. Increased activation of the Wnt/β-catenin pathway in spontaneous hepatocellular carcinoma observed in farnesoid X receptor knockout mice. *J Pharmacol Exp Ther.* (2011) 338:12–21. doi: 10.1124/jpet.111.179390
54. Liu N, Meng Z, Lou G, Zhou W, Wang X, Zhang Y, et al. Hepatocarcinogenesis in FXR-/- mice mimics human HCC progression that operates through HNF1α regulation of FXR expression. *Mol Endocrinol.* (2012) 26:775–85. doi: 10.1210/me.2011-1383
55. Reich M, Deutschmann K, Sommerfeld A, Klindt C, Kluge S, Kubitz R, et al. TGR5 is essential for bile acid-dependent cholangiocyte proliferation *in vivo* and *in vitro*. *Gut.* (2016) 65:487–501. doi: 10.1136/gutjnl-2015-309458
56. Masyuk AI, Huang BQ, Radtke BN, Gajdos GB, Splinter PL, Masyuk TV, et al. Ciliary subcellular localization of TGR5 determines the cholangiocyte functional response to bile acid signaling. *Am J Physiol Gastrointest Liver Physiol.* (2013) 304:G1013–24. doi: 10.1152/ajpgi.00383.2012
57. Liu R, Zhao R, Zhou X, Liang X, Campbell DJ, Zhang X, et al. Conjugated bile acids promote cholangiocarcinoma cell invasive growth through activation of sphingosine 1-phosphate receptor 2. *Hepatology.* (2014) 60:908–18. doi: 10.1002/hep.27085
58. Magouliotis DE, Tasiopoulou VS, Svokos AA, Svokos KA, Chatedaki C, Sioka E, et al. Ursodeoxycholic acid in the prevention of gallstone formation after bariatric surgery: an updated systematic review and meta-analysis. *Obes Surg.* (2017) 27:3021–30. doi: 10.1007/s11695-017-2924-y
59. Pares A, Caballeria L, Rodes J. Excellent long-term survival in patients with primary biliary cirrhosis and biochemical response to ursodeoxycholic acid. *Gastroenterology.* (2006) 130:715–20. doi: 10.1053/j.gastro.2005.12.029
60. Burman BE, Jhaveri MA, Kowdley KV. An update on the treatment and follow-up of patients with primary biliary cholangitis. *Clin Liver Dis.* (2017) 21:709–23. doi: 10.1016/j.cld.2017.06.005
61. Stiehl A. Ursodeoxycholic acid therapy in treatment of primary sclerosing cholangitis. *Scand J Gastroenterol Suppl.* (1994) 204:59–61. doi: 10.3109/00365529409103626
62. Lindor KD, Kowdley KV, Luketic VA, Harrison ME, McCashland T, Befeler AS, et al. High-dose ursodeoxycholic acid for the treatment of primary sclerosing cholangitis. *Hepatology.* (2009) 50:808–14. doi: 10.1002/hep.23082
63. Eaton JE, Silveira MG, Pardi DS, Sinakos E, Kowdley KV, Luketic VA, et al. High-dose ursodeoxycholic acid is associated with the development of colorectal neoplasia in patients with ulcerative colitis and primary sclerosing cholangitis. *Am J Gastroenterol.* (2011) 106:1638–45. doi: 10.1038/ajg.2011.156
64. Rudolph G, Gotthardt DN, Kloeters-Plachky P, Kulaksiz H, Schirmacher P, Stiehl A. In PSC with colitis treated with UDCA, most colonic carcinomas develop in the first years after the start of treatment. *Dig Dis Sci.* (2011) 56:3624–30. doi: 10.1007/s10620-011-1763-2
65. Fickert P, Hirschfield GM, Denk G, Marschall HU, Altorjay I, Farkkila M, et al. norUrsodeoxycholic acid improves cholestasis in primary sclerosing cholangitis. *J Hepatol.* (2017) 67:549–58. doi: 10.1016/j.jhep.2017.05.009
66. Xu Y, Li F, Zalzala M, Xu J, Gonzalez FJ, Adorini L, et al. Farnesoid X receptor activation increases reverse cholesterol transport by modulating bile acid composition and cholesterol absorption in mice. *Hepatology.* (2016) 64:1072–85. doi: 10.1002/hep.28712
67. Clinical Review Report. *Obeticholic Acid (Ocaliva): (Intercept Pharmaceuticals Canada, Inc.): Indication: for the Treatment of Primary Biliary Cholangitis (Pbc) in Combination with Ursodeoxycholic Acid (UDCA) in Adults with an Inadequate Response to UDCA or as Monotherapy in Adults Unable to Tolerate UDCA*, Ottawa, ON (2017).
68. Hirschfield GM, Mason A, Luketic V, Lindor K, Gordon SC, Mayo M, et al. Efficacy of obeticholic acid in patients with primary biliary cirrhosis and inadequate response to ursodeoxycholic acid. *Gastroenterology.* (2015) 148:751–61.e8. doi: 10.1053/j.gastro.2014.12.005
69. Bowlus CL, Pockros PJ, Kremer AE, Pares A, Forman LM, Drenth JPH, et al. Long-term obeticholic acid therapy improves histological endpoints in patients with primary biliary cholangitis. *Clin Gastroenterol Hepatol.* (2019) doi: 10.1016/j.cgh.2019.09.050. [Epub ahead of print].
70. Hameed B, Terrault NA, Gill RM, Loomba R, Chalasani N, Hoofnagle JH, et al. Clinical and metabolic effects associated with weight changes and obeticholic acid in non-alcoholic steatohepatitis. *Aliment Pharmacol Ther.* (2018) 47:645–56. doi: 10.1111/apt.14492
71. Ratziu V, Sanyal AJ, Loomba R, Rinella M, Harrison S, Anstee QM, et al. REGENERATE: design of a pivotal, randomised, phase 3 study evaluating the safety and efficacy of obeticholic acid in patients with fibrosis due to nonalcoholic steatohepatitis. *Contemp Clin Trials.* (2019) 84:105803. doi: 10.1016/j.cct.2019.06.017
72. Comerford M, Lourens S, Liangpunsakul S, Chalasani NP, Sanyal AJ, Shah VH, et al. Challenges in patient enrollment and retention in clinical studies for alcoholic hepatitis: experience of the TREAT consortium. *Alcohol Clin Exp Res.* (2017) 41:2000–6. doi: 10.1111/acer.13515
73. Pockros PJ, Fuchs M, Freilich B, Schiff E, Kohli A, Lawitz EJ, et al. CONTROL: a randomized phase 2 study of obeticholic acid and atorvastatin on lipoproteins in nonalcoholic steatohepatitis patients. *Liver Int.* (2019) 39:2082–93. doi: 10.1111/liv.14209
74. Eaton JE, Vuppalanchi R, Reddy R, Sathapathy S, Ali B, Kamath PS. Liver injury in patients with cholestatic liver disease treated with obeticholic acid. *Hepatology.* (2019) doi: 10.1002/hep.31017. [Epub ahead of print].
75. Al-Dury S, Marschall HU. Ileal bile acid transporter inhibition for the treatment of chronic constipation, cholestatic pruritus, and NASH. *Front Pharmacol.* (2018) 9:931. doi: 10.3389/fphar.2018.00931
76. Al-Dury S, Wahlstrom A, Wahlin S, Langedijk J, Elferink RO, Stahlman M, et al. Pilot study with IBAT inhibitor A4250 for the treatment of cholestatic pruritus in primary biliary cholangitis. *Sci Rep.* (2018) 8:6658. doi: 10.1038/s41598-018-25214-0
77. Hegade VS, Kendrick SF, Dobbins RL, Miller SR, Thompson D, Richards D, et al. Effect of ileal bile acid transporter inhibitor GSK2330672 on pruritus in primary biliary cholangitis: a double-blind, randomised, placebo-controlled, crossover, phase 2a study. *Lancet.* (2017) 389:1114–23. doi: 10.1016/S0140-6736(17)30319-7
78. Gelbmann CM, Schteingart CD, Thompson SM, Hofmann AF, Barrett KE. Mast cells and histamine contribute to bile acid-stimulated secretion in the mouse colon. *J Clin Invest.* (1995) 95: 2831–9. doi: 10.1172/JCI117988
79. Li WT, Luo QQ, Wang B, Chen X, Yan XJ, Qiu HY, et al. Bile acids induce visceral hypersensitivity via mucosal mast cell-to-nociceptor signaling that involves the farnesoid X receptor/nerve growth factor/transient receptor potential vanilloid 1 axis. *FASEB J.* (2019) 33:2435–50. doi: 10.1096/fj.201800935RR
80. Tang R, Wei Y, Li Y, Chen W, Chen H, Wang Q, et al. Gut microbial profile is altered in primary biliary cholangitis and partially restored after UDCA therapy. *Gut.* (2018) 67:534–41. doi: 10.1136/gutjnl-2016-313332
81. Selmi C, Balkwill DL, Invernizzi P, Ansari AA, Coppel RL, Podda M, et al. Patients with primary biliary cirrhosis react against a ubiquitous xenobiotic-metabolizing bacterium. *Hepatology.* (2003) 38:1250–7. doi: 10.1053/jhep.2003.50446
82. Song M, Ye J, Zhang F, Su H, Yang X, He H, et al. Chenodeoxycholic acid (CDCA) protects against the lipopolysaccharide-induced impairment of the intestinal epithelial barrier function via the FXR-MLCK pathway. *J Agric Food Chem.* (2019) 67:8868–74. doi: 10.1021/acs.jafc.9b03173
83. Tabibian JH, Talwalkar JA, Lindor KD. Role of the microbiota and antibiotics in primary sclerosing cholangitis. *Biomed Res Int.* (2013) 2013:389537. doi: 10.1155/2013/389537
84. Carino A, Biagioli M, Marchiano S, Fiorucci C, Zampella A, Monti MC, et al. Ursodeoxycholic acid is a GPBAR1 agonist and resets liver/intestinal FXR signaling in a model of diet-induced dysbiosis and NASH. *Biochim Biophys Acta Mol Cell Biol Lipids.* (2019) 1864:1422–37. doi: 10.1016/j.bbalip.2019.07.006
85. Friedman ES, Li Y, Shen TD, Jiang J, Chau L, Adorini L, et a. FXR-dependent modulation of the human small intestinal microbiome by the bile acid derivative obeticholic acid. *Gastroenterology.* (2018) 155:1741–52 e5. doi: 10.1053/j.gastro.2018.08.022
86. Gorbach SL, Tabaqchali S. Bacteria, bile, and the small bowel. *Gut.* (1969) 10:963–72. doi: 10.1136/gut.10.12.963

12

Bile Acids and FXR: Novel Targets for Liver Diseases

Mary Stofan[1] *and Grace L. Guo*[1,2,3*]

[1] Department of Pharmacology and Toxicology, Ernest Mario School of Pharmacy, Rutgers University, Piscataway, NJ, United States, [2] Environmental and Occupational Health Sciences Institute, Rutgers, The State University of New Jersey, Piscataway, NJ, United States, [3] VA New Jersey Health Care System, Veterans Administration Medical Center, East Orange, NJ, United States

***Correspondence:**
Grace L. Guo
guo@eohsi.rutgers.edu

Bile acids (BAs) are evolutionally conserved molecules synthesized in the liver from cholesterol and have been shown to be essential for lipid homeostasis. BAs regulate a variety of metabolic functions *via* modulating nuclear and membrane receptors. Farnesoid X receptor (FXR) is the most important nuclear receptor for maintaining BA homeostasis. FXR plays a tissue-specific role in suppressing BA synthesis and promoting BA enterohepatic circulation. Disruption of FXR in mice have been implicated in liver diseases commonly occurring in humans, including cholestasis, non-alcoholic fatty liver diseases, and hepatocellular carcinoma. Strategically targeting FXR activity has been rapidly used to develop novel therapies for the prevention and/or treatment of cholestasis and non-alcoholic steatohepatitis. This review provides an updated literature review on BA homeostasis and FXR modulator development.

Keywords: bile acids, FGF15/19, FXR, agonist, non-alcoholic fatty liver disease, species difference

INTRODUCTION

Bile acids (BAs) serve critical physiological functions, including elimination of cholesterol, absorption of fat and fat-soluble vitamins, regulation of the gut microbiome, and serving as important signaling molecules. BAs are endogenous ligands of farnesoid X receptor (FXR), Takeda G protein receptor 5 (TGR5), and sphingosine-1-phosphate receptor 2 (S1PR2). In the liver and intestine, BAs suppress their own synthesis, regulate glucose and lipid homeostasis, and inhibit inflammation and fibrogenesis. Disruption of BA homeostasis leads to severe pathological outcomes, including cholestasis, hepatic steatosis, fibrosis, and liver tumors. Regulating BA pathways has become a novel strategy to treat cholestasis and non-alcoholic steatohepatitis (NASH).

OVERVIEW OF BAS

Synthesis

BAs are amphipathic molecules synthesized from cholesterol in the liver mainly through two pathways, the classical and the alternative pathway (1). In the classical pathway, the initial and rate-limiting step is the 7α-hydroxylation of cholesterol by a cytochrome P450 enzyme, cholesterol 7α-hydroxylase (CYP7A1) (2, 3). The crucial role of CYP7A1 has been demonstrated with *Cyp7a1* knockout (KO) mice that have a high incidence of postnatal death due to abnormal neurological development following vitamin deficiencies (4). Afterwards, microsomal 3β-hydroxy-Δ^5-C27-steroid dehydroxylase (3β-HSD) converts 7α-hydroxycholesterol to 7α-hydroxy-4-cholestene-3-one (C4) (5), which can be converted by sterol 12α-hydroxylase (CYP8B1) to cholic acid

(CA) or alternatively catabolized by cytosolic Δ^4-3-oxosteroid 5β-reductase (AKR1D1) and 3α-hydroxysteroid dehydrogenase (AKR1C4), yielding a sterol intermediate, 5β-cholestan-3α,7α-diol, which is further converted to chenodeoxycholic acid (CDCA) (5, 6). *Cyp8b1* KO mice eliminated CA synthesis, suggesting that CYP8B1 is required for CA synthesis and is responsible for the CA-to-CDCA ratio in the classical pathway (7). Additionally, the C4 intermediate can be used as a serum marker for assessing BA synthesis levels *in vivo* (8).

In the alternative or acidic pathway, cholesterol is oxidized by mitochondrial sterol 27-hydroxylase (CYP27A1) to produce 27-hydroxycholesterol and 3β-hydroxy-5-cholestenoic acid, which is further hydroxylated by oxysterol 7α-hydroxylase (CYP7B1) to form the intermediate 3β, 7α-dihydroxy-5-cholestenoic acid (6, 9). Subsequent enzymatic conversions produce CDCA.

There is clear species difference of the composition of BAs between humans and mice (**Figure 1**). Human primary BAs are CA and CDCA, that form a relatively hydrophobic BA pool consisting of 40% CA, 40% CDCA, and 20% deoxycholic acid (DCA) (9). Mouse primary BAs are CA and muricholic acid (MCA) that is from 6-hydroxylation of CDCA. Hydroxylation significantly changes the physicochemical properties of BAs, resulting in a BA pool that is more hydrophilic, less potent as detergents, and cytotoxic. More significantly, this additional conversion in mice markedly changes BA signaling properties, converting the most potent endogenous FXR agonist (CDCA) to antagonists (MCAs) (9). Three seminal studies discovered the mouse 6β-hydroxylase, CYP2C70, converting CDCA to MCA (10–12). Furthermore, the DCA levels are much higher in humans than in mice because humans are unable to rehydroxylate DCA and lithocholic acid (LCA) whereas mice can. A study by Honda et al. reported that mouse CYP2A12 is the enzyme responsible for 7α-rehydroxylation of taurodeoxycholic acid (TDCA) and taurolithocholic acid (TLCA), solving another unknown of the species difference between humans and mice (12).

Conjugation is considered to be the terminal step in BA synthesis and involves the addition of an amino acid, glycine or taurine, through an amide linkage at carbon 24 (13). Humans and rodents both utilize the enzyme bile acid-CoA:amino acid *N*-acyltransferase (BAAT) for conjugation; however, primary human BAs are mainly conjugated with glycine and, to a less extent, taurine, while rodent primary BAs are taurine conjugates (14, 15). Conjugation of BAs ultimately increases their solubility and amphipathicity (13).

Enterohepatic Circulation

BAs undergo constant enterohepatic circulation. Conjugated BAs are transported across the canalicular membrane into the bile and stored in the gallbladder in both humans and mice (9). Cholecystokinin, a hormone, is secreted by the duodenum following a meal to stimulate gallbladder contraction, leading to the release of BAs into the intestine (9), where BAs help absorb dietary lipids and fat-soluble vitamins. In the ileum, about 95% BAs are reabsorbed and transported back to the liver through portal circulation (9). Daily, ~0.5 g of BAs, or 5% of the total BA pool, is excreted in the feces, with BAs being recycled 4–12 times a day; this entire process comprises the enterohepatic circulation of BAs (9).

BA transporters are responsible for dynamically moving BAs during the enterohepatic circulation. Efflux of BAs from the hepatocytes into canaliculi is mainly mediated by the bile salt export pump (BSEP; *ABCB11/Abcb11*) (16). The multidrug resistance-associated protein (MRP2; *ABCC2/Abcc2*) effluxes divalent BAs along with other organic substrates, bilirubin conjugates, glutathione, and drugs (17). Like BSEP, MRP2 is an ATP-binding cassette transporter localized to the canalicular membrane of hepatocytes (17). There seems to be a species difference between humans and mice regarding the roles of BSEP and MRP2. Mice use mainly BSEP and, to a smaller extent, MRP2, to efflux BAs into the bile, whereas humans mainly rely on BSEP to efflux BAs into the bile, which could at least partially explain the more severe cholestasis development in human patients with BSEP mutation compared to mice with BSEP deficiency (18). Mutation of the *ABCB11* gene causes BSEP deficiency and progressive familial intrahepatic cholestasis type 2 (PFIC2) (19). PFIC2 is an inherited disorder characterized by severe cholestasis beginning at infancy that can progress to cirrhosis, hepatic failure, hepatocellular carcinoma (HCC), and death (20, 21). Due to the species differences mentioned above, the PFIC2 phenotype cannot be achieved in *Abcb11* KO mice. This leaves a void for a translational model for PFIC2 to study potential therapies as the standard treatment remains to be liver transplantation.

Reabsorption of BAs in the terminal ileum mainly occurs through the uptake mediated by the apical sodium-dependent bile salt transporter (ASBT; *SLC10A2/Slc10a2*) (22), intracellular binding to intestinal bile acid-binding protein (IBABP) (23), and basolateral BA efflux into the portal circulation by the organic solute transporters OSTα and OSTβ heterodimer (24).

At the basolateral (sinusoidal) membrane of hepatocytes, the major BA uptake transporter is the sodium taurocholate co-transporting polypeptide (NTCP; *SLC10A1/Slc10a1*) (25). Interestingly, human NTCP seems to have higher affinity than does the rat transporter, allowing more efficient BA extraction

Abbreviations: ALP, Alkaline phosphatase; ALT, Alanine aminotransferase; ANIT, α-Naphthylisothiocyanate; ASBT, Apical sodium-dependent bile salt transporter; AST, Aspartate transaminase; BA, Bile acid; BDL, Bile duct ligation; BSEP, Bile salt export pump; C4, 7α-Hydroxy-4-cholesten-3-one; CA, Cholic acid; CDCA, Chenodeoxycholic acid; CY27A1, Cytochrome P450 27A1; CYP7A1, Cytochrome P450 7A1; CYP8B1, Cytochrome P450 8B1; DCA, Deoxycholic acid; FGF, Fibroblast growth factor; FGF15, Fibroblast growth factor 15; FGF19, Fibroblast growth factor 19; FGFR4, Fibroblast growth factor receptor 4; FXR, Farnesoid X receptor; GGT, Gamma-glutamyltransferase; HSC, Hepatic stellate cell; IBABP, Intestinal bile acid binding protein; iNOS, Inducible nitric oxide synthase; KO, Knockout; LCA, Lithocholic acid; LPS, Lipopolysaccharide; LT, Liver transplantation; MCA, Muricholic acid; MRP2, Multidrug resistance-associated protein 2; NASH, Non-alcoholic steatohepatitis; NR, Nuclear receptor; NTCP, Sodium taurocholate co-transporting polypeptide; OCA, Obeticholic acid; OSTα, Organic solute transporter alpha; OSTβ, Organic solute transporter beta; PBC, Primary biliary cholangitis; PFIC2, Progressive familial intrahepatic cholestasis type 2; PSC, Primary sclerosing cholangitis; PXR, Pregnane X receptor; SHP-1, Small heterodimer partner 1; UDCA, Ursodeoxycholic acid; WT, Wild type.

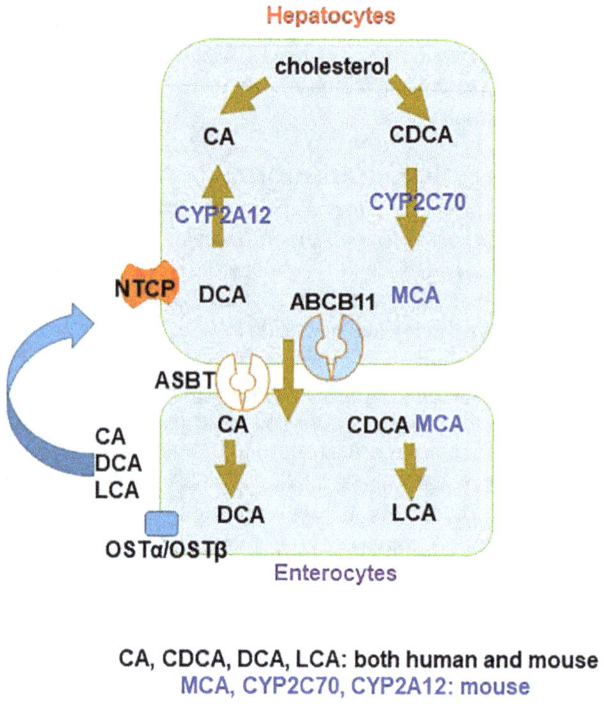

FIGURE 1 | Species difference in bile acid (BA) synthesis and composition. In hepatocytes, primary BAs, cholic acid (CA) and chenodeoxycholic acid (CDCA), are made from cholesterol. In mice, CDCA is converted to muricholic acid (MCA) by CYP2C70. CA and CDCA are conjugated and then efflux *via* ABCB11 to the intestine through the uptake transporter ASBT, where they facilitate lipid absorption. Most BAs are transported back by effluxion out of enterocytes *via* the organic solute transporter (OST)α/OSTβ complex to the liver through portal circulation and taken up into hepatocytes mainly *via* sodium taurocholate co-transporting polypeptide (NTCP), with a small amount being converted to deoxycholic acid (DCA) and lithocholic acid (LCA), the secondary BAs in the large intestine. In mice, DCA can be transported back to the liver and converted to CA by CYP2A12.

at low plasma levels (25). Sodium-independent basolateral BA uptake into hepatocytes is mediated by organic anion transporting polypeptides (OATPs) (16). Only 25% of the hepatic BA uptake is estimated to be mediated by Na^+-independent mechanism and responsible for mainly unconjugated BA uptake (16).

Although not directly involved in enterohepatic circulation, an important canalicular membrane flippase encoded by the multidrug resistance gene (*MDR3;ABCB4* in humans and *Mdr2;Abcb4* in mice) is responsible for phospholipid secretion into the bile (26, 27). Disruption of *Mdr2* prevents the secretion of phospholipids, a component of BA mixed micelles, thus increasing the concentration of free BAs that can damage the biliary epithelium (21). Defects in ABCB4 are associated with progressive familial intrahepatic cholestasis type 3 (PFIC3), intrahepatic cholestasis of pregnancy, and adult biliary cirrhosis (28, 29). *Mdr2* KO mice develop severe biliary fibrosis and are a well-established model for primary sclerosing cholangitis (PSC) (30, 31).

The gut microbiota play an important role in BA biotransformation and are responsible for secondary BA formation. Conjugated BAs that remain in the intestine are deconjugated by bacterial bile salt hydrolases (BSHs) (32). In the large intestine, bacterial 7α-dehydroxylase converts CA to DCA and CDCA to LCA through the removal of the hydroxyl group at the C-7 position (32). These secondary BAs are more cytotoxic. While LCA is highly insoluble and mostly excreted by fecal excretion, DCA can be reabsorbed through passive diffusion (33). As mentioned above, mouse hepatocytes can rehydroxylate DCA to CA by CYP2A12 (12). Species differences in the gut microbiota may affect the generation of secondary BAs and should be considered when using animal models to study human BA signaling (21).

BAs are important for the intestinal absorption of lipids and lipid-soluble nutrients, removal of excess cholesterol, regulating bile flow, modulating the gut microbiome, and modulating energy homeostasis. Many of these functions are performed by modulating a nuclear receptor (NR) FXR in a tissue-specific manner. Additional NRs and membrane-bound receptors that have been identified to be activated by BAs include pregnane X receptor (PXR), vitamin D receptor (VDR), Takeda G protein-coupled receptor (TGR5), and sphingosine-1-phosphate receptor 2 (S1PR2) (34–36).

FARNESOID X RECEPTOR

FXR is the most important NR to regulate BA homeostasis. NRs are ligand-activated transcription factors that regulate the expression of genes involved in various processes, including cell growth, differentiation, and metabolism (37). The general structure of NRs consists of an N-terminal DNA-binding domain (DBD) and a C-terminal ligand-binding domain (LBD), with the DBD being the most conserved area that contains two zinc finger motifs (9). These zinc fingers allow the NR to bind to DNA elements, known as hormone response elements (HREs), composed of direct, inverted, or everted repeats of the sequence AGGTCA and separated by a variable number of nucleotides (38). NR activation also requires either homodimerization or heterodimerization with retinoid X receptor (RXR) (39).

FXR was originally labeled as an orphan NR (38). After multiple groups demonstrated that physiological concentrations of free or conjugated BAs could activate FXR, with CDCA being the most potent, followed by DCA, CA, and LCA, BAs were recognized to be the endogenous ligands of FXR and FXR is now considered an "adopted" NR (40–42). FXR is highly expressed in the liver, ileum, kidneys, and adrenal glands (40). The most common FXR response element (FXRE) consists of an inverted AGGTCA repeat separated by one nucleotide (IR1); FXR could also bind to an everted repeat separated by two nucleotides (ER2) (43). Both steroidal and non-steroidal FXR agonists are being developed in the treatment of various liver diseases and include semi-synthetic BA obeticholic acid (OCA), cilofexor, and tropifexor,

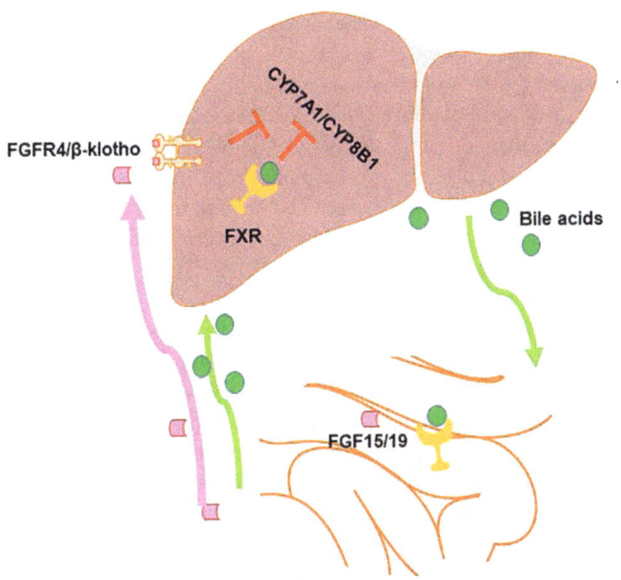

FIGURE 2 | Farnesoid X receptor (FXR) regulates bile acid (BA) synthesis in a tissue-specific manner. In the intestine, FXR activation induces fibroblast growth factor (FGF)15/19, which can go to the liver and activate the FGFR4/β-klotho dimer to activate signaling pathways in order to inhibit the expression of genes in the classical BA synthesis pathway. Hepatic FXR activation also inhibits BA synthesis, albeit to a smaller degree.

with OCA being used clinically to treat primary biliary cholangitis (PBC).

Regulation of BA Homeostasis

It has been well-established that FXR is involved in the regulation of BA homeostasis. As shown in **Figure 2**, there is a clear tissue-specific role of FXR in the liver and intestine to regulate BA synthesis (44). Activation of intestinal FXR plays a major role and activation of liver FXR serves a minor role in suppressing *CYP7A1/Cyp7a1* gene expression through the induction of the ileal hormone fibroblast growth factor 19 (FGF19) in humans and FGF15 in mice and hepatic small heterodimer partner 1 (SHP-1), respectively (42, 44–47). In contrast, *Cyp8b1* gene repression *via* FXR is almost equally dependent on both intestinal and liver FXR (44). Furthermore, FXR is critical in regulating the enterohepatic circulation of BAs by inducing the expression of BSEP, IBABP, and OSTα/β and suppressing those of NTCP and ASBT (48–52).

Regulation of Lipid and Glucose Homeostasis

FXR also shows critical effects in regulating lipid and glucose homeostasis. In general, FXR activation leads to lower lipid levels in the circulation as it suppresses *de novo* fatty acid synthesis (53, 54), decreases very low-density lipoprotein (VLDL) hepatic secretion (55), and increases triglyceride hydrolysis and clearance as well as fatty acid oxidation (56–60). Activation of FXR may reduce glucose intolerance by reducing hepatic gluconeogenesis and glycolysis and increasing glycogen synthesis (61). FXR activation may decrease gluconeogenesis *via* SHP-mediated suppression of the critical transcription factors involved in gluconeogenesis (62). In contrast, a different study utilizing human and rat hepatocytes and mouse livers showed that FXR agonism induced phosphoenolpyruvate carboxykinase (PEPCK) expression and glucose levels (63). Our genome-wide ChIP-seq analysis also suggests that FXR could regulate glucose homeostasis, but there may be species differences among humans and mice (43, 64). Despite conflicting evidence, it is apparent that FXR may play important roles in glucose homeostasis as FXR KO mice develop fatty livers, elevate circulating free fatty acids (FFAs) and serum glucose levels, and present insulin resistance (65). In both diabetic db/db and wild-type mice, FXR activation or hepatic overexpression significantly lowered the blood glucose levels, decreased the FFA levels, and increased the insulin sensitivity (66), suggesting FXR activation may improve metabolic syndrome.

Role in Inflammation and Fibrosis

During liver injury, FXR has been shown to play an anti-inflammatory role (67, 68). Monocyte chemoattractant protein-1 (MCP-1/CCL2) is a key chemokine that regulates the migration and infiltration of monocytes/macrophages (69). In the methionine/choline-deficient (MCD) diet-induced NASH model, the synthetic FXR agonist WAY-362450 decreased MCP-1 expression and significantly decreased inflammatory cell infiltration in the liver (68). Nuclear factor kappa-light-chain enhancer of activated B cell (NF-κB) is a transcription factor that induces the expression of various pro-inflammatory genes (70). FXR KO mice displayed strong hepatic inflammation after treatment with lipopolysaccharide (LPS), confirmed by massive liver necrosis and the significant increase in the hepatic cytokine signaling molecules inducible nitric oxide synthase (iNOS), cyclooxygenase-2 (COX-2), and interferon-γ (IFN-γ) (67). Ultimately, the pretreatment of HepG2 cells and mouse primary hepatocytes with FXR agonists suppressed the NF-κB-mediated inflammation in an FXR-dependent manner (67). FXR could suppress inflammation *via* an indirect mechanism by reducing cholestasis and the levels of toxic BA production and accumulation in the liver, as described above.

FXR activation suppresses the development of hepatic fibrosis. In addition to regulating hepatic lipid metabolism and reducing hepatic fibrosis, FXR seems to directly inactivate hepatic fibrosis by inducing anti-fibrotic gene expression in hepatic stellate cells (HSCs). Activation of FXR induces SHP to increase the peroxisomal proliferator-activated receptor γ (PPARγ) expression in HSCs, and PPARγ is well-known to inactivate HSCs (71, 72). Recently, we have shown that FGF15 deficiency reduces hepatic fibrosis through increasing FXR activation following loss of FGF15-mediated suppression of BA synthesis (73, 74). Interestingly, in a human HSC cell line, LX2, FGF19 does not suppress fibrogenic gene expression, but suppresses inflammation, likely through modulating the inhibitor of nuclear factor kappa B (IκB) activity (74). These studies provide another group of evidence to support the role of FXR as a homeostatic regulator to suppress liver inflammation and fibrosis.

Role in Cholestasis

There is conflicting evidence regarding the role of FXR in cholestatic diseases. In an early study, the synthetic FXR agonist GW4064 was investigated in rat models of extrahepatic and intrahepatic cholestasis through bile duct ligation (BDL) and α-naphthylisothiocyanate (ANIT) administration, respectively (75). Significant reductions in liver injury were observed in GW4064-treated animals in both cholestatic models, revealed by the reduced alanine aminotransferase (ALT) and aspartate transaminase (AST), necrosis, inflammation, and bile duct proliferation (75). The observed protective effects of GW4064 suggest that FXR agonists may be helpful in treating cholestatic diseases (75).

However, another group found that FXR KO mice were protected from obstructive cholestasis achieved through BDL (76). In FXR KO mice after BDL, mortality and liver injury were reduced as serum bilirubin was not significantly elevated (76). FXR KO mice had reduced serum total BA concentrations and had a marked induction of the basolateral transporter multidrug resistance-associated protein 4 (*Mrp4*), suggesting that these animals had a greater capacity to export BAs back into circulation and reduce hepatoxicity (76). This study supports the potential clinical use of FXR antagonists in the treatment of obstructive cholestatic diseases (76).

Looking further into the role of FXR during intrahepatic cholestasis, ANIT-induced injury was utilized in wild-type (WT), FXR KO, and PXR KO mice (77). Serum ALT, alkaline phosphatase (ALP), and bilirubin were elevated in all genotypes after ANIT administration, with the highest ALP levels seen in FXR KO mice (77). ANIT-treated FXR KO mice had higher concentrations of serum and liver unconjugated BAs across all genotypes (77). While ANIT treatment induced the messenger RNA (mRNA) expressions of *Mdr2*, *Bsep*, and ATPase, class I, type 8B and member 1 *(Atp8b1)* in WT and PXR KO mice, no upregulation was observed in FXR KOs (77). It was concluded that FXR deficiency, not PXR deficiency, was responsible for the increased susceptibility to injury in the ANIT-induced intrahepatic cholestasis model due to the reduction of hepatobiliary efflux transporters and the accumulation of unconjugated BAs (77). Furthermore, pretreatment of the FXR agonist GW4064 was also investigated in ANIT-treated WT mice (77). GW4064 treatment was shown to be protective as it reduced necrosis compared to ANIT treatment alone (77). This reproduces what Liu et al. had found in BDL and ANIT-induced injury in rats and further supports FXR as a therapeutic target for intrahepatic cholestasis (77).

Through the use of reversible BDL (rBDL) in the rat to model cholestasis, FXR activation by OCA worsened the biliary injury, shown by a considerable increase in ALT and ALP compared to the controls (78). OCA treatment in rBDL rats upregulated *Bsep*, multidrug resistance-associated protein 3 (*Mrp3*), *Mrp4*, and Ostβ transporters (78). The 8-fold induction of the FXR target gene *Bsep* was suggested to be the cause of biliary injury as BAs would be pumped *via* BSEP into an already obstructed biliary tree (78).

Cholangiocytes

Cholangiocytes are epithelial cells which line the bile ducts of the biliary tree (79). Through absorptive and secretory transport systems in cholangiocytes, bile is modified to become more fluid and alkaline (80). Bile then enters the gallbladder for concentration and storage or delivered to the intestinal lumen (80). Cholangiocytes have also been shown to be actively involved in bile homeostasis (81). Compared to hepatocytes, cholangiocytes have no or low expressions of *Cyp7a1* and *Cyp8b1*, but considerable expression of *Cyp27a1*, suggesting that cholangiocytes are involved in cholesterol metabolism (81). Measurement of the mRNA levels revealed that Fgf15 was expressed at higher levels in cholangiocytes compared to hepatocytes, while the fibroblast growth factor receptor 4 (Fgfr4) expression was lower (81). As FXR is known to regulate Fgf15/FGF19 levels, investigation of a similar regulation in cholangiocytes was achieved through treatment of rat cholangiocytes with CDCA and the FXR agonist GW4064, with both treatments inducing the expression of Fgf15 (81). Additionally, cultured human cholangiocytes treated with CDCA induced the secretion of FGF19 in the medium (81). FGF15/19-mediated repression of *Cyp27a1* in cholangiocytes was found to differ from hepatocytes and is mediated through p38 kinase (81). Ultimately, understanding BA metabolism in cholangiocytes may help provide therapeutic pathways for cholangiopathy treatments (81).

One of the most common biliary complications after liver transplantation (LT) is non-anastomotic strictures that develop after biliary epithelial damage and can result from BA toxicity (82). To investigate the mechanism of cholangiocyte BA transport following LT, a rat LT model was utilized. After transplantation, a prolonged biliary transport time of BAs was observed, while the expression of FXR was dramatically decreased and was related to cold ischemic time of the donor liver. Furthermore, *in vitro*-cultured human biliary epithelial cells under hypoxic conditions exhibited a repression of FXR expression and DNA binding activities (82). Hypoxic conditions also altered the expressions of BA transporters as hypoxia slightly induced Asbt expression and repressed both Ostα and Ostβ (82). This led to the intracellular accumulation of BAs, increased cell apoptosis, and increased expression of profibrotic factors in cholangiocytes (82). It was concluded that, after LT, repression of FXR under ischemic/hypoxic conditions led to the disruption of BA transport of cholangiocytes and, thus, biliary damage (82).

FIBROBLAST GROWTH FACTORS 15/19

Fibroblast growth factors (FGFs) make up a family of at least 22 proteins that regulate various biological processes including growth, development, and differentiation (83, 84). FGF15 and its human ortholog FGF19 belong to the subfamily of endocrine FGFs that act as hormones due to their low or no affinity for heparin sulfate, which allows them to enter systemic circulation (84, 85). FGF19 was originally identified in the fetal brain during a screen for novel FGFs (86). Although FGF15 and FGF19 are orthologs, they interestingly only share ~50% amino acid identity

(86). For high-affinity receptor binding, the endocrine FGFs require klotho proteins that interact with fibroblast growth factor receptors (FGFRs) (87). β-Klotho specifically binds to FGF15/19 which has high affinity for fibroblast growth factor receptor 4 (FGFR4) and less for fibroblast growth factor receptor 1 (FGFR1) that are highly expressed in hepatocytes and white adipose tissue (WAT), respectively (88, 89). Low levels of FGFR4 expression are also detected in other cell types, including HSCs, macrophages, and some central neurons (90). FGF15/19 is expressed in ileal enterocytes, where it is strongly induced by FXR activation (84). Once released into blood circulation, FGF15/19 acts on the liver to repress BA synthesis, as described above.

However, mouse FGFR4 does not recognized human FGF19 (91). Therefore, when using high dosage of FGF19 in mice, the observed effects may be due to the activation of FGFR1 or other FGFRs, but not FGFR4 by FGF19.

Role in Energy Expenditure

To investigate the role of FGF19 in physiological homeostasis, transgenic mice expressing human *FGF19* were utilized (92). *FGF19* transgenic mice had a significant reduction in fat mass arising from an increase in energy expenditure (92). When fed a high-fat diet, *FGF19* transgenic mice did not become obese or diabetic (92). The results suggest two mechanisms by which FGF19 may increase energy expenditure through an increase in brown adipose tissue (BAT) and through a decrease in liver enzyme acetyl CoA carboxylase 2 (ACC2) (92). Reduction in ACC2, the rate-limiting enzyme for fatty acid entry into the mitochondria, also resulted in reduced liver triglyceride levels (92). In an additional study, FGF19 increased the metabolic rate in mice fed a high-fat diet while reducing body weight and diabetes in leptin-deficient mice (93). FGF19 also acts in the central nervous system to improve insulin sensitivity by reducing hypothalamic agouti-related peptide (AGRP)/neuropeptide Y (NPY) neuron activity (94). In summary, FGF15/19 increases insulin sensitivity, thermogenesis, and weight loss and decreases serum cholesterol and triglyceride levels.

Protein and Glycogen Synthesis

FGF15/19 also regulates hepatic protein and glycogen synthesis (95). *Fgf15* KO mice were shown to be glucose-intolerant and store half as much hepatic glycogen compared to control wild-type mice (95). In diabetic mice lacking insulin, FGF19 treatment restored the hepatic glycogen concentrations to normal levels, indicating that FGF19 activates an insulin-independent pathway to regulate glycogen metabolism (95). It was determined that FGF15/19 uses a RAS/extracellular signal-regulated protein kinase (ERK)/p90RSK pathway to induce hepatic glycogen and protein synthesis *in vivo* (95). FGF19 also shows a positive effect on muscle weight, revealed by a study showing that FGF19 stimulates the phosphorylation of the ERK1/2 and the ribosomal protein S6 kinase (S6K1), an mTOR-dependent master regulator of muscle cell growth (96).

Gluconeogenesis

Energy homeostasis is additionally regulated through FGF15/19 repressing gluconeogenesis, like insulin (97). While insulin peaks in serum 15 min after feeding, FGF15/19 peaks ~45 min later due to the increase of BAs in the small intestine (97). *In vivo*, FGF15/19 blocks the expression of gluconeogenesis genes through the dephosphorylation and inactivation of the transcription factor cAMP regulatory element-binding protein (CREB) (97). This then inhibits the expression of peroxisome proliferator-activated receptor-γ coactivator-1α (PGC-1α) and other downstream hepatic metabolism genes (97).

Fatty Acid Synthesis

Lastly, FGF19 inhibits hepatic fatty acid synthesis. Primary hepatocytes incubated with recombinant FGF19 protein in the presence or absence of insulin showed that FGF19 suppressed the insulin-dependent stimulation of fatty acid synthesis (98). Similar to the SHP-mediated suppression of sterol regulatory element-binding protein 1c (SREBP1c) following FXR activation, FGF19 was shown to decrease SREBP1c through increasing the signal transducer and activator of transcription 3 (STAT3) and decreasing the peroxisome proliferator-activated receptor-γ coactivator-1β (PGC-1β), while also increasing the expression of SHP (98). This favorable inhibition of hepatic fatty acid synthesis, along with the promotion of protein and glycogen synthesis and the repression of gluconeogenesis, supports the beneficial effects of FGF15/19 on metabolic syndrome and warrants further investigation of FGF15/19 in the prevention and treatment of NASH. Indeed, modified FGF19 has been shown to be beneficial in mouse models of NASH and cholestasis (99, 100).

FXR AS DRUG TARGETS—FXR AGONISTS

There are many FXR modulators that have undergone clinical trials for the treatment of chronic liver diseases. The focus for most of these trials is the efficacy of FXR activation on cholestasis, NASH, and obesity; however, there are some studies focused on minor indications, including bile acid diarrhea or association with reactivation of latent pro-virus (clinical trials.gov). Currently, two types of FXR agonists—steroidal represented by OCA *vs.* non-steroidal represented by tropifexor—are front-runners for obtaining U.S. Food and Drug Administration (FDA) approval for the treatment of NASH.

The first FDA-approved FXR agonist for the treatment of PBC is OCA, which is a steroidal FXR agonist modified from CDCA (101). When compared to CDCA, OCA was shown to be ~100 times more potent (101). In a model of cholestasis, male Wistar rats were administered LCA through an intravenous infusion to impair bile flow. Administration of OCA alone did not induce cholestasis, while co-infusion of LCA and OCA fully reversed bile flow impairment and protected hepatocytes from necrosis (101). This initial study confirmed OCA as a selective, potent FXR agonist and warranted further investigation of additional therapeutic uses.

The traditional first-line treatment for PBC is ursodeoxycholic acid (UDCA) as it has been shown to improve liver tests and transplant-free survival with minimal side effects (102). However, not all patients respond to UDCA (102). In a randomized, double-blinded, 12-week, phase II clinical trial, the efficacy of OCA in PBC patients who did not respond favorably to

UDCA was evaluated (103). Patients ($n = 165$) were randomly assigned to receive 10, 25, or 50 mg of OCA or placebo once daily in addition to an existing dose of UDCA (103). The primary endpoint was level change of ALP from baseline until the conclusion of the study (103). All three doses significantly reduced the levels of ALP, γ-glutamyltransferase (GGT), and ALT compared to placebo. However, pruritus was reported in all groups, with severity correlating to the dose of OCA (103). Based on the efficacy and tolerability, the once daily dose of 10 mg OCA was determined to be the most effective (103).

In the randomized, double-blinded, phase III POISE trial, 217 PBC patients who had an inadequate response to UDCA were assigned to receive 10 mg OCA, 5–10 mg OCA, or placebo once daily for 12 months (104). Patients still received UCDA as a background therapy (104). The primary endpoint was a reduction in ALP from baseline and a normal total bilirubin level, which was reached in more patients in both OCA groups compared to placebo (104). As seen previously in the phase II trial, an OCA dose-dependent increase in the incidence of pruritus was reported (104). Based on the favorable effects of OCA on important biochemical markers, the FDA approved OCA for the treatment of PBC patients with an inadequate response of intolerance to UDCA in 2016 (105).

Another phase II study investigated OCA as a monotherapy in PBC patients (106). Patients received 10 mg OCA, 50 mg OCA, or placebo once daily for 3 months and then followed up for up to 6 years (106). OCA treatment as a monotherapy significantly improved ALP and other biochemical markers associated with improved clinical outcomes (106). However, severe pruritus was reported in almost all patients who received 50 mg OCA (106). Compared to UDCA co-therapy, no additional benefits for OCA as a monotherapy were reported (107).

A multiyear study (COBALT) to determine the effects of OCA in PBC patients with more advanced liver disease is ongoing (104). In 2017, after 11 cases of serious liver injury and 19 cases of death associated with OCA were reported, the FDA released a black box warning for the use of OCA in patients with decompensated cirrhosis (105). Many of the cases of increased liver injury appeared to be due to inappropriate high dosing of OCA (105).

Due to arising side effects including pruritus and increased risk of liver decompensation in cirrhotic PBC patients administered OCA, a study to determine whether OCA worsened liver injury under cholestatic conditions was carried out (108). BDL and ANIT treatment were studied in rats (108). In both models, OCA treatment exacerbated liver injury in a dose-dependent manner and downregulated the expression of basolateral transporters (108). The non-steroidal FXR agonist GW4064 was also tested in the ANIT cholestasis model. In contrast, GW4064 administration decreased the severity of cholestatic injury compared to OCA and reduced AST, ALT, GGT, and bilirubin (108). This is again consistent with the results published by Liu *et al.* (75) and suggests that the safety of FXR agonists is impacted by their pharmacokinetic properties (108). OCA, as a semi-synthetic derivative of CDCA, has a high rate of intestinal absorption, which allows it to recirculate like endogenous BAs (108). While synthetic GW4064 undergoes taurine conjugation in the liver which is then not recognized by intestinal transporters thus reducing its bioavailability (108). Under cholestatic conditions, OCA accumulates in the liver where it may reach toxic concentrations (108, 109). In mice, genetic KO of FXR or inhibition of FXR both resulted in protection from injury induced by OCA in an ANIT model of cholestasis (108). After RNAseq analysis, FXR antagonism was shown to reverse the transcription of over 2,000 genes, including V-Maf avian musculoaponeurotic fibrosarcoma oncogene homolog G (Mafg) and its partner nuclear factor erythroid 2-related factor 2 (Nrf2) (108). Mafg expression has been shown to be induced in cholestatic diseases and represses genes involved in the synthesis of antioxidant glutathione (110, 111). The modulation of these transcription factors was then investigated. Pharmacologic or genetic inhibition of Mafg prevented damage caused by ANIT and OCA, while Nrf2 induction was protective. These results support that the negative side effects of OCA treatment are FXR-mediated (108).

There is currently no approved treatment for PSC, and the efficacy of UDCA for PSC remains uncertain (112). Thus, the efficacy and safety of OCA in PSC patients were assessed in a phase II randomized, double-blind, placebo-controlled, dose-finding study (113). Patients ($n = 76$) were assigned to receive 1.5–3.0 mg OCA, 5–10 mg OCA, or placebo once daily for 24 weeks (113). At 24 weeks, treatment with 5–10 mg OCA significantly reduced serum ALP compared to placebo (113). Dose-related pruritus was reported as the most common side effect, consistent with the earlier clinical studies (113).

The safety and efficacy of the non-steroidal FXR agonist cilofexor (GS-9674) were evaluated in a phase II double-blinded, placebo-controlled study in PSC patients (114). Randomized patients received 100 mg cilofexor, 30 mg cilofexor, or placebo once daily for 12 weeks (114). Treatment with cilofexor was generally well-tolerated, safe, and improved the biochemical markers of cholestasis and inflammation (114). Significant dose-dependent reductions in serum ALP, GGT, ALT, and AST with cilofexor compared to placebo were reported (114). The effect of cilofexor on ALP was independent of UDCA use, and adverse events were similar between treatment groups (114).

Cilofexor was also evaluated in a double-blind, placebo-controlled, phase II trial in patients with NASH (115). Non-cirrhotic patients ($n = 140$) were randomized to receive 100 mg cilofexor, 50 mg cilofexor, or placebo once daily for 24 weeks (115). Cilofexor was safe and significantly improved hepatic steatosis, liver biochemistry (e.g., GGT), and bile acids (115). Compared to OCA treatment that resulted in increases in serum LDL-C and total cholesterol, cilofexor treatment had no significant effects on serum lipids (115). Moderate to severe pruritus was reported in 14% of the 100-mg cilofexor group and 4% of the 30-mg group (115). In contrast, 23% of the OCA-treated patients reported pruritus (116). However, cilofexor treatment only had modest beneficial effects on liver biochemistry compared to OCA treatment, indication of a potential limitation for efficacy (115).

To evaluate the effect of FXR activation by OCA on insulin resistance and liver lipid metabolism, Zucker (*fa*/*fa*) rats that contain a loss-of-function mutation in the hunger hormone leptin receptor were utilized (117). This mutation leads to hyperphagia and hyperleptinemia, resulting in diabetes, insulin resistance, obesity, and liver steatosis; therefore, Zucker (*fa/fa*) rats are considered a non-alcoholic fatty liver disease (NAFLD) model (117). Daily OCA treatment (10 mg/kg) over 7 weeks reversed insulin resistance and prevented body weight gain and liver fat deposition (117). Moreover, OCA treatment reduced blood triglyceride and plasma aminotransferases and improved liver histopathology (117). Reversal of insulin resistance after the administration of OCA is further supported by *in vitro* data showing that OCA significantly increases insulin secretion in mouse β-TC6 cells and human pancreatic islets (118). Additionally, OCA activation of FXR in mouse β-TC6 cells leads to AKT (protein kinase B)-dependent translocation of glucose transporter 2 (GLUT2), thus increasing the glucose uptake by these cells (118). Taken together, OCA activation of FXR improves hyperglycemia through enhanced insulin secretion and glucose uptake by the liver (118).

OCA has also been shown to exhibit anti-inflammatory and anti-fibrotic properties. While investigating the NF-κB signaling pathway, a key inflammation pathway, pretreatment of HepG2 cells with OCA (3 μM) inhibited the expression of the cytokine-inducible enzymes COX-2 and iNOS after stimulation with LPS or tumor necrosis factor alpha (TNFα) (67). Inhibition of iNOS by OCA was also confirmed in LPS-treated primary mouse hepatocytes (67).

After animal studies showed that OCA decreased insulin resistance and hepatic steatosis, the efficacy and safety of OCA were first evaluated in a phase IIa study in patients with type II diabetes and non-alcoholic fatty liver disease (119). The participants were randomly assigned to placebo ($n = 23$), 25 mg OCA ($n = 20$), or 50 mg OCA ($n = 21$) groups for the 6-week treatment period (119). Both OCA groups exhibited reduced GGT and ALT levels along with decreased bodyweight (119). Furthermore, treatment of OCA led to improved insulin sensitivity and elevated FGF19 serum levels. This, in conjunction with the decreased BA precursor C4 and endogenous BAs, again confirmed OCA's FXR agonist activity (119).

Based on previous favorable results, OCA was further investigated in the phase IIb Farnesoid X Receptor Ligand Obeticholic Acid in NASH Treatment (FLINT) trial (116). In this multicenter, double-blind, randomized clinical trial, patients with non-cirrhotic NASH were assigned to receive 25 mg OCA ($n = 141$) daily or placebo ($n = 142$) for 72 weeks (116). OCA treatment was shown to improve the biochemical and histological features of NASH when compared with placebo; specifically, 45% of OCA patients improved their NAFLD activity score by two points or greater without worsening of fibrosis compared to the 21% improvement in placebo patients (116). However, there was no significant difference in the histological resolution of NASH between the OCA-treated and placebo groups (120). Adverse outcomes of pruritus and unfavorable dyslipidemia manifested in the OCA treatment group (116). Additionally, the favorable effects on ALP, lipids, and blood glucose seen in the placebo group associated with weight loss were absent or reversed in the OCA-treated patients (120).

Currently, OCA is being evaluated by Intercept in a phase III trial REGENERATE (121). To assess OCA's effect on liver histology and clinical outcomes, 2,065 biopsy-confirmed NASH patients were randomized into a 10-mg OCA, 25-mg OCA, or placebo group (121). Total study duration is estimated to be 6 years, with interim biopsies performed after the first 18 months to evaluate improvement of fibrosis stage and resolution of NASH with no worsening fibrosis (121). Although OCA was recently approved by the FDA for treating PBC, the current American Association of the Study of Liver Diseases guidelines do not recommend the off-label treatment of OCA in NASH patients until further safety and efficacy data are available (122). In February 2019, Intercept announced that OCA achieved the primary endpoint of improving liver fibrosis without worsening of NASH after 18 months ($p = 0.0002$). This marks the first and largest successful phase 3 study in fibrosis patients due to NASH. Intercept filed a New Drug Application (NDA) with the FDA in September 2019. As of June 2020, the FDA issued a complete response letter stating that the predicted benefit of OCA did not outweigh the potential risks in patients with fibrosis due to NASH and that long-term outcome needs to be evaluated (123). Thus, accelerated approval was not granted at this time.

Tropifexor is a representative of non-steroidal FXR agonists. In mouse models of NASH, tropifexor significantly reduced oxidative stress, steatosis, inflammation, and fibrosis (124). It will be very interesting to see whether, as a non-steroidal FXR agonist, tropifexor will present similar adverse effect to the steroidal FXR agonists.

CONCLUSION

As a key regulator of BA homeostasis, FXR activation suppresses BA synthesis mainly through the induction of FGF15/19 in the gut and promotes enterohepatic BA circulation. FXR agonism also regulates lipid metabolism, reduces hepatic gluconeogenesis and glycolysis, and increases glycogen synthesis while playing an anti-inflammatory role during liver injury. FGF15/19 favorably increases energy expenditure and glycogen synthesis while decreasing gluconeogenesis and fatty acid synthesis. While FXR and FGF19 have been considered promising targets for the treatment of cholestasis and NASH, the molecular mechanism by which these two factors regulate liver BA transport, steatosis, and inflammation needs to be further determined, and most importantly, an individualized treatment plan is paramount to develop drugs and treatment strategy with better efficacy and less toxic effects.

AUTHOR CONTRIBUTIONS

MS and GG have contributed to the writing and editing of the manuscript. All authors contributed to the article and approved the submitted version.

ACKNOWLEDGMENTS

We appreciate Dr. Justin D Schumacher for his suggestions and careful review of the manuscript.

REFERENCES

1. Bloch K, Berg BN, Rittenberg D. The biological conversion of cholesterol to cholic acid. *J Biol Chem*. (1943) 149:511–7.
2. Danielsson H, Sjovall J. Bile acid metabolism. *Annu Rev Biochem*. (1975) 44:233–53. doi: 10.1146/annurev.bi.44.070175.001313
3. Myant NB, Mitropoulos KA. Cholesterol 7 alpha-hydroxylase. *J Lipid Res*. (1977) 18:135–53.
4. Ishibashi S, Schwarz M, Frykman PK, Herz J, Russell DW. Disruption of cholesterol 7alpha-hydroxylase gene in mice. I. Postnatal lethality reversed by bile acid and vitamin supplementation. *J Biol Chem*. (1996) 271:18017–23. doi: 10.1074/jbc.271.30.18017
5. Russell DW, Setchell KD. Bile acid biosynthesis. *Biochemistry*. (1992) 31:4737–49. doi: 10.1021/bi00135a001
6. Chiang JY. Regulation of bile acid synthesis: pathways, nuclear receptors, and mechanisms. *J Hepatol*. (2004) 40:539–51. doi: 10.1016/j.jhep.2003.11.006
7. Li-Hawkins J, Gafvels M, Olin M, Lund EG, Andersson U, Schuster G, et al. Cholic acid mediates negative feedback regulation of bile acid synthesis in mice. *J Clin Invest*. (2002) 110:1191–200. doi: 10.1172/JCI02 16309
8. Axelson M, Aly A, Sjovall J. Levels of 7 alpha-hydroxy-4-cholesten-3-one in plasma reflect rates of bile acid synthesis in man. *FEBS Lett*. (1988) 239:324–8. doi: 10.1016/0014-5793(88)80944-X
9. Li T, Chiang JY. Bile acid signaling in metabolic disease and drug therapy. *Pharmacol Rev*. (2014) 66:948–83. doi: 10.1124/pr.113.008201
10. Takahashi S, Fukami T, Masuo Y, Brocker CN, Xie C, Krausz KW, et al. Cyp2c70 is responsible for the species difference in bile acid metabolism between mice and humans. *J Lipid Res*. (2016) 57:2130–7. doi: 10.1194/jlr.M071183
11. de Boer JF, Verkade E, Mulder NL, de Vries HD, Huijkman N, Koehorst M, et al. A human-like bile acid pool induced by deletion of hepatic Cyp2c70 modulates effects of FXR activation in mice. *J Lipid Res*. (2020) 61:291–305. doi: 10.1194/jlr.RA119000243
12. Honda A, Miyazaki T, Iwamoto J, Hirayama T, Morishita Y, Monma T, et al. Regulation of bile acid metabolism in mouse models with hydrophobic bile acid composition. *J Lipid Res*. (2020) 61:54–69. doi: 10.1194/jlr.RA1190 00395
13. Russell DW. The enzymes, regulation, and genetics of bile acid synthesis. *Annu Rev Biochem*. (2003) 72:137–74. doi: 10.1146/annurev.biochem.72.121801.161712
14. Johnson MR, Barnes S, Kwakye JB, Diasio RB. Purification and characterization of bile acid-CoA:amino acid N-acyltransferase from human liver. *J Biol Chem*. (1991) 266:10227–33.
15. Killenberg PG, Jordan JT. Purification and characterization of bile acid-CoA:amino acid N-acyltransferase from rat liver. *J Biol Chem*. (1978) 253:1005–10.
16. Trauner M, Boyer JL. Bile salt transporters: molecular characterization, function, and regulation. *Physiol Rev*. (2003) 83:633–71. doi: 10.1152/physrev.00027.2002
17. Konig J, Nies AT, Cui Y, Leier I, Keppler D. Conjugate export pumps of the multidrug resistance protein (MRP) family: localization, substrate specificity, and MRP2-mediated drug resistance. *Biochim Biophys Acta*. (1999) 1461:377–94. doi: 10.1016/S0005-2736(99)00169-8
18. Lam P, Wang R, Ling V. Bile acid transport in sister of P-glycoprotein (ABCB11) knockout mice. *Biochemistry*. (2005) 44:12598–605. doi: 10.1021/bi050943e
19. Strautnieks SS, Bull LN, Knisely AS, Kocoshis SA, Dahl N, Arnell H, et al. A gene encoding a liver-specific ABC transporter is mutated in progressive familial intrahepatic cholestasis. *Nat Genet*. (1998) 20:233–8. doi: 10.1038/3034
20. Imagawa K, Takayama K, Isoyama S, Tanikawa K, Shinkai M, Harada K, et al. Generation of a bile salt export pump deficiency model using patient-specific induced pluripotent stem cell-derived hepatocyte-like cells. *Sci Rep*. (2017) 7:41806. doi: 10.1038/srep41806
21. Li J, Dawson PA. Animal models to study bile acid metabolism. *Biochim Biophys Acta Mol Basis Dis*. (2019) 1865:895–911. doi: 10.1016/j.bbadis.2018.05.011
22. Wong MH, Oelkers P, Craddock AL, Dawson PA. Expression cloning and characterization of the hamster ileal sodium-dependent bile acid transporter. *J Biol Chem*. (1994) 269:1340–7.
23. Gong YZ, Everett ET, Schwartz DA, Norris JS, Wilson FA. Molecular cloning, tissue distribution, and expression of a 14-kDa bile acid-binding protein from rat ileal cytosol. *Proc Natl Acad Sci USA*. (1994) 91:4741–5. doi: 10.1073/pnas.91.11.4741
24. Dawson PA, Hubbert M, Haywood J, Craddock AL, Zerangue N, Christian WV, et al. The heteromeric organic solute transporter alpha-beta, ost alpha-ost beta, is an ileal basolateral bile acid transporter. *J Biol Chem*. (2005) 280:6960–8. doi: 10.1074/jbc.M412752200
25. Hagenbuch B, Meier PJ. Molecular cloning, chromosomal localization, and functional characterization of a human liver Na+/bile acid cotransporter. *J Clin Invest*. (1994) 93:1326–31. doi: 10.1172/JCI117091
26. Smit JJ, Schinkel AH, Oude Elferink RP, Groen AK, Wagenaar E, van Deemter L, et al. Homozygous disruption of the murine mdr2 P-glycoprotein gene leads to a complete absence of phospholipid from bile and to liver disease. *Cell*. (1993) 75:451–62. doi: 10.1016/0092-8674(93)90380-9
27. Oude Elferink RP, Ottenhoff R, van Wijland M, Smit JJ, Schinkel AH, Groen AK. Regulation of biliary lipid secretion by mdr2 P-glycoprotein in the mouse. *J Clin Invest*. (1995) 95:31–8. doi: 10.1172/JCI117658
28. Vree JML, de Jacquemin E, Sturm E, Cresteil D, Bosma PJ, Aten J, et al. Mutations in the MDR3 gene cause progressive familial intrahepatic cholestasis. *Proc Natl Acad Sci USA*. (1998) 95:282–7. doi: 10.1073/pnas.95.1.282
29. Trauner M, Fickert P, Wagner M. MDR3 (ABCB4) defects: a paradigm for the genetics of adult cholestatic syndromes. *Semin Liver Dis*. (2007) 27:077–98. doi: 10.1055/s-2006-960172
30. Popov Y, Patsenker E, Fickert P, Trauner M, Schuppan D. Mdr2 (Abcb4)-/- mice spontaneously develop severe biliary fibrosis via massive dysregulation of pro- and antifibrogenic genes. *J Hepatol*. (2005) 43:1045–54. doi: 10.1016/j.jhep.2005.06.025
31. Ikenaga N, Liu SB, Sverdlov DY, Yoshida S, Nasser I, Ke Q, et al. A new Mdr2–/– mouse model of sclerosing cholangitis with rapid fibrosis progression, early-onset portal hypertension, and liver cancer. *Am J Pathol*. (2015) 185:325–34. doi: 10.1016/j.ajpath.2014.10.013
32. Ridlon JM, Kang DJ, Hylemon PB. Bile salt biotransformations by human intestinal bacteria. *J Lipid Res*. (2006) 47:241–59. doi: 10.1194/jlr.R500013-JLR200
33. Dowling RH. The enterohepatic circulation of bile acids as they relate to lipid disorders. *J Clin Pathol Suppl Assoc Clin Pathol*. (1973) 5:59–67. doi: 10.1136/jcp.s1-5.1.59
34. Guo GL, Lambert G, Negishi M, Ward JM, Brewer HBJr, Kliewer SA, et al. Complementary roles of farnesoid X receptor, pregnane X receptor, and constitutive androstane receptor in protection against bile acid toxicity. *J Biol Chem*. (2003) 278:45062–71. doi: 10.1074/jbc.M307145200
35. Maruyama T, Miyamoto Y, Nakamura T, Tamai Y, Okada H, Sugiyama E, et al. Identification of membrane-type receptor for bile acids (M-BAR). *Biochem Biophys Res Commun*. (2002) 298:714–9. doi: 10.1016/S0006-291X(02)02550-0
36. Liu R, Zhao R, Zhou X, Liang X, Campbell DJ, Zhang X, et al. Conjugated bile acids promote cholangiocarcinoma cell invasive growth through activation of sphingosine 1-phosphate receptor 2. *Hepatology*. (2014) 60:908–18. doi: 10.1002/hep.27085

37. Chawla A, Repa JJ, Evans RM, Mangelsdorf DJ. Nuclear receptors and lipid physiology: opening the X-files. *Science.* (2001) 294:1866–70. doi: 10.1126/science.294.5548.1866
38. Edwards PA, Kast HR, Anisfeld AM. BAREing it all: the adoption of LXR and FXR and their roles in lipid homeostasis. *J Lipid Res.* (2002) 43: 2–12.
39. Lu TT, Makishima M, Repa JJ, Schoonjans K, Kerr TA, Auwerx J, et al. Molecular basis for feedback regulation of bile acid synthesis by nuclear receptors. *Mol Cell.* (2000) 6:507–15. doi: 10.1016/S1097-2765(00)00050-2
40. Parks DJ, Blanchard SG, Bledsoe RK, Chandra G, Consler TG, Kliewer SA, et al. Bile acids: natural ligands for an orphan nuclear receptor. *Science.* (1999) 284:1365–8. doi: 10.1126/science.284.5418.1365
41. Wang H, Chen J, Hollister K, Sowers LC, Forman BM. Endogenous bile acids are ligands for the nuclear receptor FXR/BAR. *Mol Cell.* (1999) 3:543–53. doi: 10.1016/S1097-2765(00)80348-2
42. Makishima M, Okamoto AY, Repa JJ, Tu H, Learned RM, Luk A, et al. Identification of a nuclear receptor for bile acids. *Science.* (1999) 284:1362–5. doi: 10.1126/science.284.5418.1362
43. Thomas AM, Hart SN, Kong B, Fang J, Zhong XB, Guo GL. Genome-wide tissue-specific farnesoid X receptor binding in mouse liver and intestine. *Hepatology.* (2010) 51:1410–9. doi: 10.1002/hep.23450
44. Kim I, Ahn SH, Inagaki T, Choi M, Ito S, Guo GL, et al. Differential regulation of bile acid homeostasis by the farnesoid X receptor in liver and intestine. *J Lipid Res.* (2007) 48:2664–72. doi: 10.1194/jlr.M700330-JLR200
45. Inagaki T, Choi M, Moschetta A, Peng L, Cummins CL, McDonald JG, et al. Fibroblast growth factor 15 functions as an enterohepatic signal to regulate bile acid homeostasis. *Cell Metab.* (2005) 2:217–25. doi: 10.1016/j.cmet.2005.09.001
46. Kong B, Wang L, Chiang JY, Zhang Y, Klaassen CD, Guo GL. Mechanism of tissue-specific farnesoid X receptor in suppressing the expression of genes in bile-acid synthesis in mice. *Hepatology.* (2012) 56:1034–43. doi: 10.1002/hep.25740
47. Goodwin B, Jones SA, Price RR, Watson MA, McKee DD, Moore LB, et al. A regulatory cascade of the nuclear receptors FXR, SHP-1, and LRH-1 represses bile acid biosynthesis. *Mol Cell.* (2000) 6:517–26. doi: 10.1016/S1097-2765(00)00051-4
48. Plass JR, Mol O, Heegsma J, Geuken M, Faber KN, Jansen PL, et al. Farnesoid X receptor and bile salts are involved in transcriptional regulation of the gene encoding the human bile salt export pump. *Hepatology.* (2002) 35:589–96. doi: 10.1053/jhep.2002.31724
49. Landrier JF, Eloranta JJ, Vavricka SR, Kullak-Ublick GA. The nuclear receptor for bile acids, FXR, transactivates human organic solute transporter-alpha and -beta genes. *Am J Physiol Gastrointest Liver Physiol.* (2006) 290:G476–85. doi: 10.1152/ajpgi.00430.2005
50. Zollner G, Wagner M, Moustafa T, Fickert P, Silbert D, Gumhold J, et al. Coordinated induction of bile acid detoxification and alternative elimination in mice: role of FXR-regulated organic solute transporter-alpha/beta in the adaptive response to bile acids. *Am J Physiol Gastrointest Liver Physiol.* (2006) 290:G923–32. doi: 10.1152/ajpgi.00490.2005
51. Denson LA, Sturm E, Echevarria W, Zimmerman TL, Makishima M, Mangelsdorf DJ, et al. The orphan nuclear receptor, shp, mediates bile acid-induced inhibition of the rat bile acid transporter, ntcp. *Gastroenterology.* (2001) 121:140–7. doi: 10.1053/gast.2001.25503
52. Chen F, Ma L, Dawson PA, Sinal CJ, Sehayek E, Gonzalez FJ, et al. Liver receptor homologue-1 mediates species- and cell line-specific bile acid-dependent negative feedback regulation of the apical sodium-dependent bile acid transporter. *J Biol Chem.* (2003) 278:19909–16. doi: 10.1074/jbc.M207903200
53. Wang L, Lee Y-K, Bundman D, Han Y, Thevananther S, Kim CS, et al. Redundant pathways for negative feedback regulation of bile acid production. *Dev Cell.* (2002) 2:721–31. doi: 10.1016/S1534-5807(02)00187-9
54. Watanabe M, Houten SM, Wang L, Moschetta A, Mangelsdorf DJ, Heyman RA, et al. Bile acids lower triglyceride levels via a pathway involving FXR, SHP, and SREBP-1c. *J Clin Invest.* (2004) 113:1408–18. doi: 10.1172/JCI21025
55. Schoenfield LJ, Lachin JM. Chenodiol (chenodeoxycholic acid) for dissolution of gallstones: the National Cooperative Gallstone Study. A controlled trial of efficacy and safety. *Ann Intern Med.* (1981) 95:257–82. doi: 10.7326/0003-4819-95-3-257
56. Prieur X, Coste H, Rodriguez JC. The human apolipoprotein AV gene is regulated by peroxisome proliferator-activated receptor-alpha and contains a novel farnesoid X-activated receptor response element. *J Biol Chem.* (2003) 278:25468–80. doi: 10.1074/jbc.M301302200
57. Kast HR, Nguyen CM, Sinal CJ, Jones SA, Laffitte BA, Reue K, et al. Farnesoid X-activated receptor induces apolipoprotein C-II transcription: a molecular mechanism linking plasma triglyceride levels to bile acids. *Mol Endocrinol.* (2001) 15:1720–8. doi: 10.1210/mend.15.10.0712
58. Claudel T, Inoue Y, Barbier O, Duran-Sandoval D, Kosykh V, Fruchart J, et al. Farnesoid X receptor agonists suppress hepatic apolipoprotein CIII expression. *Gastroenterology.* (2003) 125:544–55. doi: 10.1016/S0016-5085(03)00896-5
59. Sirvent A, Claudel T, Martin G, Brozek J, Kosykh V, Darteil R, et al. The farnesoid X receptor induces very low density lipoprotein receptor gene expression. *FEBS Lett.* (2004) 566:173–7. doi: 10.1016/j.febslet.2004.04.026
60. Pineda Torra I, Claudel T, Duval C, Kosykh V, Fruchart JC, Staels B. Bile acids induce the expression of the human peroxisome proliferator-activated receptor alpha gene via activation of the farnesoid X receptor. *Mol Endocrinol.* (2003) 17:259–72. doi: 10.1210/me.2002-0120
61. Jiao Y, Lu Y, Li XY. Farnesoid X receptor: a master regulator of hepatic triglyceride and glucose homeostasis. *Acta Pharmacol Sin.* (2015) 36:44–50. doi: 10.1038/aps.2014.116
62. Yamagata K, Daitoku H, Shimamoto Y, Matsuzaki H, Hirota K, Ishida J, et al. Bile acids regulate gluconeogenic gene expression via small heterodimer partner-mediated repression of hepatocyte nuclear factor 4 and Foxo1. *J Biol Chem.* (2004) 279:23158–65. doi: 10.1074/jbc.M314322200
63. Stayrook KR, Bramlett KS, Savkur RS, Ficorilli J, Cook T, Christe ME, et al. Regulation of carbohydrate metabolism by the farnesoid X receptor. *Endocrinology.* (2005) 146:984–91. doi: 10.1210/en.2004-0965
64. Zhan L, Liu H-X, Fang Y, Kong B, He Y, Zhong X, et al. Genome-wide binding and transcriptome analysis of human farnesoid X receptor in primary human hepatocytes. *PLoS ONE.* (2014) 9:e105930. doi: 10.1371/journal.pone.0105930
65. Ma K, Saha PK, Chan L, Moore DD. Farnesoid X receptor is essential for normal glucose homeostasis. *J Clin Invest.* (2006) 116:1102–9. doi: 10.1172/JCI25604
66. Zhang Y, Lee FY, Barrera G, Lee H, Vales C, Gonzalez FJ, et al. Activation of the nuclear receptor FXR improves hyperglycemia and hyperlipidemia in diabetic mice. *Proc Natl Acad Sci USA.* (2006) 103:1006–11. doi: 10.1073/pnas.0506982103
67. Wang YD, Chen WD, Wang M, Yu D, Forman BM, Huang W. Farnesoid X receptor antagonizes nuclear factor kappaB in hepatic inflammatory response. *Hepatology.* (2008) 48:1632–43. doi: 10.1002/hep.22519
68. Zhang S, Wang J, Liu Q, Harnish DC. Farnesoid X receptor agonist WAY-362450 attenuates liver inflammation and fibrosis in murine model of non-alcoholic steatohepatitis. *J Hepatol.* (2009) 51:380–8. doi: 10.1016/j.jhep.2009.03.025
69. Daly C, Rollins BJ. Monocyte chemoattractant protein-1 (CCL2) in inflammatory disease and adaptive immunity: therapeutic opportunities and controversies. *Microcirculation.* (2003) 10:247–57. doi: 10.1080/mic.10.3-4.247.257
70. Liu T, Zhang L, Joo D, Sun SC. NF-kappaB signaling in inflammation. *Signal Transduct Target Ther.* (2017) 2:17023. doi: 10.1038/sigtrans.2017.23
71. Fiorucci S, Rizzo G, Antonelli E, Renga B, Mencarelli A, Riccardi L, et al. Cross-talk between farnesoid-X-receptor (FXR) and peroxisome proliferator-activated receptor gamma contributes to the antifibrotic activity of FXR ligands in rodent models of liver cirrhosis. *J Pharmacol Exp Ther.* (2005) 315:58–68. doi: 10.1124/jpet.105.085597
72. Renga B, Mencarelli A, Migliorati M, Cipriani S, D'Amore C, Distrutti E, et al. SHP-dependent and -independent induction of peroxisome proliferator-activated receptor-gamma by the bile acid sensor farnesoid X receptor counter-regulates the pro-inflammatory phenotype of liver myofibroblasts. *Inflamm Res.* (2011) 60:577–87. doi: 10.1007/s00011-010-0306-1
73. Schumacher JD, Kong B, Pan Y, Zhan L, Sun R, Aa J, et al. The effect of fibroblast growth factor 15 deficiency on the development of high fat diet induced non-alcoholic steatohepatitis. *Toxicol Appl Pharmacol.* (2017) 330:1–8. doi: 10.1016/j.taap.2017.06.023

74. Schumacher JD, Kong B, Wu J, Rizzolo D, Armstrong LE, Chow MD, et al. Direct and indirect effects of fibroblast growth factor (FGF) 15 and FGF19 on liver fibrosis development. *Hepatology.* (2019) 71:670–85. doi: 10.1002/hep.30810
75. Liu Y, Binz J, Numerick MJ, Dennis S, Luo G, Desai B, et al. Hepatoprotection by the farnesoid X receptor agonist GW4064 in rat models of intra- and extrahepatic cholestasis. *J Clin Invest.* (2003) 112:1678–87. doi: 10.1172/JCI18945
76. Stedman C, Liddle C, Coulter S, Sonoda J, Alvarez JG, Evans RM, et al. Benefit of farnesoid X receptor inhibition in obstructive cholestasis. *Proc Natl Acad Sci USA.* (2006) 103:11323–8. doi: 10.1073/pnas.0604772103
77. Cui YJ, Aleksunes LM, Tanaka Y, Goedken MJ, Klaassen CD. Compensatory induction of liver efflux transporters in response to ANIT-induced liver injury is impaired in FXR-null mice. *Toxicol Sci.* (2009) 110:47–60. doi: 10.1093/toxsci/kfp094
78. van Golen RF, Olthof PB, Lionarons DA, Reiniers MJ, Alles LK, Uz Z, et al. FXR agonist obeticholic acid induces liver growth but exacerbates biliary injury in rats with obstructive cholestasis. *Sci Rep.* (2018) 8:16529. doi: 10.1038/s41598-018-33070-1
79. Jones H, Alpini G, Francis H. Bile acid signaling and biliary functions. *Acta Pharm Sin B.* (2015) 5:123–8. doi: 10.1016/j.apsb.2015.01.009
80. Boyer JL. Bile formation and secretion. *Compr Physiol.* (2013) 3:1035–78. doi: 10.1002/cphy.c120027
81. Jung D, York JP, Wang L, Yang C, Zhang A, Francis HL, et al. FXR-induced secretion of FGF15/19 inhibits CYP27 expression in cholangiocytes through p38 kinase pathway. *Pflugers Arch.* (2014) 466:1011–9. doi: 10.1007/s00424-013-1364-3
82. Cheng L, Tian F, Tian F, Tang L, Chen G, Luo Z, et al. Repression of farnesoid X receptor contributes to biliary injuries of liver grafts through disturbing cholangiocyte bile acid transport. *Am J Transplant.* (2013) 13:3094–102. doi: 10.1111/ajt.12479
83. Beenken A, Mohammadi M. The FGF family: biology, pathophysiology and therapy. *Nat Rev Drug Discov.* (2009) 8:235–53. doi: 10.1038/nrd2792
84. Owen BM, Mangelsdorf DJ, Kliewer SA. Tissue-specific actions of the metabolic hormones FGF15/19 and FGF21. *Trends Endocrinol Metab.* (2015) 26:22–9. doi: 10.1016/j.tem.2014.10.002
85. Goetz R, Beenken A, Ibrahimi OA, Kalinina J, Olsen SK, Eliseenkova AV, et al. Molecular insights into the klotho-dependent, endocrine mode of action of fibroblast growth factor 19 subfamily members. *Mol Cell Biol.* (2007) 27:3417–28. doi: 10.1128/MCB.02249-06
86. Nishimura T, Utsunomiya Y, Hoshikawa M, Ohuchi H, Itoh N. Structure and expression of a novel human FGF, FGF-19, expressed in the fetal brain. *Biochim Biophys Acta.* (1999) 1444:148–51. doi: 10.1016/S0167-4781(98)00255-3
87. Potthoff MJ, Kliewer SA, Mangelsdorf DJ. Endocrine fibroblast growth factors 15/19 and 21: from feast to famine. *Genes Dev.* (2012) 26:312–24. doi: 10.1101/gad.184788.111
88. Lin BC, Wang M, Blackmore C, Desnoyers LR. Liver-specific activities of FGF19 require Klotho beta. *J Biol Chem.* (2007) 282:27277–84. doi: 10.1074/jbc.M704244200
89. Yang C, Jin C, Li X, Wang F, McKeehan WL, Luo Y. Differential specificity of endocrine FGF19 and FGF21 to FGFR1 and FGFR4 in complex with KLB. *PLoS One.* (2012) 7:e33870. doi: 10.1371/journal.pone.0033870
90. Schumacher JD, Guo GL. Pharmacologic modulation of bile acid-FXR-FGF15/FGF19 pathway for the treatment of nonalcoholic steatohepatitis. *Handb Exp Pharmacol.* (2019) 256:325–57. doi: 10.1007/164_2019_228
91. Naugler WE, Tarlow BD, Fedorov LM, Taylor M, Pelz C, Li B, et al. Fibroblast growth factor signaling controls liver size in mice with humanized livers. *Gastroenterology.* (2015) 149:728–40 e15. doi: 10.1053/j.gastro.2015.05.043
92. Tomlinson E, Fu L, John L, Hultgren B, Huang X, Renz M, et al. Transgenic mice expressing human fibroblast growth factor-19 display increased metabolic rate and decreased adiposity. *Endocrinology.* (2002) 143:1741–7. doi: 10.1210/endo.143.5.8850
93. Fu L, John LM, Adams SH, Yu XX, Tomlinson E, Renz M, et al. Fibroblast growth factor 19 increases metabolic rate and reverses dietary and leptin-deficient diabetes. *Endocrinology.* (2004) 145:2594–603. doi: 10.1210/en.2003-1671
94. Marcelin G, Jo Y-H, Li X, Schwartz GJ, Zhang Y, Dun NJ, et al. Central action of FGF19 reduces hypothalamic AGRP/NPY neuron activity and improves glucose metabolism. *Mol Metab.* (2014) 3:19–28. doi: 10.1016/j.molmet.2013.10.002
95. Kir S, Beddow SA, Samuel VT, Miller P, Previs SF, Suino-Powell K, et al. FGF19 as a postprandial, insulin-independent activator of hepatic protein and glycogen synthesis. *Science.* (2011) 331:1621–4. doi: 10.1126/science.1198363
96. Benoit B, Meugnier E, Castelli M, Chanon S, Vieille-Marchiset A, Durand C, et al. Fibroblast growth factor 19 regulates skeletal muscle mass and ameliorates muscle wasting in mice. *Nat Med.* (2017) 23:990–6. doi: 10.1038/nm.4363
97. Potthoff MJ, Boney-Montoya J, Choi M, He T, Sunny NE, Satapati S, et al. FGF15/19 regulates hepatic glucose metabolism by inhibiting the CREB-PGC-1alpha pathway. *Cell Metab.* (2011) 13:729–38. doi: 10.1016/j.cmet.2011.03.019
98. Bhatnagar S, Damron HA, Hillgartner FB. Fibroblast growth factor-19, a novel factor that inhibits hepatic fatty acid synthesis. *J Biol Chem.* (2009) 284:10023–33. doi: 10.1074/jbc.M808818200
99. Zhou M, Learned RM, Rossi SJ, DePaoli AM, Tian H, Ling L. Engineered fibroblast growth factor 19 reduces liver injury and resolves sclerosing cholangitis in Mdr2-deficient mice. *Hepatology.* (2016) 63:914–29. doi: 10.1002/hep.28257
100. Zhou M, Learned RM, Rossi SJ, DePaoli AM, Tian H, Ling L. Engineered FGF19 eliminates bile acid toxicity and lipotoxicity leading to resolution of steatohepatitis and fibrosis in mice. *Hepatol Commun.* (2017) 1:1024–42. doi: 10.1002/hep4.1108
101. Pellicciari R, Costantino G, Camaioni E, Sadeghpour BM, Entrena A, Willson TM, et al. Bile acid derivatives as ligands of the farnesoid X receptor. Synthesis, evaluation, and structure-activity relationship of a series of body and side chain modified analogues of chenodeoxycholic acid. *J Med Chem.* (2004) 47:4559–69. doi: 10.1021/jm049904b
102. Suraweera D, Rahal H, Jimenez M, Viramontes M, Choi G, Saab S. Treatment of primary biliary cholangitis ursodeoxycholic acid non-responders: a systematic review. *Liver Int.* (2017) 37:1877–86. doi: 10.1111/liv.13477
103. Hirschfield GM, Mason A, Luketic V, Lindor K, Gordon SC, Mayo M, et al. Efficacy of obeticholic acid in patients with primary biliary cirrhosis and inadequate response to ursodeoxycholic acid. *Gastroenterology.* (2015) 148:751–761.e8. doi: 10.1053/j.gastro.2014.12.005
104. Nevens F, Andreone P, Mazzella G, Strasser SI, Bowlus C, Invernizzi P, et al. A placebo-controlled trial of obeticholic acid in primary biliary cholangitis. *N Engl J Med.* (2016) 375:631–43. doi: 10.1056/NEJMoa1509840
105. Manne V, Kowdley KV. Obeticholic acid in primary biliary cholangitis: where we stand. *Curr Opin Gastroenterol.* (2019) 35:191–6. doi: 10.1097/MOG.0000000000000525
106. Kowdley KV, Luketic V, Chapman R, Hirschfield GM, Poupon R, Schramm C, et al. A randomized trial of obeticholic acid monotherapy in patients with primary biliary cholangitis. *Hepatology.* (2018) 67:1890–902. doi: 10.1002/hep.29569
107. Fiorucci S, Di Giorgio C, Distrutti E. Obeticholic acid: an update of its pharmacological activities in liver disorders. *Handb Exp Pharmacol.* (2019) 256:283–95. doi: 10.1007/164_2019_227
108. Carino A, Biagioli M, Marchianò S, Fiorucci C, Bordoni M, Roselli R, et al. Opposite effects of the FXR agonist obeticholic acid on Mafg and Nrf2 mediate the development of acute liver injury in rodent models of cholestasis. *Biochim Biophys Acta.* (2020) 1865:158733. doi: 10.1016/j.bbalip.2020.158733
109. Edwards J, LaCerte C, Peyret T, Gosselin N, Marier J, Hofmann A, et al. Modeling and experimental studies of obeticholic acid exposure and the impact of cirrhosis stage. *Clin Transl Sci.* (2016) 9:328–36. doi: 10.1111/cts.12421
110. Liu T, Yang H, Fan W, Tu J, Li TWH, Wang J, et al. Mechanisms of MAFG dysregulation in cholestatic liver injury and development of liver cancer. *Gastroenterology.* (2018) 155:557–71.e14. doi: 10.1053/j.gastro.2018.04.032
111. Yang H, Ko K, Xia M, Li TWH, Oh P, Li J, et al. Induction of avian musculoaponeurotic fibrosarcoma proteins by toxic bile acid inhibits expression of glutathione synthetic enzymes and contributes to cholestatic liver injury in mice. *Hepatology.* (2010) 51:1291–301. doi: 10.1002/hep.23471
112. Santiago P, Scheinberg A, Levy C. Cholestatic liver diseases: new targets, new therapies. *Ther Adv Gastroenterol.* (2018) 11:175628481878740. doi: 10.1177/1756284818787400

113. Kowdley KV, Vuppalanchi R, Levy C, Floreani A, Andreone P, LaRusso NF, et al. A randomized, placebo-controlled, phase II study of obeticholic acid for primary sclerosing cholangitis. *J Hepatol.* (2020) 73:94–101. doi: 10.1016/j.jhep.2020.02.033
114. Trauner M, Gulamhusein A, Hameed B, Caldwell S, Shiffman ML, Landis C, et al. The nonsteroidal farnesoid X receptor agonist cilofexor (GS-9674) improves markers of cholestasis and liver injury in patients with primary sclerosing cholangitis. *Hepatology.* (2019) 70:788–801. doi: 10.1002/hep.30509
115. Patel K, Harrison SA, Elkashab M, Trotter JF, Herring R, Rojter S, et al. Cilofexor, a nonsteroidal FXR agonist, in non-cirrhotic patients with nonalcoholic steatohepatitis: a phase 2 randomized controlled trial. *Hepatology.* (2020). 72:58–71. doi: 10.1002/hep.31205
116. Neuschwander-Tetri BA, Loomba R, Sanyal AJ, Lavine JE, Van Natta ML, Abdelmalek MF, et al. Farnesoid X nuclear receptor ligand obeticholic acid for non-cirrhotic, non-alcoholic steatohepatitis (FLINT): a multicentre, randomised, placebo-controlled trial. *Lancet.* (2015) 385:956–65. doi: 10.1016/S0140-6736(14)61933-4
117. Cipriani S, Mencarelli A, Palladino G, Fiorucci S. FXR activation reverses insulin resistance and lipid abnormalities and protects against liver steatosis in Zucker (fa/fa) obese rats. *J Lipid Res.* (2010) 51:771–84. doi: 10.1194/jlr.M001602
118. Renga B, Mencarelli A, Vavassori P, Brancaleone V, Fiorucci S. The bile acid sensor FXR regulates insulin transcription and secretion. *Biochim Biophys Acta.* (2010) 1802:363–72. doi: 10.1016/j.bbadis.2010.01.002
119. Mudaliar S, Henry RR, Sanyal AJ, Morrow L, Marschall HU, Kipnes M, et al. Efficacy and safety of the farnesoid X receptor agonist obeticholic acid in patients with type 2 diabetes and nonalcoholic fatty liver disease. *Gastroenterology.* (2013) 145:574–82 e1. doi: 10.1053/j.gastro.2013.c 05.042
120. Hameed B, Terrault NA, Gill RM, Loomba R, Chalasani N, Hoofnagle JH, et al. Clinical and metabolic effects associated with weight changes and obeticholic acid in non-alcoholic steatohepatitis. *Aliment Pharmacol Ther.* (2018) 47:645–56. doi: 10.1111/apt. 14492
121. Ratziu V, Sanyal A, Macconell L, Shringarpure R, Marmon T, Shapiro D, et al. Regenerate: a phase 3, double-blind, randomized, placebo-controlled multicenter study of obeticholic acid therapy for nonalcoholic steatohepatitis. *J Hepatol.* (2016) 64:294–5. doi: 10.1016/S0168-8278(16)00372-X
122. Chalasani N, Younossi Z, Lavine JE, Charlton M, Cusi K, Rinella M, et al. The diagnosis and management of nonalcoholic fatty liver disease: practice guidance from the American Association for the Study of Liver Diseases. *Hepatology.* (2018) 67:328–57. doi: 10.1002/hep. 29367
123. Intercept Receives Complete Response Letter from FDA for Obeticholic Acid for the Treatment of Fibrosis Due to NASH - Intercept Pharmaceuticals, Inc. *[online]*. Available online at: https://ir.interceptpharma.com/news-releases/news-release-details/intercept-receives-complete-response-letter-fda-obeticholic-acid (accessed July 6, 2020).
124. Hernandez ED, Zheng L, Kim Y, Fang B, Liu B, Valdez RA, et al. Tropifexor-mediated abrogation of steatohepatitis and fibrosis is associated with the antioxidative gene expression profile in rodents. *Hepatol Commun.* (2019) 3:1085–97. doi: 10.1002/hep 4.1368

13

Serum Metabolomic Analysis of Chronic Drug-Induced Liver Injury With or Without Cirrhosis

Shuai-shuai Chen[1,2†], Ying Huang[2†], Yu-ming Guo[2†], Shan-shan Li[2], Zhuo Shi[2], Ming Niu[3], Zheng-sheng Zou[2], Xiao-he Xiao[2*] and Jia-bo Wang[2,4*]*

[1] School of Pharmacy, Chengdu University of Traditional Chinese Medicine, Chengdu, China, [2] Department of Liver Diseases, The Fifth Medical Center of Chinese People's Liberation Army General Hospital, Beijing, China, [3] Department of Poisoning Treatment, The Fifth Medical Center of Chinese People's Liberation Army General Hospital, Beijing, China, [4] School of Traditional Chinese Medicine, Capital Medical University, Beijing, China

***Correspondence:**
Jia-bo Wang
jiabo_wang@ccmu.edu.cn
Xiao-he Xiao
pharmacy302xxh@126.com
Zheng-sheng Zou
zszou302@163.com

†These authors have contributed equally to this work

Background: Chronic drug-induced liver injury (DILI) occurs in up to 20% of all DILI patients. It presents a chronic pattern with persistent or relapsed episodes and may even progress to cirrhosis. However, its underlying development mechanism is poorly understood.

Aims: To find serum metabolite signatures of chronic DILI with or without cirrhosis, and to elucidate the underlying mechanism.

Methods: Untargeted metabolomics coupled with pattern recognition approaches were used to profile and extract metabolite signatures from 83 chronic DILI patients, including 58 non-cirrhosis (NC) cases, 14 compensated cirrhosis (CC) cases, and 11 decompensated cirrhosis (DC) cases.

Results: Of the 269 annotated metabolites associated with chronic DILI, metabolic fingerprints associated with cirrhosis (including 30 metabolites) and decompensation (including 25 metabolites), were identified. There was a significantly positive correlation between cirrhosis-associated fingerprint (eigenmetabolite) and the aspartate aminotransferase-to-platelet ratio index (APRI) ($r = 0.315$, $P = 0.003$). The efficacy of cirrhosis-associated eigenmetabolite coupled with APRI to identify cirrhosis from non-cirrhosis patients was significantly better than APRI alone [area under the curve (AUC) value 0.914 vs. 0.573]. The decompensation-associated fingerprint (eigenmetabolite) can effectively identify the compensation and decompensation periods (AUC value 0.954). The results of the metabolic fingerprint pathway analysis suggest that the blocked tricarboxylic acid cycle (TCA cycle) and intermediary metabolism, excessive accumulation of bile acids, and perturbed amino acid metabolism are potential mechanisms in the occurrence and development of chronic DILI-associated cirrhosis.

Conclusions: The metabolomic fingerprints characterize different stages of chronic DILI progression and deepen the understanding of the metabolic reprogramming mechanism of chronic DILI progression to cirrhosis.

Keywords: biomarker, chronic drug-induced liver injury, cirrhosis, fingerprint, metabolomics, signature

INTRODUCTION

DILI is one of the most common and serious adverse reactions to drugs (1–5), and an important cause of clinically acute liver injury and failure (2, 6, 7). Clinically, most patients with DILI recover after drug withdrawal. However, around 8 ~ 20% of patients progress to chronicity (2, 8–10). According to the Spanish DILI registry study (10), 8% (25/298) of DILI patients had unresolved liver injury over 1 year, and among these chronic DILI patients, 64% (16/25) did not resolve in the first 3 years. More importantly, 44% (7/16) of these chronic DILI patients who underwent liver biopsies had cirrhosis and 6% (1/16) manifested fibrosis. Collectively, a high proportion of patients with chronic DILI may progress into cirrhosis. However, the mechanism of chronic DILI progression is still unclear.

Metabolomics is the study of small molecular metabolites. It improves our understanding of the pathophysiological evolution of diseases and greatly promotes the diagnosis, treatment, and prognosis of diseases (11). Metabolic fingerprints are a cluster composed of a series of serum metabolites that highly correlate with diseases (12). They have great significance in revealing the pathophysiological mechanism of diseases and in searching for biomarkers. Metabolomic methods have been used successfully to identify biomarkers associated with DILI. Previous studies reported that metabolomic biomarkers predicted the occurrence of DILI (13, 14) and distinguished between DILI and autoimmune hepatitis (15). Xie et al. (16) reported that changes in metabolomic biomarkers, such as glycochenodeoxycholic acid, phosphatidylcholine, and two metabolomic pathways (primary bile acid biosynthesis and alpha-linolenic acid metabolism) are closely related to the severity of DILI. These studies suggest the robustness and capability of untargeted metabolomics in screening for DILI-related biomarkers. However, the metabolomics of chronic DILI progression has not been studied.

Thus, we conducted untargeted metabolomic analysis of 83 chronic DILI patients (hepatitis, compensated cirrhosis, decompensated cirrhosis) and compared three groups of serum metabolomics characteristics, to establish the metabolic fingerprint of chronic DILI-related cirrhosis, including its potential biomarkers and mechanism of occurrence and development.

MATERIALS AND METHODS

Study Design

Patients from the Fifth Medical Center of Chinese PLA General Hospital from 2015 to 2017, were enrolled. The enrolled patients were diagnosed according to DILI guidelines (2) and liver cirrhosis guidelines (17), with no age and sex restriction. A total of 83 hospitalized chronic DILI patients, including non-cirrhosis (NC, $n = 58$), compensated cirrhosis (CC, $n = 14$), and decompensated cirrhosis (DC, $n = 11$) groups were enrolled. In addition, 10 serum samples of healthy subjects (HS) were collected. This research scheme was approved by the Ethics Committee of the hospital based on the ethical principles of the Declaration of Helsinki. Also, written informed consent was obtained from all patients. Based on the utilization of untargeted metabolomics, we obtained metabolic entities (metabolome profile) with significant difference ($P < 0.05$) between cirrhosis (CC + DC) and NC groups. The differentially abundant metabolites from metabolome profiles were deemed to be cirrhosis-associated metabolome features. Similarly, the differentially abundant metabolites for comparisons between DC and CC groups were considered as decompensation-associated metabolome features. The metabolic fingerprint (a cluster of metabolites) was screened using a hierarchical cluster and heat map analysis. We mainly used unsupervised principal component analysis (PCA) for fingerprint metabolites and formed one eigenmetabolite, which is defined as the first principal component (12).

Sample Preparation and LC/MS Conditions

Serum samples from the three groups were processed using an organic solvent precipitation method, according to our previous work (14). Ten microliter from each sample was mixed and then prepared as the quality control samples (QC). Agilent ZORBAX 300 SB-C18 column (2.1 × 100 mm, 1.8 μm, Agilent Technologies, USA) was used and the temperature was maintained at 30°C. The temperature of the sample was maintained at 4°C. An optimum mobile phase was composed of water (A, containing 0.1% formic acid and 5% acetonitrile) and acetonitrile (B, containing 0.1% formic acid). The flow rate was maintained at 0.3 mL/min with gradient elution conditions set as follows: 0–1 min, A (95%); 1–9 min, B (5% to 40%); 9–19 min, B (40% to 90%); 19–21 min, B (90% to 100%); 21–25 min, B (100%). The sample injection volume was kept at 4 μL.

Mass spectrometry (MS) evaluations were conducted on an Agilent 6550 iFunnel Q-TOF LC/MS equipped with electron spray ionization (ESI). MS data in both positive and negative modes were acquired based on optimal parameters, including a mass range from m/z 50–1,200; capillary voltage of 2.2 kV (negative) and 2.5 kV (positive); cone voltage of 40 V; ion source temperature of 130°C; desolvation temperature of 350°C; cone airflow of 50 L/h; and desolvation airflow of 800 L/h.

Statistical Analysis

Mass hunter Profinder software was used for raw data pre-processing. The online analysis tool MetaboAnalyst 4.0 (https://www.metaboanalyst.ca/) was used for data filtering and normalization. The clinical data of patients was expressed as a median (p25, p75) or numerical value. Differences between groups were analyzed by the non-parametric test in SPSS software program (version 25.0, Chicago, IL, USA) and reported as statistically significant if the $P < 0.05$. PCA and orthogonal partial least square discrimination analysis (OPLS-DA) were carried out using the SIMCA-P software (version 14.1, Umetrics AB, Umea, Sweden). The MetaboAnalyst website was used to acquire AUC and the associated *P*-values of differential metabolites. The human metabolome database (HMDB, http://www.hmdb.ca) and Kyoto encyclopedia of genes and genomes (https://www.kegg.jp) were used to construct an

TABLE 1 | Clinical characteristics of chronic DILI patients in NC, CC, and DC groups.

Characteristics	NC (*n* = 58)	CC (*n* = 14)	DC (*n* = 11)	*P*-value	
				NC *vs.* CC	CC *vs.* DC
Age/year	48.0 (39.5, 55.5)	50.0 (46.0, 52.2)	59.0 (46.0, 67.0)	0.490	0.153
Sex (male/female)	11/47	4/10	2/9	–	–
Alanine aminotransferase/U·L^{-1}	35.0 (18.0, 94.0)	43.0 (17.8, 132.2)	32.0 (15.0, 41.0)	0.733	0.066
Aspartate aminotransferase/U·L^{-1}	49.5 (24.5, 117.2)	39.5 (24.5, 137.5)	53.0 (33.0, 112.0)	0.876	0.641
Alkaline phosphatase/U·L^{-1}	96.0 (77.2, 126.2)	120.0 (69.5, 195.5)	137.0 (103.0, 211.0)	0.252	0.443
Total bilirubin/μmo·L^{-1}	12.5 (8.4, 19.4)	14.9 (9.7, 35.1)	32.0 (20.4, 70.2)	0.289	0.055
Direct bilirubin/μmo·L^{-1}	4.2 (3.2, 10.4)	5.3 (4.1, 18.6)	14.8 (7.1, 49.4)	0.261	0.025
Total bile acid/μmo·L^{-1}	11.0 (5.0, 18.0)	25.0 (6.5, 40.5)	36.0 (20.0, 72.0)	0.040	0.188
International normalized ratio/IU	0.9 (0.8, 1.0)	1.0 (0.9, 1.1)	1.1 (1.0, 1.2)	0.039	0.021
γ-glutamyl transpeptidase/U·L^{-1}	57.5 (22.0, 148.5)	36.0 (14.7, 110.5)	86.0 (40.0, 140.0)	0.351	0.171
Cholinesterase/U·L^{-1}	6,212.0 (5,383.7, 7,330.0)	5,407.0 (4,653.7, 5,902.0)	3,426.0 (1,489.0, 5,910.0)	0.010	0.063
Total cholesterol/mmo·L^{-1}	4.3 (3.4, 5.1)	3.8 (3.1, 4.8)	4.5 (2.8, 4.9)	0.224	0.477
Triglyceride/mmo·L^{-1}	1.2 (1.0, 1.8)	1.36 (1.17, 1.5)	0.9 (0.8, 1.4)	0.654	0.095
Creatinine/μmol·L^{-1}	61.0 (56.0, 68.2)	63.5 (58.2, 69.5)	67.0 (54.0, 80.0)	0.555	0.381
Immunoglobulin A/g·L^{-1}	2.2 (1.6, 2.9)	2.6 (1.8, 3.5)	3.7 (2.2, 5.8)	0.164	0.192
Immunoglobulin G/g·L^{-1}	12.6 (10.5, 14.4)	14.4 (11.7, 17.1)	16.8 (13.6, 22.8)	0.191	0.099
Immunoglobulin M/g·L^{-1}	1.1 (0.8, 1.6)	1.2 (0.6, 1.7)	2.1 (1.3, 2.3)	0.976	0.034
White blood cell/10^9·L^{-1}	5.0 (3.9, 6.3)	5.8 (3.2, 7.2)	4.8 (3.6, 7.8)	0.842	1.000
Platelet/10^9·L^{-1}	204.0 (168.5, 235.0)	154.0 (109.2, 223.5)	121.0 (103.0, 182.0)	0.044	0.352
Albumin/g·L^{-1}	38.0 (35.0, 39.0)	36.5 (34.7, 39.0)	27.0 (26.0, 34.0)	0.410	0.002
Globulin/g·L^{-1}	27.0 (24.0, 31.0)	32.0 (24.7, 34.0)	33.0 (27.0, 34.0)	0.127	0.297
Albumin/Globulin ratio	1.4 (1.2, 1.5)	1.2 (1.1, 1.4)	0.9 (0.7, 1.0)	0.041	0.003
Prealbumin/mg·L^{-1}	156.0 (128.5, 206.5)	104.5 (77.5, 164.8)	81.0 (36.0, 121.0)	0.032	0.046
Roussel Uclaf causality assessment method score					
highly probable (>8)	7	3	2		
probable (6 ~ 8)	35	7	6		
possible (3 ~ 5)	16	4	3		

Data are median (p25, p75) or numerical value. P-values for comparisons were carried out by nonparametric tests.

interactive network for the metabolic fingerprint and associated metabolic pathway.

RESULTS

Demographic and Clinical Parameters of the Study Population

The demographic and clinical parameters of the three groups of study population are listed in **Table 1**, and the causative agents of DILI patients are presented in **Table 2**. Patients from NC, CC, and DC groups with no significant differences in the mean ages, with female predominance (n = 66, 79.52%) were included in this study. Comparisons between CC and NC groups were conducted and the levels of cholinesterase, platelet, albumin/globulin ratio, and pre-albumin were found to be significantly lower in CC than NC, and the reverse was true for total bile acid. Patients in the DC group showed significantly higher values of direct bilirubin, international normalized ratio, and immunoglobulin M, but significantly lower values of albumin, albumin/globulin ratio, and pre-albumin, compared to the CC group. These results suggest that a gradual disturbance of liver functions occurred during anabolism and metabolism in chronic DILI advancement.

Serum Metabolic Profiles in Chronic DILI Evolution

Significant changes in global metabolic profiles were observed in different stages of chronic DILI under both ESI$^+$ and ESI$^-$ modes (**Figures 1A–D**). This suggests that sera metabolome changed while progressing from NC to CC and DC. To explore the relationship between the evolving stages of chronic DILI and serum metabolite levels, we first screened a set of variables with significant differences (P < 0.05) between cirrhosis (CC + DC) and NC, as well as DC *vs.* CC. Of the 1,324 metabolites (including positive and negative ion modes) differentiating between cirrhosis and NC groups, 195 metabolites in the database were annotated (**Figure 1E**). This indicates that metabolites are related to cirrhosis irrespective of the status of the compensation. Similarly, a total of 465 metabolites (74 were annotated in the database)

TABLE 2 | The causative agents of enrolled DILI patients.

Classification	Ingredient	*n*
Herbal and traditional medicine (H/TM)	TM preparations (ingredient unknown)	19
	Propolis	6
	Bupleurum chinense DC	4
	Dictamnius dasycarpus Turcz.	2
	Polygonum multiflorum Thunb.	2
	Corydalis yanhusuo W. T. Wang	2
	Agrimonia pilosa Ledeb.	2
	Rubia cordifolia L.	1
	Tripterygium wilfordii Hook. f.	1
	Polygonum multiflorum Thunb./*Psoralea corylifolia* L.	1
	Bupleurum chinense DC./*Corydalis yanhusuo* W. T. Wang	1
Chemicals drugs (CDs)	Ibuprofen	6
	Amlodipine	3
	Omeprazole	3
	Amoxicillin	2
	Nitrofurantoin	2
	Phenobarbital	2
	Valproate	2
	Sulfasalazine	2
	Simvastatin	2
	Enalapril	2
	Pioglitazone	2
	Loratadine	1
	Nimesulide	1
	Nifedipine	1
	Methotrexate	1
	Metronidazole	1
	Valsartan	1
	Metronidazole/Amoxicillin	1
	Levofloxacin/Sertraline	1
	Enalapril/Simvastatin	1
	Sertraline/Valproate	1
	Isoniazid/Pyrazinamide/Rifampicin	1
Combined use of H/TM and CDs	*Bupleurum chinense* DC./Simvastatin	1
	Bupleurum chinense DC./Amoxicillin-Clavulanate	1
	Polygonum multiflorum Thunb./Amoxicillin	1

were identified and differentiated between the DC and CC groups, indicating that these findings are associated with decompensation of cirrhosis (**Figure 1F**). Then, the three-dimensional PCA scatter plot revealed good separation of 195 cirrhosis-related metabolites between cirrhosis and NC groups (**Figure 1G**) and 74 decompensation-related metabolites between CC and DC groups (**Figure 1H**). In summary, the metabolome profiles associated with cirrhosis of chronic DILI and those related to decompensation, were preliminarily found to have potential roles in the identification of cirrhosis or decompensation, respectively.

Identification of Cirrhosis-Related Metabolic Fingerprint

According to literature, the AUC and *P*-values of 195 annotated metabolites related to cirrhosis were calculated, to identify a unique metabolomic fingerprint of chronic DILI-related liver cirrhosis (12). The AUC and associated *P*-values were performed using a hierarchical cluster and heat map analysis. Next, we identified the highest relevant cluster with the top 30 metabolites, which had a highly significant association with cirrhosis (vertical violet bar, **Figure 2Ai**). The AUC and *P*-values for this cluster of metabolites are shown in **Supplementary Table 1**. Interestingly, we observed that this cluster was effective in distinguishing between CC and NC groups (**Figure 2Aii**), as well as DC *vs.* NC groups (**Figure 2Aiii**). We then performed an eigenmetabolite (12) analysis of 30-metabolite clusters by reducing the dimensions and observed that the eigenmetabolite from HS, NC, and CC to DC has been on the rise, whereas no statistically significant differences between CC and DC groups were observed (**Figure 2B**). Meanwhile, we also found that eigenmetabolite positively correlated with the fibrosis stage in liver biopsy (**Supplementary Figure 1A**). These results suggest that a single metabolomic fingerprint (30 metabolites) was associated with chronic DILI-related liver cirrhosis, regardless of the compensatory status.

Comparison of Cirrhosis-Associated Metabolic Fingerprint and APRI in the Identification of Cirrhosis and Non-Cirrhosis

Further, we observed that 30 metabolites consisting of eigenmetabolite are associated with APRI ($r = 0.315$, $P = 0.003$, **Figure 2C**). We also found that cirrhosis-associated metabolic fingerprints coupled with APRI had better ability for differentiating patients with cirrhosis from those without cirrhosis as compared to APRI alone (AUC values 0.914 *vs.* 0.573, **Figure 2D**). Collectively, these findings indicate that the 30-metabolite cluster can be used as a cirrhosis-associated fingerprint to assist the identification of cirrhosis and non-cirrhosis cases.

Identification of Decompensated Cirrhosis-Related Metabolic Fingerprint

We refined a unique metabolic fingerprint associated with decompensation among the 74 decompensation-related metabolites, in the same way. We then defined the highest relevant cluster with the top 25 metabolites (vertical blue bar, **Figure 3A**), which were highly associated with DC patients. The resulting AUC and *P*-values of this cluster are presented in **Supplementary Table 2**. Similarly, we computed an eigenmetabolite for 25-metabolite clusters. Significantly increased eigenmetabolite levels were found in DC patients

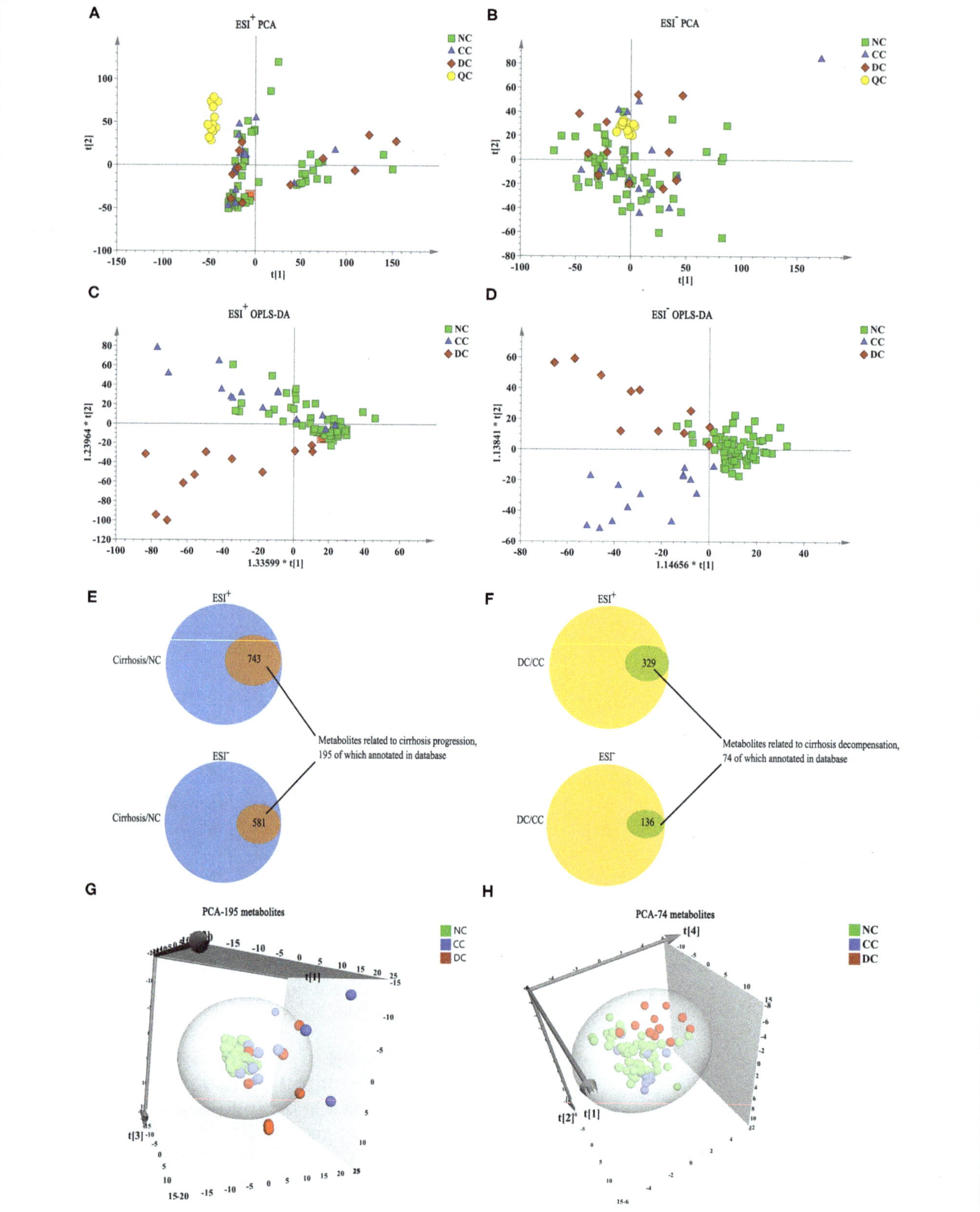

FIGURE 1 | Metabolome profile for chronic DILI with or without cirrhosis. **(A–D)** PCA, and OPLS-DA model analysis of all variables among NC group ($n = 58$, green square), CC group ($n = 14$, blue triangle), DC group ($n = 11$, red diamond), and QC ($n = 14$, yellow circle). **(E,F)** Venn diagram, the inner section of diagram has a set of variables associated with cirrhosis and decompensation, 195 and 74 metabolites annotated for metabolome feature cirrhosis and decompensation, respectively. **(G,H)** PCA 3-dimensional scatter plot of cirrhosis (CC + DC) *vs.* NC with 195 cirrhosis-related metabolites and DC *vs.* CC with 74 decompensated-related metabolites.

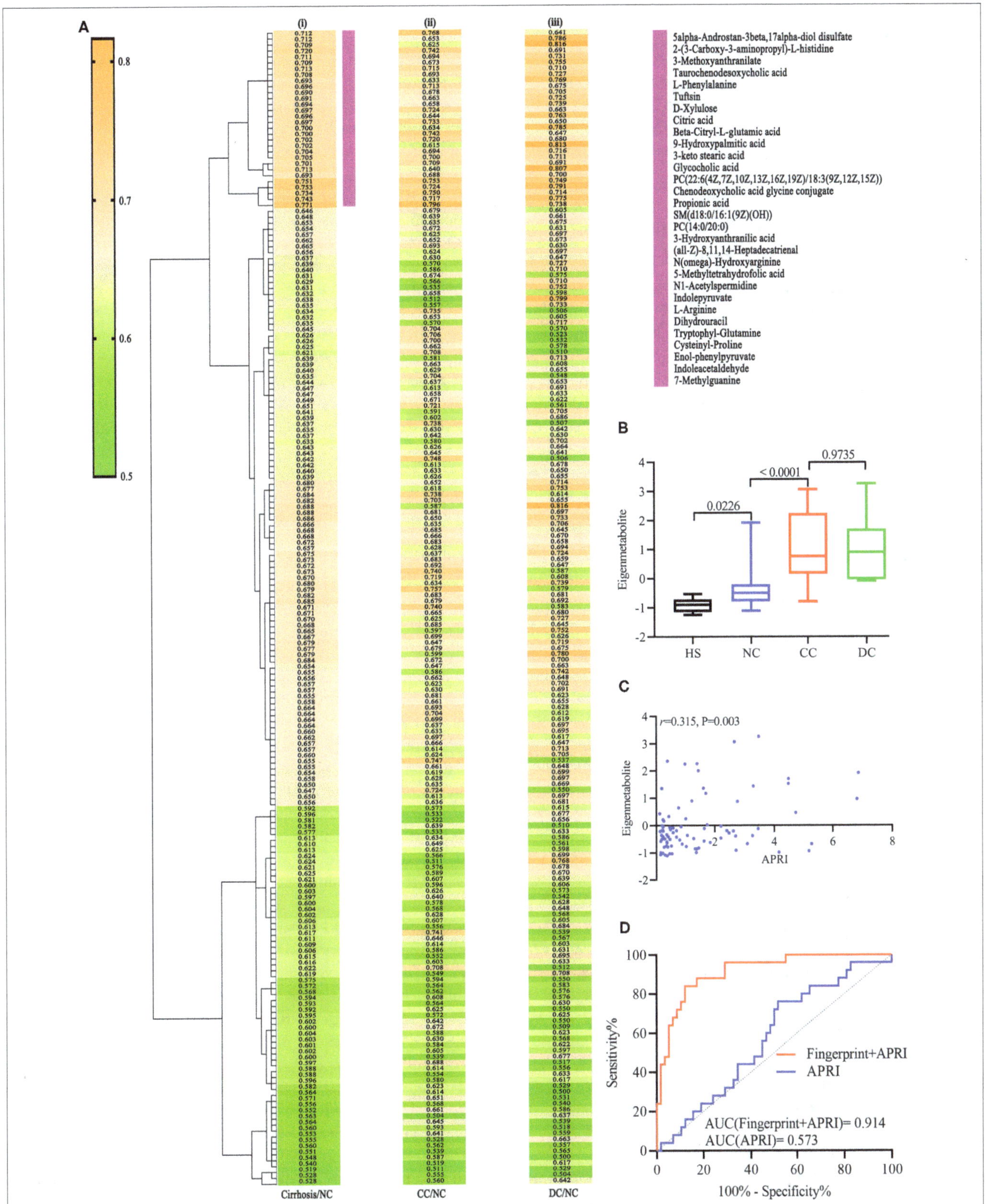

FIGURE 2 | Identification of cirrhosis-related metabolic fingerprint. **(Ai)** Hierarchical cluster analysis of AUC and P differentiation between cirrhosis and non-cirrhosis groups. **(Aii)** Corresponding metabolites in differentiating between DC and NC groups. **(Aiii)** Indicates corresponding metabolites in differentiating between DC and NC groups. **(B)** shows increasing trend of eigenmetabolite across different stages of chronic DILI, from HS to DC. **(C)** Indicates significantly positive correlation relationship between cirrhosis-associated eigenmetabolite and APRI score. **(D)** is ROC curve analysis for metabolic fingerprint (eigenmetabolite) and APRI score, in discriminating cirrhosis from non-cirrhotic patients with chronic DILI.

(**Figure 3B**) and patients with fibrosis stage 2–3 in liver biopsy (**Supplementary Figure 1B**). The 25 metabolites consisted of eigenmetabolite that could effectively discriminate patients with decompensation from those in the compensation stage (AUC value 0.954, **Figure 3C**). In summary, these findings suggest that the identified decompensation-associated metabolic fingerprint could well-discern the decompensation and compensation status in chronic DILI cases.

Metabolic Fingerprints Have Potential Pathophysiological Significance in Patients of Chronic DILI With Cirrhosis

To understand the evolution of chronic DILI, two metabolic fingerprints and the associated pathways that form an interactive network were identified, as shown in the schematic diagram (**Figure 4**). The characteristic metabolic fingerprints of chronic DILI-related cirrhosis are mainly concentrated as described below: phenylalanine and tyrosine metabolism, tryptophan metabolism, arginine and proline metabolism, TCA cycle, ubiquinone and other terpenoid-quinone biosynthesis, and bile acid biosynthesis.

DISCUSSION

This study characterizes the metabonomic profile of chronic DILI with or without cirrhosis, and reveals the metabolic fingerprints by using untargeted metabolomics and pattern recognition analysis. There are two crucial metabolic fingerprints of chronic DILI without correlation on age and sex (**Supplementary Figures 1C,D**). One is composed of 30 metabolites reflecting the cirrhosis associated characteristics (with no relationship with decompensation), the other one is decompensation-related metabolic fingerprint, composed of 25 metabolites (focus on the development from the compensated stage to the decompensated stage). Specifically, the metabolic fingerprints of chronic DILI-associated cirrhosis are mainly related to perturbed amino acid metabolism, blocked TCA cycle, intermediate metabolism, and accumulated bile acids.

Glucose metabolism of the liver is disarray in cirrhosis and depends more on proteolysis to provide energy (18–20). Two metabolic fingerprints reveal the metabolites in the amino acid metabolic pathway (phenylalanine metabolism, tryptophan metabolism, and arginine metabolism), with the elevation of proteolysis markers (tryptophyl-glutamine and cysteinyl-proline) in patients with chronic DILI-related cirrhosis (**Supplementary Table 3**). L-phenylalanine and enol-phenylpyruvate are metabolites of phenylalanine metabolism. L-phenylalanine has been reported to be positively correlated with imaging findings in liver injury patients and progression in liver cirrhosis patients (21, 22). A recent study reported that L-phenylalanine and phenylpyruvate via glycolysis inhibition affect energy metabolism of hepatocytes (23). Indolepyruvate, indole-acetaldehyde, 3-hydroxy-anthranilate, 3-methoxy-anthranilate, and quinolinic acid are metabolites of tryptophan metabolism. Tryptophan and its metabolites affect the immune and nervous system functions of patients (24). Additionally, 3-hydroxy-anthranilate has been reported to significantly provoke impairment of energy metabolism by inhibiting the activities of complexes I and II of the respiratory chain (25). Moreover, there is increased accumulation of quinolinic acid, which reflects not only the degree of liver dysfunction (26), but also inhibits the oxidative phosphorylation involved in cell energy metabolism (27). Arginine and n(omega)- hydroxyarginine are metabolites of arginine metabolism. Under cirrhosis conditions, cytokines and endotoxin may perpetuate arginine metabolism and nitric oxide (NO) generation (28). Arginine has been reported to diminish succinate dehydrogenase and complex II activities through NO formation (29). These findings suggest that energy requirements may lead to increased proteolysis to produce amino acids and their metabolites, which in turn, result in mitochondrial damage and energy metabolism dysfunction.

The disturbed TCA cycle and intermediate metabolism are some additional metabolic features of chronic DILI-associated cirrhosis. We observed a significant increase in the metabolites of TCA cycle (e.g., citric acid and 3-carboxy-1-hydroxypropylthiae diphosphate) in patients with chronic DILI-related cirrhosis (**Supplementary Table 3**). Citric acid is often revealed as a marker of hepatotoxicity (30). The TCA cycle mainly occurs in mitochondria is the core of intermediate metabolism (31). Blocked TCA cycle causes suppression of both fatty acid oxidation and carbohydrate catabolism, and leads to marked decrease of energy production from nutrients. We also observed some disorders of intermediate metabolites associated with coenzyme Q (e.g., 3-Polyprenyl-4,5-dihydroxybenzoate, menaquinol, menatetrenone), which plays a key role in the electron transport chain and in turn interferes with the electron transport chain and mitochondrial metabolism (32). Disturbed lipid metabolism has been reported as the potential biomarkers of hepatocellular, mixed, and cholestatic-type DILI (33), such as Polygonum Multiflorum-induced liver injury (34). Metabolism disorders of these lipids (e.g., phosphatidylcholine, phosphatidylethanolamine, phosphatidylserine, sphingomyelin, and ceramide; **Supplementary Table 3**) could result in hepatocyte dysfunction and liver disease progression (35, 36). The deposition of many long-chain fatty acids (e.g., 3-keto stearic acid, all-Z-8,11,14-Heptadecatrienal, 9-hydroxypalmitic acid; **Supplementary Table 3**) may indicate the inhibition of beta - oxidation in patients with chronic DILI-related cirrhosis, resulting in abnormal fat deposition and energy metabolism (37, 38). These findings therefore indicate that blocked TCA cycle and intermediary metabolism may be contributors to mitochondrial damage.

As main synthesis and metabolism in liver, bile acid is seriously affected after liver disease. We found a significant increase in conjugated bile acids (e.g., glycocholic acid, taurochenodesoxycholic acid, and chenodeoxycholic acid glycine conjugate) in patients with chronic DILI-associated cirrhosis. The excessive accumulation of chenodeoxycholic acid glycine conjugate and taurochenodesoxycholic acid promote apoptosis of liver cells and liver failure (39, 40). These abnormal accumulations of bile acids may not only be biomarkers for chronic DILI-associated cirrhosis, but also involved in

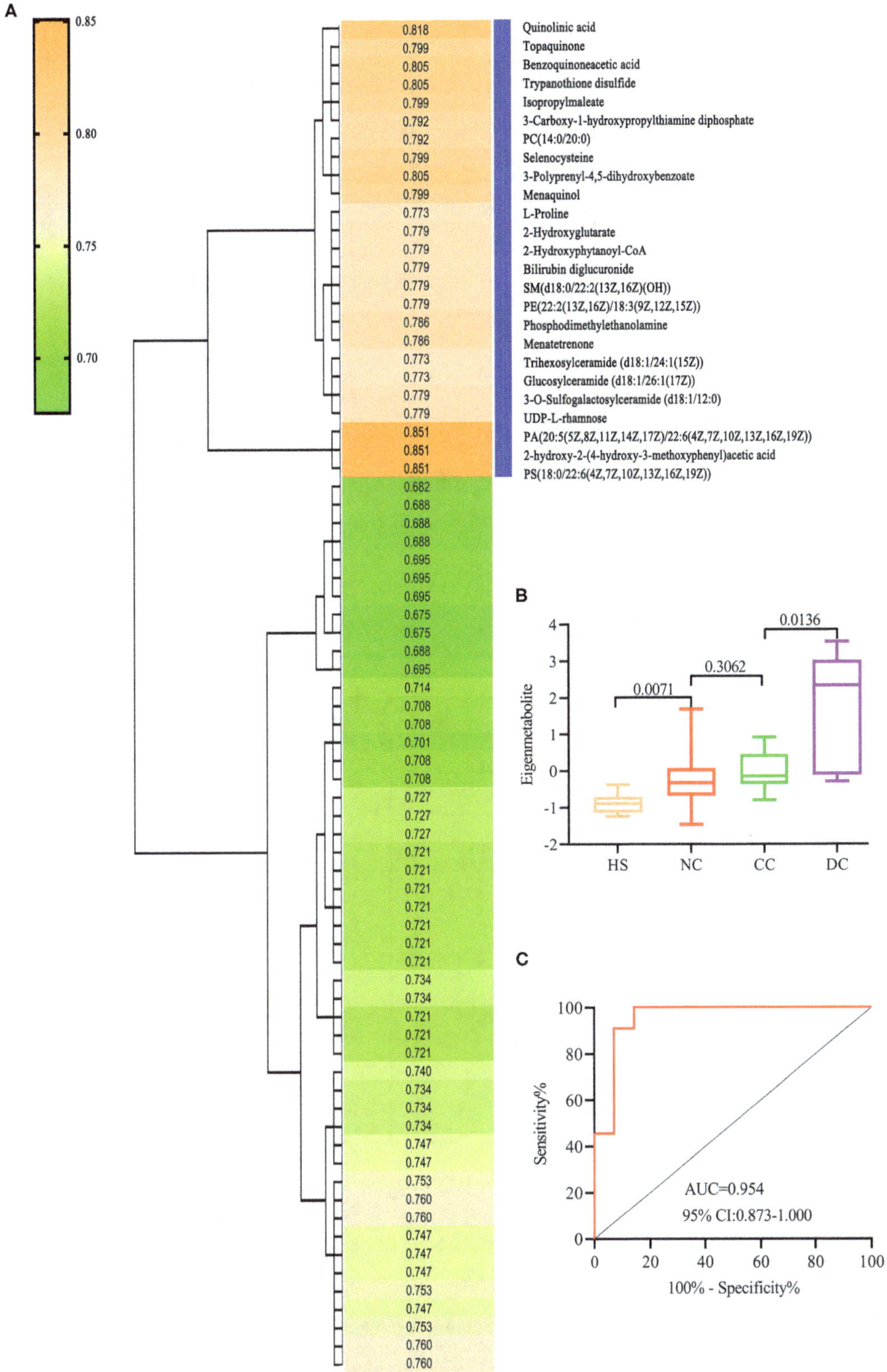

FIGURE 3 | Identification of decompensation-related metabolic fingerprint. **(A)** is a hierarchical cluster analysis of AUC and P differentiation between DC and CC groups. **(B)** shows an increasing trend of eigenmetabolite from HS, NC, and CC to DC. **(C)** ROC analysis for fingerprint (eigenmetabolite) to differentiate between DC and CC groups.

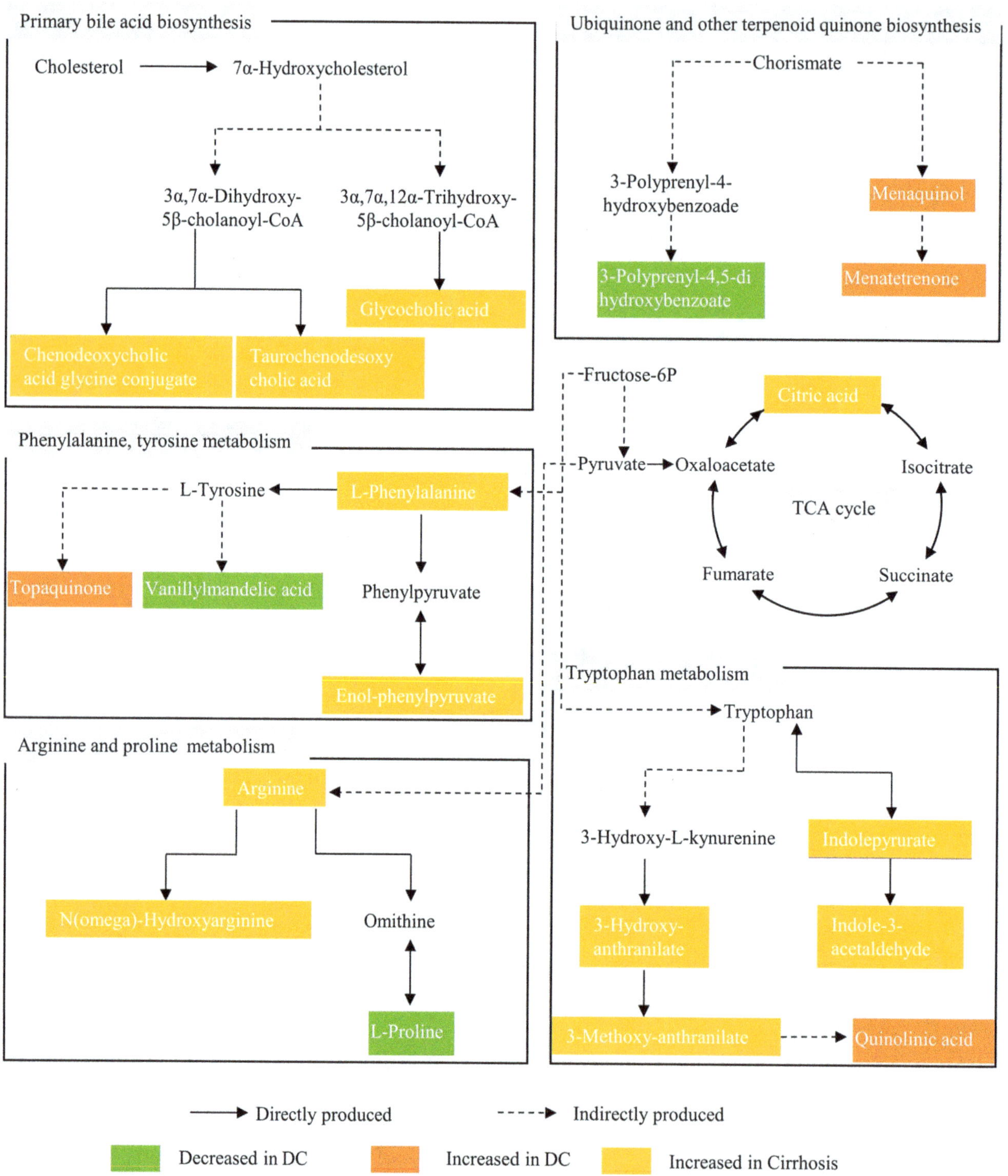

FIGURE 4 | Metabolic pathway alterations involved in chronic DILI with cirrhosis.

the development of the disease. Inhibiting accumulation of toxic bile acids in the liver may be beneficial to the clinical treatment of chronic DILI, while there are very few studies in this area, and hence it is worth exploring. Collectively, these findings indicate mitochondrial injury, lipid accumulation, and bile acid accumulation may be as mechanism implicated in DILI, which is consistent with the literature (41).

Our analysis provides novel information to further our understanding of the pathological changes of several metabolic pathways, based on serum metabolites, during the progression of chronic DILI. However, there are still a few limitations in the study. As all know, due to the abundant metabolites and biological process, the metabolomic study needs to further verify the results using animal models. And multi-center, large-sample studies could improve the application of these metabolic fingerprints to clinical DILI management in the future. Nevertheless, the study is expected to offer references for clinical diagnosis and monitoring of the occurrence and development of chronic DILI-associated cirrhosis, and to serve as a resource of metabolic adaptation and reprogramming to guide future investigations on clinical prognosis, mechanisms and novel therapeutics.

ETHICS STATEMENT

The studies involving human participants were reviewed and approved by Medical Ethics Committee of Fifth Medical Center of Chinese PLA General Hospital. The patients/participants provided their written informed consent to participate in this study.

AUTHOR CONTRIBUTIONS

J-bW, X-hX, and Z-sZ were responsible for the study concept and design. S-sC, YH, and Y-mG performed sample collection, conducted LC-MS data analysis, and manuscript preparation. S-sC and J-bW drafted the manuscript. S-sL and ZS reviewed and modified the manuscript. MN helped with data analysis. All authors contributed to the article and approved the submitted version.

SUPPLEMENTARY MATERIAL

Supplementary Figure 1 | Histological and demographic information comparison with cirrhosis and decompensation associated fingerprints. **(A,B)** Cirrhosis and decompensation associated fingerprints were positively correlated with fibrosis stage in liver biopsy. **(C,D)** Cirrhosis and decompensation associated fingerprints did not show significantly statistical difference on age and sex. S, fibrosis stage.

Supplementary Table 1 | The detailed information about 30 metabolites in metabolic fingerprint for cirrhosis.

Supplementary Table 2 | The detailed information about 25 metabolites in metabolic fingerprint for decompensation.

Supplementary Table 3 | Metabolites whose difference may affect the clinical phenotypes on cirrhosis and decompensation.

REFERENCES

1. Björnsson ES, Bergmann OM, Björnsson HK, Kvaran RB, Olafsson S. Incidence, presentation, and outcomes in patients with drug-induced liver injury in the general population of Iceland. *Gastroenterology.* (2013) 144:1419–25. doi: 10.1053/j.gastro.2013.02.006
2. Chalasani NP, Hayashi PH, Bonkovsky HL, Navarro VJ, Lee WM, Fontana RJ. ACG clinical guideline: the diagnosis and management of idiosyncratic drug-induced liver injury. *Am J Gastroenterol.* (2014) 109:950–66; quiz 67. doi: 10.1038/ajg.2014.131
3. Devarbhavi H. An update on drug-induced liver injury. *J Clin Exp Hepatol.* (2012) 2:247–59. doi: 10.1016/j.jceh.2012.05.002
4. Fontana RJ, Watkins PB, Bonkovsky HL, Chalasani N, Davern T, Serrano J, et al. Drug-Induced liver injury network (DILIN) prospective study: rationale, design and conduct. *Drug Saf.* (2009) 32:55–68. doi: 10.2165/00002018-200932010-00005
5. Miguel A, Azevedo LF, Araújo M, Pereira AC. Frequency of adverse drug reactions in hospitalized patients: a systematic review and meta-analysis. *Pharmacoepidemiol Drug Saf.* (2012) 21:1139–54. doi: 10.1002/pds.3309
6. Shen T, Liu YX, Shang J, Xie Q, Li J, Yan M, et al. Incidence and etiology of drug-induced liver injury in mainland China. *Gastroenterology.* (2019) 156:2230–41.e11. Epub 2019/02/12.
7. Navarro VJ, Senior JR. Drug-Related hepatotoxicity. *N Engl J Med.* (2006) 354:731–9. doi: 10.1056/NEJMra052270
8. Holt MP, Ju C. Mechanisms of drug-induced liver injury. *AAPS J.* (2006) 8:E48–54. doi: 10.1208/aapsj080106
9. Fontana RJ, Hayashi PH, Barnhart H, Kleiner DE, Reddy KR, Chalasani N, et al. Persistent liver biochemistry abnormalities are more common in older patients and those with cholestatic drug induced liver injury. *Am J Gastroenterol.* (2015) 110:1450–9. doi: 10.1038/ajg.2015.283
10. Medina-Caliz I, Robles-Diaz M, Garcia-Muñoz B, Stephens C, Ortega-Alonso A, Garcia-Cortes M, et al. Definition and risk factors for chronicity following acute idiosyncratic drug-induced liver injury. *J Hepatol.* (2016) 65:532–42. doi: 10.1016/j.jhep.2016.05.003
11. Wishart DS. Metabolomics for investigating physiological and pathophysiological processes. *Physiol Rev.* (2019) 99:1819–75. doi: 10.1152/physrev.00035.2018
12. Moreau R, Clària J, Aguilar F, Fenaille F, Lozano JJ, Junot C, et al. Blood metabolomics uncovers inflammation-associated mitochondrial dysfunction as a potential mechanism underlying ACLF. *J Hepatol.* (2020) 72:688–701. doi: 10.1016/j.jhep.2019.11.009
13. Kim JW, Ryu SH, Kim S, Lee HW, Lim MS, Seong SJ, et al. Pattern recognition analysis for hepatotoxicity induced by acetaminophen using plasma and urinary 1H NMR-based metabolomics in humans. *Anal Chem.* (2013) 85:11326–34. doi: 10.1021/ac402390q
14. Zhang L, Niu M, Wei AW, Tang JF, Tu C, Bai ZF, et al. Risk profiling using metabolomic characteristics for susceptible individuals of drug-induced liver injury caused by *Polygonum multiflorum*. *Arch Toxicol.* (2019) 94:245–56. doi: 10.1007/s00204-019-02595-3
15. Wang JB, Pu SB, Sun Y, Li ZF, Niu M, Yan XZ, et al. Metabolomic profiling of autoimmune hepatitis: the diagnostic utility of nuclear magnetic resonance spectroscopy. *J Proteome Res.* (2014) 13:3792–801. doi: 10.1021/pr500462f
16. Xie ZY, Chen EM, Ouyang XX, Xu XW, Ma SS, Ji FY, et al. Metabolomics and cytokine analysis for identification of severe drug-induced liver injury. *J Proteome Res.* (2019) 18:2514–24. doi: 10.1021/acs.jproteome.9b00047
17. Xu XY, Ding HG, Li WG, Xu JH, Han Y, Jia JD, et al. Chinese guidelines on the management of liver cirrhosis. *J Clin Hepatol.* (2019) 35:2408–25. doi: 10.3969/j.issn.1001-5256.2019.11.006
18. Holm E. *Encephalopathy in Chronic Liver Failure.* New York, NY: Plenum Press (1984).
19. Fischer J. *Metabolism and Nutrition in Liver Disease.* Lancaster: MTP Press (1984) 259p.
20. Meng QH, Wang JH, Yu HW, Li J, Feng YM, Hou W, et al. Resting energy expenditure and substrate metabolism in Chinese patients with acute or chronic hepatitis B or liver cirrhosis. *Inter Med.* (2010) 49:2085–91. doi: 10.2169/internalmedicine.49.3967
21. Ranjan P, Gupta A, Kumar S, Gowda GA, Ranjan A, Sonker AA, et al. Detection of new amino acid markers of liver trauma by proton

nuclear magnetic resonance spectroscopy. *Liver Int.* (2006) 26:703–7. doi: 10.1111/j.1478-3231.2006.01283.x

22. Liang KH, Cheng ML, Lo CJ, Lin YH, Lai MW, Lin WR, et al. Plasma phenylalanine and glutamine concentrations correlate with subsequent hepatocellular carcinoma occurrence in liver cirrhosis patients: an exploratory study. *Sci Rep.* (2020) 10:10926. doi: 10.1038/s41598-020-67971-x
23. Suzuki R, Sato Y, Fukaya M, Suzuki D, Yoshizawa F, Sato Y. Energy metabolism profile of the effects of amino acid treatment on hepatocytes: phenylalanine and phenylpyruvate inhibit glycolysis of hepatocytes. *Nutrition.* (2020) 82:111042. doi: 10.1016/j.nut.2020.111042
24. Lin H, Teng HL, Wu W, Li Y, Lv GF, Huang XW, et al. Pharmacokinetic and metabolomic analyses of mangiferin calcium salt in rat models of type 2 diabetes and non-alcoholic fatty liver disease. *BMC Pharmacol Toxicol.* (2020) 21:59. doi: 10.1186/s40360-020-00438-x
25. Schuck PF, Tonin A, da Costa Ferreira G, Viegas CM, Latini A, Duval Wannmacher CM, et al. Kynurenines impair energy metabolism in rat cerebral cortex. *Cell Mol Neurobiol.* (2007) 27:147–60. doi: 10.1007/s10571-006-9124-y
26. Lahdou I, Sadeghi M, Oweira H, Fusch G, Daniel V, Mehrabi A, et al. Increased serum levels of quinolinic acid indicate enhanced severity of hepatic dysfunction in patients with liver cirrhosis. *Hum Immunol.* (2013) 74:60–6. doi: 10.1016/j.humimm.2012.09.009
27. Ribeiro CA, Grando V, Dutra Filho CS, Wannmacher CM, Wajner M. Evidence that quinolinic acid severely impairs energy metabolism through activation of NMDA receptors in striatum from developing rats. *J Neurochem.* (2006) 99:1531–42. doi: 10.1111/j.1471-4159.2006.04199.x
28. La Mura V, Pasarín M, Rodriguez-Vilarrupla A, García-Pagán JC, Bosch J, Abraldes JG. Liver sinusoidal endothelial dysfunction after LPS administration: a role for inducible-nitric oxide synthase. *J Hepatol.* (2014) 61:1321–7. doi: 10.1016/j.jhep.2014.07.014
29. Delwing D, Tagliari B, Streck EL, Wannamacher CM, Wajner M, Wyse AT. Reduction of energy metabolism in rat hippocampus by arginine administration. *Brain Res.* (2003) 983:58–63. doi: 10.1016/S0006-8993(03)03029-4
30. Cuykx M, Rodrigues RM, Laukens K, Vanhaecke T, Covaci A. In vitro assessment of hepatotoxicity by metabolomics: a review. *Arch Toxicol.* (2018) 92:3007–29. doi: 10.1007/s00204-018-2286-9
31. Martínez-Reyes I, Chandel NS. Mitochondrial TCA cycle metabolites control physiology and disease. *Nat Commun.* (2020) 11:102. doi: 10.1038/s41467-019-13668-3
32. Beyer RE. The participation of coenzyme Q in free radical production and antioxidation. *Free Radic Biol Med.* (1990) 8:545–65. doi: 10.1016/0891-5849(90)90154-B
33. Saito K, Kagawa T, Tsuji K, Kumagai Y, Sato K, Sakisaka S, et al. Plasma lipid profiling of three types of drug-induced liver injury in Japanese patients: a preliminary study. *Metabolites.* (2020) 10:355. doi: 10.3390/metabo10090355
34. Wu XF, Zhang YT, Qiu JQ, Xu Y, Zhang J, Huang J, et al. Reynoutria multiflora lipidomics analysis indicates disturbed hepatocellular lipid metabolism in -induced idiosyncratic liver injury. *Front Pharmacol.* (2020) 11:569144. doi: 10.3389/fphar.2020.569144
35. Li ZY, Agellon LB, Allen TM, Umeda M, Jewell L, Mason A, et al. The ratio of phosphatidylcholine to phosphatidylethanolamine influences membrane integrity and steatohepatitis. *Cell Metab.* (2006) 3:321–31. doi: 10.1016/j.cmet.2006.03.007
36. Payne F, Lim K, Girousse A, Brown RJ, Kory N, Robbins A, et al. Mutations disrupting the Kennedy phosphatidylcholine pathway in humans with congenital lipodystrophy and fatty liver disease. *Proc Natl Acad Sci USA.* (2014) 111:8901–6. doi: 10.1073/pnas.1408523111
37. Nakamura MT, Yudell BE, Loor JJ. Regulation of energy metabolism by long-chain fatty acids. *Prog Lipid Res.* (2014) 53:124–44. doi: 10.1016/j.plipres.2013.12.001
38. Houten SM, Violante S, Ventura FV, Wanders RJ. The biochemistry and physiology of mitochondrial fatty acid β-oxidation and its genetic disorders. *Ann Rev Physiol.* (2016) 78:23–44. doi: 10.1146/annurev-physiol-021115-105045
39. Lan WF, Chen ZJ, Chen YT, Tan MD, Chen Y, Chen JW, et al. Glycochenodeoxycholic acid impairs transcription factor E3 -dependent autophagy-lysosome machinery by disrupting reactive oxygen species homeostasis in L02 cells. *Toxicol Lett.* (2020) 331:11–21. doi: 10.1016/j.toxlet.2020.05.017
40. Rust C, Bauchmuller K, Fickert P, Fuchsbichler A, Beuers U. Phosphatidylinositol 3-kinase-dependent signaling modulates taurochenodeoxycholic acid-induced liver injury and cholestasis in perfused rat livers. *Am J Physiol Gastroint Liver Physiol.* (2005) 289:G88–94. doi: 10.1152/ajpgi.00450.2004
41. Kawaguchi M, Nukaga T, Sekine S, Takemura A, Susukida T, Oeda S, et al. Mechanism-based integrated assay systems for the prediction of drug-induced liver injury. *Toxicol Appl Pharmacol.* (2020) 394:114958. doi: 10.1016/j.taap.2020.114958

14

Aging-Related Molecular Pathways in Chronic Cholestatic Conditions

Claudio Pinto, Elisabetta Ninfole, Antonio Benedetti, Luca Maroni[†] *and Marco Marzioni*[*†]

Department of Gastroenterology and Hepatology, Università Politecnica delle Marche, Ancona, Italy

***Correspondence:**
Marco Marzioni
marco.marzioni74@gmail.com

[†]*These authors share senior authorship*

Aging is commonly defined as the time-dependent functional decline of organs and tissues. Average life expectancy has increased considerably over the past century and is estimated to increase even further, consequently also the interest in understanding the aging processes. Although aging is not a disease, it is the major risk factor for the development of many chronic diseases. Pathologies, such as Primary Biliary Cholangitis (PBC) and Primary Sclerosing Cholangitis (PSC) are cholestatic liver diseases characterized by chronic inflammation, biliary damage and ultimately liver fibrosis, targeting specifically cholangiocytes. To date, the influence of aging in these biliary diseases is not fully understood. Currently, liver transplantation is the only solution because of lacking in efficiently therapies. Although liver cells have a high regenerative capacity, they undergo extensive molecular changes in response to aging. Following time-dependent damage induced by aging, the cells initially activate protective compensatory processes that, if hyperstimulated, can lead to the decline of regenerative ability and the development of pathologies. Recent studies have introduced novel therapeutic tools for cholangiopathies that have showed to have promising potential as novel therapies for PSC and PBC and for the development of new drugs. The recent advancements in understanding of molecular aging have undoubtedly the potential to unveil new pathways for selective drug treatments, but further studies are needed to deepen their knowledge.

Keywords: aging, PSC, PBC, senescence, therapeutics, inflammation, fibrosis

INTRODUCTION

The aging of a biological system is the inevitable process determined by time-dependent accumulation of damage to genetic material (1) that commonly involves DNA damage, telomere shortening, and epigenetic alterations. The functions of organs inevitably decline in time, leading to body deterioration, and increased susceptibility to death (2, 3). Average life expectancy has increased dramatically over the past century and is estimated to increase even further. However, the sharp increase in the number of elderly people suffering from chronic diseases suggests that an increase in life span does not necessarily coincide with a prolonged health span. The aging research goal focuses mainly on improving health span, given the health costs associated with the years of oldness. Although aging is not a disease, it is the major risk factor for the development of many chronic diseases (4–6), in particular chronic liver conditions (7, 8). Specific age-related hepatic changes have already been highlighted and may affect liver morphology, physiology and oxidative capacity, besides affecting the regenerative capability. Old age seems to favor non-alcoholic fatty liver disease (NAFLD), NASH, and ultimately HCC, principally caused by an increased inflammation in agreement with the inflamm-aging theory.

Pathologies affecting cholangiocytes (cholangiopathies), such as Primary Biliary Cholangitis (PBC) and Primary Sclerosing Cholangitis (PSC), are cholestatic liver diseases (targeting intra- and extra-hepatic cholangiocytes), characterized by chronic inflammation and thus biliary damage which cause proliferation and ultimately liver fibrosis, which develop and progress differently according to the patient age. Over the years, more data have been obtained regarding PSC. This pathology is characterized by destruction of intrahepatic/extrahepatic bile ducts, chronic biliary inflammation, liver fibrosis (9, 10) and is often associated with inflammatory bowel disease rising risks of developing colorectal cancer and cholangiocarcinoma (11–13). PBC, is an autoimmune disorder that specifically target cholangiocytes, characterized by the injury of small- and medium-sized bile ducts, cholestasis, and lymphocyte infiltration (14–16). Has been shown that PBC predominantly affects women, with higher incidence in patients who have a relative with PBC or any other autoimmune disorder (17). Currently, liver transplantation is the only solution for cholangiopathies because of lacking in efficiently therapies. Although new preclinical studies have provided attractive prospects for the development of new therapeutic approaches, especially for PSC, further investigation is needed in understanding mechanisms and pathophysiology of PBC to identify new candidate targets.

HALLMARKS OF AGING

Studies carried out over the years to understand typical aging processes have led to the identification of nine hallmarks that can be grouped into three main categories (3). The primary hallmarks are the cause of age-related damage, such as genomic instability, telomere attrition, epigenetic alterations and loss of proteostasis (18, 19). The response to these age-related damages, named antagonistic hallmarks, include cellular senescence, deregulated nutrient sensing and altered mitochondrial function. Finally, integrative hallmarks are the consequence of responses and responsible of aging phenotype which leads to stem cell exhaustion and altered intercellular communication.

PRIMARY HALLMARKS

The accumulation of both genomic and mitochondrial DNA damage depends on exogenous stressors (physical, chemical or biological triggers) and/or endogenous events (DNA replication errors or ROS production) (1, 20). The oldest cells are the ones with the higher genomic instability. Typical of old cells are telomers mutations and their length has been shown to be highly heritable (21). The correlations between telomeres shortening and aging has been demonstrated in different animal models (22) and in several age-related diseases (23–25). DNA methylation (epigenetic alteration that principally involve CpG islands) seems to be a predictor of human age in genome-wide methylation studies (26–28). The impairment of proteostasis (principally due to toxins or free radicals), lead to the chronic expression of unfolded or misfolded protein or to the accumulation of protein aggregates, process that has been linked to different age-related pathologies of nervous system (29–31).

ANTAGONISTIC HALLMARKS

Cell activates compensatory processes known as antagonistic hallmarks, in response to the primary hallmarks. They are initially protective processes but, when hyperstimulated, may lead to cellular aging or development of pathologies. Cellular senescence (defined as the irreversible arrest of cell growth) represents the main response to age-related damage. Senescence is associated with complex cellular changes, such as chromatin reorganization, metabolic reprogramming, increasing of autophagy and release of proinflammatory mediators and growth factors known as senescence-associated secretory phenotype (SASP) (32). Cellular senescence is not exclusively associated with aging but occurs in response to multiple inducing factors, remodeling the tissue in order to solve the damage. *In vivo* data have shown the accumulation of senescent cells in aged tissues (33, 34). The lack of balance between clearance of senescent cell and mobilization of progenitor cells, determines the accumulation of senescent cells, which contributes to aging. Nutrients sensing deregulation and mitochondrial dysfunction are also common with advancing age. The main physiologic pathway affected by aging process, in both humans and model organisms, is the growth hormone (GH)/insulin like growth factor (IGF-1) axis, that lead to impaired glucose sensing (35, 36). Others nutrient sensing systems involved in the detection of cellular energy status, such as AMPK (which detect high AMP levels) and Sirtuins (which detect high NAD^+ levels) may also play important role in aging processes (37). Finally, aging-related mitochondrial dysfunction has been associated with deletion of mtDNA, oxidation of mitochondrial proteins, destabilization of the macromolecular organization of respiratory chain complexes, alteration of lipid composition of mitochondrial membranes, defective mitophagy and imbalance between fission and fusion events (38, 39).

INTEGRATIVE HALLMARKS

As the organism ages it decreases the regenerative ability of the tissues because of depletion of stem cells niches and changes in intercellular communication (i.e., endocrine, neuroendocrine, or neuronal). For example, it is known that mesenchymal stem cell decline leads to osteoporosis, haematopoietic stem cell exhaustion results in a less production of adaptive cells (called immunosenescence) that leads to anemia and intestinal epithelial stem cell depletion causes decreased intestinal function (3). Immunosenescence and increased secretion of cytokines by adipose tissue lead to chronic inflammation (40, 41). Chronic low-grade systemic inflammation combined with immunosenescence are part of the pathogenesis of premature aging, also called inflammaging. Another physiological change that negatively influences liver function is the redistribution of adipose tissue from subcutaneous to visceral sites (42). This observation, together with the decline of immune system efficiency, accumulation of senescent cells, inflammaging, and defective autophagy, increase mortality and risk of disorders, such as hypertension, atherosclerosis, hyperlipidemia, insulin resistance, and diabetes, all of which predispose to developing NAFLD (40, 43).

MOLECULAR MECHANISMS OF AGING IN LIVER DISEASE

The liver is a pivotal organ with a wide range of functions, including detoxification, protein synthesis, regulation of energy metabolism and much more. Specific age-related hepatic changes have been reported, such as enhanced hepatocyte size, increase in the number of binucleated cells, reduction in mitochondrial number, excessive visceral fat and secretion of pro-inflammatory cytokines (44–46). These changes significantly affect liver morphology, physiology, and oxidative capacity. At molecular level, aged livers go through the loss of the regenerative capacity and may involve CCAAT/enhancer-binding protein (C/EBP) family members, glycogen synthase kinase 3 Beta (GSK3β), histone deacetylase 1 (HDAC1), and Sirtuin 1 epigenetic and signaling pathways (47–51). Age-related accumulation of lipids in the liver has also been reported (52). The resulting lipotoxicity increase the prevalence of NAFLD in elderly person (53). Furthermore, aging significantly enhance the progression to NASH and fibrosis, thus predisposing to increased mortality in elderly subjects with NAFLD (54, 55).

LIVER ENDOTHELIAL SINUSOIDAL CELLS

At the level of single-cell populations a recent study demonstrated that aging is associated with sinusoidal remodeling, both in rodents and humans (56, 57). LSECs are endothelial cells that line the hepatic sinusoids, whose main role is to facilitate bidirectional exchanges between blood and hepatocytes. LSECs also mediate endocytosis of circulating proteins, having a role in the regulation of immunotolerance, and maintaining sinusoidal microenvironment. Old rats exhibited significantly higher hepatic vascular resistance *in vivo*, with reduced liver perfusion and increased portal pressure in comparison with young ones. From a molecular point of view, sinusoidal pseudocapillarization is associated with reduced expression of VEGFR2, KLF2, and CD32b, altered expression of the von Willebrands factor, CD31 and collagen (58), and so, in a reduction in the number and size of fenestrations, thickening of the endothelium, deposition of basal lamina and collagen (56, 57) (**Figure 1**). Due to these alterations, the lipoproteins and insulin absorption is compromised causing hyperlipidemia and hepatic insulin resistance (59).

HEPATOCYTES

Age-related molecular alterations induce a reduction in the number of hepatocytes but with an increased portion of polyploid hepatocytes, along with reduced rates of DNA synthesis and repair (60). Hepatocytes, the major parenchymal cells in the liver, are the chief functional cells of the liver and perform metabolic, endocrine and secretory functions as well as protein synthesis, detoxification, activation of innate immunity and so on. Dysregulation of glycolysis, triglyceride synthesis, and lipid metabolism occurs because of decreased expression of Sirtuin1, PGC-1α, lower concentrations of NAD^+, and upregulation of the senescence marker p16 (61). On the other side, hepatocytes show to be relatively resistant to telomer shortening (62), maybe due to the high expression levels of telomerase (63). Other molecular modifications have been associated at hepatocytes aging, such as increased heterochromatin protein 1β, elevated senescence-associated-β-galactosidase activity, p21, p16, and γ-H2AX (64), but also genes involved principally in hepatic metabolism of glucose, lipids and proteins, such as PI3K/Akt, MAPK, Jak/S, NF-κB, TGFβ, IGF1, and Ca^{2+}/cAMP (65). Alterations in mitochondrial biogenesis and autophagic degradation (mitophagy) have been observed together with the presence of enlarged mitochondria (66, 67) and the reduction in hepatocytes autophagy in old livers, underlined by lowering number of autophagic vesicles (68, 69) (**Figure 1**).

HEPATIC STELLATE CELLS AND KUPFFER CELLS

Aging affects also hepatic stellate cells (HSC) and Kupffer cells (KC). HSCs are pericytes located within the space of Disse and maintain close interactions with sinusoidal endothelial cells and hepatic epithelial cells. HSCs are involved in vitamin A and lipid storage, when activated, they acquire their characteristic phenotype and produce collagen, starting the development of hepatic fibrosis. An increased expression of HSC activation markers, such as αSMA, collagen 1α1-2, and phosphorylated moesin, has been described in aged rats (70, 71). The lipid droplets in HSC significantly increase in number and size during aging, as observed in mice and non-human primates thus starting the development of hepatic fibrosis (72, 73). KCs are specialized macrophages located in the liver, lining the walls of the sinusoids, with the main function of performing phagocytic functions to remove cellular debris from the portal blood flow. KC activation is observed in most types of liver diseases and contributes to the pro-inflammatory status of the hepatic sinusoid. Phagocytic and autophagic activity of KC decline with aging, acquiring an inflammatory phenotype (71). In aged rats is increased the infiltration of $CD68^+$ cells along with significant differences in the mRNA expression of cytokines including TNFα, Mrc1, and Arg1 (70) (**Figure 1**).

LIVER PROGENITOR CELLS

Liver progenitor cells (LPCs) are quiescent cells that are activated during liver injury in order to regenerate the liver parenchyma. LPC functionality is negatively regulated by the aging process (74). LPCs in young mice could be activated and proliferate upon liver injury, whereas in old mice failed to respond and proliferate, leading to impaired liver regeneration. Levels of Reactive Oxygen Species (ROS) and neutrophils infiltration are increased in aged

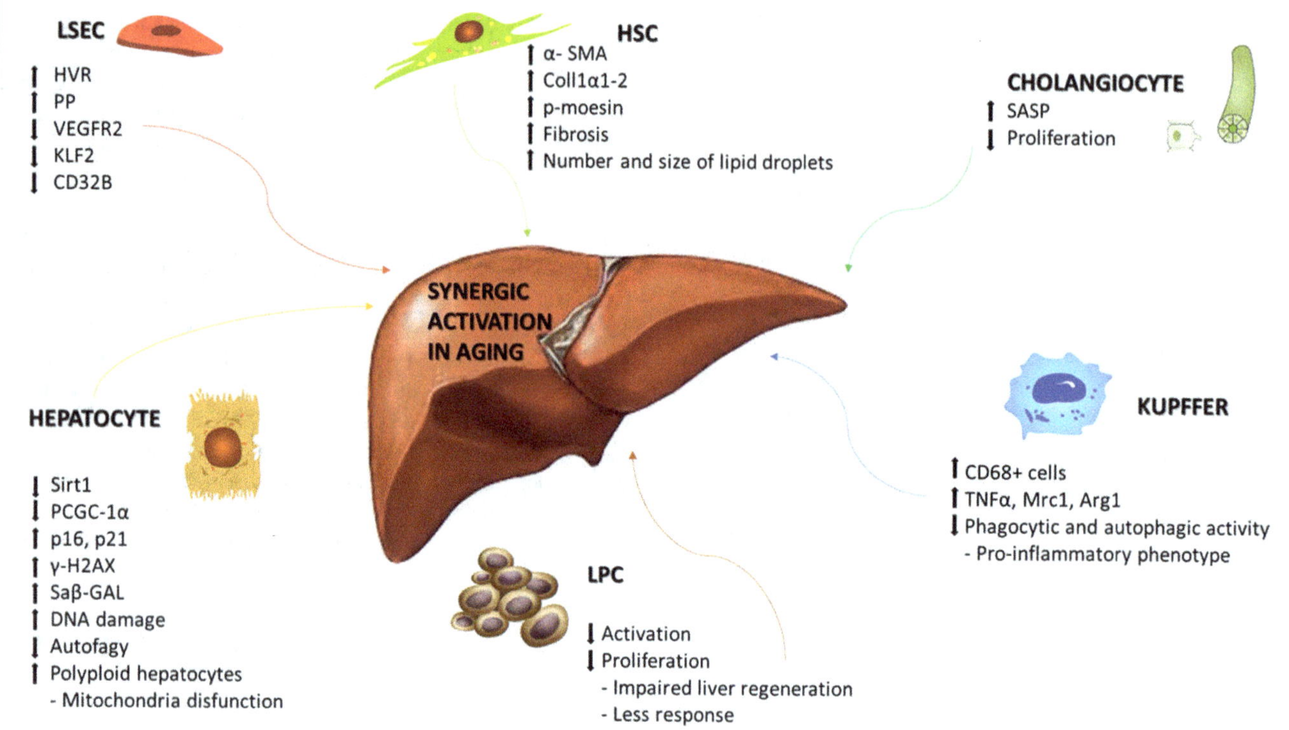

FIGURE 1 | Synergic activation of liver cells in aging. Schematic representation of the main molecular mechanisms associated with aging in liver disease. Age-related changes can include alterations that affects morphology, physiology, and oxidative capacity in the different cellular populations of the liver. HVR, Hepatic vascular resistence; PP, Portal pressure; VEGR2, Vascular endothelial growth factor receptor 2; KLF2, Krüppel-like Factor 2; Sirt1, Sirtuin1; PGC-1α, Peroxisome proliferator-activated receptor gamma coactivator 1-alpha; γ-H2AX, H2A histone family member X; Saβ-GAL, Senescence-associated beta-galactosidase; TNFα, Tumor necrosis factor alpha; Mrc1, Mannose receptor, C type 1; Arg1, Arginase 1; SASP, Senescence-associated secretory phenotype; α-SMA, Alpha smooth muscle actin; Coll1α1-2, Collagen 1α1-2; p-moesin, Phosphorylated moesin.

mice, in collaboration with chemokine production from activated HSC and decrease activation and proliferation of LPC (**Figure 1**).

CHOLANGIOCYTES AND CHOLANGIOPATHIES: FOCUS ON PSC AND PBC

Cholangiocytes are the cells lining the biliary tract and the target of cholangiopathies, such as PSC and PBC. PSC is an idiopathic, autoinflammatory disorder characterized by fibrosis and obliteration of medium and large ducts throughout the biliary epithelium. In 70% of patients is associated with inflammatory bowel disease, particularly ulcerative colitis, and it may progress in complications, such as cholestasis, hepatic failure, autoimmune disease, and cholangiocarcinoma (75, 76). PBC is an autoimmune liver disease that predominantly affects women [maybe due to the observation that 48% of PBC patients experienced prior recurrent urinary tract infections, more frequent in women and caused by *Escherichia coli* (77)], characterized by mainly portal inflammation, chronic cholestasis and destruction of small intrahepatic bile ducts that show a progressive pathogenesis from liver fibrosis to cirrhosis, portal hypertension and ultimately liver failure (78, 79). Cholestatic liver diseases are profoundly influenced by patient age. A more severe disease course in young patients affected PBC has been recently observed in a large retrospective study, showing increased risk of treatment failure, liver transplantation and death (80). In PSC, the age at diagnosis increase the risk of develop cholangiocarcinoma (21% for patients older than 60 years) (81). In elderly patients is risen the risk of complications after liver transplantation. The development of biliary complications after orthotopic liver transplantation is influenced by donor age (82), and lower survival rates in people aged more than 60 years (5-years survival rate of 59%) has been observed (83). However, the survival of recipients older than 70 years of age still remains lower than in younger patients (10-years survival of 43 vs. 64% in recipients aged 60–69 years) (84).

Important clues supporting the role of aging in shaping cholangiocyte biology in course of biliary injury are also emerging. The analysis of liver samples collected from PSC and PBC patients have shown increased expression of senescent markers and SASP components in diseased cholangiocytes (85). Furthermore, has been found a significantly increased expression of N-Ras protein co-localization with activated RAS in PSC, which was absent in PBC or control samples. These data underline the role of N-Ras protein as mediator of lipopolysaccharide-induced inflammation, further supporting a potential role for N-Ras signaling in the pathogenesis of PSC (86). In PBC seems to be more important the role of the autophagy as a necessary component to the activation of cell senescence (87). Senescent PBC cholangiocytes accumulated markers of autophagy, such as microtubule-associated proteins-light chain 3β, cathepsin D, and lysosome-associated membrane protein-1 (88). Several studies have shown as deregulated autophagy might be involved in the induction of cholangiocyte senescence in several biliary disease. The expression of autophagy markers as LC3 and p62 is significantly correlated with the expression of the known senescent markers, p16 and p21, in ductular cells in ductular reaction (DR) (89). In early and advanced stages of PBC, autophagy is frequently correlated with cellular senescence in bile ductular cells in DRs. Sasaki et al. suggests that autophagy may be involved in the pathophysiology of DRs in PBC and may precede the cellular senescence. Moreover, they have also found that deregulated autophagy may contribute to the abnormal expression of mitochondrial antigens and be involved in the autoimmune pathogenesis of bile duct lesions in PBC (89–91).

These findings are corroborated by data obtained in animal models of cholestatic liver injury. Isolated cholangiocytes from multi-drug resistance 2 knockout ($Mdr2^{-/-}$) mice develop cellular senescence (92). As a direct consequence of Mdr2 lack of expression, toxic bile acids accumulate in the bile triggering increased bile duct mass and liver fibrosis. Despite these findings demonstrate a link between senescence and disease presentation, it is unknown whether senescence is the trigger of disease or if it is a consequence of chronic damage (93, 94).

NEW POTENTIAL PATHWAYS INVOLVED IN PSC AND PBC FOR NOVEL THERAPIES

In order to identify new molecular pathways involved in course of cholangiopathies are needed adequate preclinical animal models to mimic, as much as possible, the features of relative human diseases (95–97). To date, for PSC and PBC, various genetic and chemical models are used in parallel with *in vitro* studies to resemble the pathogenesis of these pathologies (98). PSC is a heterogeneous disease, the identification of clinical endpoints and treatment goals in PSC remains difficult to determine for the complex interaction of multiple causes, such as environmental insult (99, 100), genetic susceptibility (101), dysregulation of immune signaling (102, 103) and gut microbiome derangement (104–106) (**Table 1**). New drugs that act selectively at the level of senescent cells are being evaluated for a series of human diseases, such as senolytics, inhibitor of the anti-apoptotic proteins BCL-2 and BCL-xL, inhibitor of complex that modulates SASP production (mTORC1 and JAK2/STAT3 pathway) and other alternative approaches (125). As suggested by Zhou et al. a possible pharmacological target for the treatment of cholangiopathies can lie among the mediators of Secretin/SecretinReceptor axis (107) and secretion pathway of TGF-β1 at the biliary ducts level (108), both responsible of the biliary damage and liver fibrosis regulation. In this way, another new potential target is the Substance P, a neuropeptide that plays an important role in regulating hepatic fibrosis and cellular senescence (109). In the contest of PSC and PBC, Forkhead Box A2 (FoxA2), a key transcriptional factor involved in tissue regeneration, was found upregulated in LPC and downregulated, through epigenetic mechanisms, in liver tissue (117). This reduction was associated with an exacerbation of fibrotic liver damage suggesting that, acting on an up regulation of FoxA2, could be a therapeutic strategy to reconstruct the hepatobiliary system, after a hepatic injury (**Table 1**). Recently, has been shown the role of mast cells (MCs) also in course of cholangiopathies. MCs was found surrounded bile ducts during the early stages of PSC but were located in fibrous septa in late-stage PSC (126). Their role in PSC have been studied founding that MC number and markers are increased in $Mdr2^{-/-}$ mice and PSC patients compared with controls (118). Treatment with cromolyn sodium, a MC stabilizer that blocks the release of histamine, reveled a reduction in MC indicators and PSC-associated fibrosis. Furthermore, MCs and their mediators may influence the function of cholangiocytes and hepatic bile

TABLE 1 | This table summarize both pathways and group of therapies that are currently under investigation.

Disease		References
PSC	**Features**	
	- Environmental insults	(99, 100)
	- Genetic susceptibility	(101)
	- Dysregulation of immune signaling	(102, 103)
	- Gut microbiome derangement	(104–106)
	Potential pathways	
	- Mediators of Secretin/Secretin receptor axis	(107)
	- Secretion pathway of TGF-β1 at biliary ducts level	(108)
	- Regulation of substance P	(109)
	Therapies	
	- Obeticholic acid	(110, 111)
	- Norursodeoxycholic acid, oral antibiotics, such as vancomycin and rifamixim, FXR agonist, LUM001, anti-fibrotics agents, Simtuzumab, and Cenicriviroc	(112)
PBC	**Potential pathways**	
	- Immunosuppressive and immunomodulatory agents	(113)
	Therapies	
	- Ursodeoxycholic acid	(114–116)
	- Obeticholic acid	(110, 111)
PSC and PBC	**Potential pathways**	
	- Forkhead Box A2 (FoxA2)	(117)
	- Mast Cells (MCs)	(118–121)
	- Melatonin	(122)
	- Neurokinin 1 receptor	(123)
	- Twinfilin 1	(124)

production and flow (118). Cholangiocytes secrete also stem cell factor, which is a chemoattractant for c-kit expressed on MCs. Stem cell factor was found increased in human PSC and in Mdr2$^{-/-}$ mice (119). Blocking biliary stem cell factor decreased MC migration, biliary proliferation/senescence, and HSC activation, so targeting MC infiltration may be an option to ameliorate PSC progression (119). In PBC there are minor evidence of MCs role, but is known that PBC patients often presents increased circulating bile acid pools, and it has been demonstrated that specific bile acids can alter MC activation *in vitro* (120, 121). A recent study showed that MCs are located in the portal areas and sinusoidal walls in patients with PBC and an increased expression of chymase that seems to be co-localized in areas that exhibited extensive hepatic fibrosis (127). Despite all these studies demonstrate the increased presence of MCs, and their potential in developing pharmacologic therapies, the causal effect of MCs remains to be fully examined. Other approaches concern the use of Bile acids that are already largely used in cholangiopathies therapy. Ursodeoxycholic acid (UDCA) inhibits cholangiocyte proliferation and secretion *in vivo* (114) and is an approved drug for PBC (115). UDCA stimulates secretion of bile acids from hepatocytes, preventing hepatocyte injury, apoptosis and necrosis and subsequent inflammation and fibrosis. UDCA expand the bile acid pool and induces a less toxic bile composition through the activation of AE2 transporters (116). Furthermore, UDCA administration inhibits MC activation improving liver conditions in Mdr2$^{-/-}$ mice (128), but its use for PSC treatment provided controversial results (129) (**Table 1**). Instead, there are better perspectives regarding the Obeticholic acid, which is a synthetically modified bile acid known to be a potent Farnesoid X receptor (FXR) agonist. A trial of obeticholic acid for PBC patients has demonstrated to improve serum levels of ALP and bilirubin compared to the placebo group, and long-term clinical outcomes in PBC patients (110, 111). In a clinical trial (NCT02177136), administration of obeticholic acid improved serum ALP and bilirubin levels also in PSC patients compared to the placebo group.

Others new potential pathways involved in PSC and PBC concern the Melatonin, neurokinin-1 receptor, and twinfilin-1. It has been shown how these molecules may play a role in cholangiocytes response to injury and liver fibrosis (122–124), but further studies are needed and must be deeply investigated (**Table 1**).

To date, for PSC treatment, various therapies are under investigation. Just some of this [better elucidate in a review of Rodriguez et al. (112)] include, Norursodeoxycholic acid, oral antibiotics, such as vancomycin and rifamixim, FXR agonist, LUM001, anti-fibrotic agents, Simtuzumab and Cenicriviroc. For PBC, less is known, but actually, there is good evidence concern the use of the glucocorticoid Budenoside, fibrates that act as ligand for the nuclear receptor PPAR, fenofibrates and bezafibrate, and other strategies aiming at the availment of immunosopressive and immunomodulatory agents (113) (**Table 1**). Noteworthy is a new class of drugs that aim to destroy senescent cells, called senolytics (130). The notions about these molecules are still few and need to be further tested on primates and humans, but could have great potential in improving healthspan, given the known accumulation of senescent cells in aging.

CONCLUSIONS

Cholangiopathies are deeply influenced by the aging process, and elderly patients require a careful management in clinical practice. Average life expectancy is constantly increasing, it becomes essential to understand the molecular basis of age-related modifications that are involved in disease progression. Current therapeutic approaches utilize agonists or antagonists to regulate signaling pathways involved in cholangiocyte response, particularly focused on the improve of portal fibrosis and liver inflammation and on the activation of other liver cells by cholangiocytes, such as HSCs and KC leading to further liver damage. Recently, the use of stem cells or stem cell-derived extracellular vesicles has also taken hold and together with the recent studies described above, have showed to have promising potential as novel therapies for PSC and PBC and for the development of new drugs. Such studies have undoubtedly the potential to foster a better management of patients, but further studies are needed to deepen their knowledge.

AUTHOR CONTRIBUTIONS

This work was done in full by CP. EN has processed the image and part of the contents. AB and LM have contributed to a part of the contents. MM has carried out the revision and correction of the draft.

REFERENCES

1. Moskalev AA, Shaposhnikov MV, Plyusnina EN, Zhavoronkov A, Budovsky A, Yanai H, et al. The role of DNA damage and repair in aging through the prism of Koch-like criteria. *Ageing Res Rev.* (2013) 12:661–84. doi: 10.1016/j.arr.2012.02.001
2. McHugh D, Gil J. Senescence and aging: Causes, consequences, and therapeutic avenues. *J Cell Biol.* (2018) 217:65–77. doi: 10.1083/jcb.201708092
3. Lopez-Otin C, Blasco MA, Partridge L, Serrano M, Kroemer G. The hallmarks of aging. *Cell.* (2013) 153:1194–217. doi: 10.1016/j.cell.2013.05.039
4. North BJ, Sinclair DA. The intersection between aging and cardiovascular disease. *Circ Res.* (2012) 110:1097–108. doi: 10.1161/CIRCRESAHA.111.246876
5. Querfurth HW, LaFerla FM. Alzheimer's disease. *N Engl J Med.* (2010) 362:329–44. doi: 10.1056/NEJMra0909142
6. de Magalhaes JP. How ageing processes influence cancer. *Nat Rev Cancer.* (2013) 13:357–65. doi: 10.1038/nrc3497
7. Tsochatzis EA, Bosch J, Burroughs AK. Liver cirrhosis. *Lancet.* (2014) 383:1749–61. doi: 10.1016/S0140-6736(14)60121-5
8. Sheedfar F, Di Biase S, Koonen D, Vinciguerra M. Liver diseases and aging: friends or foes? *Aging Cell.* (2013) 12:950–4. doi: 10.1111/acel.12128

9. Lazaridis KN, LaRusso NF. Primary sclerosing cholangitis. *N Engl J Med.* (2016) 375:2501–2. doi: 10.1056/NEJMra1506330
10. Sirpal S, Chandok N. Primary sclerosing cholangitis: diagnostic and management challenges. *Clin Exp Gastroenterol.* (2017) 10:265–73. doi: 10.2147/CEG.S105872
11. Dyson JK, Beuers U, Jones DEJ, Lohse AW, Hudson M. Primary sclerosing cholangitis. *Lancet.* (2018) 391:2547–59. doi: 10.1016/S0140-6736(18)30300-3
12. Karlsen TH, Folseraas T, Thorburn D, Vesterhus M. Primary sclerosing cholangitis–a comprehensive review. *J Hepatol.* (2017) 67:1298–323. doi: 10.1016/j.jhep.2017.07.022
13. Taghavi SA, Eshraghian A, Niknam R, Sivandzadeh GR, Bagheri Lankarani K. Diagnosis of cholangiocarcinoma in primary sclerosing cholangitis. *Expert Rev Gastroenterol Hepatol.* (2018) 12:575–84. doi: 10.1080/17474124.2018.1473761
14. Lleo A, Marzorati S, Anaya JM, Gershwin ME. Primary biliary cholangitis: a comprehensive overview. *Hepatol Int.* (2017) 11:485–99. doi: 10.1007/s12072-017-9830-1
15. Tsuneyama K, Baba H, Morimoto Y, Tsunematsu T, Ogawa H. Primary biliary cholangitis: its pathological characteristics and immunopathological mechanisms. *J Med Invest.* (2017) 64:7–13. doi: 10.2152/jmi.64.7
16. Gulamhusein AF, Hirschfield GM. Pathophysiology of primary biliary cholangitis. *Best Pract Res Clin Gastroenterol.* (2018) 34–35:17–25. doi: 10.1016/j.bpg.2018.05.012
17. Lindor KD, Gershwin ME, Poupon R, Kaplan M, Bergasa NV, Heathcote EJ, et al. Primary biliary cirrhosis. *Hepatology.* (2009) 50:291–308. doi: 10.1002/hep.22906
18. Lombard DB, Chua KF, Mostoslavsky R, Franco S, Gostissa M, Alt FW. DNA repair, genome stability, and aging. *Cell.* (2005) 120:497–512. doi: 10.1016/j.cell.2005.01.028
19. Aunan JR, Watson MM, Hagland HR, Soreide K. Molecular and biological hallmarks of ageing. *Br J Surg.* (2016) 103:e29–46. doi: 10.1002/bjs.10053
20. Hoeijmakers JH. DNA damage, aging, and cancer. *N Engl J Med.* (2009) 361:1475–85. doi: 10.1056/NEJMra0804615
21. Honig LS, Kang MS, Cheng R, Eckfeldt JH, Thyagarajan B, Leiendecker-Foster C, et al. Heritability of telomere length in a study of long-lived families. *Neurobiol Aging.* (2015) 36:2785–90. doi: 10.1016/j.neurobiolaging.2015.06.017
22. Armanios M, Alder JK, Parry EM, Karim B, Strong MA, Greider CW. Short telomeres are sufficient to cause the degenerative defects associated with aging. *Am J Hum Genet.* (2009) 85:823–32. doi: 10.1016/j.ajhg.2009.10.028
23. Kuszel L, Trzeciak T, Richter M, Czarny-Ratajczak M. Osteoarthritis and telomere shortening. *J Appl Genet.* (2015) 56:169–76. doi: 10.1007/s13353-014-0251-8
24. Carlquist JF, Knight S, Cawthon RM, Le VT, Jared Bunch T, Horne BD, et al. Shortened telomere length is associated with paroxysmal atrial fibrillation among cardiovascular patients enrolled in the Intermountain Heart Collaborative Study. *Heart Rhythm.* (2016) 13:21–7. doi: 10.1016/j.hrthm.2015.07.032
25. Hunt SC, Kimura M, Hopkins PN, Carr JJ, Heiss G, Province MA, et al. Leukocyte telomere length and coronary artery calcium. *Am J Cardiol.* (2015) 116:214–8. doi: 10.1016/j.amjcard.2015.03.060
26. Bocklandt S, Lin W, Sehl ME, Sánchez FJ, Sinsheimer JS, Horvath S, et al. Epigenetic predictor of age. *PLoS ONE.* (2011) 6:e14821. doi: 10.1371/journal.pone.0014821
27. Koch CM, Wagner W. Epigenetic-aging-signature to determine age in different tissues. *Aging.* (2011) 3:1018–27. doi: 10.18632/aging.100395
28. Hannum G, Guinney J, Zhao L, Zhang L, Hughes G, Sadda S, et al. Genome-wide methylation profiles reveal quantitative views of human aging rates. *Mol Cell.* (2013) 49:359–67. doi: 10.1016/j.molcel.2012.10.016
29. Koga H, Kaushik S, Cuervo AM. Protein homeostasis and aging: the importance of exquisite quality control. *Ageing Res Rev.* (2011) 10:205–15. doi: 10.1016/j.arr.2010.02.001
30. Powers ET, Morimoto RI, Dillin A, Kelly JW, Balch WE. Biological and chemical approaches to diseases of proteostasis deficiency. *Annu Rev Biochem.* (2009) 78:959–91. doi: 10.1146/annurev.biochem.052308.114844
31. Labbadia J, Morimoto RI. The biology of proteostasis in aging and disease. *Annu Rev Biochem.* (2015) 84:435–64. doi: 10.1146/annurev-biochem-060614-033955
32. Campisi J. Aging, cellular senescence, and cancer. *Annu Rev Physiol.* (2013) 75:685–705. doi: 10.1146/annurev-physiol-030212-183653
33. Hoenicke L, Zender L. Immune surveillance of senescent cells–biological significance in cancer- and non-cancer pathologies. *Carcinogenesis.* (2012) 33:1123–6. doi: 10.1093/carcin/bgs124
34. Kang TW, Yevsa T, Woller N, Hoenicke L, Wuestefeld T, Dauch D, et al. Senescence surveillance of pre-malignant hepatocytes limits liver cancer development. *Nature.* (2011) 479:547–51. doi: 10.1038/nature10599
35. Kenyon CJ. The genetics of ageing. *Nature.* (2010) 464:504–12. doi: 10.1038/nature08980
36. Barzilai N, Huffman DM, Muzumdar RH, Bartke A. The critical role of metabolic pathways in aging. *Diabetes.* (2012) 61:1315–22. doi: 10.2337/db11-1300
37. Houtkooper RH, Williams RW, Auwerx J. Metabolic networks of longevity. *Cell.* (2010) 142:9–14. doi: 10.1016/j.cell.2010.06.029
38. Sahin E, DePinho RA. Axis of ageing: telomeres, p53 and mitochondria. *Nat Rev Mol Cell. Biol.* (2012) 13:397–404. doi: 10.1038/nrm3352
39. Wang K, Klionsky DJ. Mitochondria removal by autophagy. *Autophagy.* (2011) 7:297–300. doi: 10.4161/auto.7.3.14502
40. Szarc vel Szic K, Declerck K, Vidakovic M, Vanden Berghe W. From inflammaging to healthy aging by dietary lifestyle choices: is epigenetics the key to personalized nutrition? *Clin Epigenet.* (2015) 7:33. doi: 10.1186/s13148-015-0068-2
41. Giunta S. Exploring the complex relations between inflammation and aging (inflamm-aging): anti-inflamm-aging remodelling of inflamm-aging, from robustness to frailty. *Inflamm Res.* (2008) 57:558–63. doi: 10.1007/s00011-008-7243-2
42. Tchkonia T, Morbeck DE, Von Zglinicki T, Van Deursen J, Lustgarten J, Scrable H, et al. Fat tissue, aging, and cellular senescence. *Aging Cell.* (2010) 9:667–84. doi: 10.1111/j.1474-9726.2010.00608.x
43. Tran TT, Yamamoto Y, Gesta S, Kahn CR. Beneficial effects of subcutaneous fat transplantation on metabolism. *Cell Metab.* (2008) 7:410–20. doi: 10.1016/j.cmet.2008.04.004
44. Bonomini F, Rodella LF, Rezzani R. Metabolic syndrome, aging and involvement of oxidative stress. *Aging Dis.* (2015) 6:109–20. doi: 10.14336/AD.2014.0305
45. Premoli A, Paschetta E, Hvalryg M, Spandre M, Bo S, Durazzo M. Characteristics of liver diseases in the elderly: a review. *Minerva Gastroenterol Dietol.* (2009) 55:71–8.
46. Gan L, Chitturi S, Farrell GC. Mechanisms and implications of age-related changes in the liver: nonalcoholic Fatty liver disease in the elderly. *Curr Gerontol Geriatr Res.* (2011) 2011:831536. doi: 10.1155/2011/831536
47. Gagliano N, Grizzi F, Annoni G. Mechanisms of aging and liver functions. *Dig Dis.* (2007) 25:118–23. doi: 10.1159/000099475
48. Jiang Y, Iakova P, Jin J, Sullivan E, Sharin V, Hong IH, et al. Farnesoid X receptor inhibits gankyrin in mouse livers and prevents development of liver cancer. *Hepatology.* (2013) 57:1098–106. doi: 10.1002/hep.26146
49. Jin J, Wang GL, Shi X, Darlington GJ, Timchenko NA. The age-associated decline of glycogen synthase kinase 3beta plays a critical role in the inhibition of liver regeneration. *Mol Cell Biol.* (2009) 29:3867–80. doi: 10.1128/MCB.00456-09
50. Jin J, Iakova P, Jiang Y, Medrano EE, Timchenko NA. The reduction of SIRT1 in livers of old mice leads to impaired body homeostasis and to inhibition of liver proliferation. *Hepatology.* (2011) 54:989–98. doi: 10.1002/hep.24471

51. Timchenko NA. Aging and liver regeneration. *Trends Endocrinol Metab.* (2009) 20:171–6. doi: 10.1016/j.tem.2009.01.005
52. Slawik M, Vidal-Puig AJ. Lipotoxicity, overnutrition and energy metabolism in aging. *Ageing Res Rev.* (2006) 5:144–64. doi: 10.1016/j.arr.2006.03.004
53. Floreani A. Liver diseases in the elderly: an update. *Dig Dis.* (2007) 25:138–43. doi: 10.1159/000099478
54. Regev A, Schiff ER. Liver disease in the elderly. *Gastroenterol Clin North Am.* (2001) 30:547–63, x–xi. doi: 10.1016/S0889-8553(05)70195-3
55. Frith J, Jones D, Newton JL. Chronic liver disease in an ageing population. *Age Ageing.* (2009) 38:11–8. doi: 10.1093/ageing/afn242
56. Cogger VC, Svistounov D, Warren A, Zykova S, Melvin RG, Solon-Biet SM, et al. Liver aging and pseudocapillarization in a Werner syndrome mouse model. *J Gerontol A Biol Sci Med Sci.* (2014) 69:1076–86. doi: 10.1093/gerona/glt169
57. Cogger VC, Warren A, Fraser R, Ngu M, McLean AJ, Le Couteur DG. Hepatic sinusoidal pseudocapillarization with aging in the non-human primate. *Exp Gerontol.* (2003) 38:1101–7. doi: 10.1016/j.exger.2003.07.002
58. Maeso-Diaz R, Ortega-Ribera M, Lafoz E, Lozano JJ, Baiges A, Frances R, et al. Aging influences hepatic microvascular biology and liver fibrosis in advanced chronic liver disease. *Aging Dis.* (2019) 10:684–98. doi: 10.14336/AD.2019.0127
59. Mohamad M, Mitchell SJ, Wu LE, White MY, Cordwell SJ, Mach J, et al. Ultrastructure of the liver microcirculation influences hepatic and systemic insulin activity and provides a mechanism for age-related insulin resistance. *Aging Cell.* (2016) 15:706–15. doi: 10.1111/acel.12481
60. Basso A, Piantanelli L, Rossolini G, Roth GS. Reduced DNA synthesis in primary cultures of hepatocytes from old mice is restored by thymus grafts. *J Gerontol A Biol Sci Med Sci.* (1998) 53:B111–6. doi: 10.1093/gerona/53A.2.B111
61. Blokker BA, Maijo M, Echeandia M, Galduroz M, Patterson AM, Ten A, et al. Fine-tuning of Sirtuin 1 expression is essential to protect the liver from cholestatic liver disease. *Hepatology.* (2019) 69:699–716. doi: 10.1002/hep.30275
62. Lazzerini Denchi E, Celli G, de Lange T. Hepatocytes with extensive telomere deprotection and fusion remain viable and regenerate liver mass through endoreduplication. *Genes Dev.* (2006) 20:2648–53. doi: 10.1101/gad.1453606
63. Lin S, Nascimento EM, Gajera CR, Chen L, Neuhofer P, Garbuzov A, et al. Distributed hepatocytes expressing telomerase repopulate the liver in homeostasis and injury. *Nature.* (2018) 556:244–8. doi: 10.1038/s41586-018-0004-7
64. Irvine KM, Skoien R, Bokil NJ, Melino M, Thomas GP, Loo D, et al. Senescent human hepatocytes express a unique secretory phenotype and promote macrophage migration. *World J Gastroenterol.* (2014) 20:17851–62. doi: 10.3748/wjg.v20.i47.17851
65. Aravinthan A, Shannon N, Heaney J, Hoare M, Marshall A, Alexander GJ. The senescent hepatocyte gene signature in chronic liver disease. *Exp Gerontol.* (2014) 60:37–45. doi: 10.1016/j.exger.2014.09.011
66. Daum B, Walter A, Horst A, Osiewacz HD, Kuhlbrandt W. Age-dependent dissociation of ATP synthase dimers and loss of inner-membrane cristae in mitochondria. *Proc Natl Acad Sci USA.* (2013) 110:15301–6. doi: 10.1073/pnas.1305462110
67. Hagen TM, Yowe DL, Bartholomew JC, Wehr CM, Do KL, Park JY, et al. Mitochondrial decay in hepatocytes from old rats: membrane potential declines, heterogeneity and oxidants increase. *Proc Natl Acad Sci USA.* (1997) 94:3064–9. doi: 10.1073/pnas.94.7.3064
68. Xu X, Hueckstaedt LK, Ren J. Deficiency of insulin-like growth factor 1 attenuates aging-induced changes in hepatic function: role of autophagy. *J Hepatol.* (2013) 59:308–17. doi: 10.1016/j.jhep.2013.03.037
69. Rubinsztein DC, Marino G, Kroemer G. Autophagy and aging. *Cell.* (2011) 146:682–95. doi: 10.1016/j.cell.2011.07.030
70. Maeso-Diaz R, Ortega-Ribera M, Fernandez-Iglesias A, Hide D, Munoz L, Hessheimer AJ, et al. Effects of aging on liver microcirculatory function and sinusoidal phenotype. *Aging Cell.* (2018) 17:e12829. doi: 10.1111/acel.12829
71. Hunt NJ, Kang SWS, Lockwood GP, Le Couteur DG, Cogger VC. Hallmarks of aging in the liver. *Comput Struct Biotechnol J.* (2019) 17:1151–61. doi: 10.1016/j.csbj.2019.07.021
72. Tsuchida T, Friedman SL. Mechanisms of hepatic stellate cell activation. *Nat Rev Gastroenterol Hepatol.* (2017) 14:397–411. doi: 10.1038/nrgastro.2017.38
73. Warren A, Cogger VC, Fraser R, Deleve LD, McCuskey RS, Le Couteur DG. The effects of old age on hepatic stellate cells. *Curr Gerontol Geriatr Res.* (2011) 2011:439835. doi: 10.1155/2011/439835
74. Cheng Y, Wang X, Wang B, Zhou H, Dang S, Shi Y, et al. Aging-associated oxidative stress inhibits liver progenitor cell activation in mice. *Aging.* (2017) 9:1359–74. doi: 10.18632/aging.101232
75. Saarinen S, Olerup O, Broome U. Increased frequency of autoimmune diseases in patients with primary sclerosing cholangitis. *Am J Gastroenterol.* (2000) 95:3195–9. doi: 10.1111/j.1572-0241.2000.03292.x
76. Boonstra K, Beuers U, Ponsioen CY. Epidemiology of primary sclerosing cholangitis and primary biliary cirrhosis: a systematic review. *J Hepatol.* (2012) 56:1181–8. doi: 10.1016/j.jhep.2011.10.025
77. Corpechot C, Chretien Y, Chazouilleres O, Poupon R. Demographic, lifestyle, medical and familial factors associated with primary biliary cirrhosis. *J Hepatol.* (2010) 53:162–9. doi: 10.1016/j.jhep.2010.02.019
78. Lleo A, Jepsen P, Morenghi E, Carbone M, Moroni L, Battezzati PM, et al. Evolving trends in female to male incidence and male mortality of primary biliary cholangitis. *Sci Rep.* (2016) 6:25906. doi: 10.1038/srep25906
79. Prince M, Chetwynd A, Newman W, Metcalf JV, James OF. Survival and symptom progression in a geographically based cohort of patients with primary biliary cirrhosis: follow-up for up to 28 years. *Gastroenterology.* (2002) 123:1044–51. doi: 10.1053/gast.2002.36027
80. Cheung AC, Lammers WJ, Murillo Perez CF, van Buuren HR, Gulamhusein A, Trivedi PJ, et al. Effects of age and sex of response to ursodeoxycholic acid and transplant-free survival in patients with primary biliary cholangitis. *Clin Gastroenterol Hepatol.* (2019) 17:2076–84.e2. doi: 10.1016/j.cgh.2018.12.028
81. Weismuller TJ, Trivedi PJ, Bergquist A, Imam M, Lenzen H, Ponsioen CY, et al. Patient age, sex, and inflammatory bowel disease phenotype associate with course of primary sclerosing cholangitis. *Gastroenterology.* (2017) 152:1975–84.e8. doi: 10.1053/j.gastro.2017.02.038
82. Welling TH, Heidt DG, Englesbe MJ, Magee JC, Sung RS, Campbell DA, et al. Biliary complications following liver transplantation in the model for end-stage liver disease era: effect of donor, recipient, and technical factors. *Liver Transplant.* (2008) 14:73–80. doi: 10.1002/lt.21354
83. Randall HB, Cao S, deVera ME. Transplantation in elderly patients. *Arch Surg.* (2003) 138:1089–92. doi: 10.1001/archsurg.138.10.1089
84. Mousa OY, Nguyen JH, Ma Y, Rawal B, Musto KR, Dougherty MK, et al. Evolving role of liver transplantation in elderly recipients. *Liver Transplant.* (2019) 25:1363–74. doi: 10.1002/lt.25589
85. Tabibian JH, O'Hara SP, Splinter PL, Trussoni CE, LaRusso NF. Cholangiocyte senescence by way of N-ras activation is a characteristic of primary sclerosing cholangitis. *Hepatology.* (2014) 59:2263–75. doi: 10.1002/hep.26993
86. O'Hara SP, Splinter PL, Trussoni CE, Gajdos GB, Lineswala PN, LaRusso NF. Cholangiocyte N-Ras protein mediates lipopolysaccharide-induced interleukin 6 secretion and proliferation. *J Biol Chem.* (2011) 286:30352–60. doi: 10.1074/jbc.M111.269464
87. Young AR, Narita M, Ferreira M, Kirschner K, Sadaie M, Darot JF, et al. Autophagy mediates the mitotic senescence transition. *Genes Dev.* (2009) 23:798–803. doi: 10.1101/gad.519709
88. Sasaki M, Miyakoshi M, Sato Y, Nakanuma Y. A possible involvement of p62/sequestosome-1 in the process of biliary epithelial autophagy and senescence in primary biliary cirrhosis. *Liver Int.* (2012) 32:487–99. doi: 10.1111/j.1478-3231.2011.02656.x
89. Sasaki M, Miyakoshi M, Sato Y, Nakanuma Y. Autophagy may precede cellular senescence of bile ductular cells in ductular reaction in primary biliary cirrhosis. *Dig Dis Sci.* (2012) 57:660–6. doi: 10.1007/s10620-011-1929-y
90. Sasaki M, Ikeda H, Sato Y, Nakanuma Y. Decreased expression of Bmi1 is closely associated with cellular senescence in small bile ducts in primary biliary cirrhosis. *Am J Pathol.* (2006) 169:831–45. doi: 10.2353/ajpath.2006.051237

91. Sasaki M, Miyakoshi M, Sato Y, Nakanuma Y. Increased expression of mitochondrial proteins associated with autophagy in biliary epithelial lesions in primary biliary cirrhosis. *Liver Int.* (2013) 33:312–20. doi: 10.1111/liv.12049
92. Tabibian JH, Macura SI, O'Hara SP, Fidler JL, Glockner JF, Takahashi N, et al. Micro-computed tomography and nuclear magnetic resonance imaging for noninvasive, live-mouse cholangiography. *Lab Invest.* (2013) 93:733–43. doi: 10.1038/labinvest.2013.52
93. Sasaki M, Ikeda H, Yamaguchi J, Nakada S, Nakanuma Y. Telomere shortening in the damaged small bile ducts in primary biliary cirrhosis reflects ongoing cellular senescence. *Hepatology.* (2008) 48:186–95. doi: 10.1002/hep.22348
94. Sasaki M, Miyakoshi M, Sato Y, Nakanuma Y. Modulation of the microenvironment by senescent biliary epithelial cells may be involved in the pathogenesis of primary biliary cirrhosis. *J Hepatol.* (2010) 53:318–25. doi: 10.1016/j.jhep.2010.03.008
95. Govindarajan KK. Biliary atresia: Where do we stand now? *World J Hepatol.* (2016) 8:1593–601. doi: 10.4254/wjh.v8.i36.1593
96. Liu Y, Meyer C, Xu C, Weng H, Hellerbrand C, ten Dijke P, et al. Animal models of chronic liver diseases. *Am J Physiol Gastrointest Liver Physiol.* (2013) 304:G449–68. doi: 10.1152/ajpgi.00199.2012
97. Fickert P, Pollheimer MJ, Beuers U, Lackner C, Hirschfield G, Housset C, et al. Characterization of animal models for primary sclerosing cholangitis (PSC). *J Hepatol.* (2014) 60:1290–303. doi: 10.1016/j.jhep.2014.02.006
98. Sato K, Glaser S, Kennedy L, Liangpunsakul S, Meng F, Francis H, et al. Preclinical insights into cholangiopathies: disease modeling and emerging therapeutic targets. *Expert Opin Ther Targets.* (2019) 23:461–72. doi: 10.1080/14728222.2019.1608950
99. Andersen IM, Tengesdal G, Lie BA, Boberg KM, Karlsen TH, Hov JR. Effects of coffee consumption, smoking, and hormones on risk for primary sclerosing cholangitis. *Clin Gastroenterol Hepatol.* (2014) 12:1019–28. doi: 10.1016/j.cgh.2013.09.024
100. Hagstrom H, Stal P, Stokkeland K, Bergquist A. Alcohol consumption in patients with primary sclerosing cholangitis. *World J Gastroenterol.* (2012) 18:3105–11. doi: 10.3748/wjg.v18.i24.3105
101. Liu JZ, Hov JR, Folseraas T, Ellinghaus E, Rushbrook SM, Doncheva NT, et al. Dense genotyping of immune-related disease regions identifies nine new risk loci for primary sclerosing cholangitis. *Nat Genet.* (2013) 45:670–5. doi: 10.1038/ng.2616
102. Lazaridis KN, LaRusso NF. The Cholangiopathies. *Mayo Clin Proc.* (2015) 90:791–800. doi: 10.1016/j.mayocp.2015.03.017
103. Hirschfield GM, Karlsen TH, Lindor KD, Adams DH. Primary sclerosing cholangitis. *Lancet.* (2013) 382:1587–99. doi: 10.1016/S0140-6736(13)60096-3
104. Trivedi PJ, Adams DH. Gut-liver immunity. *J Hepatol.* (2016) 64:1187–9. doi: 10.1016/j.jhep.2015.12.002
105. Tabibian JH, O'Hara SP, Lindor KD. Primary sclerosing cholangitis and the microbiota: current knowledge and perspectives on etiopathogenesis and emerging therapies. *Scand J Gastroenterol.* (2014) 49:901–8. doi: 10.3109/00365521.2014.913189
106. Kummen M, Holm K, Anmarkrud JA, Nygard S, Vesterhus M, Hoivik ML, et al. The gut microbial profile in patients with primary sclerosing cholangitis is distinct from patients with ulcerative colitis without biliary disease and healthy controls. *Gut.* (2017) 66:611–9. doi: 10.1136/gutjnl-2015-310500
107. Zhou T, Wu N, Meng F, Venter J, Giang TK, Francis H, et al. Knockout of secretin receptor reduces biliary damage and liver fibrosis in $Mdr2^{-}/^{-}$ mice by diminishing senescence of cholangiocytes. *Lab Invest.* (2018) 98:1449–64. doi: 10.1038/s41374-018-0093-9
108. Wu N, Meng F, Zhou T, Venter J, Giang TK, Kyritsi K, et al. The Secretin/Secretin receptor axis modulates ductular reaction and liver fibrosis through changes in transforming growth factor-beta1-mediated biliary senescence. *Am J Pathol.* (2018) 188:2264–80. doi: 10.1016/j.ajpath.2018.06.015
109. Wan Y, Meng F, Wu N, Zhou T, Venter J, Francis H, et al. Substance P increases liver fibrosis by differential changes in senescence of cholangiocytes and hepatic stellate cells. *Hepatology.* (2017) 66:528–41. doi: 10.1002/hep.29138
110. Nevens F, Andreone P, Mazzella G, Strasser SI, Bowlus C, Invernizzi P, et al. A placebo-controlled trial of obeticholic acid in primary biliary cholangitis. *N Engl J Med.* (2016) 375:631–43. doi: 10.1056/NEJMoa1509840
111. Kowdley KV, Luketic V, Chapman R, Hirschfield GM, Poupon R, Schramm C, et al. A randomized trial of obeticholic acid monotherapy in patients with primary biliary cholangitis. *Hepatology.* (2018) 67:1890–902. doi: 10.1002/hep.29569
112. Rodriguez EA, Carey EJ, Lindor KD. Emerging treatments for primary sclerosing cholangitis. *Expert Rev Gastroenterol Hepatol.* (2017) 11:451–9. doi: 10.1080/17474124.2017.1293524
113. Harms MH, van Buuren HR, van der Meer AJ. Improving prognosis in primary biliary cholangitis–therapeutic options and strategy. *Best Pract Res Clin Gastroenterol.* (2018) 34–35:85–94. doi: 10.1016/j.bpg.2018.06.004
114. Alpini G, Baiocchi L, Glaser S, Ueno Y, Marzioni M, Francis H, et al. Ursodeoxycholate and tauroursodeoxycholate inhibit cholangiocyte growth and secretion of BDL rats through activation of PKC alpha. *Hepatology.* (2002) 35:1041–52. doi: 10.1053/jhep.2002.32712
115. Gong Y, Huang Z, Christensen E, Gluud C. Ursodeoxycholic acid for patients with primary biliary cirrhosis: an updated systematic review and meta-analysis of randomized clinical trials using Bayesian approach as sensitivity analyses. *Am J Gastroenterol.* (2007) 102:1799–807. doi: 10.1111/j.1572-0241.2007.01235.x
116. Beuers U. Drug insight: mechanisms and sites of action of ursodeoxycholic acid in cholestasis. *Nat Clin Pract Gastroenterol Hepatol.* (2006) 3:318–28. doi: 10.1038/ncpgasthep0521
117. McDaniel K, Meng F, Wu N, Sato K, Venter J, Bernuzzi F, et al. Forkhead box A2 regulates biliary heterogeneity and senescence during cholestatic liver injury in micedouble dagger. *Hepatology.* (2017) 65:544–59. doi: 10.1002/hep.28831
118. Jones H, Hargrove L, Kennedy L, Meng F, Graf-Eaton A, Owens J, et al. Inhibition of mast cell-secreted histamine decreases biliary proliferation and fibrosis in primary sclerosing cholangitis $Mdr2^{-}/^{-}$ mice. *Hepatology.* (2016) 64:1202–16. doi: 10.1002/hep.28704
119. Meadows V, Kennedy L, Hargrove L, Demieville J, Meng F, Virani S, et al. Downregulation of hepatic stem cell factor by vivo-morpholino treatment inhibits mast cell migration and decreases biliary damage/senescence and liver fibrosis in $Mdr2^{-}/^{-}$ mice. *Biochim Biophys Acta Mol Basis Dis.* (2019) 1865:165557. doi: 10.1016/j.bbadis.2019.165557
120. Quist RG, Ton-Nu HT, Lillienau J, Hofmann AF, Barrett KE. Activation of mast cells by bile acids. *Gastroenterology.* (1991) 101:446–56. doi: 10.1016/0016-5085(91)90024-F
121. Yamazaki K, Suzuki K, Nakamura A, Sato S, Lindor KD, Batts KP, et al. Ursodeoxycholic acid inhibits eosinophil degranulation in patients with primary biliary cirrhosis. *Hepatology.* (1999) 30:71–8. doi: 10.1002/hep.510300121
122. Baiocchi L, Zhou T, Liangpunsakul S, Ilaria L, Milana M, Meng F, et al. Possible application of melatonin treatment in human diseases of the biliary tract. *Am J Physiol Gastrointest Liver Physiol.* (2019) 317:G651–60. doi: 10.1152/ajpgi.00110.2019
123. Glaser S, Gaudio E, Renzi A, Mancinelli R, Ueno Y, Venter J, et al. Knockout of the neurokinin-1 receptor reduces cholangiocyte proliferation in bile duct-ligated mice. *Am J Physiol Gastrointest Liver Physiol.* (2011) 301:G297–305. doi: 10.1152/ajpgi.00418.2010
124. Maroni L, Pinto C, Giordano DM, Saccomanno S, Banales JM, Spallacci D, et al. aging-related expression of twinfilin-1 regulates cholangiocyte biological response to injury. *Hepatology.* (2019) 70:883–98. doi: 10.1002/hep.30466
125. Aravinthan AD, Alexander GJM. Senescence in chronic liver disease: is the future in aging? *J Hepatol.* (2016) 65:825–34. doi: 10.1016/j.jhep.2016.05.030
126. Tsuneyama K, Saito K, Ruebner BH, Konishi I, Nakanuma Y, Gershwin ME. Immunological similarities between primary sclerosing cholangitis and chronic sclerosing sialadenitis: report of the overlapping of these two autoimmune diseases. *Dig Dis Sci.* (2000) 45:366–72. doi: 10.1023/A:1005429130150
127. Satomura K, Yin M, Shimizu S, Kato Y, Nagano T, Komeichi H, et al. Increased chymase in livers with autoimmune disease: colocalization with fibrosis. *J Nippon Med Sch.* (2003) 70:490–5. doi: 10.1272/jnms.70.490

128. Meng F, Kennedy L, Hargrove L, Demieville J, Jones H, Madeka T, et al. Ursodeoxycholate inhibits mast cell activation and reverses biliary injury and fibrosis in Mdr2^{-}/$^{-}$ mice and human primary sclerosing cholangitis. *Lab Invest.* (2018) 98:1465–77. doi: 10.1038/s41374-018-0101-0
129. Lindor KD, Dickson ER, Baldus WP, Jorgensen RA, Ludwig J, Murtaugh PA, et al. Ursodeoxycholic acid in the treatment of primary biliary cirrhosis. *Gastroenterology.* (1994) 106:1284–90. doi: 10.1016/0016-5085(94)90021-3
130. Zhu Y, Tchkonia T, Pirtskhalava T, Gower AC, Ding H, Giorgadze N, et al. The Achilles' heel of senescent cells: from transcriptome to senolytic drugs. *Aging Cell.* (2015) 14:644–58. doi: 10.1111/acel.12344

15

Hepatic Autonomic Nervous System and Neurotrophic Factors Regulate the Pathogenesis and Progression of Non-alcoholic Fatty Liver Disease

Muhammad Amir [1], Michael Yu [2], Peijian He [1] and Shanthi Srinivasan [1,3]*

[1] *Division of Digestive Diseases, Department of Medicine, Emory University School of Medicine, Atlanta, GA, United States,* [2] *Department of Medicine, Emory University School of Medicine, Atlanta, GA, United States,* [3] *Research-Gastroenterology, Atlanta VA Health Care System, Decatur, GA, United States*

***Correspondence:**
Shanthi Srinivasan
ssrini2@emory.edu

Non-alcoholic fatty liver disease represents a continuum of excessive hepatic steatosis, inflammation and fibrosis. It is a growing epidemic in the United States of America and worldwide. Progression of non-alcoholic fatty liver disease can lead to morbidity and mortality due to complications such as cirrhosis or hepatocellular carcinoma. Pathogenesis of non-alcoholic fatty liver disease is centered on increased hepatic lipogenesis and decreased hepatic lipolysis in the setting of hepatic and systemic insulin resistance. Adipose tissue and hepatic inflammation can further perpetuate the severity of illness. Currently there are no approved therapies for non-alcoholic fatty liver disease. Most of the drugs being explored for non-alcoholic fatty liver disease focus on classical pathogenic pathways surrounding hepatic lipid accumulation, inflammation or fibrosis. Studies have demonstrated that the autonomic nervous system innervating the liver plays a crucial role in regulation of hepatic lipid homeostasis, inflammation and fibrosis. Additionally, there is growing evidence that neurotrophic factors can modulate all stages of non-alcoholic fatty liver disease. Both the autonomic nervous system and neurotrophic factors are altered in patients and murine models of non-alcoholic fatty liver disease. In this review we focus on the pathophysiological role of the autonomic nervous system and neurotrophic factors that could be potential targets for novel therapeutic approaches to treat non-alcoholic fatty liver disease.

Keywords: autonomic nervous system, fibrosis, GDNF, NAFLD, NASH, neurotrophic factors

INTRODUCTION

Non-alcoholic fatty liver disease (NAFLD) is rapidly becoming a significant global burden by affecting over 25% of the adult population (1). NAFLD encompasses a continuous range of liver conditions covering steatosis, steatohepatitis, fibrosis, and cirrhosis (2). It is projected to be the leading indication for liver transplantation in the next 20 years (3). The pathogenesis of NAFLD remains poorly understood and therapeutic approaches are still being explored. Currently there is no approved drug therapy for NAFLD by the Food and Drug Administration. Mechanisms for hepatic steatosis involve insulin resistance, an excess influx of fatty acids into the liver, enhanced *de novo* lipogenesis, impaired lipophagy and resultant triglyceride accumulation in hepatocytes (2, 4). Steatosis progresses to non-alcoholic steatohepatitis (NASH) when inflammation develops due to mitochondrial dysfunction, endoplasmic reticulum stress, activation of the innate immune system, and dysregulation of autophagy (2, 3). Fibrosis is primarily mediated by hepatic stellate cells (HSCs), which are mesenchymal cells and part of the repair system of injured liver. Stellate cells are quiescent in homeostatic condition, but are transformed to myofibroblast-like cells in response to oxidative stress, lipopolysaccharide (LPS), apoptotic bodies and paracrine stimuli from neighboring cells. Activated stellate cells are the main source of extracellular fibrous matrix in the development of fibrosis and cirrhosis (5–7).

Both murine and primate livers are innervated by autonomic nervous system (ANS). Sympathetic and parasympathetic branches of ANS play critical roles in energy homeostasis, liver injury and repair (8–10). Both parenchymal and non-parenchymal cells in liver express receptors for common neurotransmitters (11–14). HSCs are considered as resident hepatic neuroglia functioning as neuroendocrine cells in close proximity with hepatic nervous system. HSCs express various neuroglial marker proteins such as nestin, neural cell adhesion molecule, glial acidic fibrillary protein, and synaptophysin. HSCs also express receptors for serotonin, adrenergic or muscarinic neurotransmitters, cannabinoids and opioids (15). Despite the rich hepatic supply by ANS and its interactions with hepatic cells, its role in the pathogenesis and progression of NAFLD remains elusive.

Neurotrophic factors play an integral role in the development and function of nervous system, and are involved in pathogenesis of neurodegenerative and psychiatric disorders (16). Consequently, various neurotrophic factors have been explored as therapeutic agents in treatment of neurological disorders (17, 18). Several neurotrophic factors and their receptors are expressed in various hepatic cell types (19–21), and regulate insulin sensitivity, lipid homeostasis, cellular injury and fibrosis of the liver (22–26). However, their potential in management of liver diseases including NAFLD remains mostly unexplored. This review summarizes current knowledge about the role of ANS and neurotrophic factors in modulation of hepatic steatosis, NASH, and NASH-associated hepatic fibrosis.

HEPATIC NERVOUS SYSTEM

The liver is regulated by both sympathetic and parasympathetic branches of the central nervous system using aminergic, peptinergic, adrenergic, and cholinergic nerve endings (8). Sympathetic nerve fibers supply the liver via the splanchnic nerve and start in celiac and superior mesenteric ganglia that are under influence of intermediolateral column of spinal cord (8, 9). In rodents, sympathetic nerves have been detected only up to the portal tracts surrounding hepatic artery and portal veins (27). It is postulated that connecting gap junctions further transmit electrical signals between the hepatocytes in rodents (28) as well as in humans (8, 9). Sympathetic nerve fibers directly supply nerve endings to hepatic lobules and along hepatic sinusoids in humans and guinea-pigs. Sympathetic nerve fibers however are absent in regenerating nodules in livers affected by cirrhosis (27, 29). The Vagus nerve supplies parasympathetic neurons originating in dorsal motor nucleus and relays their nerve endings directly to the liver or indirectly via hepatic hilar ganglia (8, 9, 30). Like sympathetic nerve fibers, parasympathetic or cholinergic fibers penetrate deep into hepatic parenchyma (31). Cholinergic fibers directly interact with HSCs and the quantity of these nerve fibers increases in fibrous septa in livers of carbon tetrachloride (CCl_4)-treated rats (32, 33). Alpha/beta-adrenergic receptors and muscarinic cholinergic receptors are expressed by hepatocytes and HSCs (11, 12, 34–37), while nicotinic acetylcholine receptors are present in hepatocytes, Kupffer cells, macrophages, and dendritic cells (13, 14). Overall, sympathetic and parasympathetic nerve endings can relay signals to liver cells through three different mechanisms: (1) direct innervation onto or near cells by secreting norepinephrine, acetylcholine and neuropeptides such as galanin, neuropeptide Y, etc.; (2) spreading of ions or small molecules using gap junctions; (3) innervation of sinusoidal endothelial and Kupffer cells which communicate with hepatocytes via eicosanoids, cytokines, endothelin, and nitric oxide (38).

Afferent fibers of the sympathetic nervous system (SNS) and parasympathetic nervous system (PSNS) sense levels of ions, glucose, free fatty acids, cytokines as well as hormones such as glucagon like peptide-1 and cholecystokinin. This sensory information is then relayed to the hypothalamus, which in turn modulates sympathetic or parasympathetic outflow to control hepatic energy homeostasis (8, 9). Activation of SNS leads to increased gluconeogenesis and decreased glycogenesis, whereas parasympathetic activation plays an opposite role. In addition, hepatic sympathetic supply also regulates lipoprotein secretion, beta oxidation, ketone body synthesis and release (30).

Sympathetic Nervous System and Non-alcoholic Steatohepatitis

Limited investigations have been done to study the role of SNS in pathogenesis of NASH. Overexpression of adrenergic β-receptors in cultured hepatocytes from rats or mice causes an increase in lipid accumulation (39). Hurr et al. showed that sympathetic nerve activity doubled after 10 weeks of high-fat diet (HFD) feeding in mice. Chemical ablation of sympathetic nerves significantly reversed steatosis in just 3 days with improvement in hepatomegaly and hepatic triglyceride content without affecting food intake, energy expenditure or body mass. Whole body chemical sympathectomy lowered hepatic expression of gluconeogenic enzymes and peroxisome proliferator activated receptor (PPAR) alpha (40). PPARs such as PPARα and PPARγ are transcription factors that are central in the regulation of lipid, glucose and amino acid metabolism, maintaining the homeostasis of adipose tissue and hepatocytes (41, 42). Selective hepatic sympathetic denervation using phenol also resulted in similar impact on hepatic gluconeogenic enzymes and led to almost complete resolution of hepatic steatosis in 1 week (40). Mechanistically, hepatic denervation attenuated HFD-increased hepatic expression of *CD36* (a fatty acid transporter), *PPARα*, and *Diacyl-glycerol O-acyltransferase (DGAT) 1* and *DGAT2*, which encode critical enzymes catalyzing the final step of triglyceride synthesis. Hepatic denervation however did not affect mitochondrial or peroxiosomal β-oxidation of fatty acids (40). Hepatic β-adrenergic activity increases with aging in murine models (39), and aging itself is linked with development of NASH (43). Ghosh et al. reported that older rats accumulated even more fat in livers as compared to younger rats with pharmacologic β-adrenergic stimulation (39). Age-related increase in sympathetic activity may thus be a critical link toward development of NASH. In summary, HFD and aging increase hepatic sympathetic activity elevating hepatic lipid burden, whereas surgical or pharmacological ablation of hepatic sympathetic supply ameliorates hepatic steatosis.

Sympathetic Nervous System and Hepatic Fibrosis

SNS is overly activated in humans with advanced fibrosis or cirrhosis and in animal models of liver fibrosis. Patients with cirrhosis elicit increased levels of catecholamines in blood and enhanced sympathetic nerve activity (44, 45). In mice, over-activity of SNS worsens CCl_4-mediated fibrosis, whereas dampened sympathetic tone renders lowered susceptibility (46). Norepinephrine, a type of catecholamine, increases the proliferation of cultured HSCs, which is inhibited by alpha- and beta-adrenergic receptor antagonists. Moreover, murine HSCs produce catecholamine and norepinephrine (12). Norepinephrine promotes HSC proliferation likely through the activation of PI3K and MAPK/ERK signaling cascades. Norepinephrine also induces HSC expression of collagen (12, 47). Oben et al. further showed that treatment with norepinephrine induces proliferation of HSCs *in vivo* in *ob/ob* mice. This catecholamine stimulation also results in increased expression of transforming growth factor beta (TGF-β) along with accentuated fibrosis (12). The above stimulatory effects of catecholamines on HSC proliferation as well as the expression of collagen and TGF-β were also found in cultured human HSCs as reported by Sigala et al. (48). Thus, the SNS branch of ANS is pro-fibrogenic in nature. These findings implicate that pharmacological or surgical disruption of sympathetic supply may be effective in preventing the progression to steatohepatitis and fibrosis.

Parasympathetic Nervous System and Non-alcoholic Steatohepatitis

Anti-inflammatory effects of the PSNS was first demonstrated in a landmark paper by Borovikova et al. They identified that nicotine, acetylcholine and cholinergic agonist carbachol inhibit LPS-mediated production of tumor necrosis factor (TNF) by peripheral blood macrophages. In addition, acetylcholine can inhibit the release of several other pro-inflammatory cytokines including IL-1β, IL-6, and IL-18, but not anti-inflammatory cytokine IL-10. Their work further revealed that electrical stimulation of vagus nerve decreases LPS-mediated hepatic TNF production whereas vagotomy stimulates TNF production (49). This inhibitory effect of vagal electrical stimulation or acetylcholine receptor (AChR) agonism on hepatic TNF production was validated in ischemia/reperfusion injury model. Inhibition of TNF production was at least in part mediated by decreased nuclear translocation of NF-κB (13). Li et al. reported that vagus nerve flow suppresses LPS/galactosamine-induced hepatocyte injury by attenuation of Kupffer cell activation through the activation of nicotinic α7nAchR receptors (50). PSNS also elicits anti-inflammatory effects in *db/db* and HFD-fed obese mice. Low dose nicotine improved insulin resistance in these mice whereas knockout of α7nAChR exacerbated insulin resistance with pro-inflammatory M1 macrophages infiltrating white adipose tissue (WAT). Nicotine also attenuated the production of pro-inflammatory cytokines in peritoneal macrophages induced by stearic acid or TNF (51).

Direct evidence of the role of parasympathetic anti-inflammatory pathway in NAFLD comes from work done by Nishio et al. They demonstrated that hepatic vagotomy worsened methionine-choline deficient diet induced steatohepatitis. Moreover, vagotomy led to activation of Kupffer cells along with downregulation of hepatic PPARα and an aggravated hepatic pro-inflammatory cytokine profile. Beneficial effect of cholinergic stimulation was mediated by activation of STAT3 pathway and inhibition of nuclear translocation of NF-κB. Chimeric mice with α7nAChR deficiency in Kupffer cells had significant aggravation of steatohepatitis. These mice had increased expression levels of enzymes responsible for fatty acid synthesis such as fatty acid synthase (FASN) (52). Galantamine is a cholinergic activator with a unique dual-mode of action via inhibition of acetylcholinesterase and by modulation of nicotinic acetylcholine receptors, and has been used in patients with Alzheimer's disease (53). Galantamine improves insulin resistance and serum lipid profile in streptozotocin-induced diabetic rats (54). HFD-fed mice treated by galantamine show decreased bodyweight and expression of pro-inflammatory cytokines as well as improved insulin resistance. These changes are accompanied by significant reduction in hepatic triglyceride content and marked improvement in hepatic steatosis and inflammation (55).

Taken together, PSNS plays anti-inflammatory role in multiple sites of the body including the liver primarily through modulation of cytokine production in macrophages and via reduction in hepatic lipid content.

Parasympathetic Nervous System and Hepatic Fibrosis

The role of PSNS in modulation of hepatic fibrosis remains mostly unclear due to limited number of studies. Given the anti-inflammatory role of PSNS in the setting of NAFLD, it is postulated that PSNS is anti-fibrotic indirectly by inhibition of HSC activation. However, Oben et al. showed that PSNS exerts pro-fibrotic effects. Treatment of HSCs in culture with acetylcholine increases the proliferation and collagen expression of HSCs whereas mecamylamine, an inhibitor of nAChRs receptor, abolishes this response (33). Luo et al. demonstrated that treatment with anisodamine, a non-specific cholinergic inhibitor, improves hepatic inflammation, accompanied by decreased production of TGF-β1, malondialdehyde, and hydroxyproline in the liver of CCl_4-treated mice (56). Of note, anisodamine is also an anti-oxidant agent (57). Thus, it is unclear whether anisodamine's effects attribute to decreased activity of the PSNS or inhibition of oxidative stress. Further studies are warranted toward a better understanding of the role of PSNS in the pathogenesis and progression of hepatic fibrosis.

NEUROTROPHIC FACTORS

Neurotrophic factors are small proteins or polypeptides that play crucial roles in the development, differentiation, migration, and survival of various neurons in central and peripheral nervous system (17, 58, 59). Major families of neurotrophic factors include neurotrophins or nerve growth factors (NGF), ciliary neurotrophic family (CNTF), glial cell line-derived neurotrophic factor (GDNF) family, and neuropoietic cytokines (17, 60). Early studies demonstrated the important role of neurotrophic factors in neuronal regeneration in neurodegenerative diseases (59, 60). Recent evidence has identified extra-neuronal role of neurotrophic factors in many other tissues, such as the liver, pancreas, heart, breast, lung, testis, ovary, etc. (61). Neurotrophic factors also regulate systemic energy homeostasis and insulin sensitivity. GDNF, brain-derived neurotrophic factor (BDNF, a NGF family member), CNTF and Neuregulin-4 (NRG4) are among the most studied neurotrophic factors in the context of NAFLD, and their roles are discussed below.

Glial Cell-Line Derived Neurotrophic Factor

GDNF is the most studied neurotrophic factor in GDNF family of proteins. Other members include neurturin, artemin and persephin (62). GDNF is a glycosylated, disulfide-bonded homodimer that has distant relation with TGF-β superfamily (63). It binds its cognate GDNF family receptor α_1 (GFRα1) (64, 65) stimulating intracellular PI3K/AKT and Ras/MAPK pathways (66). GDNF promotes the survival and differentiation of dopaminergic neurons (59, 63). GDNF also acts on non-neuronal cells by regulating spermatogenesis, salivary stem cell survival, and ureteral budding in embryonic kidney (67, 68). Our work has shown that GDNF and its cognate receptor are expressed in white adipose tissue (WAT), brown adipose tissue and the liver, playing an important role in lipid metabolism and the progression of NAFLD (69).

Glial Cell-Line Derived Neurotrophic Factor and Non-alcoholic Steatohepatitis

Hepatic deposition of fat leads to an increase in hepatic infiltration by inflammatory cells along with increased synthesis of cytokines such as TNF, IL-1β, and IL-6 (70–72). Thus, tight regulation of lipid metabolism in the liver has an important role in the progression of NAFLD. We used a transgenic mouse strain that overexpresses GDNF in central nervous system, enteric nervous system, WAT, brown adipose tissue and liver as described earlier. We have shown that GDNF has a protective effect on HFD induced obesity and hepatic steatosis (69). *GDNF* transgenic mice are resistant to HFD-induced obesity as well as insulin and leptin resistance. *GDNF* transgenic mice are also protected from developing hepatic steatosis as manifested by decreased steatosis and substantially lower triglyceride accumulation in the liver as compared to controls (20, 69). Mechanistically, overexpression of GDNF in transgenic mice reduced the expression of master regulators of lipid homeostasis, including sterol regulatory element binding transcription factor 1 (*SREBF1*), *PPARα*, *PPARγ*, and carnitine palmitoyltransferase 1 (*CPT1*), all of which are elevated in models of NAFLD. Specific analysis of *PPARγ* promoter has revealed an inhibitory effect of GDNF on *PPARγ* promoter activity in HepG2 cells (20). The *CD 36* gene, which encodes fatty acid translocase mediating fatty acid uptake in hepatocytes, is under direct control by transcription factor PPARα and PPARγ (42, 73). Transgenic expression of *GDNF* abrogated HFD-induced expression of CD 36 protein. *De novo* lipogenesis machinery was also diminished in *GDNF* transgenic mice as seen by significant reduction in the mRNA levels of *FASN*, stearoyl-CoA desaturase (*SCD-1*) and *DGAT2* while on HFD (20). The protective role of transgenic expression of GDNF against hepatic steatosis was recapitulated in a more therapeutic approach by using GDNF-loaded nanoparticles. Direct role of GDNF in improving hepatic lipid homeostasis has also been confirmed in heterozygous GFRα1 receptor-knockout mice, whereby the expression of *PPARα*, *PPARγ*, *CD36*, *FASN*, *DGAT2*, and *SCD-1* are all increased (20). Autophagy maintains insulin sensitivity, regulates lipid stores, and protects against the development of inflammation (4). Work in our lab has demonstrated a stimulatory effect of GDNF on hepatic macroautophagy (20, 74). As compared to HFD-fed WT mice, *GDNF* transgenic mice displayed reduced expression of autophagic marker p62/sequestosome-1 and increased expression of autophagy related 5 (Atg5), Beclin 1 and microtubule-associated protein-1 light chain 3 (20). This *in vivo* effect of GDNF was further confirmed by *in vitro* analysis of autophagic flux in primary mouse hepatocytes and secondary rat cell line (74).

In line with reduced hepatic steatosis, *GDNF* transgenic mice resist the development of hepatic inflammation when challenged with HFD (20, 69). GDNF-loaded nanoparticles also successfully attenuated hepatic inflammation in HFD-fed mice (20). Overall, these findings have revealed that GDNF plays a crucial role in HFD-induced hepatic steatosis through its effect on autophagy and critical transcription factors such as PPARα, PPARγ, and Srebf1. Thus, GDNF may be a therapeutic agent in reversing steatosis and steatohepatitis (20, 69). It however remains unexplored as to the source of GDNF in native hepatic tissues. Regardless, it is possible that GDNF functions as a trophic factor for hepatic neurons as well as executing direct effects on hepatic parenchymal and possibly non-parenchymal cells. Tao et al. analyzed human liver tissue specimens and primary cell lines from human livers, and showed that GDNF is likely present in human HSCs as it is colocalized with α-smooth muscle actin positive cells (21).

Glial Cell-Line Derived Neurotrophic Factor and Hepatic Fibrosis

Hepatic *GDNF* expression is elevated in patients with advanced liver fibrosis in conditions including NASH, alcoholic liver disease or hepatitis B virus infection. Serum GDNF level is increased in a stepwise fashion with the advancement of fibrosis stages. Similar results were seen in mouse fibrosis models. *GDNF* expression in the liver was increased by 2–4-folds in mice which received bile duct ligation or were fed with methionine-choline deficient diet, and by almost 13-fold in mice treated with CCl_4 (21). Whether the increase in GDNF plays a protective or exacerbating role in the pathogenesis of hepatic fibrosis remains elusive, and results are conflicting. Work from our laboratory has shown that GDNF negates hepatic fibrogenesis in HFD-fed mice. HFD-fed mice with administration of GDNF-loaded nanoparticles exhibited 4.5-fold less fibrosis as compared to control nanoparticles-treated mice (20). It is unclear if this modulation of hepatic fibrosis by GDNF was due to decreased hepatocyte injury or direct inhibition of HSC activation. Conversely, in the study by Tao et al. mice treated with GDNF-expressing adenovirus showed worsened fibrosis and increased hepatic expression of pro-inflammatory and pro-fibrotic genes in bile duct ligation and CCl_4 fibrotic models; whereas, GDNF knockdown lowered fibrosis burden. The same study showed that GDNF activated mouse HSCs *in vitro*. This pro-fibrotic role of GDNF in CCl_4 and bile duct ligation models of hepatic fibrosis is opposite to what was seen in our study with HFD-fed model of NAFLD (20). Although Tao et al. showed increased expression of hepatic *GDNF* in human and animal models of NASH, they did not determine the role of GDNF in the progression or prevention of NASH associated fibrosis. Further work is warranted to clarify the precise role of GDNF in the pathogenesis of liver fibrosis associated with NASH.

Brain-Derived Neurotrophic Factor

BDNF, a member of neurotrophin family, is the most studied neurotrophic factor due to its abundance in nervous system and brain. BDNF plays important roles in development, differentiation, maintenance, and regeneration of neurons (75, 76). It signals through p75 neurotrophin receptor and tropomyosin receptor kinases (77), which are expressed primarily in neurons as well as in a variety of tissues including the liver, pancreas, colon, breast, immune system, muscles, and prostrate. Multiple studies have shown that BDNF regulates energy homeostasis and the development of NAFLD. BDNF improves blood glucose and insulin resistance as well as hepatomegaly and inflammation in *db/db* mice (78–80). Tsuchida et al. showed that subcutaneous administration of BDNF to *db/db* mice decreased dyslipidemia, hepatic triglyceride content and hepatic steatosis (81). Comparison of BDNF with thiazolidinediones in *db/db* mice revealed that BDNF was superior to thiazolidinediones in decreasing food intake, reducing body weight, and ameliorating hepatic steatosis and hepatomegaly (82). These findings point toward the role of BDNF in improving dysregulated energy homeostasis, insulin resistance and hepatic steatosis. Thus, BDNF could potentially be used as an agent to treat hepatic steatosis. Further studies are needed to establish the beneficial effects of BDNF in the treatment of hepatic steatosis in other models of hepatic steatosis than *db/db* mice.

Ciliary Neurotrophic Factor

CNTF is a well-studied neurotrophic factor that is structurally related to IL-6 and is highly expressed in central and peripheral nervous system including PSNS. Its attachment to cognate CNTFα receptor initiates heterodimerization of leukemia inhibitory factor and gp130 receptors (83). This heterodimer then transduces signals intracellularly though JAK/STAT or Ras/MAPK pathways (84). CNTF also signals through IL-6 receptor, at least in humans (85). CNTF prevents degeneration and cell death of neuroglia, sensory, motor, hippocampal and cerebellar neurons (83). Nonogaki et al. showed that treatment of rats with CNTF promoted lipolysis and lipid export from liver (86). Sleeman et al. demonstrated that CNTF treatment increased basal metabolic rate of HFD-fed *db/db* mice. CNTF improved hepatomegaly, hepatic steatosis, and inflammation. These effects were associated with decreased hepatic expression of *SCD-1* and *glycerol-3-phosphate acyltransferase 1* that mediate *de novo* lipogenesis as well as increased expression of *PPARα* and *CPT-1* that promote mitochondrial β-oxidation (87). Cui et al. studied effects of recombinant human CNTF in HFD-fed rat model of obesity and hepatic steatosis. Treatment with CNTF significantly improved hepatic steatosis and serum markers of hepatic inflammation. In *in vitro* cultured HepG2 cells, CNTF increased the levels of *PPARα* and *CPT-1* and reduced the expression of *FASN*, *SCD-1*, and *SREBF1*. Overall these changes elucidated a peripheral role of CNTF in decreasing *de novo* lipogenesis and enhancing lipolysis in hepatocytes (88). Despite somewhat discouraging clinical outcomes of CNTF in the treatment of obesity due to various adverse effects and lack of long term effect, it remains an exciting and novel therapeutic agent to modulate hepatic steatosis (84). Modifications of CNTF molecule to improve its pharmacokinetics, efficacy, and reduction of immunogenicity could reignite its role in clinical applications.

Neuregulin-4

NRG4 is a neurotrophic factor that belongs to Neuregulin family of epidermal growth factor-like ligands and signals through tyrosinase kinase receptor members of the ErbB family (89). It regulates neuron development, adipocyte differentiation, brown adipose tissue thermogenesis, and energy homeostasis (90–92). It is also produced in both brown and white adipose tissues and then transduces signal to hepatocytes in an endocrine fashion through ErbB4 receptors. Expression of NRG4 is significantly higher in brown adipose tissues and expression of NRG4 in adipose tissues is inversely related with obesity in mice and human adipose tissue (92, 93). Decreased production of NRG4 in obesity is likely due to direct impact of pro-inflammatory cytokines produced in obesity such as TNF-α and IL-1β (92, 94). Wang et al. showed that HFD-fed *NRG4* knockout mice had increased adiposity, hypertriglyceridemia and increased insulin resistance (92). These mice also manifested more pronounced hepatic steatosis and increased serum markers of hepatic inflammation as compared to WT mice. Knockout mice had increased hepatic expression of genes associated with *de novo* lipogenesis and inflammation along with increased *SREBF1* expression, whereas the expression of genes associated with beta oxidation of fatty acids and gluconeogenesis was unchanged (92, 95). NRG4 attenuated lipogenesis in cultured hepatocytes *in vitro*. On the other hand, transgenic expression of NRG4 in adipose tissues rendered mice resistant to HFD-induced weight gain as compared to WT mice. These mice also had significantly less hepatic steatosis, inflammation and fibrosis (92, 95), along with increased hepatic beta oxidation of fatty acids and increased ketogenesis (94). Moreover, NRG4 directly affects hepatocyte cell death *in vivo* through downregulation of proteasomal degradation of c-FLIP, a major anti-apoptotic/necrotic protein. *NRG4* knockout mice had decreased hepatic c-FLIP levels whereas *NRG4* transgenic mice had elevated c-FLIP levels. Restoration of hepatic c-FLIP expression in HFD-fed *NRG4* knockout mice using adenovirus blocked the progression of hepatic steatosis to NASH (95). In multiple cross-sectional studies of adults and children with NAFLD, serum NRG4 levels were significantly lower when compared to healthy controls, suggesting an important role of NRG4 in human NALFD as well (96–98). Collectively, these studies demonstrate that adipose tissue-derived NRG4, via an endocrine fashion, can improve hepatic steatosis, inflammation and fibrosis.

CONCLUSIONS

In conclusion, changes in SNS and PSNS activity as well as the expression of neurotrophic factors play significant roles in the pathogenesis of NAFLD and its progression to NASH and cirrhosis. Activation of SNS and adrenergic signaling promotes steatosis and hepatic fibrosis, whereas stimulation of PSNS improves NASH with its effects on hepatic fibrosis remaining unclear. Increased expression of neurotrophic factors including GDNF, CNTF, BDNF, and NRG4 all alleviate hepatic steatosis. BDNF, CNTF, and NRG4 decrease inflammation, but only

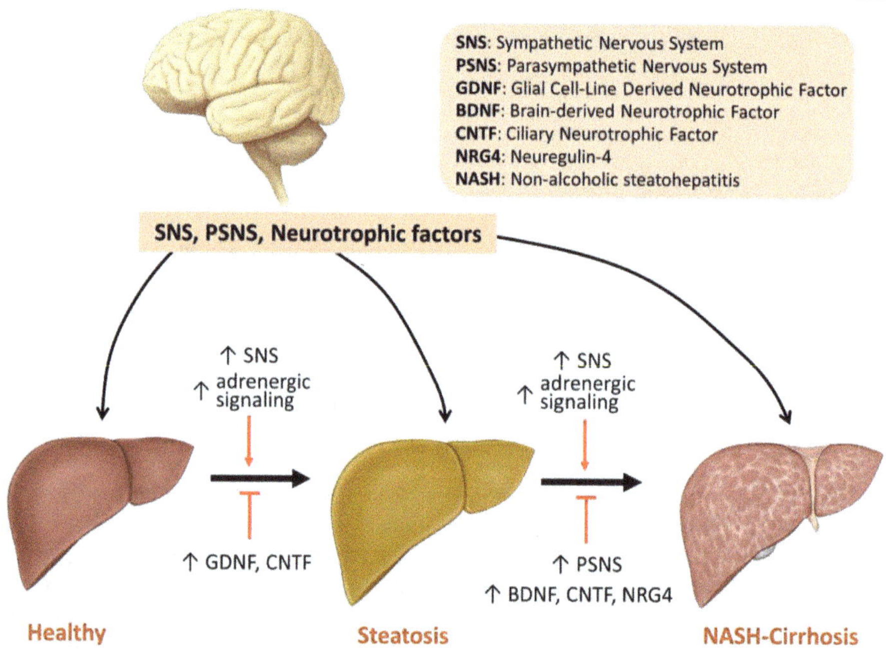

FIGURE 1 | Model of the regulation of steatosis, NASH, and fibrosis by SNS, PSNS and neurotrophic factors.

TABLE 1 | Key References.

	Conclusions	Models	References
Sympathetic nervous system	Pharmacological sympathetic agonism induces hepatic fibrosis by promoting HSC proliferation	Mouse model of obesity	Oben et al. (12)
	Pharmacological β-adrenergic agonism promotes steatosis	Mouse and rat model of NAFLD	Ghosh et al. (39)
	HFD increases sympathetic activity, and surgical or chemical ablation of hepatic sympathetic supply improves steatosis	Mouse model of NAFLD	Hurr et al. (40)
Parasympathetic nervous system	Pharmacological or electrical parasympathetic agonism dampens proinflammatory cytokine production	Rat model of endotoxemia	Borovikova et al. (49)
	Vagotomy exacerbates steatosis and hepatic inflammation	Mouse model of NASH	Nishio et al. (52)
Neurotrophic factors	GDNF overexpression renders resistance to development of obesity and steatosis	Mouse model of obesity	Mwangi et al. (69)
	BDNF improves steatohepatitis	Mouse model of diabetes	Tonra JR et al. (79)
	CNTF improves hepatic steatosis and inflammation	Mouse model of diabetes	Sleeman et al. (87)
	NRG4 prevents development of steatohepatitis and fibrosis	Mouse model of NASH	Guo et al. (95)

NRG4 improves fibrosis (**Figure 1**, **Table 1**). The following is a point-by-point summary of the roles of SNS, PSNS, and neurotrophic factors.

- Modulation of the hepatic nervous system and neurotrophic factors play significant roles in management of hepatic steatosis, NASH and hepatic fibrosis.
- SNS is over-activated in the setting of aging, HFD-induced steatosis and advanced hepatic fibrosis.
- SNS stimulation promotes hepatic steatosis whereas surgical or chemical inhibition of SNS improves steatosis.
- SNS activation promotes hepatic fibrosis by enhancing proliferation and activation of HSCs along with increased signaling of TGF-β.
- PSNS activation improves NASH by decreasing hepatic lipid content and by reducing proinflammatory cytokine production in liver. This can be achieved by vagus stimulation or chemical agonism of PSNS.
- Role of PSNS in modulation of hepatic fibrosis remains unclear, with limited data indicating a promoting effect.
- GDNF, CNTF, BDNF, and NRG4 improve insulin resistance and alleviate hepatic steatosis by reducing hepatic lipogenesis and improving β-oxidation.
- GDNF's effects on liver fibrosis are contradictory by playing antifibrotic and profibrotic roles in different models. NRG4 has been shown to ameliorate fibrosis. The role of CNTF and BDNF in hepatic fibrosis is not understood.
- Further studies are needed to better understand the roles of neurotrophic factors and the hepatic nervous system in modulation of NAFLD.

AUTHOR CONTRIBUTIONS

MA wrote most of the paper and organized final draft. MY wrote the initial section of the paper. MA, PH, and SS edited and revised the paper.

ACKNOWLEDGMENTS

The authors would like to thank Brian C. Brockway, MS for his help with drawing the figure.

REFERENCES

1. Estes C, Razavi H, Loomba R, Younossi Z, Sanyal AJ. Modeling the epidemic of nonalcoholic fatty liver disease demonstrates an exponential increase in burden of disease. *Hepatology*. (2018) 67:123–33. doi: 10.1002/hep.29466
2. Arab JP, Arrese M, Trauner M. Recent insights into the pathogenesis of nonalcoholic fatty liver disease. *Annu Rev Pathol*. (2018) 13:321–50. doi: 10.1146/annurev-pathol-020117-043617
3. Benedict M, Zhang X. Non-alcoholic fatty liver disease: an expanded review. *World J Hepatol*. (2017) 9:715–32. doi: 10.4254/wjh.v9.i16.715
4. Amir M, Czaja MJ. Autophagy in nonalcoholic steatohepatitis. *Expert Rev Gastroenterol Hepatol*. (2011) 5:159–66. doi: 10.1586/egh.11.4
5. Manne V, Handa P, Kowdley KV. Pathophysiology of nonalcoholic fatty liver disease/nonalcoholic steatohepatitis. *Clin Liver Dis*. (2018) 22:23–37. doi: 10.1016/j.cld.2017.08.007
6. Yin C, Evason KJ, Asahina K, Stainier DY. Hepatic stellate cells in liver development, regeneration, and cancer. *J Clin Invest*. (2013) 123:1902–10. doi: 10.1172/JCI66369
7. Friedman SL. Mechanisms of hepatic fibrogenesis. *Gastroenterology*. (2008) 134:1655–69. doi: 10.1053/j.gastro.2008.03.003
8. Taher J, Farr S, Adeli K. Central nervous system regulation of hepatic lipid and lipoprotein metabolism. *Curr Opin Lipidol*. (2017) 28:32–8. doi: 10.1097/MOL.0000000000000373
9. Jensen KJ, Alpini G, Glaser S. Hepatic nervous system and neurobiology of the liver. *Compr Physiol*. (2013) 3:655–65. doi: 10.1002/cphy.c120018
10. Das UN. Obesity: genes, brain, gut, and environment. *Nutrition*. (2010) 26:459–73. doi: 10.1016/j.nut.2009.09.020
11. Exton JH. Mechanisms involved in alpha-adrenergic phenomena: role of calcium ions in actions of catecholamines in liver and other tissues. *Am J Physiol*. (1980) 238:E3–12. doi: 10.1152/ajpendo.1980.238.1.E3
12. Oben JA, Roskams T, Yang S, Lin H, Sinelli N, Torbenson M, et al. Hepatic fibrogenesis requires sympathetic neurotransmitters. *Gut*. (2004) 53:438–45. doi: 10.1136/gut.2003.026658
13. Metz CN, Pavlov VA. Vagus nerve cholinergic circuitry to the liver and the gastrointestinal tract in the neuroimmune communicatome. *Am J Physiol Gastrointest Liver Physiol*. (2018) 315:G651–8. doi: 10.1152/ajpgi.00195.2018
14. Kalashnyk OM, Gergalova GL, Komisarenko SV, Skok MV. Intracellular localization of nicotinic acetylcholine receptors in human cell lines. *Life Sci*. (2012) 91:1033–7. doi: 10.1016/j.lfs.2012.02.005
15. Schachtrup C, Le Moan N, Passino MA, Akassoglou K. Hepatic stellate cells and astrocytes: stars of scar formation and tissue repair. *Cell Cycle*. (2011) 10:1764–71. doi: 10.4161/cc.10.11.15828
16. Mitre M, Mariga A, Chao MV. Neurotrophin signalling: novel insights into mechanisms and pathophysiology. *Clin Sci*. (2017) 131:13–23. doi: 10.1042/CS20160044
17. Razavi S, Nazem G, Mardani M, Esfandiari E, Salehi H, Esfahani SH. Neurotrophic factors and their effects in the treatment of multiple sclerosis. *Adv Biomed Res*. (2015) 4:53. doi: 10.4103/2277-9175.151570
18. Evans JR, Barker RA. Neurotrophic factors as a therapeutic target for Parkinson's disease. *Expert Opin Ther Targets*. (2008) 12:437–47. doi: 10.1517/14728222.12.4.437
19. Cassiman D, Denef C, Desmet VJ, Roskams T. Human and rat hepatic stellate cells express neurotrophins and neurotrophin receptors. *Hepatology*. (2001) 33:148–58. doi: 10.1053/jhep.2001.20793
20. Mwangi SM, Peng S, Nezami BG, Thorn N, Farris AB III, Jain S, et al. Glial cell line-derived neurotrophic factor protects against high-fat diet-induced hepatic steatosis by suppressing hepatic PPAR-gamma expression. *Am J Physiol Gastrointest Liver Physiol*. (2016) 310:G103–16. doi: 10.1152/ajpgi.00196.2015
21. Tao L, Ma W, Wu L, Xu M, Yang Y, Zhang W, et al. Glial cell line-derived neurotrophic factor (GDNF) mediates hepatic stellate cell activation via ALK5/Smad signalling. *Gut*. (2019) 68:2214–27. doi: 10.1136/gutjnl-2018-317872
22. Ji H, Zhang Y, Shen XD, Gao F, Huang CY, Abad C, et al. Neuropeptide PACAP in mouse liver ischemia and reperfusion injury: immunomodulation by the cAMP-PKA pathway. *Hepatology*. (2013) 57:1225–37. doi: 10.1002/hep.25802
23. Li JF, Shu JC, Tang SH, Deng YM, Fu MY, Lv X. β-Nerve growth factor attenuates hepatocyte injury induced by D-galactosamine *in vitro* via TrkA NGFR. *Mol Med Rep*. (2013) 8:813–7. doi: 10.3892/mmr.2013.1590

24. Kendall TJ, Hennedige S, Aucott RL, Hartland SN, Vernon MA, Benyon RC, et al. p75 neurotrophin receptor signaling regulates hepatic myofibroblast proliferation and apoptosis in recovery from rodent liver fibrosis. *Hepatology.* (2009) 49:901–10. doi: 10.1002/hep.22701
25. Nakagawa T, Tsuchida A, Itakura Y, Nonomura T, Ono M, Hirota F, et al. Brain-derived neurotrophic factor regulates glucose metabolism by modulating energy balance in diabetic mice. *Diabetes.* (2000) 49:436–44. doi: 10.2337/diabetes.49.3.436
26. Rezende LF, Santos GJ, Santos-Silva JC, Carneiro EM, Boschero AC. Ciliary neurotrophic factor (CNTF) protects non-obese Swiss mice against type 2 diabetes by increasing beta cell mass and reducing insulin clearance. *Diabetologia.* (2012) 55:1495–504. doi: 10.1007/s00125-012-2493-5
27. Fukuda Y, Imoto M, Koyama Y, Miyazawa Y, Hayakawa T. Demonstration of noradrenaline-immunoreactive nerve fibres in the liver. *J Int Med Res.* (1996) 24:466–72. doi: 10.1177/030006059602400603
28. Taba Taba Vakili S, Kailar R, Rahman K, Nezami BG, Mwangi SM, Anania FA, et al. Glial cell line-derived neurotrophic factor-induced mice liver defatting: a novel strategy to enable transplantation of steatotic livers. *Liver Transpl.* (2016) 22:459–67. doi: 10.1002/lt.24385
29. Miyazawa Y, Fukuda Y, Imoto M, Koyama Y, Nagura H. Immunohistochemical studies on the distribution of nerve fibers in chronic liver diseases. *Am J Gastroenterol.* (1988) 83:1108–14.
30. Mizuno K, Ueno Y. Autonomic nervous system and the liver. *Hepatol Res.* (2017) 47:160–5. doi: 10.1111/hepr.12760
31. Thoene M, Rytel L, Dzika E, Wlodarczyk A, Kruminis-Kaszkiel E, Konrad P, et al. Bisphenol a Causes liver damage and selectively alters the neurochemical coding of intrahepatic parasympathetic nerves in juvenile porcine models under physiological conditions. *Int J Mol Sci.* (2017) 18:2726. doi: 10.3390/ijms18122726
32. Akiyoshi H, Terada T. Mast cell, myofibroblast and nerve terminal complexes in carbon tetrachloride-induced cirrhotic rat livers. *J Hepatol.* (1998) 29:112–9. doi: 10.1016/S0168-8278(98)80185-2
33. Oben JA, Yang S, Lin H, Ono M, Diehl AM. Acetylcholine promotes the proliferation and collagen gene expression of myofibroblastic hepatic stellate cells. *Biochem Biophys Res Commun.* (2003) 300:172–7. doi: 10.1016/S0006-291X(02)02773-0
34. Cardani R, Zavanella T. Immunohistochemical localization of beta 1-adrenergic receptors in the liver of male and female F344 rat. *Histochem Cell Biol.* (2001) 116:441–5. doi: 10.1007/s00418-001-0340-8
35. Luo L, Xu T, Wang P, Mao L, Xi C, Huang J, et al. Expression of muscarinic acetylcholine receptors in hepatocytes from rat fibrotic liver. *Exp Toxicol Pathol.* (2017) 69:73–81. doi: 10.1016/j.etp.2016.11.005
36. Bockx I, Vander Elst I, Roskams T, Cassiman D. The hepatic vagus nerve stimulates hepatic stellate cell proliferation in rat acute hepatitis via muscarinic receptor type 2. *Liver Int.* (2010) 30:693–702. doi: 10.1111/j.1478-3231.2010.02229.x
37. Li JH, Gautam D, Han SJ, Guettier JM, Cui Y, Lu H, et al. Hepatic muscarinic acetylcholine receptors are not critically involved in maintaining glucose homeostasis in mice. *Diabetes.* (2009) 58:2776–87. doi: 10.2337/db09-0522
38. Streba LA, Vere CC, Ionescu AG, Streba CT, Rogoveanu I. Role of intrahepatic innervation in regulating the activity of liver cells. *World J Hepatol.* (2014) 6:137–43. doi: 10.4254/wjh.v6.i3.137
39. Ghosh PM, Shu ZJ, Zhu B, Lu Z, Ikeno Y, Barnes JL, et al. Role of beta-adrenergic receptors in regulation of hepatic fat accumulation during aging. *J Endocrinol.* (2012) 213:251–61. doi: 10.1530/JOE-11-0406
40. Hurr C, Simonyan H, Morgan DA, Rahmouni K, Young CN. Liver sympathetic denervation reverses obesity-induced hepatic steatosis. *J Physiol.* (2019) 597:4565–80. doi: 10.1113/JP277994
41. Wahli W, Braissant O, Desvergne B. Peroxisome proliferator activated receptors: transcriptional regulators of adipogenesis, lipid metabolism and more. *Chem Biol.* (1995) 2:261–6. doi: 10.1016/1074-5521(95)90045-4
42. Kersten S. Integrated physiology and systems biology of PPARα. *Mol Metab.* (2014) 3:354–71. doi: 10.1016/j.molmet.2014.02.002
43. Fontana L, Zhao E, Amir M, Dong H, Tanaka K, Czaja MJ. Aging promotes the development of diet-induced murine steatohepatitis but not steatosis. *Hepatology.* (2013) 57:995–1004. doi: 10.1002/hep.26099
44. Henriksen JH, Moller S, Ring-Larsen H, Christensen NJ. The sympathetic nervous system in liver disease. *J Hepatol.* (1998) 29:328–41. doi: 10.1016/S0168-8278(98)80022-6
45. Esler M, Dudley F, Jennings G, Debinski H, Lambert G, Jones P, et al. Increased sympathetic nervous activity and the effects of its inhibition with clonidine in alcoholic cirrhosis. *Ann Intern Med.* (1992) 116:446–55. doi: 10.7326/0003-4819-116-6-446
46. Oben JA, Diehl AM. Sympathetic nervous system regulation of liver repair. *Anat Rec A Discov Mol Cell Evol Biol.* (2004) 280:874–83. doi: 10.1002/ar.a.20081
47. Oben JA, Yang S, Lin H, Ono M, Diehl AM. Norepinephrine and neuropeptide Y promote proliferation and collagen gene expression of hepatic myofibroblastic stellate cells. *Biochem Biophys Res Commun.* (2003) 302:685–90. doi: 10.1016/S0006-291X(03)00232-8
48. Sigala B, McKee C, Soeda J, Pazienza V, Morgan M, Lin CI, et al. Sympathetic nervous system catecholamines and neuropeptide Y neurotransmitters are upregulated in human NAFLD and modulate the fibrogenic function of hepatic stellate cells. *PLoS ONE.* (2013) 8:e72928. doi: 10.1371/journal.pone.0072928
49. Borovikova LV, Ivanova S, Zhang M, Yang H, Botchkina GI, Watkins LR, et al. Vagus nerve stimulation attenuates the systemic inflammatory response to endotoxin. *Nature.* (2000) 405:458–62. doi: 10.1038/35013070
50. Li Y, Xu Z, Yu Y, Yuan H, Xu H, Zhu Q, et al. The vagus nerve attenuates fulminant hepatitis by activating the Src kinase in Kuppfer cells. *Scand J Immunol.* (2014) 79:105–12. doi: 10.1111/sji.12141
51. Wang X, Yang Z, Xue B, Shi H. Activation of the cholinergic antiinflammatory pathway ameliorates obesity-induced inflammation and insulin resistance. *Endocrinology.* (2011) 152:836–46. doi: 10.1210/en.2010-0855
52. Nishio T, Taura K, Iwaisako K, Koyama Y, Tanabe K, Yamamoto G, et al. Hepatic vagus nerve regulates Kupffer cell activation via alpha7 nicotinic acetylcholine receptor in nonalcoholic steatohepatitis. *J Gastroenterol.* (2017) 52:965–76. doi: 10.1007/s00535-016-1304-z
53. Lilienfeld S. Galantamine–a novel cholinergic drug with a unique dual mode of action for the treatment of patients with Alzheimer's disease. *CNS Drug Rev.* (2002) 8:159–76. doi: 10.1111/j.1527-3458.2002.tb00221.x
54. Ali MA, El-Abhar HS, Kamel MA, Attia AS. Antidiabetic effect of galantamine: novel effect for a known centrally acting drug. *PLoS ONE.* (2015) 10:e0134648. doi: 10.1371/journal.pone.0134648
55. Satapathy SK, Ochani M, Dancho M, Hudson LK, Rosas-Ballina M, Valdes-Ferrer SI, et al. Galantamine alleviates inflammation and other obesity-associated complications in high-fat diet-fed mice. *Mol Med.* (2011) 17:599–606. doi: 10.2119/molmed.2011.00083
56. Luo L, Zhou A. Antifibrotic activity of anisodamine *in vivo* is associated with changed intrahepatic levels of matrix metalloproteinase-2 and its inhibitor tissue inhibitors of metalloproteinases-2 and transforming growth factor beta1 in rats with carbon tetrachloride-induced liver injury. *J Gastroenterol Hepatol.* (2009) 24:1070–6. doi: 10.1111/j.1440-1746.2008.05756.x
57. Poupko JM, Baskin SI, Moore E. The pharmacological properties of anisodamine. *J Appl Toxicol.* (2007) 27:116–21. doi: 10.1002/jat.1154
58. Gordon T. The role of neurotrophic factors in nerve regeneration. *Neurosurg Focus.* (2009) 26:E3. doi: 10.3171/FOC.2009.26.2.E3
59. Xiao N, Le QT. Neurotrophic factors and their potential applications in tissue regeneration. *Arch Immunol Ther Exp.* (2016) 64:89–99. doi: 10.1007/s00005-015-0376-4
60. Weissmiller AM, Wu C. Current advances in using neurotrophic factors to treat neurodegenerative disorders. *Transl Neurodegener.* (2012) 1:14. doi: 10.1186/2047-9158-1-14
61. Zhao P, Qiao J, Huang S, Zhang Y, Liu S, Yan LY, et al. Gonadotrophin-induced paracrine regulation of human oocyte maturation by BDNF and GDNF secreted by granulosa cells. *Hum Reprod.* (2011) 26:695–702. doi: 10.1093/humrep/deq390
62. Fielder GC, Yang TW, Razdan M, Li Y, Lu J, Perry JK, et al. The GDNF family: a role in cancer? *Neoplasia.* (2018) 20:99–117. doi: 10.1016/j.neo.2017.10.010
63. Lin LF, Doherty DH, Lile JD, Bektesh S, Collins F. GDNF: a glial cell line-derived neurotrophic factor for midbrain dopaminergic neurons. *Science.* (1993) 260:1130–2. doi: 10.1126/science.8493557
64. Airaksinen MS, Saarma M. The GDNF family: signalling, biological functions and therapeutic value. *Nat Rev Neurosci.* (2002) 3:383–94. doi: 10.1038/nrn812

65. Uesaka T, Jain S, Yonemura S, Uchiyama Y, Milbrandt J, Enomoto H. Conditional ablation of GFRalpha1 in postmigratory enteric neurons triggers unconventional neuronal death in the colon and causes a Hirschsprung's disease phenotype. *Development.* (2007) 134:2171–81. doi: 10.1242/dev.001388
66. Takahashi M. The GDNF/RET signaling pathway and human diseases. *Cytokine Growth Fact Rev.* (2001) 12:361–73. doi: 10.1016/S1359-6101(01)00012-0
67. Meng X, Lindahl M, Hyvonen ME, Parvinen M, de Rooij DG, Hess MW, et al. Regulation of cell fate decision of undifferentiated spermatogonia by GDNF. *Science.* (2000) 287:1489–93. doi: 10.1126/science.287.5457.1489
68. Xiao N, Lin Y, Cao H, Sirjani D, Giaccia AJ, Koong AC, et al. Neurotrophic factor GDNF promotes survival of salivary stem cells. *J Clin Invest.* (2014) 124:3364–77. doi: 10.1172/JCI74096
69. Mwangi SM, Nezami BG, Obukwelu B, Anitha M, Marri S, Fu P, et al. Glial cell line-derived neurotrophic factor protects against high-fat diet-induced obesity. *Am J Physiol Gastrointest Liver Physiol.* (2014) 306:G515–25. doi: 10.1152/ajpgi.00364.2013
70. Shoelson SE, Herrero L, Naaz A. Obesity, inflammation, and insulin resistance. *Gastroenterology.* (2007) 132:2169–80. doi: 10.1053/j.gastro.2007.03.059
71. Siersbaek R, Nielsen R, Mandrup S. PPARgamma in adipocyte differentiation and metabolism–novel insights from genome-wide studies. *FEBS Lett.* (2010) 584:3242–9. doi: 10.1016/j.febslet.2010.06.010
72. Pan H, Guo J, Su Z. Advances in understanding the interrelations between leptin resistance and obesity. *Physiol Behav.* (2014) 130:157–69. doi: 10.1016/j.physbeh.2014.04.003
73. Motojima K, Passilly P, Peters JM, Gonzalez FJ, Latruffe N. Expression of putative fatty acid transporter genes are regulated by peroxisome proliferator-activated receptor alpha and gamma activators in a tissue- and inducer-specific manner. *J Biol Chem.* (1998) 273:16710–4. doi: 10.1074/jbc.273.27.16710
74. Mwangi SM, Li G, Ye L, Liu Y, Reichardt F, Yeligar SM, et al. Glial cell line-derived neurotrophic factor enhances autophagic flux in mouse and rat hepatocytes and protects against palmitate lipotoxicity. *Hepatology.* (2019) 69:2455–70. doi: 10.1002/hep.30541
75. Binder DK, Scharfman HE. Brain-derived neurotrophic factor. *Growth Fact.* (2004) 22:123–31. doi: 10.1080/08977190410001723308
76. McGregor CE, English AW. The role of BDNF in peripheral nerve regeneration: activity-dependent treatments and val66Met. *Front Cell Neurosci.* (2018) 12:522. doi: 10.3389/fncel.2018.00522
77. Tsuchida A, Nakagawa T, Itakura Y, Ichihara J, Ogawa W, Kasuga M, et al. The effects of brain-derived neurotrophic factor on insulin signal transduction in the liver of diabetic mice. *Diabetologia.* (2001) 44:555–66. doi: 10.1007/s001250051661
78. Ono M, Ichihara J, Nonomura T, Itakura Y, Taiji M, Nakayama C, et al. Brain-derived neurotrophic factor reduces blood glucose level in obese diabetic mice but not in normal mice. *Biochem Biophys Res Commun.* (1997) 238:633–7. doi: 10.1006/bbrc.1997.7220
79. Tonra JR, Ono M, Liu X, Garcia K, Jackson C, Yancopoulos GD, et al. Brain-derived neurotrophic factor improves blood glucose control and alleviates fasting hyperglycemia in C57BLKS-Lepr(db)/lepr(db) mice. *Diabetes.* (1999) 48:588–94. doi: 10.2337/diabetes.48.3.588
80. Ono M, Itakura Y, Nonomura T, Nakagawa T, Nakayama C, Taiji M, et al. Intermittent administration of brain-derived neurotrophic factor ameliorates glucose metabolism in obese diabetic mice. *Metabolism.* (2000) 49:129–33. doi: 10.1016/S0026-0495(00)90988-0
81. Tsuchida A, Nonomura T, Nakagawa T, Itakura Y, Ono-Kishino M, Yamanaka M, et al. Brain-derived neurotrophic factor ameliorates lipid metabolism in diabetic mice. *Diabetes Obes Metab.* (2002) 4:262–9. doi: 10.1046/j.1463-1326.2002.00206.x
82. Yamanaka M, Itakura Y, Tsuchida A, Nakagawa T, Noguchi H, Taiji M. Comparison of the antidiabetic effects of brain-derived neurotrophic factor and thiazolidinediones in obese diabetic mice. *Diabetes Obes Metab.* (2007) 9:879–88. doi: 10.1111/j.1463-1326.2006.00675.x
83. Richardson PM. Ciliary neurotrophic factor: a review. *Pharmacol Ther.* (1994) 63:187–98. doi: 10.1016/0163-7258(94)90045-0
84. Pasquin S, Sharma M, Gauchat JF. Ciliary neurotrophic factor (CNTF): new facets of an old molecule for treating neurodegenerative and metabolic syndrome pathologies. *Cytokine Growth Fact Rev.* (2015) 26:507–15. doi: 10.1016/j.cytogfr.2015.07.007
85. Schuster B, Kovaleva M, Sun Y, Regenhard P, Matthews V, Grotzinger J, et al. Signaling of human ciliary neurotrophic factor (CNTF) revisited. The interleukin-6 receptor can serve as an alpha-receptor for CTNF. *J Biol Chem.* (2003) 278:9528–35. doi: 10.1074/jbc.M210044200
86. Nonogaki K, Pan XM, Moser AH, Shigenaga J, Staprans I, Sakamoto N, et al. LIF and CNTF, which share the gp130 transduction system, stimulate hepatic lipid metabolism in rats. *Am J Physiol.* (1996) 271:E521–8. doi: 10.1152/ajpendo.1996.271.3.E521
87. Sleeman MW, Garcia K, Liu R, Murray JD, Malinova L, Moncrieffe M, et al. Ciliary neurotrophic factor improves diabetic parameters and hepatic steatosis and increases basal metabolic rate in db/db mice. *Proc Natl Acad Sci USA.* (2003) 100:14297–302. doi: 10.1073/pnas.2335926100
88. Cui MX, Yang LN, Wang XX, Wang L, Li RL, Han W, et al. Alleviative effect of ciliary neurotrophic factor analogue on high fat-induced hepatic steatosis is partially independent of the central regulation. *Clin Exp Pharmacol Physiol.* (2017) 44:395–402. doi: 10.1111/1440-1681.12709
89. Britsch S. The neuregulin-I/ErbB signaling system in development and disease. *Adv Anat Embryol Cell Biol.* (2007) 190:1–65. doi: 10.1007/978-3-540-37107-6_1
90. Paramo B, Wyatt S, Davies AM. An essential role for neuregulin-4 in the growth and elaboration of developing neocortical pyramidal dendrites. *Exp Neurol.* (2018) 302:85–92. doi: 10.1016/j.expneurol.2018.01.002
91. Paramo B, Wyatt S, Davies AM. Neuregulin-4 is required for the growth and elaboration of striatal medium spiny neuron dendrites. *J Neuropathol Exp Neurol.* (2019) 78:725-34. doi: 10.1093/jnen/nlz046
92. Wang GX, Zhao XY, Meng ZX, Kern M, Dietrich A, Chen Z, et al. The brown fat-enriched secreted factor Nrg4 preserves metabolic homeostasis through attenuation of hepatic lipogenesis. *Nat Med.* (2014) 20:1436–43. doi: 10.1038/nm.3713
93. Khan RS, Newsome PN. NAFLD in 2017: novel insights into mechanisms of disease progression. *Nat Rev Gastroenterol Hepatol.* (2018) 15:71–2. doi: 10.1038/nrgastro.2017.181
94. Chen Z, Wang GX, Ma SL, Jung DY, Ha H, Altamimi T, et al. Nrg4 promotes fuel oxidation and a healthy adipokine profile to ameliorate diet-induced metabolic disorders. *Mol Metab.* (2017) 6:863–72. doi: 10.1016/j.molmet.2017.03.016
95. Guo L, Zhang P, Chen Z, Xia H, Li S, Zhang Y, et al. Hepatic neuregulin 4 signaling defines an endocrine checkpoint for steatosis-to-NASH progression. *J Clin Invest.* (2017) 127:4449–61. doi: 10.1172/JCI96324
96. Cai C, Lin M, Xu Y, Li X, Yang S, Zhang H. Association of circulating neuregulin 4 with metabolic syndrome in obese adults: a cross-sectional study. *BMC Med.* (2016) 14:165. doi: 10.1186/s12916-016-0703-6
97. Yan P, Xu Y, Wan Q, Feng J, Li H, Yang J, et al. Plasma neuregulin 4 levels are associated with metabolic syndrome in patients newly diagnosed with type 2 diabetes mellitus. *Dis Markers.* (2018) 2018:6974191. doi: 10.1155/2018/6974191
98. Wang R, Yang F, Qing L, Huang R, Liu Q, Li X. Decreased serum neuregulin 4 levels associated with non-alcoholic fatty liver disease in children with obesity. *Clin Obes.* (2019) 9:e12289. doi: 10.1111/cob.12289

16

Distinct EpCAM-Positive Stem Cell Niches are Engaged in Chronic and Neoplastic Liver Diseases

Samira Safarikia[1†], Guido Carpino[2†], Diletta Overi[3], Vincenzo Cardinale[4], Rosanna Venere[1], Antonio Franchitto[3], Paolo Onori[3], Domenico Alvaro[1] and Eugenio Gaudio[3]*

[1] *Department of Precision and Translational Medicine, Sapienza University of Rome, Rome, Italy,* [2] *Department of Movement, Human and Health Sciences, Division of Health Sciences, University of Rome "Foro Italico," Rome, Italy,* [3] *Department of Anatomical, Histological, Forensic Medicine and Orthopedic Sciences, Sapienza University of Rome, Rome, Italy,* [4] *Department of Medico-Surgical Sciences and Biotechnologies, Sapienza University of Rome, Latina, Italy*

***Correspondence:**
Guido Carpino
guido.carpino@uniroma1.it

† These authors have contributed equally to this work

In normal human livers, EpCAM^{pos} cells are mostly restricted in two distinct niches, which are (i) the bile ductules and (ii) the mucous glands present inside the wall of large intrahepatic bile ducts (the so-called peribiliary glands). These EpCAM^{pos} cell niches have been proven to harbor stem/progenitor cells with great importance in liver and biliary tree regeneration and in the pathophysiology of human diseases. The EpCAM^{pos} progenitor cells within bile ductules are engaged in driving regenerative processes in chronic diseases affecting hepatocytes or interlobular bile ducts. The EpCAM^{pos} population within peribiliary glands is activated when regenerative needs are finalized to repair large intra- or extra-hepatic bile ducts affected by chronic pathologies, including primary sclerosing cholangitis and ischemia-induced cholangiopathies after orthotopic liver transplantation. Finally, the presence of distinct EpCAM^{pos} cell populations may explain the histological and molecular heterogeneity characterizing cholangiocarcinoma, based on the concept of multiple candidate cells of origin. This review aimed to describe the precise anatomical distribution of EpCAM^{pos} populations within the liver and the biliary tree and to discuss their contribution in the pathophysiology of human liver diseases, as well as their potential role in regenerative medicine of the liver.

Keywords: progenitor cells, liver, biliary tree, cholangiopathy, cholangiocarcinoma

INTRODUCTION

In the adult liver and biliary tree, mature parenchymal cells (i.e., hepatocytes and cholangiocytes) are characterized by remarkable proliferative capabilities, which support the regenerative needs of these organs in physiological conditions (1). According to that, lineage tracing studies indicated that hepatocytes are able to restore hepatic parenchyma after subcritical liver resection and regenerate cell loss after acute and chronic damage; furthermore, studies on cell plasticity in rodents indicated the potential of hepatocytes to differentiate toward biliary cells after injury (1–5). Therefore, conflicting evidence is present in scientific literature regarding the existence and function of a distinct stem/progenitor cell population capable of participating in liver regeneration (6). Nonetheless, experimental models characterized by an extensive (or prolonged over time) liver injury, which mimic the natural history of human liver diseases, demonstrated the contribution of stem/progenitor cells in the regenerative response (7, 8).

Recent single cell transcriptomic studies turned the spotlight on the EpCAM^{pos} cell fraction within the liver as a candidate progenitor cell population (9, 10). The epithelial cell adhesion molecule (EpCAM) is a surface epithelial marker selectively expressed in the biliary tree, where it individuates the stem/progenitor cell fraction from mature cholangiocytes (1, 11); differently, mature hepatocytes within the hepatic lobule do not express EpCAM (11). The elegant single-cell transcriptomic atlas compiled by Aizarani et al. produced a comprehensive depiction of liver cell populations, including hepatocytes, biliary epithelial cells, endothelial cells, macrophages, and inflammatory cells (9). The authors revealed the presence of transcriptomic heterogeneity in the EpCAM^{pos} population and, within this population, identified the cell fraction with the highest potential to form liver organoids and to putatively serve as a stem cell compartment. In parallel, the study by Segal et al. individuated, by using a similar approach, a unique gene expression profile within the EpCAM^{pos} cell population in human fetal livers: in particular, they individuated a distinct *EpCAM^{pos}* cell fraction which has bi-potential capability, is distinguishable from hepatocytes and cholangiocytes, and persists in the adult organ (10). Besides some discrepancies in cell phenotype, both studies individuated the *EpCAM^{pos}* population within the intrahepatic biliary tree as a strong candidate stem/progenitor cell compartment with regenerative potential for the liver and biliary tree.

The present review aimed to discuss the phenotype and the precise anatomical distribution of EpCAM^{pos} cell populations within the liver and the biliary tree, to describe their changes induced by human liver diseases, and to highlight their role as a potential source for regenerative medicine.

THE HETEROGENEITY OF EPCAM^{POS} CELL POPULATIONS IN HUMAN LIVER

In human livers, EpCAM^{pos} cells are localized and organized in two distinct anatomical niches (**Figure 1**), namely, bile ductules and peribiliary glands (PBGs).

The intrahepatic biliary tree begins with the canals of Hering, which represent the point of junction between the hepatocyte canalicular system and the biliary tree (12, 13). The canals of Hering are located at the interface between the portal tract and the hepatic parenchyma and continue into the bile ductules, with tortuous conduits draining into the interlobular bile ducts inside the portal space. A population of EpCAM^{pos} cells has been identified within the canals of Hering and the bile ductules, serving as facultative bipotent progenitors (Hepatic Stem/progenitor Cells: HpSCs) capable to differentiate into hepatocytes and cholangiocytes (**Figure 2**, panel A) (9, 14, 15), and represents the remnant of the ductal plate in the adult liver (10, 16, 17). Morphologically, HpSCs are small cells characterized by a high nucleus-to-cytoplasm ratio and expressing a large variety of markers, which include stem cell markers [e.g., EpCAM, neural cell adhesion molecule (NCAM), transcription factor Sox9, CD44, and CD133], biliary cytokeratins (CK7/19), and hepatocellular traits (e.g., albumin, CK18, hepatocyte nuclear factor 4 alpha) (10, 18). While differentiating toward a mature fate, the progeny of HpSCs is characterized by the progressive loss of EpCAM and NCAM expression and the acquirement of mature hepatocyte or cholangiocyte traits (10, 14, 19, 20). Recently, this EpCAM^{pos} cellular population has been further characterized by single-cell transcriptomic, with the identification of an *EpCAM^{pos}/NCAM^{pos}* fraction which also displays prominent stem cell features *in vitro* (10).

Notably, a second EpCAM^{pos} cell niche is endowed in PBGs located inside the walls of large (i.e., segmental and area) intrahepatic bile ducts and along the entire extrahepatic biliary tree (21). PBGs are tubulo-alveolar mucous glands, in continuity with the surface epithelium of the bile duct (22, 23). Intriguingly, the EpCAM^{pos} cell population within PBGs showed stem/progenitor properties, including organoid formation and plasticity to differentiate into hepatocytes, cholangiocytes, and endocrine pancreatic cells (**Figure 2**, panel B) (21, 24, 25). PBG cells have been collectively named biliary tree stem/progenitor cells (BTSC) and, embryologically, they represent the remnant of the common bilio-pancreatic progenitors of the ventral endoderm (23, 24). Phenotypically, mucin family genes (e.g., *MUC5A* and *MUC6*) are largely expressed in this anatomical niche (23); moreover, the EpCAM^{pos} cell pool within PBGs shows a heterogeneous profile and a radial axis (depth-to-surface) organization: EpCAM^{pos} cells are mostly found at the bottom of PBGs, where a subpopulation of them co-expresses markers of pluripotency (i.e., Oct4, Sox2, and Nanog) (23); a transit-amplifying (i.e., proliferating) population is located in the middle portion of the glands; finally, cells with a more mature phenotype [e.g., expressing secretin receptor, cystic fibrosis transmembrane conductance receptor (CFTR), mucins, and Trop2] are located in direct continuity with the surface epithelium (23, 26, 27). Altogether, these findings are confirmed by single-cell transcriptomic analysis in human, with the identification of an *EpCAM^{pos}/TROP2^{int}/MUC6^{high}* progenitor compartment with prominent stem cell features (9). Moreover, the contribution of PBG cells in the regeneration of mature biliary epithelium has been demonstrated in experimental conditions and by an *ex vivo* human model of biliary regeneration, which have disclosed that PBG cells can repopulate the surface epithelium of bile ducts by proliferation and differentiation into mature cholangiocytes (25, 28, 29).

In the light of these findings, one of the main aspects to be considered when interpreting transcriptomic analysis of liver samples resides in the fact that PBGs and bile ductules are two anatomically distinct compartments which, however, can be found in strict spatial proximity within the same

Abbreviations: BTSC, biliary tree stem/progenitor cell; CD, cluster differentiation; CFTR, cystic fibrosis transmembrane conductance receptor; CK, cytokeratin; DR, ductular reaction; EpCAM, epithelial cell adhesion molecule; GMP, good manufacturing practice; HpSC, hepatic stem/progenitor cell; MUC, mucin; NAFLD, non-alcoholic fatty liver disease; NCAM, neural cell adhesion molecule; PBC, primary biliary cholangitis; PBG, peribiliary gland; PSC, primary sclerosing cholangitis.

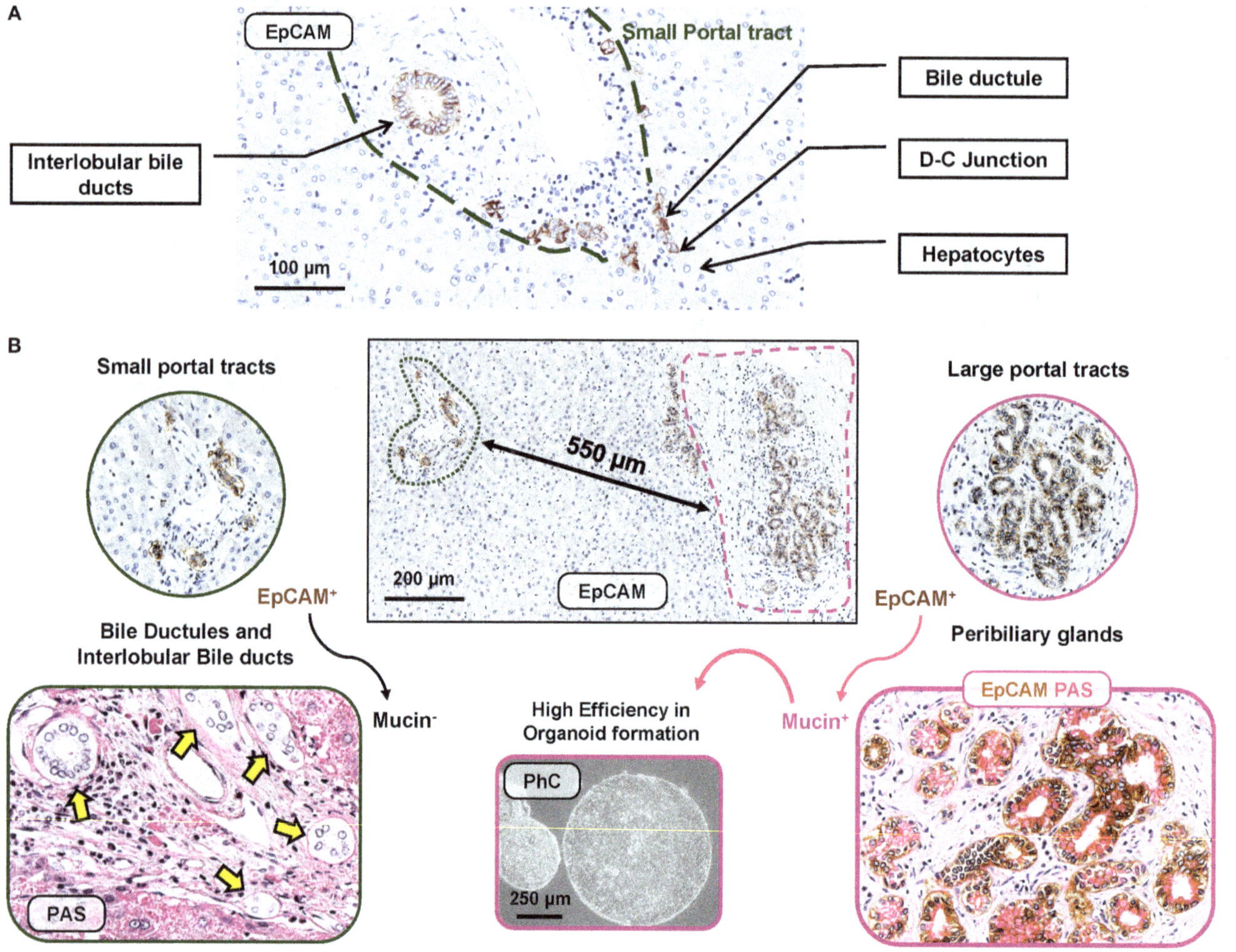

FIGURE 1 | EpCAM^{pos} cell niches in human liver fragments obtained from normal subjects. **(A)** EpCAM^{pos} cells are present in small portal tracts and are endowed in interlobular bile ducts and bile ductules up to the ductular-canalicular (D-C) junction. Hepatocytes are constantly negative for EpCAM. **(B)** Large portal tracts can be present together with small ones in the same liver fragment, given their close proximity in sectional histology. Large intrahepatic bile ducts (i.e., segmental and area bile ducts) contain an EpCAM^{pos} cell niche endowed in the mucous glands present inside their walls (so-called peribiliary glands). Mucin positivity is typically present in EpCAM^{pos} peribiliary gland cells (on the right) but not in bile ductules and interlobular bile ducts at small portal tracts (on the left). Once isolates from peribiliary glands, EpCAM^{pos} cells showed progenitor cell features, including high efficiency in organoid formation *in vitro*. Histologic images are representatives of human liver fragments obtained from liver donors ($N = 5$). Specimens were stained by immunohistochemistry for EpCAM and periodic acid-Schiff (PAS) for mucins. EpCAM immunohistochemistry is counterstained with hematoxylin or with PAS. Organoids were generated by EpCAM^{pos} peribiliary gland cells isolated from the human common hepatic duct obtained from organ donors (routinely discarded in orthotopic liver transplantation procedures); the phase contrast (PhC) microscopic image is representative of at least $N = 3$ biological replicates.

liver fragment (**Figure 1**, panel B). Thus, the transcriptomic heterogeneity in the EpCAM^{pos} population revealed by single cell approaches could be due to the collection of one or both of these distinct progenitor cell compartments from the same specimen. EpCAM^{pos} progenitor cells within bile ductules are characterized by a distinct signature identifying them from mature cholangiocytes, immature hepatocytes, and mature hepatocytes, based on *NCAM*^{pos}/*TROP2*^{neg} expression (**Figure 2**). Therefore, these cells could be distinguished from cholangiocytes that populate interlobular bile ducts, the latter expressing *TROP2* and mucin family genes. However, a *TROP*^{int} cell fraction among the EpCAM^{pos} compartment was proven to have high stemness properties; thus, this fraction resides more likely into peribiliary glands than in bile ductules, given also its high mucin family gene expression (e.g., *MUC5A* and *MUC6)* and low CK19 and CFTR levels (25, 30).

Understanding the phenotypes of distinct biliary populations and their anatomical niches is crucial when considering that the pathophysiology of hepatic and biliary diseases is often hindered by difficulties in identifying regenerative pathways. Interestingly, the EpCAM^{pos} population exhibited only a stochastic expression of proliferation markers (9). This finding strengthens the concept of a facultative progenitor compartment that is only engaged by the regenerative needs and trajectories required after prolonged chronic or acute massive damage (8).

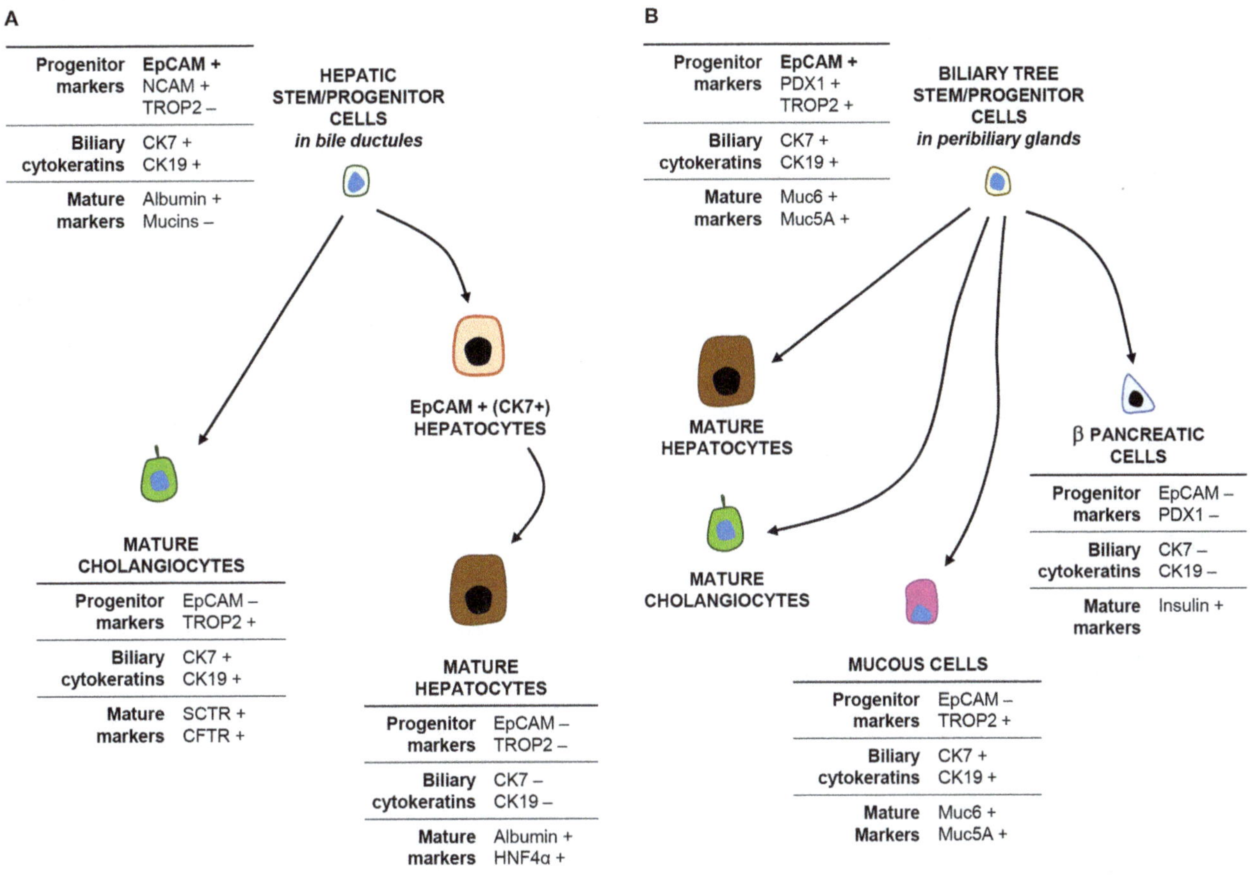

FIGURE 2 | EpCAM^{pos} cells within the liver and biliary tree and their progeny. The cartoon shows the phenotype (main markers) of EpCAM^{pos} stem/progenitor cells within the bile ductules **(A)** and the peribiliary glands **(B)** and their differentiative capabilities.

EPCAM^{POS} CELL POPULATIONS IN CHRONIC HUMAN DISEASES OF THE LIVER AND BILIARY TREE

In human liver diseases, the phenotypic and transcriptomic profiles of liver cells change noticeably. In this context, taking into account the heterogeneity within the EpCAM^{pos} progenitor population is a crucial prerequisite to understand the specific contribution of different hepatic regenerative pathways in human disease progression. Chronic prolonged diseases affecting hepatocytes or interlobular bile ducts could engage HpSCs within bile ductules (**Figure 3**, panel A) (19); differently, PBGs and their EpCAM^{pos} cell fraction (i.e., BTSCs) could be activated when the disease leads to the damage of large intrahepatic (or extra-hepatic) bile ducts (**Figure 3**, panel B) (30, 31).

EpCAM^{pos} Cell Fraction in Bile Ductules: Ductular Reaction and Chronic Liver Diseases

In a number of different chronic liver diseases, EpCAM^{pos} HpSCs within the canals of Hering and the bile ductules represent the source of a prominent ductular reaction (DR) (**Figure 3**, panel A) (19, 32). The phenotype and the behavior of EpCAM^{pos} DR have been extensively characterized in liver diseases affecting hepatocytes (19). In these conditions, DR appearance is associated with the emergence of a unique EpCAM^{pos} hepatocyte population, which localizes periportally and is characterized by the co-expression of biliary cytokeratins (11, 19, 33). Detailed studies of liver samples obtained from cirrhotic patients allowed accurately describing the expansion of DR and the emergence of an EpCAM^{pos} hepatocyte population, able to regenerate large portions of liver parenchyma (34, 35).

In chronic liver diseases, the expansion of DR is secondary to the prolonged exposure of hepatocytes to pathogenetic insults, which leads to the progressive loss of hepatocyte replicative capability and induces hepatocellular senescence. For example, in non-alcoholic fatty liver disease (NAFLD), hepatocyte regenerative capabilities are highly impaired due to progressive lipotoxicity and lobular inflammation (36, 37); this induces a prominent EpCAM^{pos} DR, followed by the appearance of EpCAM^{pos} hepatocytes at the periportal zone (37–42). In NAFLD, DR correlates with disease activity and NASH onset; interestingly, DR extent also correlates with periportal fibrogenesis and is predictive of fibrosis stage

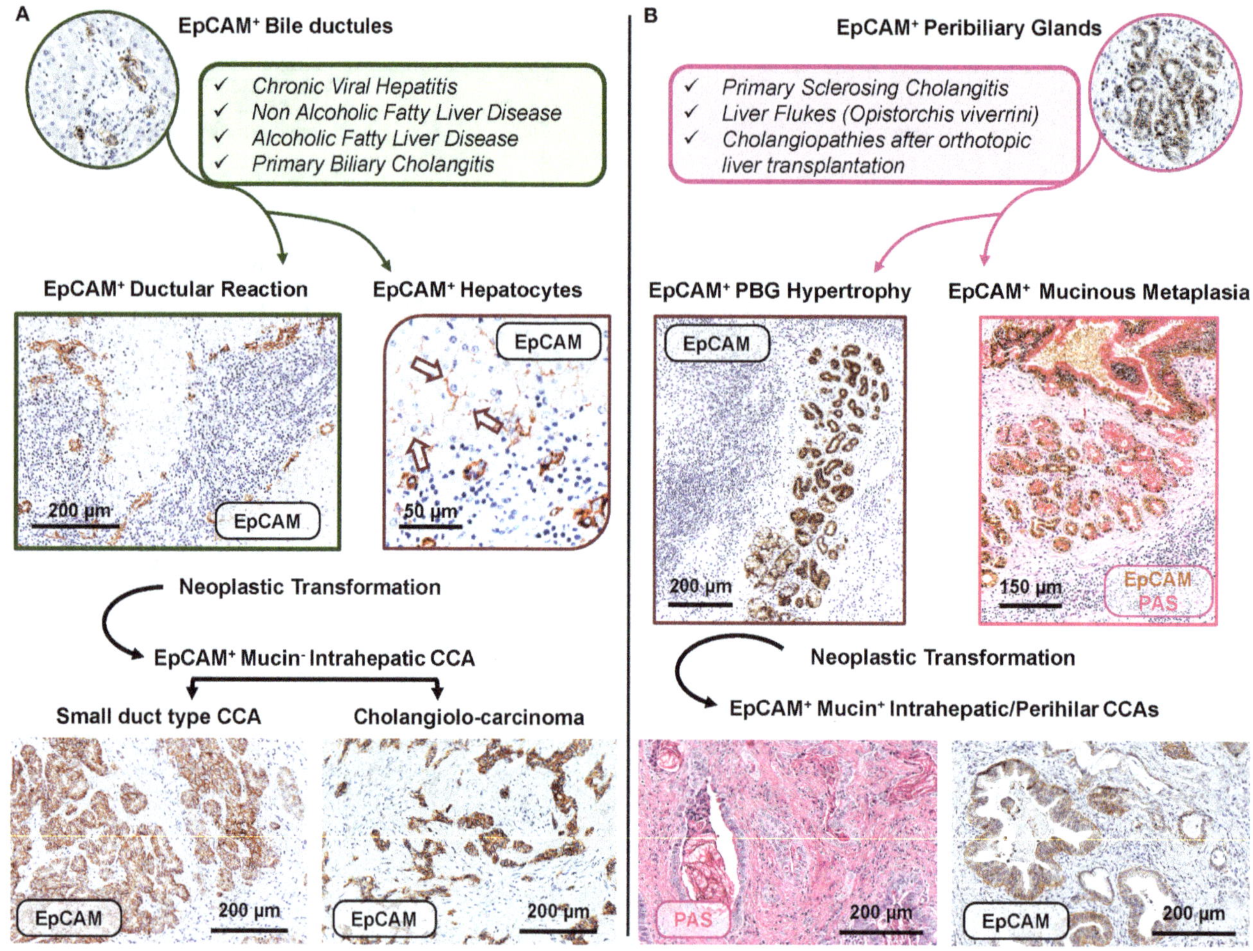

FIGURE 3 | Distinct EpCAM^{pos} cell niches are engaged by specific human diseases based on regenerative needs and may represent the cell of origin of specific subtypes of cholangiocarcinoma. **(A)** Regenerative pathways engage EpCAM^{pos}/MUC6^{neg} progenitors within bile ductules in chronic human diseases affecting hepatocytes and/or interlobular bile ducts. In these diseases, an expansion of the EpCAM^{pos} cell population is present and includes the emergence of ductular reaction and the appearance of EpCAM^{pos} hepatocytes (arrows). Two subtypes of EpCAM^{pos} cholangiocarcinoma (CCA) may derive from the neoplastic transformation of EpCAM^{pos} interlobular cholangiocytes (small duct type CCA) and bile ductules (cholangiolo-carcinoma). **(B)** The EpCAM^{pos}/MUC6^{pos} population within peribiliary glands (PBGs) could be engaged when regenerative needs are finalized to repair large intra- or extrahepatic bile ducts affected by chronic pathologies, including primary sclerosing cholangitis. The EpCAM^{pos} PBG cell population response is characterized by hypertrophy and mucinous metaplasia of this compartment. The onset of mucinous CCAs could be due to the neoplastic transformation of the EpCAM^{pos} PBG niche, through the sequence hypertrophy-metaplasia-dysplasia-cancer. Histologic images in **(A)** are representative of human liver fragments obtained from patients affected by chronic viral hepatitis, primary biliary cholangitis, and CCA. In **(B)**, specimens were obtained from patients affected by primary sclerosing cholangitis and CCA. Specimens were stained by immunohistochemistry for EpCAM and periodic acid-Schiff (PAS) for mucins. EpCAM immunohistochemistry is counterstained with hematoxylin or with PAS.

(43, 44). Parallel studies confirmed this role of DR also in pediatric subjects affected by NASH (39, 45). Moreover, DR is associated with systemic oxidative stress levels (38) and extra-hepatic clinical manifestations such as obstructive sleep apnea syndrome (46).

Extensive EpCAM^{pos} DR can also be triggered by a severe hepatocyte loss as a consequence of acute liver injury. In alcoholic hepatitis, a relevant cause of morbidity and mortality in heavy drinkers with alcoholic liver disease (47), DR extension is correlated with the severity of the damage and can predict short-term mortality (47, 48). In this setting, patients responding to first-line steroid therapy were characterized by higher DR (49); differently, in non-responders, cells within DR do not show signs of differentiation into hepatocytes, which correlates with a less favorable outcome (19, 50–53).

A prominent EpCAM^{pos} DR also appears in chronic diseases affecting the biliary tree (i.e., cholangiopathies) and acquires a peculiar phenotype, which reflects the pathophysiology of the disease. Primary biliary cholangitis (PBC) is a chronic, autoimmune cholangiopathy, characterized by the damage of interlobular bile ducts, leading to impaired bile duct flow into the biliary tree (54). In patients affected by PBC, DR is composed of cells expressing stem cell markers (EpCAM, NCAM, Sox9, and CD133) and displaying a variable degree of cholangiocyte differentiation signs, together with Notch pathway activation (19, 33, 55, 56). Disease severity and stage are correlated with the extent of DR, which might serve as prognostic marker for the development of clinical symptoms, patient prognosis, and response to therapy (55, 57). Differently from PBC, patients affected by primary sclerosing cholangitis (PSC) show a unique DR phenotype. In PSC, chronic inflammatory damage targets large intrahepatic bile ducts and mostly spares interlobular bile ducts; the development of fibrotic strictures and consequent cholestatic injury of the liver parenchyma trigger DR which, however, is less prominent compared to PBC and is characterized by the expression of hepatocellular traits, with the appearance of numerous EpCAM^{pos} hepatocytes (55).

In summary, liver diseases induce a substantial modification of the EpCAM^{pos} fraction within the liver; these changes are strongly influenced by the etiology of liver diseases and the specific regenerative needs. Remarkably, liver diseases further re-shape the non-parenchymal cell fractions (i.e., macrophages and hepatic stellate cells), inducing an inflammatory and fibrogenetic response (**Table 1**) (37, 40). In turn, these changes influence the EpCAM^{pos} cell compartment and support the vicious cycle which promotes and sustains liver fibrosis (58, 59). This represents the rationale for the strong correlation between EpCAM^{pos} fraction activation and clinical outcomes in human diseases (40, 57).

EpCAM^{pos} Cells Within PBGs in Human Cholangiopathies

The EpCAM^{pos} cell population in PBGs is implicated in human diseases affecting large intrahepatic and extrahepatic bile ducts (**Figure 3**, panel B) (1). Indeed, in PSC samples, progressive hyperplasia, and mucinous metaplasia of PBGs characterize fibrotic large bile ducts. Hyperplasia of PBGs is determined by the expansion of BTSCs, which also contributes to biliary fibrosis trough epithelial-to-mesenchymal transition and is sustained by the signaling pathway mediated by hedgehog ligands (**Table 1**) (30, 55). Interestingly, in PSC patients, the expansion of PBG mass correlated with the severity of the histological stage of liver cirrhosis and with the clinical stages according the Mayo score (30). It is worth noting that the histopathology of large bile duct fibrosis (which is at the basis of biliary strictures development in PSC) was understudied for years, although a consensus on PSC animal models highlighted the need to study large bile ducts and associated PBGs (60). In PSC and in pathologies of large bile ducts and in extrahepatic cholestasis, indeed, inflammation mostly spares the interlobular bile ducts within the liver parenchyma, whereas ductular reaction and fibrosis are present (55). These observations indicate that parenchymal injury in PSC is the consequence of ascending cholestasis. Differently, in PBC patients, the histomorphological study of bile ducts and livers demonstrated no activation of the PBG niche, thus indicating that the EpCAM^{pos} BTSCs endowed in large intrahepatic and extrahepatic bile ducts are elicited by the injury of this portion of the biliary tree (as in PSC) but not in diseases affecting occurring interlobular bile ducts (i.e., PBC) (30).

Other than PSC, PBGs are involved in the turnover and regeneration of biliary epithelia in sclerosing reactions in secondary sclerosing cholangitis and hepatolithiasis (22, 61). Cystic changes in PBGs can occur *de novo*, as part of a congenital syndrome, or secondarily to insults such as alcoholic cirrhosis (61). Interestingly, the systematic examination of bile ducts of liver grafts revealed the relationship between the degree of ischemic-based PBG injuries and the future development of non-anastomotic strictures (28, 62). Moreover, using an *ex vivo* model based on precision-cut slices of extrahepatic human bile ducts obtained from discarded donor livers, the spatiotemporal differentiation and migration of PBG cells after severe biliary injury was recently studied; this approach revealed that human PBGs contain biliary progenitor cells and are able to respond to bile duct epithelial loss with proliferation, differentiation, and maturation to restore epithelial integrity, providing evidence for a pivotal role of PBGs in biliary regeneration after severe injury (28).

Although normal PBGs themselves are particularly small structures that cannot be recognized using any of the currently available imaging modalities, these glands are closely associated with several diseases which have typical imaging features. The knowledge of the basic pathophysiology of PBGs could be helpful for depicting innovative diagnostic modalities and endpoints in biliary diseases associated with PBG injury (61). Since human BTSC activation in fibrotic large duct pathologies is associated with PBGs hyperplasia/metaplasia and dysplasia, in the future, histomorphology and radiology correlation studies are needed in order to envision innovative PBG imaging tools.

Mechanisms underlying the repair of extrahepatic biliary tree after injury have been scarcely explored. We have recently shown that the Wnt signaling pathway triggers human BTSC proliferation *in vitro* and influences PBG hyperplasia *in vivo* in a mouse biliary injury model (25). In particular, Notch signaling pathway activation induces BTSC differentiation *in vitro* toward mature cholangiocytes, in parallel with the observation of Notch pathway activation within PBGs in a mouse model; moreover, in human PSC, inflammatory and stromal cells trigger PBG activation through the upregulation of the Wnt and Notch signaling pathways (25). Considering these findings, the demonstration of the involvement of PBG cells in regenerating the injured biliary epithelium and identifying the signaling pathways driving BTSC activation could have relevant implications on the treatment of cholangiopathies.

The EpCAM^{pos} (MUC6^{high}) cell population may even respond to systemic stimuli, like hyperglycemia. In experimental and human diabetes, EpCAM^{pos}/MUC6^{high} cell population in PBGs respond to diabetes with proliferation and differentiation toward insulin-producing cells, indicating that PBG niches may rescue pancreatic islet impairment in diabetes (63). These findings offer important implications for the pathophysiology and complications of this disease, comprising the understanding of the paramount role of type II diabetes in cholangiocarcinoma risk nowadays (see the next paragraph) (63).

TABLE 1 | Summary of the main signaling pathways involved in EpCAM^{pos} niches of the liver and biliary tree.

Pathway	Secreted ligand	Receptor	Intracellular effector	Function
Notch	Jagged 1 Source: HSCs/MFs	Notch	Notch intra-cellular domain	Cholangiocyte fate
Wnt/β-catenin	Wnt1/Wnt3a Source: macrophages	P-β-Catenin	β-Catenin	Proliferation Hepatocyte fate
Hedgehog	Hh Source: EpCAM^{pos} stem/progenitor cells	Patched	Gli-1	Fibrogenesis EMT
Wnt/planar cell polarity	Wnt5a Source: HSCs/MFs	VANGL2	JNK/JUN	Modulation of niche microenvironment

EMT, epithelial/mesenchymal transition; HSC, hepatic stellate cell; MF, myofibroblast.

EPCAM^{POS} CELL POPULATIONS IN CHOLANGIOCARCINOMA

The recent focus on the EpCAM^{pos}/MUC6^{high} cell population residing in large intrahepatic and extrahepatic bile ducts sheds light on the clinical management of malignancies arising in this organ, which are collectively termed cholangiocarcinoma (30, 31). From an anatomical point of view, cholangiocarcinoma can be classified as intrahepatic, perihilar, or distal (64); however, growing evidence suggests that distinct cells of origin within an organ, particularly tissue-specific stem cells, may give rise to different cancer subtypes (**Figure 3**) (65). In this context, certain subtypes of intrahepatic cholangiocarcinoma (small bile duct type and cholangiolo-carcinoma) are constituted by mucin^{neg} cells and could originate from small cholangiocytes or from the EpCAM^{pos}/MUC6^{neg} population located in ductules and/or interlobular bile ducts. In keeping, chronic liver diseases and cirrhosis represent specific risk factors for these tumor subtypes, and the surrounding parenchyma is generally characterized by a marked EpCAM^{pos}/mucin^{neg} DR (40, 57). The division rate of stem cells is linearly correlated with the lifetime risk of developing primary liver cancer (66).

Intriguingly, mucinous intrahepatic (large bile duct type) and perihilar cholangiocarcinoma show a similar phenotype, with mucin^{pos} cells occupying the entire neoplastic mass, and are characterized by a similar clinical course (67); such tumors could arise from PBGs and, likely, from the EpCAM^{pos}/TROP2^{int}/MUC6^{high} compartment (31). PSC and liver flukes represent well-recognized risk factors for these tumor subtypes (67); these diseases chronically affect large intrahepatic and extrahepatic bile ducts and determine hyperplasia, mucinous metaplasia, and dysplasia in PBGs (30). The expansion of the EpCAM^{pos}/MUC6^{high} compartment within PBGs represents an attempt to restore epithelial integrity as a response to chronic bile duct damage (25). However, the continuous exposure to harmful stimuli leads to a progressively uncontrolled response, and dysplasia-to-cancer progression takes place diffusely within bile ducts with multiple neoplastic foci, mimicking field cancerization (31).

The inter-tumor heterogeneity of cholangiocarcinoma might be due to the interplay of distinct tissues/cells of origin, the underlying disease, and the associated molecular clustering based on driver mutations which shape the pathobiological features of the different cholangiocarcinoma subtypes. In keeping with that, intrahepatic cholangiocarcinoma can be distinguished into two main subtypes (small and large bile duct type) based on its origin and histomorphologic features. Remarkably, these tumor subtypes have distinct cancer stem cell profiles (68), thus suggesting a putative different cell of origin (HpSCs vs. BTSCs). These subtypes also differ in terms of gross growth pattern, genetic signatures, and driver mutations (e.g., IDH1/2 in small bile duct type and KRAS in large bile duct type), and prognosis. With this latter regard, the large bile duct cholangiocarcinoma subtype is a highly aggressive cancer, characterized by a low disease-free and overall survival. This tumor typically arises in patients with PSC and has been proved to derive from dysplastic EpCAM^{pos} PBGs both in humans (31) and in experimental models (69).

Emphasizing the role of the different tissues/cells of origin on the complex pathogenesis of cholangiocarcinoma, also in the picture of EpCAM^{pos} cell niches, could have implications on preventive strategies and early diagnosis in patients with underlying clinical or subclinical hepatobiliary disease, shedding new light on dissecting cholangiocarcinoma heterogeneity and allowing a rational approach to personalized medicine for this devastating cancer (67, 70).

PERSPECTIVES AND APPLICATIONS OF EPCAM^{POS} CELLS IN REGENERATIVE MEDICINE

Orthotopic liver transplantation represents the main curative option for the majority of chronic liver diseases. In this context, the shortage of organ donors represents a severe limitation to patients' treatment, which results in many patients dying while waiting for transplantation. For these patients, the development of effective strategies for cell therapy could represent a promising approach to the treatment of liver diseases, also as a bridge to liver transplantation.

Therefore, different strategies of cell therapy have been attempted (71, 72). Hepatocyte transplantation represents the proof of concept of liver cell therapy but it is limited by the scarcity of donor organs, the low cell engraftment, difficulties in cryopreservation, and the necessity of long-term immunosuppression (72–74). Mesenchymal-derived stem cells, comprising hematopoietic stem cells and mesenchymal stem cells, have been largely applied for liver regenerative medicine purposes in a number of clinical trials throughout the world (71, 75–79). Although autologous transplantation of hematopoietic and mesenchymal stem cells is clinically safe, the recent negative results of randomized clinical trials limit the future application of this strategy (75–79). Clinical applications of pluripotent stem cells in hepatology are actually null; this is due to the teratocarcinogenic risk and the ethical concerns for the use of embryonic stem cells and to the possibility of tumorigenic expansion of reprogrammed induced pluripotent stem cells (72).

In this scenario, the hepatic EpCAM^{pos} cell fractions could represent an important alternative source, currently under investigation worldwide. Other than case reports concerning the use of EpCAM^{pos} HpSCs in biliary atresia and inborn errors of metabolism (80, 81), a non-randomized clinical trial of 25 subjects and 25 controls with decompensated liver cirrhosis due to various causes undergoing human fetal EpCAM^{pos} HpSCs infusion into the liver via the hepatic artery has been reported (82). At 6-months follow-up, multiple diagnostic and biochemical parameters showed improvement, with a significant decrease in the patients' MELD (model for end-stage liver disease) scores (82). In western countries, Pietrosi et al. performed an intrasplenic infusion of a total cell population obtained from the fetal liver in nine patients affected by end-stage liver disease, demonstrating that the procedure was safe and well-tolerated in all patients (83). Similar to HpSCs, EpCAM^{pos} BTSCs could represent a possible source for stem/progenitor cells for liver regenerative medicine, as they are readily available from the biliary tree of adult or fetal organ donors and from cholecystectomized patients (84–87). In the past, we reported a preliminary experience in treating patients with advanced cirrhosis by the infusion via hepatic artery of human EpCAM^{pos} BTSCs (84). This report represents the proof of concept that EpCAM^{pos} BTSCs are a suitable source for the cell therapy of liver cirrhosis and represents the basis for an ongoing controlled clinical trial (84). Moreover, cells are routinely isolated in good manufacturing practices (GMP) conditions, and all required media are available in GMP-grade (84). Finally, the EpCAM-based sorting procedure is highly standardized and has been already used in clinical program (11, 84, 88, 89).

3D organoids represent an advanced culture technology in the field of stem cells and regenerative medicine, recapitulating embryonic development and the physiology of the tissue of origin. So far, organoid cultures have been developed for the adult intestine (90), stomach (91), and pancreas (92) of different species, like mouse and human. When cultured as organoids, cells can expand long term in culture, maintain the genetic stability, and spontaneously self-organize into structures that resemble the *in vivo* tissue in terms of cellular composition and function.

Organoid techniques have been largely applied to human liver, in particular to its EpCAM^{pos} stem/progenitor compartments. Under defined culture conditions, EpCAM^{pos} HpSCs from adult liver can be expanded for months (>1 year) in culture, showing an exponential rate of proliferation and genetic stability (92). HpSCs can readily be expanded as bipotent stem cells into 3D organoids and differentiate into functional hepatocyte cells both *in vitro* and *in vivo* upon transplantation (93, 94). Noteworthily, single isolated EpCAM^{pos} cells develop into organoid with high colony forming efficiency, while EpCAM^{neg} cells failed to create organoids (93). Moreover, the engraftment and differentiation of organoids was demonstrated in mouse models of acute liver injury; in these mice, a stable expression of human hepatocyte markers was observed in recipient serum for more than 4 months, and cell engraftment was confirmed by immunohistochemistry for human albumin (93).

The application of the organoid technique is feasible to obtain long-term expansion of BTSCs, maintaining stem cell markers and genetic stability over months (24, 87, 95). Interestingly, Sampaziotis et al. have demonstrated that cells isolated from the extrahepatic biliary tree can be expanded *in vitro* in long-term 3D organoid culture, while maintaining the biliary transcriptional signature and functional characteristics; this culture can be propagated as a potential system for the application of regenerative medicine in the field of cholangiopathies and *in vitro* common bile duct disease modeling (96).

Overall, organoid cultures derived from patients' liver could represent a relevant system to study human biology, physiology, and the regeneration and development of the liver and biliary tree (97). In addition, 3D organoid cultures enable the study of molecular mechanism driving liver diseases, comprising cholangiopathies (98) and primary liver cancers including cholangiocarcinoma (99); at the same time, this technique can provide potential tools to manipulating genomes and facilitate gene correction for regenerative medicine and autologous therapy (97). Recently, a specific interest has increased for the genetic modification of liver organoids to create disease-specific models in settings where providing a patient's material is challenging (100).

Liver organoids facilitate the study of human liver diseases and regeneration and open the way to expand human liver cells *in vitro* in the field of personalized medicine or drug testing for biliary and liver disease. The effective application of organoid-derived hepatocytes and cholangiocytes to humans needs to face important technical issues related to the *in vitro* manipulation and the large use of non-clinical-grade GMP substances necessary to promote and sustain long-term 3D growth.

CONCLUSION

The liver and the biliary tree harbor two EpCAM^{pos} stem/progenitor cell niches, both yielding high regenerative capabilities and the potential to differentiate into mature hepatocytes and cholangiocytes, but displaying distinct localization and phenotype and peculiar behavior and role in the physio-pathogenesis of liver and biliary diseases.

EpCAM^{pos} HpSCs are located at the canals of Hering and in the bile ductules; these cells are recruited in human acute and chronic liver diseases affecting hepatocytes, contributing to liver regeneration and being implicated in the fibrogenetic processes. HpSCs are also elicited in cholangiopathies affecting interlobular bile ducts (i.e., primary biliary cholangitis). EpCAM^{pos} BTSCs can be found in the PBGs of large intrahepatic or extrahepatic bile ducts and participate in regenerative responses following cholangiopathies affecting large ducts. Their activation is key in the pathogenesis of biliary strictures in primary sclerosing cholangitis, and their injury is implicated in the onset of non-anastomotic strictures following orthotropic liver transplantation.

Both niches could contribute to the development of cholangiocarcinoma due to their prominent activation occurring in pre-neoplastic conditions, and their distinct phenotype could explain, at least in part, the heterogeneity observed in cholangiocarcinoma subtypes.

Finally, due to their stem cell properties and safety of use, they represent a valid cell source for regenerative medicine of the liver.

AUTHOR CONTRIBUTIONS

SS: study concept, design, and drafting of the manuscript. GC: study concept, design, drafting of the manuscript, figure preparation, and study supervision. DO, AF, and VC acquisition of images, figure preparation, drafting of the manuscript, and critical revision of the manuscript for important intellectual content. PO, DA, and EG critical revision of the manuscript for important intellectual content, obtained funding, and study supervision. All authors contributed to the article and approved the submitted version.

REFERENCES

1. Lanzoni G, Cardinale V, Carpino G. The hepatic, biliary, and pancreatic network of stem/progenitor cell niches in humans: a new reference frame for disease and regeneration. *Hepatology.* (2016) 64:277–86. doi: 10.1002/hep.28326
2. Malato Y, Naqvi S, Schurmann N, Ng R, Wang B, Zape J, et al. Fate tracing of mature hepatocytes in mouse liver homeostasis and regeneration. *J Clin Invest.* (2011) 121:4850–60. doi: 10.1172/JCI59261
3. Yanger K, Knigin D, Zong Y, Maggs L, Gu G, Akiyama H, et al. Adult hepatocytes are generated by self-duplication rather than stem cell differentiation. *Cell Stem Cell.* (2014) 15:340–9. doi: 10.1016/j.stem.2014.06.003
4. Chen F, Jimenez RJ, Sharma K, Luu HY, Hsu BY, Ravindranathan A, et al. Broad distribution of hepatocyte proliferation in liver homeostasis and regeneration. *Cell Stem Cell.* (2020) 26:27–33 e4. doi: 10.1016/j.stem.2019.11.001
5. Matsumoto T, Wakefield L, Tarlow BD, Grompe M. *In vivo* lineage tracing of polyploid hepatocytes reveals extensive proliferation during liver regeneration. *Cell Stem Cell.* (2020) 26:34–47 e3. doi: 10.1016/j.stem.2019.11.014
6. Aleksieva N, Forbes SJ. Biliary-derived hepatocytes in chronic liver injury: bringing new troops to the battlefield? *J Hepatol.* (2019) 70:1051–3. doi: 10.1016/j.jhep.2019.03.015
7. Choi TY, Ninov N, Stainier DY, Shin D. Extensive conversion of hepatic biliary epithelial cells to hepatocytes after near total loss of hepatocytes in zebrafish. *Gastroenterology.* (2014) 146:776–88. doi: 10.1053/j.gastro.2013.10.019
8. Russell JO, Lu WY, Okabe H, Abrams M, Oertel M, Poddar M, et al. Hepatocyte-specific beta-catenin deletion during severe liver injury provokes cholangiocytes to differentiate into hepatocytes. *Hepatology.* (2019) 69:742–59. doi: 10.1002/hep.30270
9. Aizarani N, Saviano A, Sagar, Mailly L, Durand S, Herman JS, et al. A human liver cell atlas reveals heterogeneity and epithelial progenitors. *Nature.* (2019) 572:199–204. doi: 10.1038/s41586-019-1373-2
10. Segal JM, Kent D, Wesche DJ, Ng SS, Serra M, Oules B, et al. Single cell analysis of human foetal liver captures the transcriptional profile of hepatobiliary hybrid progenitors. *Nat Commun.* (2019) 10:3350. doi: 10.1038/s41467-019-11266-x
11. Yoon SM, Gerasimidou D, Kuwahara R, Hytiroglou P, Yoo JE, Park YN, et al. Epithelial cell adhesion molecule (EpCAM) marks hepatocytes newly derived from stem/progenitor cells in humans. *Hepatology.* (2011) 53:964–73. doi: 10.1002/hep.24122
12. Gaudio E, Carpino G, Cardinale V, Franchitto A, Onori P, Alvaro D. New insights into liver stem cells. *Dig Liver Dis.* (2009) 41:455–62. doi: 10.1016/j.dld.2009.03.009
13. Alvaro D, Gaudio E. Liver capsule: biliary tree stem cell subpopulations. *Hepatology.* (2016) 64:644. doi: 10.1002/hep.28546
14. Roskams TA, Theise ND, Balabaud C, Bhagat G, Bhathal PS, Bioulac-Sage P, et al. Nomenclature of the finer branches of the biliary tree: canals, ductules, and ductular reactions in human livers. *Hepatology.* (2004) 39:1739–45. doi: 10.1002/hep.20130
15. Schmelzer E, Zhang L, Bruce A, Wauthier E, Ludlow J, Yao HL, et al. Human hepatic stem cells from fetal and postnatal donors. *J Exp Med.* (2007) 204:1973–87. doi: 10.1084/jem.20061603
16. Carpentier R, Suner RE, Van Hul N, Kopp JL, Beaudry JB, Cordi S, et al. Embryonic ductal plate cells give rise to cholangiocytes, periportal hepatocytes, and adult liver progenitor cells. *Gastroenterology.* (2011) 141:1432–8. doi: 10.1053/j.gastro.2011.06.049
17. Turner R, Lozoya O, Wang Y, Cardinale V, Gaudio E, Alpini G, et al. Human hepatic stem cell and maturational liver lineage biology. *Hepatology.* (2011) 53:1035–45. doi: 10.1002/hep.24157
18. Libbrecht L, Desmet V, Van Damme B, Roskams T. The immunohistochemical phenotype of dysplastic foci in human liver: correlation with putative progenitor cells. *J Hepatol.* (2000) 33:76–84. doi: 10.1016/S0168-8278(00)80162-2
19. Spee B, Carpino G, Schotanus BA, Katoonizadeh A, Vander Borght S, Gaudio E, et al. Characterisation of the liver progenitor cell niche in liver diseases: potential involvement of Wnt and Notch signalling. *Gut.* (2010) 59:247–57. doi: 10.1136/gut.2009.188367
20. Deng X, Zhang X, Li W, Feng RX, Li L, Yi GR, et al. Chronic liver injury induces conversion of biliary epithelial cells into hepatocytes. *Cell Stem Cell.* (2018) 23:114–22 e3. doi: 10.1016/j.stem.2018.05.022
21. Cardinale V, Wang Y, Carpino G, Cui CB, Gatto M, Rossi M, et al. Multipotent stem/progenitor cells in human biliary tree give rise to hepatocytes, cholangiocytes, and pancreatic islets. *Hepatology.* (2011) 54:2159–72. doi: 10.1002/hep.24590
22. Igarashi S, Sato Y, Ren XS, Harada K, Sasaki M, Nakanuma Y. Participation of peribiliary glands in biliary tract pathophysiologies. *World J Hepatol.* (2013) 5:425–32. doi: 10.4254/wjh.v5.i8.425
23. Carpino G, Cardinale V, Onori P, Franchitto A, Berloco PB, Rossi M, et al. Biliary tree stem/progenitor cells in glands of extrahepatic and intraheptic bile ducts: an anatomical *in situ* study yielding evidence of maturational lineages. *J Anatomy.* (2012) 220:186–99. doi: 10.1111/j.1469-7580.2011.01462.x
24. Carpino G, Cardinale V, Gentile R, Onori P, Semeraro R, Franchitto A, et al. Evidence for multipotent endodermal stem/progenitor cell populations in human gallbladder. *J Hepatol.* (2014) 60:1194–202. doi: 10.1016/j.jhep.2014.01.026
25. Carpino G, Nevi L, Overi D, Cardinale V, Lu WY, Di Matteo S, et al. Peribiliary gland niche participates in biliary tree regeneration in mouse and in human primary sclerosing cholangitis. *Hepatology.* (2020) 71:972–89. doi: 10.1002/hep.30871
26. Cardinale V, Wang Y, Carpino G, Mendel G, Alpini G, Gaudio E, et al. The biliary tree–a reservoir of multipotent stem cells. *Nat Rev Gastroenterol Hepatol.* (2012) 9:231–40. doi: 10.1038/nrgastro.2012.23

27. Matsui S, Harada K, Miyata N, Okochi H, Miyajima A, Tanaka M. Characterization of peribiliary gland-constituting cells based on differential expression of trophoblast cell surface protein 2 in biliary tract. *Am J Pathol.* (2018) 188:2059–73. doi: 10.1016/j.ajpath.2018.05.016
28. de Jong IEM, Matton APM, van Praagh JB, van Haaften WT, Wiersema-Buist J, van Wijk LA, et al. Peribiliary glands are key in regeneration of the human biliary epithelium after severe bile duct injury. *Hepatology.* (2019) 69:1719–34. doi: 10.1002/hep.30365
29. DiPaola F, Shivakumar P, Pfister J, Walters S, Sabla G, Bezerra JA. Identification of intramural epithelial networks linked to peribiliary glands that express progenitor cell markers and proliferate after injury in mice. *Hepatology.* (2013) 58:1486–96. doi: 10.1002/hep.26485
30. Carpino G, Cardinale V, Renzi A, Hov JR, Berloco PB, Rossi M, et al. Activation of biliary tree stem cells within peribiliary glands in primary sclerosing cholangitis. *J Hepatol.* (2015) 63:1220–8. doi: 10.1016/j.jhep.2015.06.018
31. Carpino G, Cardinale V, Folseraas T, Overi D, Grzyb K, Costantini D, et al. Neoplastic transformation of the peribiliary stem cell niche in cholangiocarcinoma arisen in primary sclerosing cholangitis. *Hepatology.* (2019) 69:622–38. doi: 10.1002/hep.30210
32. Pepe-Mooney BJ, Dill MT, Alemany A, Ordovas-Montanes J, Matsushita Y, Rao A, et al. Single-cell analysis of the liver epithelium reveals dynamic heterogeneity and an essential role for YAP in homeostasis and regeneration. *Cell Stem Cell.* (2019) 25:23–38 e8. doi: 10.1016/j.stem.2019.04.004
33. Gouw AS, Clouston AD, Theise ND. Ductular reactions in human liver: diversity at the interface. *Hepatology.* (2011) 54:1853–63. doi: 10.1002/hep.24613
34. Stueck AE, Wanless IR. Hepatocyte buds derived from progenitor cells repopulate regions of parenchymal extinction in human cirrhosis. *Hepatology.* (2015) 61:1696–707. doi: 10.1002/hep.27706
35. Dezso K, Rokusz A, Bugyik E, Szucs A, Szuak A, Dorogi B, et al. Human liver regeneration in advanced cirrhosis is organized by the portal tree. *J Hepatol.* (2017) 66:778–86. doi: 10.1016/j.jhep.2016.11.014
36. Schuster S, Cabrera D, Arrese M, Feldstein AE. Triggering and resolution of inflammation in NASH. *Nat Rev Gastroenterol Hepatol.* (2018) 15:349–64. doi: 10.1038/s41575-018-0009-6
37. Overi D, Carpino G, Franchitto A, Onori P, Gaudio E. Hepatocyte injury and hepatic stem cell niche in the progression of non-alcoholic steatohepatitis. *Cells.* (2020) 9:30590. doi: 10.3390/cells9030590
38. Carpino G, Pastori D, Baratta F, Overi D, Labbadia G, Polimeni L, et al. PNPLA3 variant and portal/periportal histological pattern in patients with biopsy-proven non-alcoholic fatty liver disease: a possible role for oxidative stress. *Sci Rep.* (2017) 7:15756. doi: 10.1038/s41598-017-15943-z
39. Nobili V, Carpino G, De Peppo F, Caccamo R, Mosca A, Romito I, et al. Laparoscopic sleeve gastrectomy improves nonalcoholic fatty liver disease-related liver damage in adolescents by reshaping cellular interactions and hepatic adipocytokine production. *J Pediatr.* (2018) 194:100–8 e3. doi: 10.1016/j.jpeds.2017.10.036
40. Gadd VL, Skoien R, Powell EE, Fagan KJ, Winterford C, Horsfall L, et al. The portal inflammatory infiltrate and ductular reaction in human nonalcoholic fatty liver disease. *Hepatology.* (2014) 59:1393–405. doi: 10.1002/hep.26937
41. Guldiken N, Kobazi Ensari G, Lahiri P, Couchy G, Preisinger C, Liedtke C, et al. Keratin 23 is a stress-inducible marker of mouse and human ductular reaction in liver disease. *J Hepatol.* (2016) 65:552–9. doi: 10.1016/j.jhep.2016.04.024
42. Franchitto A, Carpino G, Alisi A, De Peppo F, Overi D, De Stefanis C, et al. The contribution of the adipose tissue-liver axis in pediatric patients with nonalcoholic fatty liver disease after laparoscopic sleeve gastrectomy. *J Pediatr.* (2020) 216:117–27 e2. doi: 10.1016/j.jpeds.2019.07.037
43. Carpino G, Del Ben M, Pastori D, Carnevale R, Baratta F, Overi D, et al. Increased liver localization of lipopolysaccharides in human and experimental non-alcoholic fatty liver disease. *Hepatology.* (2019). doi: 10.1002/hep.31056. [Epub ahead of print].
44. Richardson MM, Jonsson JR, Powell EE, Brunt EM, Neuschwander-Tetri BA, Bhathal PS, et al. Progressive fibrosis in nonalcoholic steatohepatitis: association with altered regeneration and a ductular reaction. *Gastroenterology.* (2007) 133:80–90. doi: 10.1053/j.gastro.2007.05.012
45. Nobili V, Carpino G, Alisi A, Franchitto A, Alpini G, De Vito R, et al. Hepatic progenitor cells activation, fibrosis, and adipokines production in pediatric nonalcoholic fatty liver disease. *Hepatology.* (2012) 56:2142–53. doi: 10.1002/hep.25742
46. Nobili V, Alisi A, Cutrera R, Carpino G, De Stefanis C, D'Oria V, et al. Altered gut-liver axis and hepatic adiponectin expression in OSAS: novel mediators of liver injury in paediatric non-alcoholic fatty liver. *Thorax.* (2015) 70:769–81. doi: 10.1136/thoraxjnl-2015-206782
47. Sancho-Bru P, Altamirano J, Rodrigo-Torres D, Coll M, Millan C, Jose Lozano J, et al. Liver progenitor cell markers correlate with liver damage and predict short-term mortality in patients with alcoholic hepatitis. *Hepatology.* (2012) 55:1931–41. doi: 10.1002/hep.25614
48. Aguilar-Bravo B, Rodrigo-Torres D, Arino S, Coll M, Pose E, Blaya D, et al. Ductular reaction cells display an inflammatory profile and recruit neutrophils in alcoholic hepatitis. *Hepatology.* (2019) 69:2180–95. doi: 10.1002/hep.30472
49. Lanthier N, Rubbia-Brandt L, Lin-Marq N, Clement S, Frossard JL, Goossens N, et al. Hepatic cell proliferation plays a pivotal role in the prognosis of alcoholic hepatitis. *J Hepatol.* (2015) 63:609–21. doi: 10.1016/j.jhep.2015.04.003
50. Dubuquoy L, Louvet A, Lassailly G, Truant S, Boleslawski E, Artru F, et al. Progenitor cell expansion and impaired hepatocyte regeneration in explanted livers from alcoholic hepatitis. *Gut.* (2015) 64:1949–60. doi: 10.1136/gutjnl-2014-308410
51. Odena G, Chen J, Lozano JJ, Altamirano J, Rodrigo-Torres D, Affo S, et al. LPS-TLR4 pathway mediates ductular cell expansion in alcoholic hepatitis. *Sci Rep.* (2016) 6:35610. doi: 10.1038/srep35610
52. Rastogi A, Maiwall R, Bihari C, Trehanpati N, Pamecha V, Sarin SK. Two-tier regenerative response in liver failure in humans. *Virchows Arch.* (2014) 464:565–73. doi: 10.1007/s00428-014-1547-0
53. Dezso K, Nagy P, Paku S. Human liver regeneration following massive hepatic necrosis: two distinct patterns. *J Gastroenterol Hepatol.* (2020) 35:124–34. doi: 10.1111/jgh.14721
54. Lindor KD, Bowlus CL, Boyer J, Levy C, Mayo M. Primary biliary cholangitis: 2018 practice guidance from the American Association for the Study of Liver Diseases. *Hepatology.* (2019) 69:394–419. doi: 10.1002/hep.30145
55. Carpino G, Cardinale V, Folseraas T, Overi D, Floreani A, Franchitto A, et al. Hepatic stem/progenitor cell activation differs between primary sclerosing and primary biliary cholangitis. *Am J Pathol.* (2018) 188:627–39. doi: 10.1016/j.ajpath.2017.11.010
56. Kennedy L, Francis H, Invernizzi P, Venter J, Wu N, Carbone M, et al. Secretin/secretin receptor signaling mediates biliary damage and liver fibrosis in early-stage primary biliary cholangitis. *FASEB J.* (2019) 33:10269–79. doi: 10.1096/fj.201802606R
57. Carbone M, Nardi A, Flack S, Carpino G, Varvaropoulou N, Gavrila C, et al. Pretreatment prediction of response to ursodeoxycholic acid in primary biliary cholangitis: development and validation of the UDCA Response Score. *Lancet Gastroenterol Hepatol.* (2018) 3:626–34. doi: 10.1016/S2468-1253(18)30163-8
58. Wilson DH, Jarman EJ, Mellin RP, Wilson ML, Waddell SH, Tsokkou P, et al. Non-canonical Wnt signalling regulates scarring in biliary disease via the planar cell polarity receptors. *Nat Commun.* (2020) 11:445. doi: 10.1038/s41467-020-14283-3
59. Planas-Paz L, Sun T, Pikiolek M, Cochran NR, Bergling S, Orsini V, et al. YAP, but not RSPO-LGR4/5, signaling in biliary epithelial cells promotes a ductular reaction in response to liver injury. *Cell Stem Cell.* (2019) 25:39–53 e10. doi: 10.1016/j.stem.2019.04.005
60. Fickert P, Pollheimer MJ, Beuers U, Lackner C, Hirschfield G, Housset C, et al. Characterization of animal models for primary sclerosing cholangitis (PSC). *J Hepatol.* (2014) 60:1290–303. doi: 10.1016/j.jhep.2014.02.006
61. Matsubara T, Kozaka K, Matsui O, Nakanuma Y, Uesaka K, Inoue D, et al. Peribiliary glands: development, dysfunction, related conditions and imaging findings. *Abdom Radiol.* (2020) 45:416–36. doi: 10.1007/s00261-019-02298-4
62. Franchitto A, Overi D, Mancinelli R, Mitterhofer AP, Muiesan P, Tinti F, et al. Peribiliary gland damage due to liver transplantation involves peribiliary vascular plexus and vascular endothelial growth factor. *Eur J Histochem.* (2019) 63:3022. doi: 10.4081/ejh.2019.3022

63. Carpino G, Puca R, Cardinale V, Renzi A, Scafetta G, Nevi L, et al. Peribiliary glands as a niche of extrapancreatic precursors yielding insulin-producing cells in experimental and human diabetes. *Stem Cells.* (2016) 34:1332–42. doi: 10.1002/stem.2311
64. Kendall T, Verheij J, Gaudio E, Evert M, Guido M, Goeppert B, et al. Anatomical, histomorphological and molecular classification of cholangiocarcinoma. *Liver Int.* (2019) 39(Suppl.1):7–18. doi: 10.1111/liv.14093
65. Hoadley KA, Yau C, Hinoue T, Wolf DM, Lazar AJ, Drill E, et al. Cell-of-origin patterns dominate the molecular classification of 10,000 tumors from 33 types of cancer. *Cell.* (2018) 173:291–304 e6. doi: 10.1016/j.cell.2018.03.022
66. Tomasetti C, Vogelstein B. Cancer etiology. Variation in cancer risk among tissues can be explained by the number of stem cell divisions. *Science.* (2015) 347:78–81. doi: 10.1126/science.1260825
67. Banales JM, Cardinale V, Carpino G, Marzioni M, Andersen JB, Invernizzi P, et al. Expert consensus document: cholangiocarcinoma: current knowledge and future perspectives consensus statement from the European Network for the Study of Cholangiocarcinoma (ENS-CCA). *Nat Rev Gastroenterol Hepatol.* (2016) 13:261–80. doi: 10.1038/nrgastro.2016.51
68. Cardinale V, Renzi A, Carpino G, Torrice A, Bragazzi MC, Giuliante F, et al. Profiles of cancer stem cell subpopulations in cholangiocarcinomas. *Am J Pathol.* (2015) 185:1724–39. doi: 10.1016/j.ajpath.2015.02.010
69. Nakagawa H, Suzuki N, Hirata Y, Hikiba Y, Hayakawa Y, Kinoshita H, et al. Biliary epithelial injury-induced regenerative response by IL-33 promotes cholangiocarcinogenesis from peribiliary glands. *Proc Natl Acad Sci USA.* (2017) 114:E3806–15. doi: 10.1073/pnas.1619416114
70. Carnevale G, Carpino G, Cardinale V, Pisciotta A, Riccio M, Bertoni L, et al. Activation of Fas/FasL pathway and the role of c-FLIP in primary culture of human cholangiocarcinoma cells. *Sci Rep.* (2017) 7:14419. doi: 10.1038/s41598-017-14838-3
71. Lanzoni G, Oikawa T, Wang Y, Cui CB, Carpino G, Cardinale V, et al. Concise review: clinical programs of stem cell therapies for liver and pancreas. *Stem Cells.* (2013) 31:2047–60. doi: 10.1002/stem.1457
72. Qi X, Guo X, Su C. Clinical outcomes of the transplantation of stem cells from various human tissue sources in the management of liver cirrhosis: a systematic review and meta-analysis. *Curr Stem Cell Res Ther.* (2015) 10:166–80. doi: 10.2174/1574888X09666141112114011
73. Lee CA, Sinha S, Fitzpatrick E, Dhawan A. Hepatocyte transplantation and advancements in alternative cell sources for liver-based regenerative medicine. *J Mol Med.* (2018) 96:469–81. doi: 10.1007/s00109-018-1638-5
74. Fox IJ, Chowdhury JR, Kaufman SS, Goertzen TC, Chowdhury NR, Warkentin PI, et al. Treatment of the Crigler-Najjar syndrome type I with hepatocyte transplantation. *N Engl J Med.* (1998) 338:1422–6. doi: 10.1056/NEJM199805143382004
75. An SY, Jang YJ, Lim HJ, Han J, Lee J, Lee G, et al. Milk fat globule-EGF factor 8, secreted by mesenchymal stem cells, protects against liver fibrosis in mice. *Gastroenterology.* (2017) 152:1174–86. doi: 10.1053/j.gastro.2016.12.003
76. Lanthier N, Lin-Marq N, Rubbia-Brandt L, Clement S, Goossens N, Spahr L. Autologous bone marrow-derived cell transplantation in decompensated alcoholic liver disease: what is the impact on liver histology and gene expression patterns? *Stem Cell Res Ther.* (2017) 8:88. doi: 10.1186/s13287-017-0541-2
77. Newsome PN, Fox R, King AL, Barton D, Than NN, Moore J, et al. Granulocyte colony-stimulating factor and autologous CD133-positive stem-cell therapy in liver cirrhosis (REALISTIC): an open-label, randomised, controlled phase 2 trial. *Lancet Gastroenterol Hepatol.* (2018) 3:25–36. doi: 10.1016/S2468-1253(17)30326-6
78. Peng L, Xie DY, Lin BL, Liu J, Zhu HP, Xie C, et al. Autologous bone marrow mesenchymal stem cell transplantation in liver failure patients caused by hepatitis B: short-term and long-term outcomes. *Hepatology.* (2011) 54:820–8. doi: 10.1002/hep.24434
79. Spahr L, Chalandon Y, Terraz S, Kindler V, Rubbia-Brandt L, Frossard JL, et al. Autologous bone marrow mononuclear cell transplantation in patients with decompensated alcoholic liver disease: a randomized controlled trial. *PLoS ONE.* (2013) 8:e53719. doi: 10.1371/journal.pone.0053719
80. Khan AA, Parveen N, Mahaboob VS, Rajendraprasad A, Ravindraprakash HR, Venkateswarlu J, et al. Treatment of Crigler-Najjar Syndrome type 1 by hepatic progenitor cell transplantation: a simple procedure for management of hyperbilirubinemia. *Transplant Proc.* (2008) 40:1148–50. doi: 10.1016/j.transproceed.2008.03.022
81. Lysy PA, Najimi M, Stephenne X, Bourgois A, Smets F, Sokal EM. Liver cell transplantation for Crigler-Najjar syndrome type I: update and perspectives. *World J Gastroenterol.* (2008) 14:3464–70. doi: 10.3748/wjg.14.3464
82. Khan AA, Shaik MV, Parveen N, Rajendraprasad A, Aleem MA, Habeeb MA, et al. Human fetal liver-derived stem cell transplantation as supportive modality in the management of end-stage decompensated liver cirrhosis. *Cell Transplant.* (2010) 19:409–18. doi: 10.3727/096368909X484707a
83. Pietrosi G, Vizzini G, Gerlach J, Chinnici C, Luca A, Amico G, et al. Phases I-II matched case-control study of human fetal liver cell transplantation for treatment of chronic liver disease. *Cell Transplant.* (2015) 24:1627–38. doi: 10.3727/096368914X682422
84. Cardinale V, Carpino G, Gentile R, Napoletano C, Rahimi H, Franchitto A, et al. Transplantation of human fetal biliary tree stem/progenitor cells into two patients with advanced liver cirrhosis. *BMC Gastroenterol.* (2014) 14:204. doi: 10.1186/s12876-014-0204-z
85. Nevi L, Cardinale V, Carpino G, Costantini D, Di Matteo S, Cantafora A, et al. Cryopreservation protocol for human biliary tree stem/progenitors, hepatic and pancreatic precursors. *Sci Rep.* (2017) 7:6080. doi: 10.1038/s41598-017-05858-0
86. Nevi L, Carpino G, Costantini D, Cardinale V, Riccioni O, Di Matteo S, et al. Hyaluronan coating improves liver engraftment of transplanted human biliary tree stem/progenitor cells. *Stem Cell Res Ther.* (2017) 8:68. doi: 10.1186/s13287-017-0492-7
87. Costantini D, Overi D, Casadei L, Cardinale V, Nevi L, Carpino G, et al. Simulated microgravity promotes the formation of tridimensional cultures and stimulates pluripotency and a glycolytic metabolism in human hepatic and biliary tree stem/progenitor cells. *Sci Rep.* (2019) 9:5559. doi: 10.1038/s41598-019-41908-5
88. Carpino G, Renzi A, Franchitto A, Cardinale V, Onori P, Reid L, et al. Stem/progenitor cell niches involved in hepatic and biliary regeneration. *Stem Cells Int.* (2016) 2016:3658013. doi: 10.1155/2016/3658013
89. Semeraro R, Carpino G, Cardinale V, Onori P, Gentile R, Cantafora A, et al. Multipotent stem/progenitor cells in the human foetal biliary tree. *J Hepatol.* (2012) 57:987–94. doi: 10.1016/j.jhep.2012.07.013
90. Sato T, Vries RG, Snippert HJ, van de Wetering M, Barker N, Stange DE, et al. Single Lgr5 stem cells build crypt-villus structures *in vitro* without a mesenchymal niche. *Nature.* (2009) 459:262–5. doi: 10.1038/nature07935
91. Barker N, Huch M, Kujala P, van de Wetering M, Snippert HJ, van Es JH, et al. Lgr5(+ve) stem cells drive self-renewal in the stomach and build long-lived gastric units *in vitro*. *Cell Stem Cell.* (2010) 6:25–36. doi: 10.1016/j.stem.2009.11.013
92. Huch M, Dorrell C, Boj SF, van Es JH, Li VS, van de Wetering M, et al. *In vitro* expansion of single Lgr5+ liver stem cells induced by Wnt-driven regeneration. *Nature.* (2013) 494:247–50. doi: 10.1038/nature11826
93. Huch M, Gehart H, van Boxtel R, Hamer K, Blokzijl F, Verstegen MM, et al. Long-term culture of genome-stable bipotent stem cells from adult human liver. *Cell.* (2015) 160:299–312. doi: 10.1016/j.cell.2014.11.050
94. Aloia L, McKie MA, Vernaz G, Cordero-Espinoza L, Aleksieva N, van den Ameele J, et al. Epigenetic remodelling licences adult cholangiocytes for organoid formation and liver regeneration. *Nat Cell Biol.* (2019) 21:1321–33. doi: 10.1038/s41556-019-0402-6
95. Rimland CA, Tilson SG, Morell CM, Tomaz RA, Lu WY, Adams SE, et al. Regional differences in human biliary tissues and corresponding *in vitro* derived organoids. *Hepatology.* (2020). doi: 10.1002/hep.31252. [Epub ahead of print].
96. Sampaziotis F, Justin AW, Tysoe OC, Sawiak S, Godfrey EM, Upponi SS, et al. Reconstruction of the mouse extrahepatic biliary tree using primary human extrahepatic cholangiocyte organoids. *Nat Med.* (2017) 23:954–63. doi: 10.1038/nm.4360
97. Kruitwagen HS, Oosterhoff LA, Vernooij I, Schrall IM, van Wolferen ME, Bannink F, et al. Long-term adult feline liver organoid cultures for disease modeling of hepatic steatosis. *Stem Cell Rep.* (2017) 8:822–30. doi: 10.1016/j.stemcr.2017.02.015

98. Soroka CJ, Assis DN, Boyer JL. Patient-derived organoids from human bile: an *in vitro* method to study cholangiopathies. *Methods Mol Biol.* (2019) 1981:363–72. doi: 10.1007/978-1-4939-9420-5_24
99. Broutier L, Mastrogiovanni G, Verstegen MM, Francies HE, Gavarro LM, Bradshaw CR, et al. Human primary liver cancer-derived organoid cultures for disease modeling and drug screening. *Nat Med.* (2017) 23:1424–35. doi: 10.1038/nm.4438
100. Schwank G, Koo BK, Sasselli V, Dekkers JF, Heo I, Demircan T, et al. Functional repair of CFTR by CRISPR/Cas9 in intestinal stem cell organoids of cystic fibrosis patients. *Cell Stem Cell.* (2013) 13:653–8. doi: 10.1016/j.stem.2013.11.002

17

Neddylation: A Versatile Pathway Takes on Chronic Liver Diseases

*Jiping Yao, Xue Liang, Yanning Liu and Min Zheng**

The State Key Laboratory for Diagnosis and Treatment of Infectious Diseases, National Clinical Research Center for Infectious Diseases, Collaborative Innovation Center for Diagnosis and Treatment of Infectious Diseases, The First Affiliated Hospital, College of Medicine, Zhejiang University, Hangzhou, China

Correspondence:
Min Zheng
minzheng@zju.edu.cn

Neddylation is a ubiquitin-like posttranslational modification that conjugates neural precursor cell expressed developmentally downregulated-8 (Nedd8) to specific substrates for regulation of protein activity. In light of current researches, the neddylation pathway is aberrant in the pathogenesis of many diseases. In our review, we summarize the versatile roles of neddylation in chronic liver diseases (CLDs). CLDs are one of the leading causes of chronic disease-associated deaths worldwide. There are diverse etiologic agents causing CLDs, mainly including hepatitis B virus (HBV) infection, nonalcoholic fatty liver disease (NAFLD), chronic exposure to alcohol or drugs, and autoimmune causes. So far, however, there remains a paucity of effective therapeutic approach to CLDs. In this review, we summarized the role of the neddylation pathway which runs through the chronic hepatitis B/NAFLD–liver fibrosis–cirrhosis–hepatocellular carcinoma (HCC) axis, a canonical pattern in the process of CLD development and progression. The dysregulation of neddylation may provide a better understanding of CLD pathology and even a novel therapeutic strategy. Correspondingly, inhibiting neddylation via MLN4924, a small molecule compound targeting NEDD8-activating enzyme (NAE), can potently alleviate CLD progression and improve the outcome. On this basis, profiling and characterization of the neddylation pathway can provide new insights into the CLD pathology as well as novel therapeutic strategies, independently of the etiology of CLD.

Keywords: neddylation, HBV, NAFLD, liver fibrosis, HCC, therapy, MLN4924

INTRODUCTION

Chronic liver disease (CLD) is posing a significant public health problem worldwide for it causes ~2 million deaths annually. It is desperately needed to pay high attention to it (1). There are diverse etiologic agents causing CLDs, primarily including chronic infection of hepatitis B or C viruses (HBV or HCV), chronic aberrant metabolic conditions [nonalcoholic fatty liver disease (NAFLD)], chronic consumption of alcohol or drugs, and abnormal autoimmunity (2, 3). Further, the onset, development, and deterioration of CLD are progressive processes. A variety of factors are involved in them, such as inflammatory cell infiltration, liver tissue reconstruction, fibrogenesis, and extracellular matrix (ECM) deposition (4, 5). Therefore, the pathological process of CLD is complicated, characterized by pan-cellular and pan-pathway mechanisms. Recently, more and more attention has been paid to the ubiquitination pathway due to its potential role in the therapy of CLD, particularly hepatocellular carcinoma (HCC), the advanced stage of CLD.

A new insight into the CLD field is the emerging role of the neddylation pathway. Neddylation is a ubiquitination-like modification. However, unlike ubiquitination that mainly targets proteins doomed to be degraded, neddylation regulates proteins' function and stability (6). The best-known physiological substrates of neddylation are the cullin family, the crucial component of cullin-RING ligases (CRLs). CRL is the largest family of ubiquitination E3 ligases (7) and responsible for about 20% of cellular protein degradation via proteasome (8). Neddylation of cullin activates CRLs (9) and promotes the ubiquitination of substrates (10). Hence, neddylation modulates the cellular function in some degree via manipulating ubiquitination E3 ligases behind the scene. Previous researches demonstrated that neddylation inhibition can inactivate CRLs (11) and then results in accumulation of their substrates, such candidates including chromatin licensing and DNA replication factor 1 (CDT1) (12), p21 (13), and nuclear factor erythroid 2-related factor 2 (NRF2) (14, 15). Most substrates of CRLs are tumor suppressors (16). The consequence of neddylation inhibition is cell apoptosis, cell autophagy, cell senescence, and ultimately cancer suppression (17) (**Table 1**). Current researches of noncullin substrates of neddylation uncover that neddylation might participate in additional biological process of cells (41) (**Table 2**). On this basis, recent studies have uncovered that neddylation inhibition can repress HBV survival (64), alleviate steatosis (65), reduce liver fibrosis (66), and restrain pro-tumor inflammation (67). Considering the progress that has been made to understand the role of neddylation, it is worthy to explore and conclude the relevance between neddylation and CLD. In this review, we particularly focus on the role of the neddylation pathway in CLD pathology and assess the therapeutic approach targeting neddylation in CLD.

NEDDYLATION IN CLD

Overactivation of Neddylation

Deregulation of the neddylation pathway has been described in various pathological conditions. Focusing on the CLD context like liver fibrosis and HCC, both NAE1 and global protein neddylation expressions are upregulated (66, 68). However, the initial triggering mechanism that overactivates neddylation pathways during CLD is not understood exactly. Significantly, a previous study demonstrated that diverse stress conditions such as heat shock and oxidative stress may lead to an entire increase of the neddylation pathway *in vitro*. Under the stress circumstance, the ubiquitin E1 enzyme Ubel, rather than NAE1, regulates the conjugation of the NEDD8 (69, 70). Further analysis reveals that the crosstalk between NEDD8 and ubiquitin causes a prompt and dramatic amplification of the NEDD8 proteome under stress conditions. In addition, neddylation of the substrate competing with its ubiquitination upon stress could stabilize its protein level and prevent its degradation (69). Subsequently, accumulated substrates mediate vital biological processes and trigger diverse cellular responses, which may result in multiple hepatic dysfunctions eventually. Besides, in HCC, a decrease in deneddylating enzyme NEDP1 with a concomitant increase of NEDD8 conjugates leads to the inhibition of ATPase activity of heat shock protein 70 (HSP70) (71). As a result, the formation of the apoptosome is disturbed, and subsequently, the apoptosis resistance of hepatoma cells is elevated (72).

NEDDYLATION AND HBV INFECTION

HBV chronic infection is a primary pathogeny leading to CLDs, especially cirrhosis and HBV-related HCC (64). HBV-encoded X protein (HBx) is a small regulatory protein that exhibits pleiotropic activities, including affecting transcription, DNA repair, cell growth, and apoptotic cell death (73). HBx can interact with various cellular proteins to influence its own activity. Among all these HBx-interacting proteins, the damage-specific DNA binding protein 1 (DDB1) is a well-characterized HBx binding partner (74). This interaction is worthy of attention because DDB1 is the adaptor protein of CRL4 ubiquitin E3 ligase. Previous researches reported that HBx–DDB1 interaction is indispensable in HBx-induced viral genome replication and affects cell viability. An interesting structural study revealed that HBx contains an α-helical motif termed the H-box, which is shared by several DDB1–CUL4-associated factor (DCAF) proteins (75). DCAF proteins act as well-known CRL4 substrate acceptors. According to the above, it is possible that HBx assembles an HBx–DDB1–CUL4–ROC1 E3 ligase complex (CRL^{HBx}) as CRL4 and HBx plays the role of substrate receptor. HBx targets host proteins that suppress HBV genome replication, and CRL^{HBx} promotes their ubiquitylation and degradation

Abbreviations: CLD, chronic liver diseases; MDM2, murine double minute-2; NEDD8, neural precursor cell expressed developmentally downregulated-8; HBV, hepatitis B virus; HCV, hepatitis C virus; HCC, hepatocellular carcinoma; HBx, HBV-encoded X protein; HSC, hepatic stellate cell; NAE, NEDD8-activating enzyme; E2F-1, E2F transcription factor 1; ECM, extracellular matrix; CRL, cullin-RING ligases; VHL, von Hippel-Lindau; RBX, RING box protein-1; SKP, S-phase kinase-associated protein; CDT1, chromatin licensing and DNA replication factor; CDT2, chromatin licensing and DNA replication factor 2; NRF2, nuclear factor erythroid 2-related factor 2; NF-κB, the nuclear factor kappa-light-chain-enhancer of activated B cells; ATF4, activating transcription factor 4; βTrCP, beta-transducin repeat containing protein; DCN1, defective in cullin neddylation 1; ROS, reactive oxygen species; mTORC, mammalian target of rapamycin complex; NASH, nonalcoholic steatohepatitis; NAFLD, nonalcoholic fatty liver disease; TRIM40, tripartite motif containing 40; BCA3, breast cancer-associated protein 3; FBXO11, F-box protein 11; HuR, Hu antigen R; TGFβ-RII, transforming growth factor β type II receptor; AICD, APP intracellular domain; EGFR, epidermal growth factor receptor; BRAP2, BRCA1-associated protein 2; SCF, Skp1, cullin, and F-box protein; RTK, receptor tyrosine kinase; cccDNA, covalently closed circular DNA; IL-8, interleukin-8; MMP9, matrix metalloproteinase-9; DEPTOR, DEP domain containing mTOR-interacting protein; HIFα, hypoxia-inducible factor-α; DCAF, DDB1-CUL4-associated factor; IFNα, interferon-α; Collα1, collagen type I alpha 1; TGFβ, transforming growth factor; TNFα, tumor necrosis factor α; IL-6, interleukin-6; Cxcl, the chemokine (C-X-C motif) ligand; Ccl, the chemokine (C-C motif) ligand; Ccr, the C-C chemokine receptors; c-Cbl, Casita B-lineage lymphoma; pVHL, Von-Hippel-Lindau protein; DDB1, the damage-specific DNA binding protein 1; SARM, sterile α and HEAT/armadillo-motif-containing protein; Bax, Bcl-2 associated protein X; CUL, cullin; KC, Kupffer cells; CCl4, carbon tetrachloride; JNK, c-Jun N-terminal kinase; Bcl-2, β-cell lymphoma 2; SMC, the structural maintenance of chromosomes; ETFs, electron transfer flavoproteins; SRSF3, serine-rich splicing factor 3; BDL, bile duct ligation; CCl4, carbon tetrachloride; HSP70, heat shock protein 70; SREBP1c, sterol regulatory element-binding protein 1c; HDM2, human homolog of mouse double minute 2; LKB1, liver kinase B1; AGEs, advanced glycation end products; WIPI2, WD repeat domain, phosphoinositide interacting 2.

TABLE 1 | Neddylation inhibition and CRL inactivation.

Response	Substrate	CRL	Function	Reference
Apoptosis	CDT1	$CRL1^{SKP}/CRL4^{CDT2}$	DNA damage	(12, 18, 19)
	pIkBα	$CRL1^{\beta-Trcp}$	NF-κB inactivation	(17, 20, 21)
	NOXA	RBX2-associated CRLs	DNA damage	(22–24)
	ATF4	RBX1-CRL1	DR5 expression	(25–28)
Autophagy	DEPTOR	$CRL1^{\beta-Trcp}$	mTORC1 inactivation	(29–31)
	HIF1α	$CRL2^{VHL}$	mTORC1 inactivation	(32–34)
Senescence	p21	$CRL1^{SKP2}/CRL4^{CDT2}$	G2 (or G2/M) phase arrest	(13, 35–37)
	P27	$CRL1^{SKP2}$	G2 (or G2/M) phase arrest	(38)
	WEE1	CRL1	G2 (or G2/M) phase arrest	(39)
Redox Homeostasis	NRF2	CRL1/CRL3	scavenging ROS	(14, 15, 40)

TABLE 2 | Neddylation pathway substrates.

Type		Substrates	E3 ligases	Function of neddylation	References
Ubiquitin E3 ligases		CRLs	RBX1/2 and/or DCN1	Increases CRL activity	(42)
		Smurf	Smurf	Increases Smurf activity	(43)
		Parkin		Increases parkin activity	(44)
		VHL		Promotes VHL association with fibronectin	(45)
		BRAP2		Inhibits NF-κB-mediated transcription	(46)
		MDM2	MDM2	Increases MDM2 stability	(47)
Transcription regulation		p53	MDM2 and SCF^{FBXO11}	Inhibits p53 transcriptional activity	(47)
		p73	MDM2	Inhibits p73 transcriptional activity	(48)
		IKKγ	TRIM40	Inhibits NF-κB activity	(49)
		BCA3		Inhibits NF-κB-mediated transcription	(50)
		E2F1		Reduces E2F-1 stability	(51)
		APP/AICD		Inhibits AICD-mediated transcriptional activation	(52)
		HIF1α/HIF2α		Increases protein stability	(53)
		HuR	Mdm2	Increases stability and nuclear localization	(54)
Signaling pathways	RTK signaling	EGFR	c-CBL	Facilitates EGFR degradation	(55)
		TGFβRII	c-CBL	Increases TGF-βRII stability	(56)
		SHC		Promotes Erk activation	(57)
	Apoptosis	drICE		Inhibits apoptosis	(58)
		Caspases/IAPs/RIP1		Suppresses caspase activity	(59)
	DNA damage	Histone H4	RNF111	Activates DNA damage-induced ubiquitination	(60)
	Nucleolar stress signaling	L11	MDM2	Increase stability and nucleolar	(61)
		S14		localization	(62)
	Oxidative/calcium stress	RCAN1		Increase RCAN1 stability	(63)

via the proteasome pathway (75–77). Neddylation activates $CRL4^{HBx}$ via conjugating Nedd8 to the cullin protein's conserved lysine residues to affect HBV replication indirectly.

Liu et al. also found that HBx can be neddylated by the Nedd8 E3 ligase human homolog of mouse double minute 2 (HDM2). Neddylation modification alters HBx's half-life and enhances its stability. Moreover, it also increases HBx's chromatin localization and the binding with DDB1 (64). Previous researches show that HBx is ubiquitylated by E3 ligase Siah-1 to induce HBx degradation (78). Interestingly, Liu and his colleagues found that the mechanism of HDM2-mediated neddylation modification increases HBx stability by preventing its ubiquitination-induced degradation (64). These processes ultimately favor HBx's activity of transcriptional regulation, cell proliferation, and HBV-driven tumor growth. In conclusion, it provides an insight into the neddylation's role in HBV invasion. Further study found that HDM2's expression is positively correlated with HBx expression in HBV-related HCC samples (**Figure 1**). HDM2 has the potential to act as a new prognostic marker for HBV-related HCC. Inhibition of the neddylation pathway may provide us with a novel therapeutic method for HBV-related HCC.

NEDDYLATION AND NAFLD

NAFLD is an increasingly prevalent CLD and has become a prominent healthy concern globally due to dietary structure change and lifestyle change (79). NAFLD is characterized by steatosis, a pathologic phenomenon of excessive triglyceride accumulation in hepatocytes. NAFLD will frequently progress to its more severe form called nonalcoholic steatohepatitis (NASH), which consists of hepatic steatosis, inflammation, and fibrosis. NASH accompanied with advanced fibrosis may eventually lead to cirrhosis and even HCC (80, 81). Recently, more and more insight has been shed on the association between NAFLD and neddylation.

Neddylation plays a crucial physiological role in lipid metabolism. Recent research reported that liver-specific deficiency of NEDD8 or UBA3 causes neonatal death with spontaneous fatty liver in mouse models. Interestingly, electron transfer flavoproteins (ETFs), whose defects can lead to fatty acid oxidation disorder in glutaric aciduria type II (GA-II), are neddylation substrates. Hepatic neddylation modification can stabilize ETFs and even enhance ETF expression via suppressing their ubiquitination, which prevents fasting-induced steatosis (82).

Furthermore, another research of serine-rich splicing factor 3 (SRSF3) illuminates that neddylation is involved in the pathology of NAFLD and NASH. It suggested that the low expression of SRSF3 is correlated with an increased risk of NAFLD, NASH, or cirrhosis. In the condition of oxidative stress, SRSF3 could be modified by the NEDD8 protein at lysine 11, which results in the degradation of SRSF3 via proteasome (83). On this basis, the result above implies that intervening with the neddylation of SRSF3 contributes to its stability and accumulation, which is beneficial for preventing hepatic steatosis, fibrosis, and inflammation.

Recently, it was reported that sterol regulatory element-binding protein 1c (SREBP1c), a critical role in maintaining lipid homeostasis, is upregulated in liver to contribute to the progress of hepatic steatosis. However, unlike SRSF3, neddylation of SREBP1c competing with its ubiquitination facilitates its stability and, rather than promoting its degradation via proteasome, eventually contributes to hepatic steatosis. Further, SREBP1c can be neddylated by NEDD8 E3 ligase HDM2, which can also mediate the neddylation of HBx as described above (84).

Additionally, Dehnad et al. revealed that advanced glycation end product (AGE) clearance receptor AGER1 was decreased

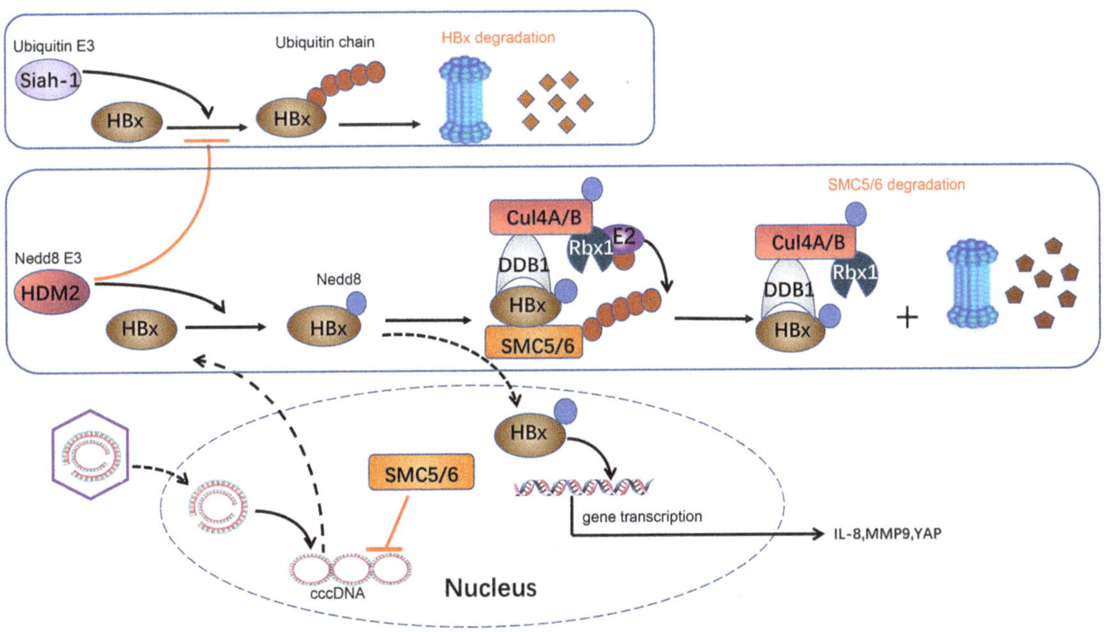

FIGURE 1 | Neddylation and HBV infection. HBV is a DNA virus carrying a 3.2-kb genome. Following entry into the host cell, the 3.2-kb genome is transported into the nucleus and converted to a cccDNA, which serves as a crucial template for HBV transcription. HBx is transcripted from cccDNA and serves as a transcriptional activator to promote the expression of IL-8, MMP9, and YAP, which are implicated in HCC development. HBx in cytoplasm is ubiquitylated by E3 ligase Siah-1 to induce HBx degradation through proteasome. HBx can be neddylated by Nedd8 E3 ligase HDM2 in the cytoplasm. HDM2-mediated neddylation modification increases HBx stability by preventing its ubiquitination-induced degradation. Meanwhile, HBx plays a role as a substrate acceptor and assembles CRL4^{HBx} ubiquitin E3 ligases. HBx targets SMC5/6, a host protein that suppresses HBV genome replication, and CRL4^{HBx} promotes its ubiquitylation and degradation via proteasome. Besides, neddylation activates CRL4^{HBx} via conjugating Nedd8 to cullin protein's conserved lysine residues to affect HBV replication indirectly.

in NASH. Further analysis demonstrated that exposure to high AGEs promotes an AGER1/RAGE imbalance and subsequently promotes NRF2 degradation via neddylation of cullin3, which eventually causes downregulation of AGER1 (85).

Taken together, these studies come to the conclusion that a neddylation-dependent pathway is implicated in liver steatosis and fibrosis mainly via regulating the stability of its substrates, which function as critical regulators in the process of liver steatosis. Revealing the role of neddylation in hepatic lipid metabolism and fibrosis progression may pave the way for a novel therapeutic approach in NAFLD and NASH (65).

NEDDYLATION AND LIVER FIBROSIS

Liver fibrosis is a continuous wound-healing progress leading to sustained scarring response (86). Liver fibrosis can be triggered by underlying etiologies of CLDs, such as viral infection, alcohol, and NASH (87). The pathology progress is a dynamic and reversible response that can be regulated by halting or reversing the fibrosis to cirrhosis and HCC (3). To date, specific therapies validated as being effective for liver fibrosis have primarily been etiology induced. However, there is no thoroughly validated antifibrosis therapy that is independent of the underlying etiology in the clinic.

More recently, deregulated neddylation is founded in liver fibrosis (66). Firstly, neddylation inhibition decreases liver inflammation. It is reported that neddylation inhibition reduces the expression level of pro-inflammatory cytokines and chemokines, such as tumor necrosis factor α (TNFα), interleukin-6 (IL-6) and its receptor, the tumor necrosis factor alpha receptor (TNFR1) (88), the chemokine (C-X-C motif) ligand 1 (Cxcl1), the chemokine (C-X-C motif) ligand 2 (Cxcl2), the chemokine (C-C motif) ligand 2 (Ccl2), and the C-C chemokine receptors (Ccr) (Ccr1, Ccr2, and Ccr5) (89). Secondly, neddylation plays a role in hepatic stellate cell activation. In bile duct ligation (BDL) and carbon tetrachloride (CCl_4)-induced injury rodents, neddylation inhibition decreases HSC activation and collagen accumulation, certified by reduced levels of the pro-fibrogenic factor, transforming growth factor (TGFβ), and the expression of collagen type I alpha 1 (Col1α1) (90). Thirdly, neddylation inhibition decreases fibrosis by inducing HSC apoptosis due to c-Jun accumulation. c-Jun, associated with apoptosis in several types of cells, such as HSC, could be targeted by neddylated cullins for degradation via the ubiquitin proteasome system. This provides a critical clue that neddylation inhibition could somehow modulate c-Jun levels and concomitant apoptosis (91).

Moreover, there are another two possible regulated mechanisms of neddylation in liver fibrogenesis. The transcription factor NF-κB mediates transcription of genes, such as pro-inflammation cytokines involved in the inflammation progress of fibrogenesis (92). Neddylation functions on NF-κB activation by promoting its nuclear translocation via activating $SCF^{\beta TrCP}$'s cullin. $SCF^{\beta TrCP}$ is a CRL that targets the NF-κB inhibitory protein IκBα for degradation via proteasome (93). It is reasonable to believe that neddylation inhibition could ameliorate inflammation and fibrosis via reducing specific NF-κB target genes' expressions. Another possible mechanism is associated with TGFβ. TGFβ is significantly important in HSC activation and involved in Smad2 signaling through transmembrane receptor serine/threonine kinases (94). An intriguing research shows that Casita B-lineage lymphoma (c-Cbl) can function as a Nedd8 E3 ligase of the type II receptor (TGFβ-RII) beyond CRL (56). The neddylation modification of TGFβ-RII interferes with its ubiquitination–proteasome degradation in blood cells. Therefore, we can speculate that the neddylation modification of TGFβ-RII stabilizes its function and thereby promotes TGFβ signaling, playing a key role in HSC activation (66, 95).

NEDDYLATION AND HCC

HCC, the most common and frequent primary liver cancer, is the advanced stage of CLD. Although some alteration of signal molecules involved in HCC progression is discovered, the high mortality and the poor prognosis make it the third malignancy that leads to cancer-related death globally (96). Recently, it was reported that the dysregulation of the neddylation pathway is associated with HCC. The whole neddylation pathway including NEDD8; NEDD8-specific E1, E2, and E3; and even deneddylation enzymes was upregulated in HCC (97).

Inhibiting the neddylation pathway can significantly suppress HCC cell proliferation and migration, induce apoptosis, and eventually inhibit HCC growth and metastasis (98). Nieves Embade and his colleagues found that Hu antigen R (HuR) was implicated in the above process. HuR plays a critical role in hepatocyte proliferation, survival, differentiation, and HCC transformation via enhancing the stability of target mRNAs (92). The stability of HuR itself in cells is attributed to Mdm2-mediated neddylation. The neddylation modification of HuR promotes its nuclear localization and reduces its degradation (54, 99). SREBP-1 is not merely a critical regulator of lipid metabolism but is also associated with cancer metabolism. In metastatic HCC samples, SREBP-1 is upregulated with a concomitant increase of UBC12. Recently, it was reported that SREBP-1 can be neddylated by NEDD8 E3 ligase UBC12. Consequently, neddylation of SREBP-1 competing with its ubiquitination promotes the stability of SREBP-1 (68). Otherwise, liver kinase B1 (LKB1) and Akt kinases, critical regulators in proliferative metabolism of the liver, could be neddylated to enhance their stability. Inhibition of neddylation leads to metabolic reprogramming and concomitant apoptosis of liver cancer cells via altering the stability of LKB1 and Akt (100).

Importantly, neddylation is closely related to regulation of autophagy in liver cancer cells (101). Autophagy is a cellular biological process in response to various stresses to maintain cellular homeostasis. Several researches have reported that autophagy could play a pro-survival role in cancer cells. Inhibition of neddylation would induce autophagy to promote survival of cancer cell and thus result in drug resistance. Mechanistically, suppressing neddylation causes inactivation of $CRL1^{\beta-TrCP}$ and $CRL2^{VHL}$ and subsequently contributes to the accumulation of their substrates: DEPTOR and HIF1α.

DEPTOR and the HIF1–REDD1–TSC1 axis would induce mTOR inactivation, which partially leads to autophagy (34, 102, 103). Additionally, increased level of reactive oxygen species (ROS) and activating transcription factor 3 (ATF3) could also trigger autophagy in the circumstance of neddylation inhibition (104). Recently, it was reported that inactivation of CRL4 would block polyubiquitination and proteasomal degradation of the WD repeat domain, phosphoinositide interacting 2 (WIPI2) via inhibition of neddylation, which eventually induces autophagy during mitosis (105).

Moreover, neddylation also regulates pro-tumorigenic inflammation in liver cancer cells. Hypoxia-inducible factor-1 (HIF1), an oxygen homeostasis transcription factor, provides anti-inflammation activity under hypoxia conditions (106). The alpha subunit of HIF1 (HIF1α) can be targeted by the Von-Hippel-Lindau protein (pVHL), a substrate receptor of CRL2 (107). Under normoxic conditions, HIF1α prefers to be hydroxylated and then recognized by pVHL, which mediates the degradation of hydroxylated HIF1α by the UPS pathway (32, 33). Under hypoxic conditions, HIF1α tends to translocate to the nucleus and form a heterodimer with a HIF1β subunit and transcriptionally regulates a wide spectrum of genes significant for the anti-inflammatory response (108). Likewise, neddylation modification of cullin2 alters the activity of CRL2 and eventually influences the stability of HIF1α (109) (**Figure 2**). Recently, Cannito et al. (110) have suggested that SerpinB3, a serine protease inhibitor, can stimulate proliferation of hepatic tumor cells and subsequently facilitate HCC progression by enhancing the stabilization of HIF2α by promoting the direct and selective neddylation of HIF2α (111).

Further analysis elucidates that the role of neddylation poses a profound effect not only on liver cancer cells but also on immune cells. In macrophages, blocking neddylation regulates NF-κB signaling and eventually causes the downregulation of proinflammatory cytokines. Besides, further research reveals that the sensitive to apoptosis gene (SAG), a neddylation E3 ligase, collaborates with UPS to promote survival of infectious macrophages via degrading proapoptotic Bax and sterile α and HEAT/armadillo-motif-containing protein (SARM) (112). SAG also affects cytokine secretion of macrophages (113). Similar to innate immune cells, SAG-deficient T cells also show decreased proliferation, reduced production of cytokines, and diminished release of the T-cell lineage. Besides, knockdown of Ubc12 in CD4+ T cells caused impaired T-cell receptor/CD28-induced proliferation because T cells were arrested in the G0/G1 phase of the cell cycle (113). Moreover, cytokine production like IL-2 and the differentiation of CD4+ T cells into effector Th-cell subsets are decreased when the expression of Ubc12 is reduced. The neddylation pathway regulates various aspects of CD4+ T-cell function. However, the exact mechanism remains to be investigated. A similar result was found in B cells (114–116).

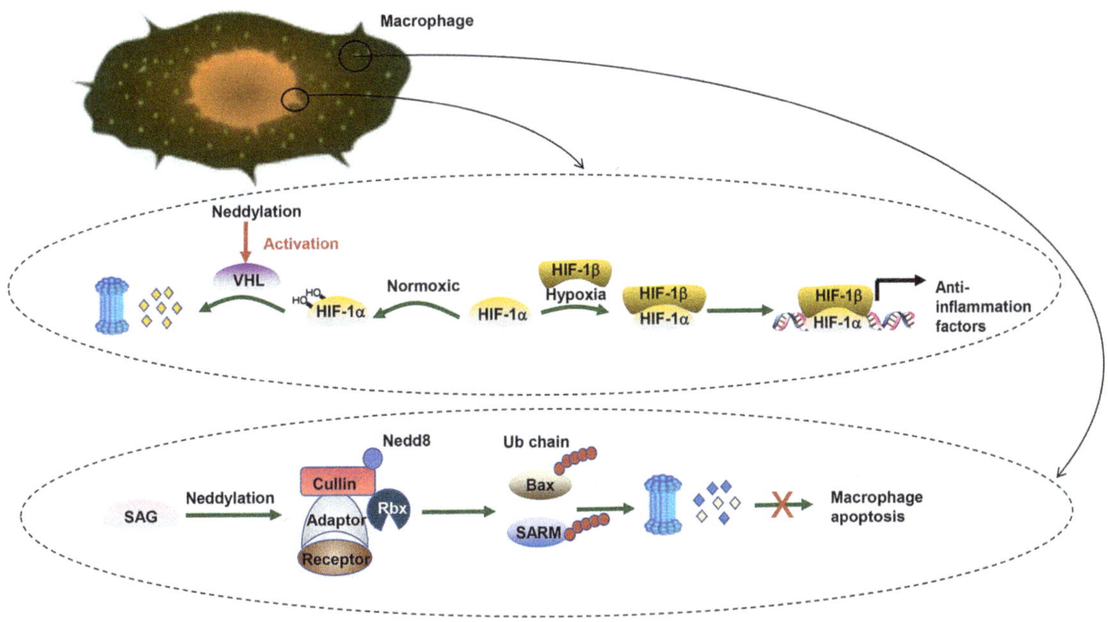

FIGURE 2 | Neddylation and HCC. There are two biological processes taking place in pro-inflammation macrophages. One is related to the transcription factor HIF. HIF-1α can be targeted by pVHL, a substrate receptor of CRL2. Under normoxic conditions, HIF-1α prefers to be hydroxylated and then recognized by pVHL for degradation via the UPS pathway. Under hypoxic conditions, HIFα tends to translocate to the nucleus and form a heterodimer with a HIF1β subunit and transcriptionally regulates a wide spectrum of genes significant for the anti-inflammatory response. The other is about the apoptosis inhibition of pro-inflammation macrophages. SAG, a neddylation E3 ligase, collaborates with UPS to promote survival of infectious macrophages via ubiquitination of Bax and SARM. In contrast, SAG knockdown leads to the accumulation of proapoptotic Bax and SARM and breaks the balance between antiapoptotic Bcl-2 and Bax in the mitochondria, which induces the death of macrophages.

THERAPEUTIC STRATEGIES TARGETING NEDDYLATION

MLN4924 (pevonedistat), a small molecule inhibitor of NAE, disrupts CRL-mediated protein turnover; causes restraining tumor cell growth by inducing apoptosis, senescence, and autophagy; and causes sensitization to chemoradiation therapies in a cellular context-dependent manner (8). Currently, MLN4924 is being evaluated in several phase Ib/II/III clinical trials (https://www.clinicaltrials.gov/). Among these clinical trials, five completed phase I clinical trials in solid tumors and hematological malignancies have verified that MLN4924 is safe and feasible. Several phase II clinical trials are under way. Particularly, a phase III clinical trial of MLN4924 combined with azacytidine is currently recruiting volunteers with hematological malignancies. Previous researches suggested that MLN4924 is a potent and selective inhibitor in hematological neoplasms as well as many solid neoplasms, including HCC. Given that the summaries about previous studies of MLN4924 in HCC are relatively sufficient, we primarily demonstrate the use of MLN4924 in HBV infectious, NAFLD, and liver fibrosis.

Currently, although nucleoside or nucleoside analogs can suppress new viral DNA replication, they are unable to eradicate the cccDNA from infected hepatocytes thoroughly (117). This is the most critical reason resulting in HBV rebound and obstinacy. Recently, it is reported that MLN4924 can suppress HBV transcription and protein expression significantly via restoring the structural maintenance of chromosome (SMC) complex protein (SMC5/6) levels (118). Murphy et al. (119) identified that SMC5/6, a host restriction that restricts HBV replication by inhibiting HBV gene expression, is the substrate of CRL^{HBx} (120). HBx targets SMC5/6 for degradation by the ubiquitin–proteasome system, and subsequently, the transcription from cccDNA is elevated (**Figure 1**). Neddylation of cullin is necessary for activation of CRL^{HBx}. MLN4924 inhibits the neddylation process, promotes SMC5/6 accumulation, and ultimately leads to restriction of viral transcription and HBV DNA level, particularly cccDNA (118). Thereby, the neddylation pathway is a potential target for HBV treatment. MLN4924 may become a novel anti-HBV agent, though evidence is far from being enough.

In view of the role of neddylation in regulating stabilization of SRSF3, MLN4924 can repress the degradation of SRSF3 and reduce the accumulation of SREBP1c, which alleviate the steatosis and prevent the progression of NAFLD (65). Serrano-Macia et al. have found that β-oxidation activity and ketone body levels were enhanced after treatment. On the contrary, the levels of lipid peroxidation and ROS are significantly reduced after MLN4924 treatment. Further study suggests that in a NASH mouse model, MLN4924 treatment can reverse steatosis, inflammation, and fibrosis. Hence, inhibition of neddylation via MLN4924 is a potent therapeutic option because it can ameliorate fatty acid metabolism (121).

Similarly, using the pharmacological inhibitor MLN4924 could protect liver from injury, inflammation, and fibrosis via regulating the function of hepatocytes. To be more specific, MLN4924 treatment reduces the expression of pro-inflammatory cytokines previously associated with liver damage and, therefore, ameliorate the inflammation after liver injury (122). In agreement, pro-fibrogenic factors implicated in liver fibrosis, such as TGFβ, COL1α1, matrix metalloproteinase-9 (MMP9), and interferon-α (IFNα), are consistently decreased after using MLN4924. More importantly, MLN4924 diminishes the activation of HSC (66). Together, these results highlight that MLN4924 treatment is pointed out as a potential antifibrosis therapy that is independent of the underlying etiology in the clinic.

In this review, we conclude that inhibition of neddylation pharmacologically via MLN4924 can significantly alleviate CLD exacerbation and progression in view of recent researches (8). Given its well-tolerated toxicity and potent antitumor activity

TABLE 3 | Neddylation in CLDs.

CLD	Substrate	CRL/E3 ligase	Function	Reference
Hepatitis B	SMC5/6	$CRL4^{HBx}$/HDM2	Promotes HBV replication	(77, 78)
NAFLD/NASH	ETFs	?	Promotes hepatic steatosis	(82)
	SRSF	?		(83)
	SREBP1c	HDM2		(84)
	NRF2	CRL3		(85)
Liver fibrosis	c-Jun	CRL?	Promotes activation of HSC and inflammation	(91)
	IkBα	$CRL1^{\beta-Trcp}$		(93)
	TGFb-RII	c-CBL		(56)
HCC	HuR	Mdm2	Promotes proliferation, survival and metastasis of cancer cells	(54, 99)
	SREBP1	?	Regulates pro-tumorigenic	(68)
	LKB1	?	inflammation Regulates the function of immune cells	(100)
	Akt	?		(100)
	HIF1a	$CRL2^{VHL}$		(106–109)
	HIF2a	?		(110)
	Bax/SARM	SAG		(112)

in preclinical trails, MLN4924 is anticipated to be a promising therapeutic approach for CLD. However, there still remains some challenges for final application of MLN4924 in the clinic. Due to the treatment-emergent NAEb mutations, resistance to MLN4924 during therapy will appear, which subsequently reduces the effectiveness of this medicine (123). Therefore, it is indispensable to design next-generation NAE inhibitors that can overcome treatment-emergent resistance.

CONCLUSIONS AND PERSPECTIVES

Chronic hepatitis/NAFLD–liver fibrosis–cirrhosis–HCC axis is a canonical pattern in the process of CLD progression (124). Recent studies in the neddylation pathway provides us with crucial clues that neddylation is a versatile pathway that takes on various aspects and phases of CLD (**Table 3**). Although the complicated mechanism underlying the overactivation of the neddylation pathway during CLD still remains elusive, there are several notable features of neddylation in CLD. First, the NEDD8 and NAE1 expressions are upregulated significantly in NAFLD, liver fibrosis, and HCC, and the components of the neddylation pathway like Nedd8, E1 (NAE), E2, and E3 may become novel biomarkers for CLD diagnosis. Second, under stress conditions, neddylation modification directly or by activating CRL indirectly promotes the stability of the substrate (promotes degradation in rare cases), and the accumulated substrate functions as a crucial molecule to facilitate the development of CLD. Third, MLN4924 could inhibit the overactivation of neddylation during CLD and thus alleviates the pathological process.

However, there remain several issues that need to be further explained correspondingly. First, the underlying mechanism by which the neddylation pathway is overactivated in CLD has not been demonstrated clearly so far. Second, besides HSC and cancer cells, whether and how the upregulated neddylation pathway plays a significant role in hepatic parenchyma, Kupffer cells, and tumor microenvironment require further exploration. Third, MLN4924 suppresses the whole neddylation pathway and may cause potential unforeseeable secondary effects. Moreover, MLN4924 would induce autophagy that acts as a pro-survival signal in cancer cells. Given this situation, it is probably sensible to be cautious about using MLN4924 for CLD therapy.

Notably, sumoylation, another important ubiquitin-like posttranslational modification, is identified as a double-edged sword in CLD while neddylation generally causes pathological consequences. Inhibition of the global sumoylation pathway might not always be an optimal therapeutic strategy due to its "two faces" in CLD (125–128). Therefore, targeting the neddylation pathway holds promise for the therapy of CLD. On the context of drug discovery, it is highly anticipated that more specific and safer small molecule inhibitors aiming at special targets such as specific E3 Nedd8 ligases or deneddylase enzymes should be discovered as novel therapeutic approaches for CLD.

AUTHOR CONTRIBUTIONS

JY wrote the manuscript and prepared figures: MZ, YL, and XL provided expert comments and edits. All authors contributed to the article and approved the submitted version.

REFERENCES

1. Global, regional, and national age-sex specific all-cause and cause-specific mortality for 240 causes of death, 1990-2013: a systematic analysis for the Global Burden of Disease Study 2013. *Lancet.* (2015) 385:117–71. doi: 10.1016/S0140-6736(14)61682-2
2. Parola M, Pinzani M. Liver fibrosis: pathophysiology, pathogenetic targets and clinical issues. *Mol Aspects Med.* (2019) 65:37–55. doi: 10.1016/j.mam.2018.09.002
3. Trautwein C, Friedman SL, Schuppan D, Pinzani M. Hepatic fibrosis: concept to treatment. *J Hepatol.* (2015) 62:S15–S24. doi: 10.1016/j.jhep.2015.02.039
4. Lee YA, Wallace MC, Friedman SL. Pathobiology of liver fibrosis: a translational success story. *Gut.* (2015) 64:830–41. doi: 10.1136/gutjnl-2014-306842
5. Rosselli M, MacNaughtan J, Jalan R, Pinzani M. Beyond scoring: a modern interpretation of disease progression in chronic liver disease. *Gut.* (2013) 62:1234–41. doi: 10.1136/gutjnl-2012-302826
6. Kamitani T, Kito K, Nguyen HP, Yeh ETH. Characterization of NEDD8, a developmentally down-regulated ubiquitin-like protein. *J Biol Chem.* (1997) 272:28557–62. doi: 10.1074/jbc.272.45.28557
7. Pan ZQ, Kentsis A, Dias DC, Yamoah K, Wu K. Nedd8 on cullin: building an expressway to protein destruction. *Oncogene.* (2004) 23:1985–97. doi: 10.1038/sj.onc.1207414
8. Soucy TA, Smith PG, Milhollen MA, Berger AJ, Gavin JM, Adhikari S, et al. An inhibitor of NEDD8-activating enzyme as a new approach to treat cancer. *Nature.* (2009) 458:732–6. doi: 10.1038/nature07884
9. Huang DT, Ayrault O, Hunt HW, Taherbhoy AM, Duda DM, Scott DC, et al. E2-RING expansion of the NEDD8 cascade confers specificity to cullin modification. *Mol Cell.* (2009) 33:483–95. doi: 10.1016/j.molcel.2009.01.011
10. Saha A, Deshaies RJ. Multimodal activation of the ubiquitin ligase SCF by Nedd8 conjugation. *Mol Cell.* (2008) 32:21–31. doi: 10.1016/j.molcel.2008.08.021
11. Brownell JE, Sintchak MD, Gavin JM, Liao H, Bruzzese FJ, Bump NJ, et al. Substrate-assisted inhibition of ubiquitin-like protein-activating enzymes: the NEDD8 E1 inhibitor MLN4924 forms a NEDD8-AMP mimetic *in situ*. *Mol Cell.* (2010) 37:102–11. doi: 10.1016/j.molcel.2009.12.024
12. Hu J, McCall CM, Ohta T, Xiong Y. Targeted ubiquitination of CDT1 by the DDB1-CUL4A-ROC1 ligase in response to DNA damage. *Nat Cell Biol.* (2004) 6:1003–9. doi: 10.1038/ncb1172
13. Abbas T, Sivaprasad U, Terai K, Amador V, Pagano M, Dutta A. PCNA-dependent regulation of p21 ubiquitylation and degradation via the CRL4Cdt2 ubiquitin ligase complex. *Genes Dev.* (2008) 22:2496–506. doi: 10.1101/gad.1676108
14. Rada P, Rojo AI, Chowdhry S, McMahon M, Hayes JD, Cuadrado A. SCF/{beta}-TrCP promotes glycogen synthase kinase 3-dependent degradation of the Nrf2 transcription factor in a Keap1-independent manner. *Mol Cell Biol.* (2011) 31:1121–33. doi: 10.1128/MCB.01204-10
15. Rada P, Rojo AI, Evrard-Todeschi N, Innamorato NG, Cotte A, Jaworski T, et al. Structural and functional characterization of Nrf2 degradation

by the glycogen synthase kinase 3/beta-TrCP axis. *Mol Cell Biol.* (2012) 32:3486–99. doi: 10.1128/MCB.00180-12
16. Welcker M, Orian A, Jin JP, Grim JE, Harper JW, Eisenman RN, et al. The Fbw7 tumor suppressor regulates glycogen synthase kinase 3 phosphorylation-dependent c-Myc protein degradation (vol 101, pg 9085, 2004). *Proc Natl Acad Sci U S A.* (2006) 103:504. doi: 10.1073/pnas.0402770101
17. Milhollen MA, Traore T, Adams-Duffy J, Thomas MP, Berger AJ, Dang L, et al. MLN4924, a NEDD8-activating enzyme inhibitor, is active in diffuse large B-cell lymphoma models: rationale for treatment of NF-{kappa}B-dependent lymphoma. *Blood.* (2010) 116:1515–23. doi: 10.1182/blood-2010-03-272567
18. Li X, Zhao Q, Liao R, Sun P, Wu X. The SCF(Skp2) ubiquitin ligase complex interacts with the human replication licensing factor Cdt1 and regulates Cdt1 degradation. *J Biol Chem.* (2003) 278:30854–8. doi: 10.1074/jbc.C300251200
19. Blank JL, Liu XJ, Cosmopoulos K, Bouck DC, Garcia K, Bernard H, et al. Novel DNA damage checkpoints mediating cell death induced by the NEDD8-activating enzyme inhibitor MLN4924. *Cancer Res.* (2013) 73:225–34. doi: 10.1158/0008-5472.CAN-12-1729
20. Godbersen JC, Humphries LA, Danilova OV, Kebbekus PE, Brown JR, Eastman A, et al. The Nedd8-activating enzyme inhibitor MLN4924 thwarts microenvironment-driven NF-κB activation and induces apoptosis in chronic lymphocytic leukemia B cells. *Clin Cancer Res.* (2014) 20:1576–89. doi: 10.1158/1078-0432.CCR-13-0987
21. Swords RT, Kelly KR, Smith PG, Garnsey JJ, Mahalingam D, Medina E, et al. Inhibition of NEDD8-activating enzyme: a novel approach for the treatment of acute myeloid leukemia. *Blood.* (2010) 115:3796–800. doi: 10.1182/blood-2009-11-254862
22. Tan M, Li Y, Yang R, Xi N, Sun Y. Inactivation of SAG E3 ubiquitin ligase blocks embryonic stem cell differentiation and sensitizes leukemia cells to retinoid acid. *PLoS One.* (2011) 6:e27726. doi: 10.1371/journal.pone.0027726
23. Jia L, Yang J, Hao X, Zheng M, He H, Xiong X, et al. Validation of SAG/RBX2/ROC2 E3 ubiquitin ligase as an anticancer and radiosensitizing target. *Clin Cancer Res.* (2010) 16:814–24. doi: 10.1158/1078-0432.CCR-09-1592
24. Wei D, Li H, Yu J, Sebolt JT, Zhao L, Lawrence TS, et al. Radiosensitization of human pancreatic cancer cells by MLN4924, an investigational NEDD8-activating enzyme inhibitor. *Cancer Res.* (2012) 72:282–93. doi: 10.1158/0008-5472.CAN-11-2866
25. Chen P, Hu T, Liang Y, Li P, Chen X, Zhang J, et al. Neddylation inhibition activates the extrinsic apoptosis pathway through ATF4-CHOP-DR5 axis in human esophageal cancer cells. *Clin Cancer Res.* (2016) 22:4145–57. doi: 10.1158/1078-0432.CCR-15-2254
26. Knorr KL, Schneider PA, Meng XW, Dai H, Smith BD, Hess AD, et al. MLN4924 induces Noxa upregulation in acute myelogenous leukemia and synergizes with Bcl-2 inhibitors. *Cell Death Differ.* (2015) 22:2133–42. doi: 10.1038/cdd.2015.74
27. Pike LR, Phadwal K, Simon AK, Harris AL. ATF4 orchestrates a program of BH3-only protein expression in severe hypoxia. *Mol Biol Rep.* (2012) 39:10811–22. doi: 10.1007/s11033-012-1975-3
28. Liu X, Jiang Y, Wu J, Zhang W, Liang Y, Jia L, et al. NEDD8-activating enzyme inhibitor, MLN4924 (Pevonedistat) induces NOXA-dependent apoptosis through up-regulation of ATF-4. *Biochem Biophys Res Commun.* (2017) 488:1–5. doi: 10.1016/j.bbrc.2017.04.122
29. Duan S, Skaar JR, Kuchay S, Toschi A, Kanarek N, Ben-Neriah Y, et al. mTOR generates an auto-amplification loop by triggering the βTrCP- and CK1α-dependent degradation of DEPTOR. *Mol Cell.* (2011) 44:317–24. doi: 10.1016/j.molcel.2011.09.005
30. Gao D, Inuzuka H, Tan MK, Fukushima H, Locasale JW, Liu P, et al. mTOR drives its own activation via SCF(betaTrCP)-dependent degradation of the mTOR inhibitor DEPTOR. *Mol Cell.* (2011) 44:290–303. doi: 10.1016/j.molcel.2011.08.030
31. Zhao Y, Xiong X, Sun Y. DEPTOR, an mTOR inhibitor, is a physiological substrate of SCF(betaTrCP) E3 ubiquitin ligase and regulates survival and autophagy. *Mol Cell.* (2011) 44:304–16. doi: 10.1016/j.molcel.2011.08.029
32. Ivan M, Kondo K, Yang H, Kim W, Valiando J, Ohh M, et al. HIFalpha targeted for VHL-mediated destruction by proline hydroxylation: implications for O2 sensing. *Science.* (2001) 292:464–8. doi: 10.1126/science.1059817
33. Jaakkola P, Mole DR, Tian YM, Wilson MI, Gielbert J, Gaskell SJ, et al. Targeting of HIF-alpha to the von Hippel-Lindau ubiquitylation complex by O_2-regulated prolyl hydroxylation. *Science.* (2001) 292:468–72. doi: 10.1126/science.1059796
34. Zhao Y, Xiong X, Jia L, Sun Y. Targeting Cullin-RING ligases by MLN4924 induces autophagy via modulating the HIF1-REDD1-TSC1-mTORC1-DEPTOR axis. *Cell Death Dis.* (2012) 3:e386. doi: 10.1038/cddis.2012.125
35. Jia L, Li H, Sun Y. Induction of p21-dependent senescence by an NAE inhibitor, MLN4924, as a mechanism of growth suppression. *Neoplasia.* (2011) 13:561–9. doi: 10.1593/neo.11420
36. Kim Y, Starostina NG, Kipreos ET. The CRL4Cdt2 ubiquitin ligase targets the degradation of p21Cip1 to control replication licensing. *Genes Dev.* (2008) 22:2507–19. doi: 10.1101/gad.1703708
37. Yu ZK, Gervais JL, Zhang H. Human CUL-1 associates with the SKP1/SKP2 complex and regulates p21(CIP1/WAF1) and cyclin D proteins. *Proc Natl Acad Sci U S A.* (1998) 95:11324–9. doi: 10.1073/pnas.95.19.11324
38. Zhao Y, Morgan MA, Sun Y. Targeting Neddylation pathways to inactivate cullin-RING ligases for anticancer therapy. *Antioxid Redox Signal.* (2014) 21:2383–400. doi: 10.1089/ars.2013.5795
39. Mackintosh C, Garcia-Dominguez DJ, Ordonez JL, Ginel-Picardo A, Smith PG, Sacristan MP, et al. WEE1 accumulation and deregulation of S-phase proteins mediate MLN4924 potent inhibitory effect on Ewing sarcoma cells. *Oncogene.* (2013) 32:1441–51. doi: 10.1038/onc.2012.153
40. Chowdhry S, Zhang Y, McMahon M, Sutherland C, Cuadrado A, Hayes JD. Nrf2 is controlled by two distinct beta-TrCP recognition motifs in its Neh6 domain, one of which can be modulated by GSK-3 activity. *Oncogene.* (2013) 32:3765–81. doi: 10.1038/onc.2012.388
41. Batuello CN, Hauck PM, Gendron JM, Lehman JA, Mayo LD. Src phosphorylation converts Mdm2 from a ubiquitinating to a neddylating E3 ligase. *Proc Natl Acad Sci U S A.* (2015) 112:1749–54. doi: 10.1073/pnas.1416656112
42. Abidi N, Xirodimas DP. Regulation of cancer-related pathways by protein NEDDylation and strategies for the use of NEDD8 inhibitors in the clinic. *Endocr Relat Cancer.* (2015) 22:T55–70. doi: 10.1530/ERC-14-0315
43. Xie P, Zhang M, He S, Lu K, Chen Y, Xing G, et al. The covalent modifier Nedd8 is critical for the activation of Smurf1 ubiquitin ligase in tumorigenesis. *Nat Commun.* (2014) 5:3733. doi: 10.1038/ncomms4733
44. Choo YS, Vogler G, Wang D, Kalvakuri S, Iliuk A, Tao WA, et al. Regulation of parkin and PINK1 by neddylation. *Hum Mol Genet.* (2012) 21:2514–23. doi: 10.1093/hmg/dds070
45. Russell RC, Ohh M. NEDD8 acts as a 'molecular switch' defining the functional selectivity of VHL. *EMBO Rep.* (2008) 9:486–91. doi: 10.1038/embor.2008.19
46. Takashima O, Tsuruta F, Kigoshi Y, Nakamura S, Kim J, Katoh MC, et al. Brap2 regulates temporal control of NF-kappaB localization mediated by inflammatory response. *PLoS One.* (2013) 8:e58911. doi: 10.1371/journal.pone.0058911
47. Xirodimas DP, Saville MK, Bourdon JC, Hay RT, Lane DP. Mdm2-mediated NEDD8 conjugation of p53 inhibits its transcriptional activity. *Cell.* (2004) 118:83–97. doi: 10.1016/j.cell.2004.06.016
48. Watson IR, Blanch A, Lin DC, Ohh M, Irwin MS. Mdm2-mediated NEDD8 modification of TAp73 regulates its transactivation function. *J Biol Chem.* (2006) 281:34096–103. doi: 10.1074/jbc.M603654200
49. Noguchi K, Okumura F, Takahashi N, Kataoka A, Kamiyama T, Todo S, et al. TRIM40 promotes neddylation of IKKgamma and is downregulated in gastrointestinal cancers. *Carcinogenesis.* (2011) 32:995–1004. doi: 10.1093/carcin/bgr068
50. Gao F, Cheng J, Shi T, Yeh ET. Neddylation of a breast cancer-associated protein recruits a class III histone deacetylase that represses NFκB-dependent transcription. *Nat Cell Biol.* (2006) 8:1171–7. doi: 10.1038/ncb1483
51. Loftus SJ, Liu G, Carr SM, Munro S, La Thangue NB. NEDDylation regulates E2F-1-dependent transcription. *EMBO Rep.* (2012) 13:811–8. doi: 10.1038/embor.2012.113
52. Lee MR, Lee D, Shin SK, Kim YH, Choi CY. Inhibition of APP intracellular domain (AICD) transcriptional activity via covalent

conjugation with Nedd8. *Biochem Biophys Res Commun.* (2008) 366:976–81. doi: 10.1016/j.bbrc.2007.12.066

53. Ryu JH, Li SH, Park HS, Park JW, Lee B, Chun YS. Hypoxia-inducible factor alpha subunit stabilization by NEDD8 conjugation is reactive oxygen species-dependent. *J Biol Chem.* (2011) 286:6963–70. doi: 10.1074/jbc.M110.188706
54. Embade N, Fernandez-Ramos D, Varela-Rey M, Beraza N, Sini M, Gutierrez de Juan V, et al. Murine double minute 2 regulates Hu antigen R stability in human liver and colon cancer through NEDDylation. *Hepatology.* (2012) 55:1237–48. doi: 10.1002/hep.24795
55. Oved S, Mosesson Y, Zwang Y, Santonico E, Shtiegman K, Marmor MD, et al. Conjugation to Nedd8 instigates ubiquitylation and down-regulation of activated receptor tyrosine kinases. *J Biol Chem.* (2006) 281:21640–51. doi: 10.1074/jbc.M513034200
56. Zuo W, Huang F, Chiang YJ, Li M, Du J, Ding Y, et al. c-Cbl-mediated neddylation antagonizes ubiquitination and degradation of the TGF-β type II receptor. *Mol Cell.* (2013) 49:499–510. doi: 10.1016/j.molcel.2012.12.002
57. Jin HS, Liao L, Park Y, Liu YC. Neddylation pathway regulates T-cell function by targeting an adaptor protein Shc and a protein kinase Erk signaling. *Proc Natl Acad Sci U S A.* (2013) 110:624–9. doi: 10.1073/pnas.1213819110
58. Nagano T, Hashimoto T, Nakashima A, Kikkawa U, Kamada S. X-linked inhibitor of apoptosis protein mediates neddylation by itself but does not function as a NEDD8-E3 ligase for caspase-7. *FEBS Lett.* (2012) 586:1612–6. doi: 10.1016/j.febslet.2012.04.056
59. Broemer M, Tenev T, Rigbolt KT, Hempel S, Blagoev B, Silke J, et al. Systematic in vivo RNAi analysis identifies IAPs as NEDD8-E3 ligases. *Mol Cell.* (2010) 40:810–22. doi: 10.1016/j.molcel.2010.11.011
60. Ma T, Chen Y, Zhang F, Yang CY, Wang S, Yu X. RNF111-dependent neddylation activates DNA damage-induced ubiquitination. *Mol Cell.* (2013) 49:897–907. doi: 10.1016/j.molcel.2013.01.006
61. Sundqvist A, Liu G, Mirsaliotis A, Xirodimas DP. Regulation of nucleolar signalling to p53 through NEDDylation of L11. *EMBO Rep.* (2009) 10:1132–9. doi: 10.1038/embor.2009.178
62. Zhang J, Bai D, Ma X, Guan J, Zheng X. hCINAP is a novel regulator of ribosomal protein-HDM2-p53 pathway by controlling NEDDylation of ribosomal protein S14. *Oncogene.* (2014) 33:246–54. doi: 10.1038/onc.2012.560
63. Noh EH, Hwang HS, Hwang HS, Min B, Im E, Chung KC. Covalent NEDD8 conjugation increases RCAN1 protein stability and potentiates its inhibitory action on calcineurin. *PLos One.* (2012) 7:e0048315. doi: 10.1371/journal.pone.0048315
64. Liu N, Zhang J, Yang X, Jiao T, Zhao X, Li W, et al. HDM2 promotes NEDDylation of Hepatitis B virus HBx to enhance its stability and function. *J Virol.* (2017) 91:e00340-17. doi: 10.1128/JVI.00340-17
65. Kumar D, Das M, Sauceda C, Ellies LG, Kuo K, Parwal P, et al. Degradation of splicing factor SRSF3 contributes to progressive liver disease. *J Clin Invest.* (2019) 130:4477–91. doi: 10.1172/JCI127374
66. Zubiete-Franco I, Fernandez-Tussy P, Barbier-Torres L, Simon J, Fernandez-Ramos D, Lopitz-Otsoa F, et al. Deregulated neddylation in liver fibrosis. *Hepatology.* (2017) 65:694–709. doi: 10.1002/hep.28933
67. Mathewson N, Toubai T, Kapeles S, Sun Y, Oravecz-Wilson K, Tamaki H, et al. Neddylation plays an important role in the regulation of murine and human dendritic cell function. *Blood.* (2013) 122:2062–73. doi: 10.1182/blood-2013-02-486373
68. Heo MJ, Kang SH, Kim YS, Lee JM, Yu J, Kim HR, et al. UBC12-mediated SREBP-1 neddylation worsens metastatic tumor prognosis. *Int J Cancer.* (2020) 147:2550–63. doi: 10.1002/ijc.33113
69. Leidecker O, Matic I, Mahata B, Pion E, Xirodimas DP. The ubiquitin E1 enzyme Ube1 mediates NEDD8 activation under diverse stress conditions. *Cell Cycle.* (2012) 11:1142–50. doi: 10.4161/cc.11.6.19559
70. Schmidt MHH, Dikic I. Ubiquitin and NEDD8: brothers in arms. *Sci STKE.* (2006) 2006:.pe50. doi: 10.1126/stke.3622006pe50
71. Richter K, Haslbeck M, Buchner J. The heat shock response: life on the verge of death. *Mol Cell.* (2010) 40:253–66. doi: 10.1016/j.molcel.2010.10.006
72. Bailly AP, Perrin A, Serrano-Macia M, Maghames C, Leidecker O, Trauchessec H, et al. The balance between mono- and NEDD8-chains controlled by NEDP1 upon DNA damage is a regulatory module of the HSP70 ATPase activity. *Cell Rep.* (2019) 29:212–24.e8. doi: 10.1016/j.celrep.2019.08.070
73. Slagle BL, Bouchard MJ. Hepatitis B virus X and regulation of viral gene expression. *Cold Spring Harb Perspect Med.* (2016) 6:a021402. doi: 10.1101/cshperspect.a021402
74. Guo L, Wang X, Ren L, Zeng M, Wang S, Weng Y, et al. HBx affects CUL4-DDB1 function in both positive and negative manners. *Biochem Biophys Res Commun.* (2014) 450:1492–7. doi: 10.1016/j.bbrc.2014.07.019
75. Li T, Robert EI, van Breugel PC, Strubin M, Zheng N. A promiscuous alpha-helical motif anchors viral hijackers and substrate receptors to the CUL4-DDB1 ubiquitin ligase machinery. *Nat Struct Mol Biol.* (2010) 17:105–11. doi: 10.1038/nsmb.1719
76. Hodgson AJ, Hyser JM, Keasler VV, Cang Y, Slagle BL. Hepatitis B virus regulatory HBx protein binding to DDB1 is required but is not sufficient for maximal HBV replication. *Virology.* (2012) 426:73–82. doi: 10.1016/j.virol.2012.01.021
77. Leupin O, Bontron S, Schaeffer C, Strubin M. Hepatitis B virus X protein stimulates viral genome replication via a DDB1-dependent pathway distinct from that leading to cell death. *J Virol.* (2005) 79:4238–45. doi: 10.1128/JVI.79.7.4238-4245.2005
78. Zhao J, Wu J, Cai H, Wang D, Yu L, Zhang WH. E3 ubiquitin ligase siah-1 is down-regulated and fails to target natural HBx truncates for degradation in hepatocellular carcinoma. *J Cancer.* (2016) 7:418–26. doi: 10.7150/jca.13019
79. Younossi Z, Anstee QM, Marietti M, Hardy T, Henry L, Eslam M, et al. Global burden of NAFLD and NASH: trends, predictions, risk factors and prevention. *Nat Rev Gastroenterol Hepatol.* (2018) 15:11–20. doi: 10.1038/nrgastro.2017.109
80. Chalasani N, Younossi Z, Lavine JE, Charlton M, Cusi K, Rinella M, et al. The diagnosis and management of nonalcoholic fatty liver disease: practice guidance from the American Association for the Study of Liver Diseases. *Hepatology.* (2018) 67:328–57. doi: 10.1002/hep.29367
81. Fabbrini E, Sullivan S, Klein S. Obesity and nonalcoholic fatty liver disease: biochemical, metabolic, and clinical implications. *Hepatology.* (2010) 51:679–89. doi: 10.1002/hep.23280
82. Zhang X, Zhang Y-L, Qiu G, Pian L, Guo L, Cao H, et al. Hepatic neddylation targets and stabilizes electron transfer flavoproteins to facilitate fatty acid beta-oxidation. *Proc Natl Acad Sci U S A.* (2020) 117:2473–83. doi: 10.1073/pnas.1910765117
83. Sen S, Langiewicz M, Jumaa H, Webster NJG. Deletion of serine/arginine-rich splicing factor 3 in hepatocytes predisposes to hepatocellular carcinoma in mice. *Hepatology.* (2015) 61:171–83. doi: 10.1002/hep.27380
84. Ju UI, Jeong DW, Seo J, Park JB, Park JW, Suh KS, et al. Neddylation of sterol regulatory element-binding protein 1c is a potential therapeutic target for nonalcoholic fatty liver treatment. *Cell Death Dis.* (2020) 11:283. doi: 10.1038/s41419-020-2472-6
85. Dehnad A, Fan W, Jiang JX, Fish SR, Li Y, Das S, et al. AGER1 downregulation associates with fibrosis in nonalcoholic steatohepatitis and type 2 diabetes. *J Clin Invest.* (2020) 130:4320–30. doi: 10.1172/JCI133051
86. Pinzani M, Rombouts K. Liver fibrosis: from the bench to clinical targets. *Dig Liver Dis.* (2004) 36:231–42. doi: 10.1016/j.dld.2004.01.003
87. Schuppan D, Kim YO. Evolving therapies for liver fibrosis. *J Clin Invest.* (2013) 123:1887–901. doi: 10.1172/JCI66028
88. Leist M, Gantner F, Bohlinger I, Tiegs G, Germann PG, Wendel A. Tumor necrosis factor-induced hepatocyte apoptosis precedes liver failure in experimental murine shock models. *Am J Pathol.* (1995) 146:1220–34.
89. Saiman Y, Friedman SL. The role of chemokines in acute liver injury. *Front Physiol.* (2012) 3:213. doi: 10.3389/fphys.2012.00213
90. Mederacke I, Hsu CC, Troeger JS, Huebener P, Mu X, Dapito DH, et al. Fate tracing reveals hepatic stellate cells as dominant contributors to liver fibrosis independent of its aetiology. *Nat Commun.* (2013) 4:2823. doi: 10.1038/ncomms3823
91. Wertz IE, O'Rourke KM, Zhang Z, Dornan D, Arnott D, Deshaies RJ, et al. Human De-etiolated-1 regulates c-Jun by assembling a CUL4A ubiquitin ligase. *Science.* (2004) 303:1371–4. doi: 10.1126/science.1093549
92. Collins PE, Mitxitorena I, Carmody RJ. The ubiquitination of NF-κB subunits in the control of transcription. *Cells.* (2016) 5:23. doi: 10.3390/cells5020023

93. Sasaki R, Kanda T, Nakamura M, Nakamoto S, Haga Y, Wu S, et al. Possible involvement of Hepatitis B virus infection of hepatocytes in the attenuation of apoptosis in hepatic stellate cells. *PLoS One.* (2016) 11:e0146314. doi: 10.1371/journal.pone.0146314
94. Hellerbrand C, Stefanovic B, Giordano F, Burchardt ER, Brenner DA. The role of TGFβ1 in initiating hepatic stellate cell activation *in vivo*. *J Hepatol.* (1999) 30:77–87. doi: 10.1016/S0168-8278(99)80010-5
95. Troeger JS, Mederacke I, Gwak G-Y, Dapito DH, Mu X, Hsu CC, et al. Deactivation of hepatic stellate cells during liver fibrosis resolution in mice. *Gastroenterology.* (2012) 143:1073–83.e22. doi: 10.1053/j.gastro.2012.06.036
96. Tapper EB, Parikh ND. Mortality due to cirrhosis and liver cancer in the United States, 1999-2016: observational study. *BMJ Br Med J.* (2018) 362:k2817. doi: 10.1136/bmj.k2817
97. Yu J, Huang WL, Xu QG, Zhang L, Sun SH, Zhou WP, et al. Overactivated neddylation pathway in human hepatocellular carcinoma. *Cancer Med.* (2018) 7:3363–72. doi: 10.1002/cam4.1578
98. Yang Z, Zhang J, Lin X, Wu D, Li G, Zhong C, et al. Inhibition of neddylation modification by MLN4924 sensitizes hepatocellular carcinoma cells to sorafenib. *Oncol Rep.* (2019) 41:3257–69. doi: 10.3892/or.2019.7098
99. McLarnon A. Cancer: Mdm2-regulated stabilization of HuR by neddylation in HCC and colon cancer–a possible target for therapy. *Nat Rev Gastroenterol Hepatol.* (2011) 9:4. doi: 10.1038/nrgastro.2011.241
100. Barbier-Torres L, Delgado TC, García-Rodríguez JL, Zubiete-Franco I, Fernández-Ramos D, Buqué X, et al. Stabilization of LKB1 and Akt by neddylation regulates energy metabolism in liver cancer. *Oncotarget.* (2015) 6:2509–23. doi: 10.18632/oncotarget.3191
101. Zhou L, Zhang W, Sun Y, Jia L. Protein neddylation and its alterations in human cancers for targeted therapy. *Cell Signal.* (2018) 44:92–102. doi: 10.1016/j.cellsig.2018.01.009
102. Luo Z, Yu G, Lee HW, Li L, Wang L, Yang D, et al. The Nedd8-activating enzyme inhibitor MLN4924 induces autophagy and apoptosis to suppress liver cancer cell growth. *Cancer Res.* (2012) 72:3360–71. doi: 10.1158/0008-5472.CAN-12-0388
103. Zhao Y, Sun Y. Targeting the mTOR-DEPTOR pathway by CRL E3 ubiquitin ligases: therapeutic application. *Neoplasia.* (2012) 14:360–7. doi: 10.1593/neo.12532
104. Liang Y, Jiang Y, Jin X, Chen P, Heng Y, Cai L, et al. Neddylation inhibition activates the protective autophagy through NF-κB-catalase-ATF3 Axis in human esophageal cancer cells. *Cell Commun Signal.* (2020) 18:72. doi: 10.1186/s12964-020-00576-z
105. Lu G, Yi J, Gubas A, Wang YT, Wu Y, Ren Y, et al. Suppression of autophagy during mitosis via CUL4-RING ubiquitin ligases-mediated WIPI2 polyubiquitination and proteasomal degradation. *Autophagy.* (2019) 15:1917–34. doi: 10.1080/15548627.2019.1596484
106. Gorlach A, Bonello S. The cross-talk between NF-kappaB and HIF-1: further evidence for a significant liaison. *Biochem J.* (2008) 412:e17–9. doi: 10.1042/BJ20080920
107. Hon WC, Wilson MI, Harlos K, Claridge TDW, Schofield CJ, Pugh CW, et al. Structural basis for the recognition of hydroxyproline in alpha IF-1 alpha by pVHL. *Nature.* (2002) 417:975–8. doi: 10.1038/nature00767
108. Zhang W, Shi X, Peng Y, Wu M, Zhang P, Xie R, et al. HIF-1α promotes epithelial-mesenchymal transition and metastasis through direct regulation of ZEB1 in colorectal cancer. *PLoS One.* (2015) 10:e0129603. doi: 10.1371/journal.pone.0129603
109. Walmsley SR, Print C, Farahi N, Peyssonnaux C, Johnson RS, Cramer T, et al. Hypoxia-induced neutrophil survival is mediated by HIF-1α-dependent NF-κB activity. *J Exp Med.* (2005) 201:105–15. doi: 10.1084/jem.20040624
110. Cannito S, Foglia B, Villano G, Turato C, Delgado TC, Morello E, et al. SerpinB3 differently up-regulates hypoxia inducible factors-1 alpha and-2 alpha in hepatocellular carcinoma: mechanisms revealing novel potential therapeutic targets. *Cancers.* (2019) 11:1933. doi: 10.3390/cancers11121933
111. Belaiba RS, Bonello S, Zahringer C, Schmidt S, Hess J, Kietzmann T, et al. Hypoxia up-regulates hypoxia-inducible factor-1alpha transcription by involving phosphatidylinositol 3-kinase and nuclear factor κB in pulmonary artery smooth muscle cells. *Mol Biol Cell.* (2007) 18:4691–7. doi: 10.1091/mbc.e07-04-0391
112. Chang SC, Ding JL. Ubiquitination by SAG regulates macrophage survival/death and immune response during infection. *Cell Death Differ.* (2014) 21:1388–98. doi: 10.1038/cdd.2014.54
113. Mathewson ND, Fujiwara H, Wu SR, Toubai T, Oravecz-Wilson K, Sun Y, et al. SAG/Rbx2-dependent neddylation regulates T-cell responses. *Am J Pathol.* (2016) 186:2679–91. doi: 10.1016/j.ajpath.2016.06.014
114. Wang Y, Luo Z, Pan Y, Wang W, Zhou X, Jeong LS, et al. Targeting protein neddylation with an NEDD8-activating enzyme inhibitor MLN4924 induced apoptosis or senescence in human lymphoma cells. *Cancer Biol Ther.* (2015) 16:420–9. doi: 10.1080/15384047.2014.1003003
115. Godbersen JC, Paiva C, Danilova OV, Berger A, Brown JR, Danilov AV. Targeting neddylation effectively antagonizes nuclear factor-κB in chronic lymphocytic leukemia B-cells. *Leuk Lymphoma.* (2015) 56:1566–9. doi: 10.3109/10428194.2014.990901
116. Paiva C, Godbersen JC, Berger A, Brown JR, Danilov AV. Targeting neddylation induces DNA damage and checkpoint activation and sensitizes chronic lymphocytic leukemia B cells to alkylating agents. *Cell Death Dis.* (2015) 6:e1807. doi: 10.1038/cddis.2015.161
117. Brenner C, Galluzzi L, Kepp O, Kroemer G. Decoding cell death signals in liver inflammation. *J Hepatol.* (2013) 59:583–94. doi: 10.1016/j.jhep.2013.03.033
118. Sekiba K, Otsuka M, Ohno M, Yamagami M, Kishikawa T, Seimiya T, et al. Pevonedistat, a neuronal precursor cell-expressed developmentally down-regulated protein 8–activating enzyme inhibitor of hepatitis B virus. *Hepatology.* (2019) 69, 1903–15. doi: 10.1002/hep.30491
119. Murphy CM, Xu Y, Li F, Nio K, Reszka-Blanco N, Li X, et al. Hepatitis B virus X protein promotes degradation of SMC5/6 to enhance HBV replication. *Cell Rep.* (2016) 16:2846–54. doi: 10.1016/j.celrep.2016.08.026
120. Decorsiere A, Mueller H, Van Breugel PC, Abdul F, Gerossier L, Beran RK, et al. Hepatitis B virus X protein identifies the Smc5/6 complex as a host restriction factor. *Nature.* (2016) 531:386–9. doi: 10.1038/nature17170
121. Serrano-Macia M, Azkargorta M, Simon J, Lopitz Otsoa F, Cardoso Delgado T, Fernandez Ramos D, et al. NEDDylation inhibition as a new potential therapy of nonalcoholic fatty liver disease. *J Hepatol.* (2019) 70:E546. doi: 10.1016/S0618-8278(19)31082-5
122. Chang F-M, Reyna SM, Granados JC, Wei S-J, Innis-Whitehouse W, Maffi SK, et al. Inhibition of neddylation represses lipopolysaccharide-induced proinflammatory cytokine production in macrophage cells. *J Biol Chem.* (2012) 287:35756–67. doi: 10.1074/jbc.M112.397703
123. Milhollen MA, Thomas MP, Narayanan U, Traore T, Riceberg J, Amidon BS, et al. Treatment-emergent mutations in NAE beta confer resistance to the NEDD8-activating enzyme inhibitor MLN4924. *Cancer Cell.* (2012) 21:388–401. doi: 10.1016/j.ccr.2012.02.009
124. Dawkins J, Webster RM. The hepatocellular carcinoma market. *Nat Rev Drug Discov.* (2019) 18:13–4. doi: 10.1038/nrd.2018.146
125. Bu FT, Chen Y, Yu HX, Chen X, Yang Y, Pan XY, et al. SENP2 alleviates CCl(4)-induced liver fibrosis by promoting activated hepatic stellate cell apoptosis and reversion. *Toxicol Lett.* (2018) 289:86–98. doi: 10.1016/j.toxlet.2018.03.010
126. Ramani K, Tomasi ML, Yang H, Ko K, Lu SC. Mechanism and significance of changes in glutamate-cysteine ligase expression during hepatic fibrogenesis. *J Biol Chem.* (2012) 287:36341–55. doi: 10.1074/jbc.M112.370775
127. Lachiondo-Ortega S, Mercado-Gómez M, Serrano-Maciá M, Lopitz-Otsoa F, Salas-Villalobos TB, Varela-Rey M, et al. Ubiquitin-like post-translational modifications (Ubl-PTMs): small peptides with huge impact in liver fibrosis. *Cells.* (2019) 8:1575. doi: 10.3390/cells8121575
128. Stein S, Lemos V, Xu P, Demagny H, Wang X, Ryu D, et al. Impaired SUMOylation of nuclear receptor LRH-1 promotes nonalcoholic fatty liver disease. *J Clin Invest.* (2017) 127:583–92. doi: 10.1172/JCI85499

18

Does Mechanocrine Signaling by Liver Sinusoidal Endothelial Cells Offer New Opportunities for the Development of Anti-fibrotics?

Sumeyye Soydemir [1†], Olivia Comella [1†], Dina Abdelmottaleb [1,2] and James Pritchett [1,2]*

[1] Department of Life Sciences, Faculty of Science and Engineering, Manchester Metropolitan University, Manchester, United Kingdom, [2] Centre for Bioscience, Faculty of Science and Engineering, Manchester Metropolitan University, Manchester, United Kingdom

Keywords: liver, endothelial, LSEC, PIEZO, HSC, fibrosis, ECM, mechanocrine

***Correspondence:**
James Pritchett
j.pritchett@mmu.ac.uk

† These authors have contributed equally to this work

INTRODUCTION

Liver sinusoidal endothelial cells (LSECs) are specialized endothelial cells that have essential roles in normal liver homeostasis, and are also involved in disease processes. The importance of LSEC biology has recently been extensively reviewed (1, 2). LSECs line the walls of the hepatic sinusoid (**Figure 1**) where they scavenge blood borne macromolecules. LSECs are constantly exposed to antigens carried from the gastrointestinal tract by the portal vein. LSECs therefore have a crucial role, alongside Kupffer cells, as gate keepers for liver immunomodulation. If LSEC immune responses are dysregulated, the result is chronic inflammation which can drive the development of fibrosis (2).

LSECs maintain a perforated plasma membrane to form fenestrations ranging between 50 and 300 nm in diameter (3). In a healthy, functioning liver, blood enters the sinusoids via the portal vein and hepatic artery, thus enabling oxygen and macromolecules to be transferred across the endothelial barrier to hepatocytes, facilitated by the LSEC fenestrae (1).

Due to their location lining the sinusoid LSECs (**Figure 1**) are in direct contact with blood flow and therefore exposed to changes in both shear stress and blood pressure. Numerous researchers have made this observation, however recent reviews of LSEC biology (1, 2) also illustrate how little is known about mechano-sensing pathways in LSECs. A recent article by Hilscher et al. (4) has now highlighted how mechano-sensitive pathways in LSECs can drive recruitment of circulating blood cells to drive portal hypertension. Mechanocrine signaling by LSECs can orchestrate complex responses across cell types and tissues. This article will highlight the importance of mechano-biology in LSECs during liver disease and point out important gaps in knowledge. This exciting research topic has the potential to reveal novel targets for the development of urgently needed anti-fibrotics.

Importantly LSECs are able to modulate phenotypic changes in hepatic stellate cells (HSCs) (5–7). HSCs are responsible for the altered extracellular matrix (ECM) production characteristic of liver fibrosis (8). In the healthy liver HSCs reside in the space of disse between the endothelial (LSEC) layer and epithelial (hepatocyte) layer. In response to fibrogenic cues, including inflammatory signals from hepatocytes or LSECs, HSCs alter their phenotype to become activated myofibroblasts. Activated HSCs are proliferative, migratory, and contractile cells that secrete fibrotic ECM (9). This means that mechanically induced changes in LSECs have the potential to rapidly alter HSC phenotype and drive fibrogenesis. The fact that LSEC dysfunction precedes the

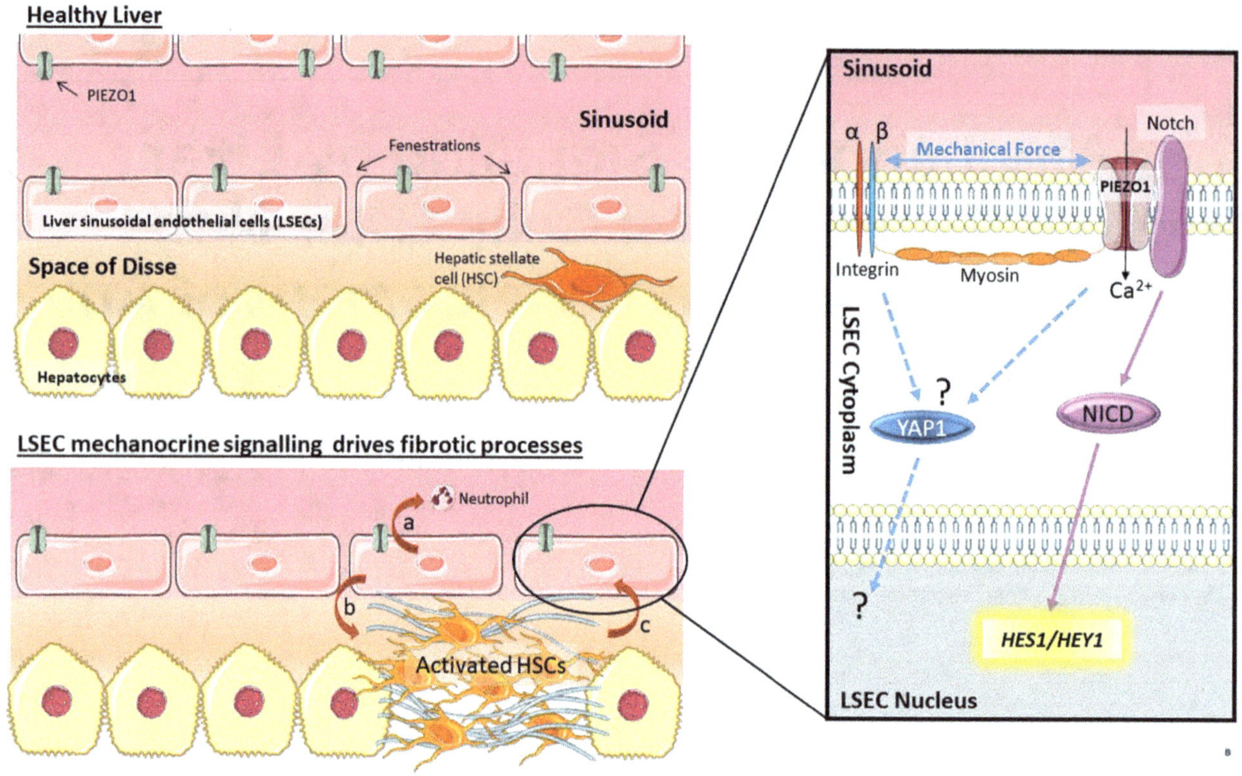

FIGURE 1 | Mechano-sensing by LSECs drives fibrotic processes. LSECs can respond to changes in shear stress and pressure in the sinusoid through activation of PIEZO channels. Data by Hilscher et al. (4) suggests this is triggered by integrins and myosin filaments. PIEZO channel activation drives cleavage of Notch to release NICD, and transcription of Notch pathway genes *HES1* and *HEY1*. Activation of this mechanism results in chemokine secretion (CXCL1) which recruits neutrophils (a). Signaling by LSECs is also known to trigger HSC activation (b) which leads to stiffening of the ECM, potentially driving activation of other mechano-sensitive pathways (c) such as YAP1.

development of fibrosis in non-alcoholic liver disease (10) supports the hypothesis that signals from LSECs may be one of the earliest triggers of HSC activation. There is also the potential for the establishment of a positive feedback loop in which mechanically activated LSECs trigger mechanocrine signaling that activates HSCs. In turn, activated HSCs alter the ECM to increase tissue stiffness, driving further mechano-activation of both LSECs and HSCs. Drugs that in some way break this mechanocrine feedback loop could have great therapeutic potential for the treatment of fibrotic disease.

MECHANO-BIOLOGY IN LIVER DISEASE

Key experiments by Rebecca Wells's group clearly showed that liver stiffness changes very early following hepatic injury (11), and that increased substrate stiffness is necessary for HSC activation (12, 13), a key step in fibrogenesis This raises the question of whether increased hepatic stiffness is a symptom or a driver of liver disease. Or both? Mechanical force across a tissue can change due to fluctuations in blood pressure, the behavior of contractile cells (e.g., HSCs) and changes in the ECM. Following liver injury changes in hepatic blood pressure occur rapidly (11, 14), and hypertension in the context of non-alcoholic fatty liver disease appears to increase the risk of fibrosis (15, 16).

Interest in mechano-sensing during fibrotic liver disease has largely focused on HSCs (12, 17, 18), and several mechanically sensitive signaling pathways have been shown to function in HSCs. Latent TGFbeta, a pro-fibrotic cytokine (19), is released from the ECM by contractile force transmitted from HSCs via the α_V integrin subunit (20). Furthermore, the mechano-sensitive transcriptional regulator Yes Associated Protein 1 (YAP1) (21) is activated in HSCs by increased substrate stiffness (22, 23). YAP1 can be inhibited using verteporfin (24) to reduce fibrosis *in vivo* (23). By contrast, relatively little is known about how LSECs sense and respond to external mechanical cues.

Portal Hypertension and Regulation of Sinusoidal Tone

Changes in vascular tone cause rapid changes in blood pressure, shear forces and the overall mechanical stiffness of the liver (14). LSECs regulate vascular tone by releasing vasoconstrictors, e.g., cyclooxygenase 1 (COX1) and thromboxane A2 (TXA2); and vasodilators, e.g., NO which act on HSCs to modulate their contraction and therefore regulate sinusoidal pressure (25). Some studies suggest that endothelin, a potent vasoconstrictor, has an important role in driving portal hypertension, as patients with cirrhosis have an increased circulating ET-1 (26). When liver injury occurs, HSCs secrete Endothelin-1 (ET-1), establishing an autocrine loop contributing to increased blood pressure (14, 27, 28). Intriguingly, recent data suggests that ET-1 activates YAP-1 in ovarian cancer cells (29). Tocci and co-workers showed that beta-arrestin, functioning downstream of ET_AR, physically interacts with YAP1 to increase nuclear shuttling.

Research is now beginning to reveal how LSECs detect and respond to changes in hepatic blood flow and altered ECM stiffness.

POTENTIAL FOR MECHANO-SIGNALING BY LSECS

LSECs are exposed to mechanical cues derived from both blood flow/pressure changes and changes in the surrounding ECM of the liver during fibrotic disease. Endothelial cell populations in other vascular beds are able to detect and respond to mechanical cues, so it seems reasonable to suggest similar mechanisms would exist in LSECs. Several different mechano-signaling pathways, including Neurogenic locus notch homolog (Notch) 1 (30), PIEZO channels (31–33) and YAP1 (34), have all been shown to function in endothelial cells. Furthermore, as described above, ET-1 can drive YAP1 nuclear shuttling (29). This makes possible a positive feedback loop where HSCs activated by mechanical cues release ET-1, which could have a dual function. (1) Autocrine constriction of activated HSCs, contributing to portal hypertension and increased liver stiffness; and (2) YAP1 activation in both HSCs and LSECs, due to ET-1 signaling, *and* increased mechanical stiffness.

Notch

Notch proteins are transmembrane proteins that undergo proteolytic cleavage upon ligand binding. Notch ligands are themselves membrane bound proteins from the jagged and delta families. Upon binding to jagged or delta proteins presented by neighboring cells, Notch proteins are cleaved to release an intracellular domain (NICD) that translocates to the nucleus to orchestrate transcriptional regulation (35). This highly conserved mechanism allows cell-to-cell contact to regulate key processes such as proliferation, cell fate, differentiation, and cell death.

Notch proteins are expressed by vascular endothelial cells (36), and play a critical role in development of the vascular system (37). Mechanical force is necessary to reveal the Notch cleavage site and allow release of NICD (38, 39). It has recently been shown that Notch1 localization in endothelial cells is polarized by shear force. Notch1 protein polarization occurs in the direction of flow, and Notch1 is aligned with the downstream direction of flow across the endothelial cell layer (30). Furthermore, levels of nuclear NICD increased in a step wise fashion as shear stress induced by flow increased, providing compelling evidence that endothelial Notch is a mechano-sensor (30) that regulates endothelial function and phenotype in response to changes in shear stress.

In the liver Notch is expressed by LSECs (40, 41). Targeted deletion of *Notch1*, or the canonical notch effector *Rbpj1*, specifically in LSECs, caused dilated sinusoids and portal hypertension in adult mice (42). When Notch1 protein expression was disrupted in LSECs at birth, development of the liver vasculature was severely disrupted (42). Conversely, forced Notch pathway activation by endothelial specific overexpression of NICD also disrupted normal liver homeostasis, with expanded sinusoids, reduced hepatocyte proliferation and increased hepatocyte cell death. LSECs appeared to become dedifferentiated, and the fibrogenic response to CCl4 induced liver injury was increased (43).

These findings highlight the importance of tightly regulated Notch1 signaling in LSECs for normal liver function. Mechanical regulation of Notch1 could play a critical role in normal liver homeostasis, and in the response to liver injury. Intriguingly, recent data (4) shows that the Notch1 pathway in LSECs is sensitive to mechanical cues. Hilscher et al. (4) suggest that stretch activated PIEZO cation channels activate Notch signaling which drives recruitment of neutrophils and formation of neutrophil extracellular traps that cause portal hypertension.

PIEZO Channels

PIEZO proteins form mechano-sensitive cation channels in the plasma membrane (44, 45). PIEZO1 is essential for correct vascular development, and global knockout of *PIEZO1* is lethal (31, 32). PIEZO1 channels are present in the plasma membrane of endothelial cells and activated by shear stress to trigger Calcium influx into the cell (31, 32). Since their initial discovery, it has been shown that PIEZO1 is also critical for normal vascular homeostasis. Endothelial cells respond to changes in shear forces via PIEZO1. PIEZO1 induced signaling elicits downstream changes in vascular tone and blood pressure. In mice with endothelial specific PIEZO1 deficiency the ability of endothelial cells to respond to changes in flow by releasing NO to trigger vasodilation was lost, resulting in hypertension (33).

PIEZO channels are present on LSECs (31), and, as mentioned above, Hilscher et al. have recently highlighted how PIEZO1 channels modulate Notch pathway activity in response to changes in blood pressure (4). In their experimental model of cyclic stretch, integrins transmitted changes in mechanical force to activate PIEZO1 cation channels, possibly via myosin (46, 47). Similarly, force transmitted via non-muscle myosin has recently been shown to be involved in the ligand-activated cleavage of Notch (48). In LSECs the integrin-activated PIEZO1 channels interact with the Notch1 receptor to activate Notch target genes via production of the transcription factors Hes1 and Hey1 (4). Future experiments are necessary to establish whether myosin filaments in LSECs can interact directly with Notch1, or via PIEZO1, to drive notch cleavage and downstream signaling. It is also important to note that the actomyosin cytoskeleton has a crucial role in maintaining the fenestrated plasma membrane characteristic of healthy LSECs (49–51). This adds further complexity to the interplay between external and internal mechanical forces. How are changes in external force transmitted into LSECs? How do changes in external force affect the LSEC cytoskeleton? Could external mechanical cues have a direct influence on the maintenance of the fenestrated plasma membrane?

YAP1

Another mechanism for mechano-signaling in LSECs is YAP1, which has recently been shown to be sensitive to shear forces in zebrafish endothelial cells (34). Nuclear YAP1 is also present in primary LSECs isolated from murine livers (52). YAP1 can be activated downstream of PIEZO1 (46). Further work is therefore necessary to confirm YAP1 expression and function in mammalian LSECs, and whether YAP1 status in LSECs can be regulated by PIEZO channel activation. Current understanding of YAP1 function in the liver has recently been extensively reviewed (53).

THERAPEUTIC POTENTIAL

LSEC phenotype restoration through inhibition of mechano-sensitive pathways provides an intriguing therapeautic strategy for the treatment, and even reversal, of liver fibrosis. Compelling evidence that LSECs signal to neighboring cells in a context dependent manner to drive either tissue regeneration or fibrosis (7) provides strong support for the targeting of LSECs as a means to drive fibrosis regression. As many of the pathways discussed are not specific to LSECs, or even to endothelial cells, a means of delivering a therapy specifically to LSECs is desirable. Nano-particles targeting LSECs for the regulation of auto-immunity have already been developed (54). Similar approaches could be used to deliver molecules targeting mechano-sensing pathways specifically to LSECs. Timing of therapy will be crucial. Early intervention would arguably provide more chance of success, but this is made challenging due to issues with late diagnosis. However, clearance of hepatitis C infection leads to fibrosis regression, and clearly shows that human liver fibrosis is reversible at later stages than previously thought (55).

Targeting Notch

Two classes of drug that target notch signaling are currently in clinical trials as cancer therapies (56). (1) Gamma-secretase inhibitors (GSIs) target the enzymes responsible for cleavage of Notch and block release of NICD. (2) Monoclonal antibodies block notch-ligand receptor interactions. Both classes of drug have dose limiting side effects linked to normal notch function in the gastrointestinal tract. Successful adoption of notch inhibition as a therapeutic strategy for liver fibrosis would therefore require cellular targeting to avoid severe side effects. As mentioned previously (section NOTCH), Notch has diverse functions during liver development, homeostasis and disease (57). In hepatocytes (58) or LSECs (43) Notch signaling can induce HSC activation and promotes fibrosis. It has been demonstrated that inhibition of Notch signaling using a GSI *in vivo* ameliorated fibrosis in a CCl4 pre-clinical model (59). Therefore, therapeutic targeting of Notch would impact multiple pro-fibrotic mechanisms, potentially including mechano-crine signaling by LSECs (4).

Targeting PIEZO Channels

Yoda1 was the first molecule identified which could artificially regulate PIEZO channel activity (60). However, Yoda1 functions as an agonist and causes activation of PIEZO1. Based on the evidence from Hilscher et al. activating PIEZO1 would have a negative impact on liver fibrosis (4). Dooku is a more recently identified analog of Yoda1, which appears to function as a Yoda1 antagonist (61). Importantly this molecule only inhibits Yoda1 induced PIEZO channel activation. As yet, no small molecule antagonists of PIEZO channel mechano-activation have been discovered. It is interesting to speculate what effect PIEZO channel inhibitors might have on liver fibrosis, especially if they could be delivered specifically to LSECs. As PIEZO receptors are widely expressed across endothelial cell types, long term global treatment with a PIEZO antagonist would likely have undesirable side effects.

Integrins

Hilscher et al. demonstrate that PIEZO channel mechano-activation is triggered by integrin signaling; treatment of cells with arginine-glycine-aspartate (RGD) peptide inhibited stretch-induced transcription of Notch target genes (4). Identification and targeting of the integrin heterodimers (62) involved in this mechanism could be a strategy for developing anti-fibrotics. The integrin subunits present in the LSEC cell membrane are yet to be fully characterized. Mass spectrometry showed that integrin beta 3 is expressed by LSECs following partial hepatectomy (63). Candidate integrin alpha subunits include alphaV and alphaIIb, both of which partner with the beta3 subunit to facilitate interactions between LSECs and platelets (64).

Targeting YAP1?

Verteporfin (tradename Visudyne, Novartis) was originally developed as a light activated treatment for neovascular macular degeneration (65). Verteporfin's ability to inhibit YAP1 activity was identified by screening for compounds able to disrupt the interaction between YAP-1 and it's DNA binding partner TEAD1 (24). Mice tolerate verteporfin treatment via intraperitoneal injection over 3 weeks (23). However, further studies are needed to assess its specificity and potential for development as a long term therapeutic strategy. In light of this it is important to note that more specific alternatives to verteporfin have already been developed and tested *in vitro* (66).

DISCUSSION

The data presented by Hilscher et al. (4) is compelling: mechanical cues alter LSEC function. In response to mechanical stretch PIEZO channels activate the notch pathway to trigger secretion of the chemokine CXCL1 by LSECs. CXCL1 release recruits neutrophils that drive microthrombi formation and promote portal hypertension. This is the first direct evidence of mechano-sensing by LSECs, and links PIEZO channels with notch-signaling, both of which are known to be mechanically activated in other contexts. It is reasonable to expect that integrins will also be involved in the detection of mechanical cues by LSECs. For other mechanosensitive pathways such as YAP/TAZ there is potential for involvement in LSEC biology as YAP1 responds to shear stress in a zebrafish model (34). Another area of interest is how actomyosin contractility responds to and generates force to regulate LSEC shape (fenestrae) and integrate external and internal cues via PIEZO (47), notch (48), or YAP1 (67). The next challenge will be to harness our improving understanding of the importance of mechanobiology in LSECs to attempt to develop novel therapies for liver disease. Breaking the positive feedback loop set in motion when mechanical cues cause LSECs to trigger neutrophil recruitment, and potentially HSC activation, could be a successful therapeutic strategy.

AUTHOR CONTRIBUTIONS

SS and OC researched the topic and prepared draft text and figure. DA edited the text and provided feedback. JP supervised, SS and OC managed the preparation of the manuscript, researched the topic, and prepared the final text.

ACKNOWLEDGMENTS

We acknowledge the support of the Center for Bioscience and Department of Life Sciences at Manchester Metropolitan University. We used The SMART Medical Art platform (https://smart.servier.com/) for figure design.

REFERENCES

1. Poisson J, Lemoinne S, Boulanger C, Durand F, Moreau R, Valla D, et al. Liver sinusoidal endothelial cells: physiology and role in liver diseases. *J Hepatol.* (2017) 66:212–27. doi: 10.1016/j.jhep.2016.07.009
2. Shetty S, Lalor PF, Adams DH. Liver sinusoidal endothelial cells - gatekeepers of hepatic immunity. *Nat Rev.* (2018) 15:555–67. doi: 10.1038/s41575-018-0020-y
3. Cogger VC, McNerney GP, Nyunt T, DeLeve LD, McCourt P, Smedsrød B, et al. Three-dimensional structured illumination microscopy of liver sinusoidal endothelial cell fenestrations. *J Struct Biol.* (2010) 171:382–8. doi: 10.1016/j.jsb.2010.06.001
4. Hilscher MB, Sehrawat T, Arab JP, Zeng Z, Gao J, Liu M, et al. Mechanical stretch increases expression of CXCL1 in liver sinusoidal endothelial cells to recruit neutrophils, generate sinusoidal microthombi, and promote portal hypertension. *Gastroenterology.* (2019) 15:193–209.e199. doi: 10.1053/j.gastro.2019.03.013
5. Xie G, Wang X, Wang L, Atkinson RD, Kanel GC, Gaarde WA, et al. Role of differentiation of liver sinusoidal endothelial cells in progression and regression of hepatic fibrosis in rats. *Gastroenterology.* (2012) 14:918–27.e916. doi: 10.1053/j.gastro.2011.12.017
6. Marrone G, Russo L, Rosado E, Hide D, Garcia-Cardena G, Garcia-Pagan JC, et al. The transcription factor KLF2 mediates hepatic endothelial protection and paracrine endothelial-stellate cell deactivation induced by statins. *J Hepatol.* (2013) 5:98–103. doi: 10.1016/j.jhep.2012.08.026
7. Ding BS, Cao Z, Lis R, Nolan DJ, Guo P, Simons M, et al. Divergent angiocrine signals from vascular niche balance liver regeneration and fibrosis. *Nature.* (2014) 50:97–102. doi: 10.1038/nature12681
8. Tsuchida T, Friedman SL. Mechanisms of hepatic stellate cell activation. *Nat Rev.* (2017) 14:397–411. doi: 10.1038/nrgastro.2017.38
9. Hernandez-Gea V, Friedman SL. Pathogenesis of liver fibrosis. *Annu. Rev. Pathol.* (2011) 6:425–56. doi: 10.1146/annurev-pathol-011110-130246
10. Pasarín M, La Mura V, Gracia-Sancho J, García-Calderó H, Rodríguez-Vilarrupla A, García-Pagán JC, et al. Sinusoidal endothelial dysfunction precedes inflammation and fibrosis in a model of NAFLD. *PLoS ONE.* (2012) 7:e32785. doi: 10.1371/journal.pone.0032785
11. Georges PC, Hui JJ, Gombos Z, McCormick ME, Wang AY, Uemura M, et al. Increased stiffness of the rat liver precedes matrix deposition: implications for fibrosis. *Am J Physiol Gastrointest. Liver Physiol.* (2007) 293:G1147–54. doi: 10.1152/ajpgi.00032.2007
12. Wells RG. The role of matrix stiffness in hepatic stellate cell activation and liver fibrosis. *J Clin Gastroenterol.* (2005) 3:S158–61. doi: 10.1097/01.mcg.0000155516.02468.0f
13. Olsen AL, Bloomer SA, Chan EP, Gaca MDA, Georges PC, Sackey B, et al. Hepatic stellate cells require a stiff environment for myofibroblastic differentiation. *Am J Physiol Gastrointest Liver Physiol.* (2011) 30:G110–18. doi: 10.1152/ajpgi.00412.2010
14. Rockey DC. Hepatic blood flow regulation by stellate cells in normal and injured liver. *Semin Liver Dis.* (2001) 2:337–49. doi: 10.1055/s-2001-17551
15. Dixon JB, Bhathal PS, O'Brien PE. Nonalcoholic fatty liver disease: predictors of nonalcoholic steatohepatitis and liver fibrosis in the severely obese. *Gastroenterology.* (2001) 12:91–100. doi: 10.1053/gast.2001.25540
16. Arima S, Uto H, Ibusuki R, Kumamoto R, Tanoue S, Mawatari S, et al. Hypertension exacerbates liver injury and hepatic fibrosis induced by a choline-deficient L-amino acid-defined diet in rats. *Int J Mol Med.* (2014) 3:68–76. doi: 10.3892/ijmm.2013.1544
17. Wells RG. Tissue mechanics and fibrosis. *Biochim Biophys Acta.* (2013) 183:884–90. doi: 10.1016/j.bbadis.2013.02.007
18. Daniel JT, Giovanni L, Moira BH, Vijay HS. Mechanosensing and fibrosis. *J. Clin. Invest.* (2018) 12:74–84. doi: 10.1172/JCI93561
19. Gressner AM, Weiskirchen R, Breitkopf K, Dooley S. Roles of TGF-beta in hepatic fibrosis. *Front Biosci.* 7:D793–807. doi: 10.2741/A812
20. Henderson N, Arnold T, Katamura Y, Giacomini M, Rodriguez J, McCarty J, et al. Targeting of αv integrin identifies a core molecular pathway that regulates fibrosis in several organs. *Nat Med.* (2013) 19:1617–24. doi: 10.1038/nm.3282
21. Dupont S, Morsut L, Aragona M, Enzo E, Giulitti S, Cordenonsi M, et al. Role of YAP/TAZ in mechanotransduction. *Nature.* (2011) 47:179–83. doi: 10.1038/nature10137
22. Mannaerts I, Leite SB, Verhulst S, Claerhout S, Eysackers N, Thoen LFR, et al. The Hippo pathway effector YAP controls mouse hepatic stellate cell activation. *J Hepatol.* (2015) 6:679–88. doi: 10.1016/j.jhep.2015.04.011
23. Martin K, Pritchett J, Llewellyn J, Mullan AF, Athwal VS, Dobie R, et al. PAK proteins and YAP-1 signalling downstream of integrin beta-1 in myofibroblasts promote liver fibrosis. *Nat Commun.* (2016) 7:12502. doi: 10.1038/ncomms12502
24. Liu-Chittenden Y, Huang B, Shim JS, Chen Q, Lee SJ, Anders RA, et al. Genetic and pharmacological disruption of the TEAD-YAP complex suppresses the oncogenic activity of YAP. *Genes Dev.* (2012) 26:1300–5. doi: 10.1101/gad.192856.112
25. Gracia-Sancho J, Marrone G, Fernández-Iglesias A. Hepatic microcirculation and mechanisms of portal hypertension. *Nat Rev*

Gastroenterol Hepatol. (2019) 16:221–34. doi: 10.1038/s41575-018-0097-3

26. Trevisani F, Colantoni A, Gerbes AL, Gülberg V, Sica G, Caraceni P, et al. Daily profile of plasma endothelin-1 and−3 in pre-ascitic cirrhosis: relationships with the arterial pressure and renal function. *J Hepatol.* (1997) 26:808–15. doi: 10.1016/S0168-8278(97)80246-2
27. Gandhi CR, Sproat LA, Subbotin VM. Increased hepatic endothelin-1 levels and endothelin receptor density in cirrhotic rats. *Life Sci.* (1996) 58:55–62. doi: 10.1016/0024-3205(95)02255-4
28. Cho TJ, Kim HJ, Cho J. Endothelin-converting enzyme-1 expression in acute and chronic liver injury in fibrogenesis. *Anim Cells Syst.* (2019) 23:170–5. doi: 10.1080/19768354.2019.1595141
29. Tocci P, Cianfrocca R, Di Castro V, Rosano L, Sacconi A, Donzelli S, et al. β-arrestin1/YAP/mutant p53 complexes orchestrate the endothelin A receptor signaling in high-grade serous ovarian cancer. *Nat Commun.* (2019) 10:3196. doi: 10.1038/s41467-019-11045-8
30. Mack JJ, Mosqueiro TS, Archer BJ, Jones WM, Sunshine H, Faas GC, et al. NOTCH1 is a mechanosensor in adult arteries. *Nat Commun.* (2017) 8:1620. doi: 10.1038/s41467-017-01741-8
31. Li J, Hou B, Tumova S, Muraki K, Bruns A, Ludlow MJ, et al. Piezo1 integration of vascular architecture with physiological force. *Nature.* (2014) 515:279–82. doi: 10.1038/nature13701
32. Ranade SS, Qiu Z, Woo SH, Hur SS, Murthy SE, Cahalan SM, et al. Piezo1, a mechanically activated ion channel, is required for vascular development in mice. *Proc Natl Acad Sci USA.* (2014) 111:10347–52. doi: 10.1073/pnas.1409233111
33. Wang S, Chennupati R, Kaur H, Iring A, Wettschureck N, Offermanns S. Endothelial cation channel PIEZO1 controls blood pressure by mediating flow-induced ATP release. *J Clin Invest.* (2016) 126:4527–36. doi: 10.1172/JCI87343
34. Nakajima H, Yamamoto K, Agarwala S, Terai K, Fukui H, Fukuhara S, et al. Flow-Dependent endothelial YAP regulation contributes to vessel maintenance. *DevCell.* (2017) 40:523–36.e6. doi: 10.1016/j.devcel.2017.02.019
35. Kopan R. Notch signaling. *Cold Spring Harb Perspect Biol.* (2012) 4:a011213. doi: 10.1101/cshperspect.a011213
36. Del Amo FF, Smith DE, Swiatek PJ, Gendron-Maguire M, Greenspan RJ, McMahon AP, et al. Expression pattern of Motch, a mouse homolog of Drosophila Notch, suggests an important role in early postimplantation mouse development. *Development.* (1992) 115:737–44.
37. Krebs LT, Xue Y, Norton CR, Shutter JR, Maguire M, Sundberg JP, et al. Notch signaling is essential for vascular morphogenesis in mice. *Genes Dev.* (2000) 14:1343–52. doi: 10.1101/gad.14.11.1343
38. Gordon WR, Vardar-Ulu D, Histen G, Sanchez-Irizarry C, Aster JC, Blacklow SC. Structural basis for autoinhibition of Notch. *Nat Struct Mol Biol.* (2007) 14:295–300. doi: 10.1038/nsmb1227
39. Wang X, Ha T. Defining single molecular forces required to activate integrin and Notch signaling. *Science.* (2013) 340:991–4. doi: 10.1126/science.1231041
40. Loomes KM, Taichman DB, Glover CL, Williams PT, Markowitz JE, Piccoli DA, et al. Characterization of Notch receptor expression in the developing mammalian heart and liver. *Am J Med Genet.* (2002) 112:181–9. doi: 10.1002/ajmg.10592
41. Köhler C, Bell AW, Bowen WC, Monga SP, Fleig W, Michalopoulos GK. Expression of Notch-1 and its ligand Jagged-1 in rat liver during liver regeneration. *Hepatology.* (2004) 39:1056–65. doi: 10.1002/hep.20156
42. Cuervo H, Nielsen CM, SimonettoDA, Ferrell L, Shah VH, Wang RA. Endothelial Notch signaling is essential to prevent hepatic vascular malformations in mice. *Hepatology.* (2016) 64:1302–16. doi: 10.1002/hep.28713
43. Duan JL, Ruan B, Yan XC, Liang L, Song P, Yang ZY, et al. Endothelial Notch activation reshapes the angiocrine of sinusoidal endothelia to aggravate liver fibrosis and blunt regeneration in mice. *Hepatology.* (2018) 68:677–90. doi: 10.1002/hep.29834
44. Coste B, Mathur J, Schmidt M, Earley TJ, Ranade S, Petrus MJ, et al. Piezo1 and Piezo2 are essential components of distinct mechanically activated cation channels. *Science.* (2010) 330:55–60. doi: 10.1126/science.1193270
45. Coste B, Xiao B, Santos JS, Syeda R, Grandl J, Spencer KS, et al. Piezo proteins are pore-forming subunits of mechanically activated channels. *Nature.* (2012) 483:176–81. doi: 10.1038/nature10812
46. Pathak MM, Nourse JL, Tran T, Hwe J, Arulmoli J, Le DTT, et al. Stretch-activated ion channel Piezo1 directs lineage choice in human neural stem cells. *Proc. Natl. Acad. Sci. USA.* (2014) 111:16148–53. doi: 10.1073/pnas.1409802111
47. Quintanilla MA, Hammer JA, Beach JR. Pulling in new directions: Myosin 2, Piezo, and metabolism [version 1; peer review: 3 approved]. *F1000Res.* (2019) 8:1486. doi: 10.12688/f1000research.18856.1
48. Hunter GL, He L, Perrimon N, Charras G, Giniger E, Baum B. A role for actomyosin contractility in Notch signaling. *BMC Biol.* (2019) 17:12. doi: 10.1186/s12915-019-0625-9
49. Yokomori H, Yoshimura K, Funakoshi S, Nagai T, Fujimaki K, Nomura M, et al. Rho modulates hepatic sinusoidal endothelial fenestrae via regulation of the actin cytoskeleton in rat endothelial cells. *Lab Invest.* (2004) 84:857–64. doi: 10.1038/labinvest.3700114
50. Yokomori H. New insights into the dynamics of sinusoidal endothelial fenestrae in liver sinusoidal endothelial cells. *Med Mol Morphol.* (2008) 41:1–4. doi: 10.1007/s00795-007-0390-7
51. Venkatraman L, Tucker-Kellogg L. The CD47-binding peptide of thrombospondin-1 induces defenestration of liver sinusoidal endothelial cells. *Liver Int.* (2013) 33:1386–97. doi: 10.1111/liv.12231
52. Zhang C, Bian M, Chen X, Jin H, Zhao S, Yang X, et al. Oroxylin A prevents angiogenesis of LSECs in liver fibrosis via inhibition of YAP/HIF-1α signaling. *J Cell Biochem.* (2018) 119:2258–68. doi: 10.1002/jcb.26388
53. Manmadhan S, Ehmer U. Hippo signaling in the liver - a long and ever-expanding story. *Front Cell Dev Biol.* (2019) 7:33. doi: 10.3389/fcell.2019.00033
54. Carambia A, Freund B, Schwinge D, Bruns OT, Salmen SC, Ittrich H, et al. Nanoparticle-based autoantigen delivery to Treg-inducing liver sinusoidal endothelial cells enables control of autoimmunity in mice. *J Hepatol.* (2015) 62:1349–56. doi: 10.1016/j.jhep.2015.01.006
55. van der Meer AJ, Berenguer M. Reversion of disease manifestations after HCV eradication. *J Hepatol.* (2016) 65:S95–108. doi: 10.1016/j.jhep.2016.07.039
56. Venkatesh V, Nataraj R, Thangaraj GS, Karthikeyan M, Gnanasekaran A, Kaginelli SB, et al. Targeting Notch signalling pathway of cancer stem cells. *Stem Cell Investig.* (2018) 5:5. doi: 10.21037/sci.2018.02.02
57. Adams JM, Jafar-Nejad H. The roles of Notch signaling in liver development and disease. *Biomolecules.* (2019) 9:E608. doi: 10.3390/biom9100608
58. Zhu C, Kim K, Wang X, Bartolome A, Salomao M, Dongiovanni P, et al. Hepatocyte Notch activation induces liver fibrosis in nonalcoholic steatohepatitis. *Sci Transl Med.* (2018) 10:eaat0344. doi: 10.1126/scitranslmed.aat0344
59. Chen Y, Zheng S, Qi D, Zheng S, Guo J, Zhang S, et al. Inhibition of Notch signaling by a γ-secretase inhibitor attenuates hepatic fibrosis in rats. *PLoS ONE.* (2012) 7:e46512. doi: 10.1371/journal.pone.0046512
60. Syeda R, Xu J, Dubin AE, Coste B, Mathur J, Huynh T, et al. Chemical activation of the mechanotransduction channel Piezo1. *Elife.* (2015) 4:e07369. doi: 10.7554/eLife.07369.008
61. Evans EL, Cuthbertson K, Endesh N, Rode B, Blythe NM, Hyman AJ, et al. Yoda1 analogue (Dooku1) which antagonizes Yoda1-evoked activation of Piezo1 and aortic relaxation. *Br J Pharmacol.* (2018) 175:1744–59. doi: 10.1111/bph.14188
62. Raab-Westphal S, Marshall JF, Goodman SL. Integrins as therapeutic targets: successes and cancers. *Cancers.* (2017) 9:E110. doi: 10.3390/cancers9090110
63. Li X, Xiong L, Xie C, Cao J, Deng H, Lin Y, et al. Proteomics analysis of plasma membrane from liver sinusoidal endothelial cells after partial hepatectomy by an improved two-dimensional electrophoresis. *Mol Cell Biochem.* (2010) 344:137–50. doi: 10.1007/s11010-010-0537-z
64. Lalor PF, Herbert J, Bicknell R, Adams DH. Hepatic sinusoidal endothelium avidly binds platelets in an integrin-dependent manner, leading to platelet and endothelial activation and leukocyte recruitment. *Am J Physiol.* (2013) 304:G469–78. doi: 10.1152/ajpgi.00407.2012

65. Michels S, Schmidt-Erfurth U. Photodynamic therapy with verteporfin: a new treatment in ophthalmology. *Semin Ophthalmol.* (2001) 16:201–6. doi: 10.1076/soph.16.4.201.10298
66. Smith SA, Sessions RB, Shoemark DK, Williams C, Ebrahimighaei R, McNeill MC, et al. Antiproliferative and antimigratory effects of a novel YAP-TEAD interaction inhibitor identified using in silico molecular docking. *J Med Chem.* (2019) 62:1291–305. doi: 10.1021/acs.jmedchem.8b01402
67. Mana-Capelli S, Paramasivam M, Dutta S, McCollum D. Angiomotins link F-actin architecture to Hippo pathway signaling. *Mol Biol Cell.* (2014) 25:1676–85. doi: 10.1091/mbc.e13-11-0701

19

Inflammation and Progression of Cholangiocarcinoma: Role of Angiogenic and Lymphangiogenic Mechanisms

*Sukanya Roy, Shannon Glaser and Sanjukta Chakraborty**

Department of Medical Physiology, Texas A&M Health Science Center College of Medicine, Bryan, TX, United States

***Correspondence:**
Sanjukta Chakraborty
schakraborty@tamu.edu

Cholangiocarcinoma (CCA), or cancer of the biliary epithelium is a relatively rare but aggressive form of biliary duct cancer which has a 5-year survival rate post metastasis of 2%. Although a number of risk factors are established for CCA growth and progression, a careful evaluation of the existing literature on CCA reveals that an inflammatory environment near the biliary tree is the most common causal link between the risk factors and the development of CCA. The fact that inflammation predisposes affected individuals to CCA is further bolstered by multiple observations where the presence and maintenance of an inflammatory microenvironment at the site of the primary tumor plays a significant role in the development and metastasis of CCA. In addition, mechanisms activating the tumor vasculature and enhancing angiogenesis and lymphangiogenesis significantly contribute to CCA aggressiveness and metastasis. This review aims to address the role of an inflammatory microenvironment-CCA crosstalk and will present the basic concepts, observations, and current perspectives from recent research studies in the field of tumor stroma of CCA.

Keywords: microenvironment, inflammatory signaling, cholangiocarcinoma, tumor lymphangiogenesis, angiogenesis

INTRODUCTION

Cholangiocarcinoma (CCA) is a term used to define a group of different biliary epithelial cancers and is the second most common type of liver cancer. This group of primary biliary malignancy represents three different classically recognized kinds of biliary tree cancers, classified on the basis of anatomical point of origin in the bile duct, intrahepatic CCA (iCCA), perihilar CCA (pCCA), and distal CCA (dCCA) (1). Among these three types, iCCA originates in the intrahepatic ducts and represents the second most prevalent type of primary liver malignancy (about 10% of primary liver malignancies are iCCA). Duration of survival post-resection in intrahepatic CCA is 12.4 months (2). The most common type of CCA, is the pCCA, constituting ~50–60% of all recorded cases. pCCA comprises tumor arising from the emergence of left/right hepatic ducts at liver hilum to the confluence of cystic duct with common hepatic duct (choledocus formation) while distal CCA representing 20–30% of CCA occurs in the epithelial cells of the extra hepatic bile ducts (3). Although iCCA represents only about 5–10% of all CCA cases there is an increase in the number of iCCA among the three CCA types being observed recently (4). Internationally, CCA cases have increased since the past decade, in United States ~5,000 new cases are diagnosed each year (5). The incidence of CCA is highest among Hispanics and Asians (2.8–3.3/100,000) and lowest (2.1/100,000) among non-hispanics and African Americans (6). With a 5 year mortality rate post metastasis of 2%, CCA, originally described as a rare form of cancer is receiving more attention compared to the past decades due to its high mortality rate (1).

ETIOLOGY

The number of people afflicted with CCA differs geographically primarily because of the difference in the presence of the risk factors that predispose an individual toward CCA. The number of CCA cases is higher in Asian countries (7). CCA also shows a slight bias toward the male gender (7). The number of risk factors and their extent of influence on CCA predisposition, is not as high as in other malignancies. This could be partially due to the limited number of studies focused on identifying risk factors of CCA. Presence of bile duct cysts, primary sclerosing cholangitis, liver cirrhosis, hepatobiliary parasitic infections such as with liver fluke, hepatolithiasis, and thorotrast exposure, are the most common risk factors. Further complicating this scenario is the fact that a majority of CCA cases develop without the presence of any of the above-mentioned risk factors (8). Hence, there is a need to look at new prognostic factors that will aid in predicting the surgical eligibility, outcome and survival of CCA patients. This has opened up new avenues in research and has identified the critical role of different inflammatory cytokines, increased lymphangiogenesis, relatively low angiogenesis, cancer associated fibroblasts (CAFs), mesenchymal stem cells (MSCs), and other factors, in the growth and progression of the different types of CCA. In the next section we will review some of these risk factors.

Primary Sclerosing Cholangitis (PSC)

Inflammation and inflammatory mediators form a key underlying basis for several risk factors significantly associated with CCA (9). An inflammatory and obstructive autoimmune disease of the bile ducts, PSC is one of the most important risk factors of CCA. Patients with PSC have a 400-fold higher chance of developing CCA than those without PSC. Interestingly, majority of PSC patients are between the ages of 30 and 40 (in general CCA has a reported age specificity of 60–70 years in age) at the time of diagnosis (9). Up to 50% of these cases are recorded in the first year of diagnosis of PSC (10). The presence of chronic inflammation of bile ducts typically associated with PSC is thought to be one of the reasons for this heightened risk (11–13). Other factors that serve as the link between PSC and CCA include increased proliferation of the epithelial cells of the biliary tree, cholestasis in the ducts leading to the liver and presence of mutagens produced in the bile (10, 11). The role of inflammation in the growth and rapid development of CCA is also underscored by studies that identify inflammatory bowel disease (IBD) as one of the risk factors of CCA (12, 13).

Cirrhosis

Liver cirrhosis develops as a consequence of liver diseases and/or conditions such as alcoholism and hepatitis. As a result, the liver parenchyma is dominated by fibrosis/scarring of liver tissue resulting in disruption and eventual loss of normal liver function. Cirrhosis is an important risk factor for iCCA (14) and shows high degree of association, especially, in Asian populations (15). Similar to PSC, this too has an inflammatory stimulus and a sudden rise in epithelial proliferation, presence of pro-inflammatory cytokines and chemokines and the generation of fibrotic nodules in liver, mediates a link between cirrhosis and CCA (3).

Liver Fluke Infections

Liver fluke (*Clonorchis sinensis*, *Opisthorchis viverrini*) infections have been identified as critical risk factors for CCA especially in eastern Asian countries where these infections are deemed to be endemic (16). In fact, the recognition of *O. viverrini* as a cancer-inducing parasite by IARC (International Agency for research on Cancer) is due to its role in the development of CCA in affected individuals. These infections are associated with a rise in inflammation, generation of fibrotic nodules, obstruction of bile ducts and/or cholestasis. Chronic inflammation in the biliary tree in *O. viverrini* infected patients (especially in the background of gene polymorphisms and exposure to other environmental factors) leads to CCA development (17, 18).

Viral Infections

Viral infections such as hepatitis B and C (HBV and HCV, respectively), serve as important risk factors for CCA (19). While HBV infection is endemic to Asian countries and thus serves as the stronger risk factor for iCCA (20), HCV is the primary causative agent for iCCA in western countries (14). Cirrhosis is a common manifestation of hepatitis and leads to the development of the chronic inflammatory background that predisposes to CCA. However, the role of hepatitis viruses in causing proliferation of the hepatic epithelium is also considered to be a reason for CCA incidence in hepatitis patients (21).

Choledocholithiasis and Hepatolithiasis

Choledolithiasis and cholelithiasis are conditions that involve the presence of stones in the gall bladder and common bile ducts. The presence of these gall stones causes biliary obstruction resulting in cholestasis and serve especially as a risk factor for extrahepatic CCA (22). The presence of stones or calcium deposition inside the intrahepatic bile ducts also leads to cholestasis and chronic inflammation, ultimately serving as a risk factor for CCA. In the Asian population, 5–13% of patients with hepatolithiasis develop iCCA (15, 23).

Other Inflammatory Conditions

Chronic pancreatitis is a strong risk factor for extrahepatic CCA with an odds ratio of 6.61 (95% CI 5.21–8.40) in comparison to the 2.66 odds ratio of iCCA (95% CI, 1.72–4.10). In chronic pancreatitis too, cholestasis and inflammation may arise leading to CCA (24). Also, the presence of cysts in the bile ducts (intrahepatic and extrahepatic) when left untreated leads to the development of iCCA and eCCA tumors, because of biliary duct obstruction and dilatation leading to cholestasis and inflammation

(24, 25). Thus, it is evident that inflammation forms an underlying theme in the predisposition and development of CCA.

CELLULAR ORIGIN OF CCA

Role of Cell of Origin

As CCAs originate from cholangiocytes from different anatomical locations of the biliary tree, they also exhibit considerable tumor heterogeneity that points to the possibility of diverse cellular origins (1, 26). In general, CCA originates from the peribiliary gland (PBG) lining epithelium of intra- and extra- hepatic ducts (IH and EH, respectively) of the biliary tree (27). Additionally, cholangiocytes and hepatocytes originating from canals of Herring can undergo mutation to give rise to tumors having varying phenotypes (28). Based on the wide range of these phenotypes, pCCA and dCCA have been characterized as adenocarcinomas mucinous in nature, while iCCA has two subtypes: iCCA arising from small bile ducts, mixed in histological phenotype and those arising directly from large intrahepatic bile duct, mucinous in histology (29, 30). While bile ductular type iCCA has been recognized to be associated with solid tumor formation not having preneoplastic lesions, iCCA arising from large intrahepatic bile duct is one which is distinctly preceded by preneoplastic lesions (biliary intraepithelial/intraductal papillary neoplasm). Additionally, bile ductular type iCCA has been correlated with chronic liver disease cases such as cirrhosis in contrast to bile duct type iCCA which is mostly correlated with PSC. These differences in histology point to the role of different cells of origin of CCA (29, 30).

Stem Cell/Progenitor Niches for CCA Development

The undeniable role of stem cells in CCA development and origin is proven by the fact that human hepatic stem cells (hHPSCs) are the progenitor cells giving rise to cholangiocytes and hepatocytes that mutate to give rise to CCA (28). The PBG niche starts at septal-segmental bile ducts and ends near duodenal area at hepatic pancreatic common duct. PBG niche thus distributed all across the biliary tree has a significant role in harboring a multipotent stem cell niche which forms the source of the endodermal hepatic mucinous cells that ultimately give rise to the mucinous CCA subtypes of dCCA, pCCA and bile duct type iCCA (27, 30–32). Cancer stem cells (CSCs) are more generally characterized as cellular subset that maintains tumor growth, such CSCs are recognized by the expression of extracellular markers like CD 24, CD44, CD133, epithelial cell adhesion molecule (EpCAM) etc. in liver malignancies (33). In CCA, more of these studies identifying the specific roles of CSCs are needed. As such two distinct stem cell niches are recognized for CCA development: BTSCs (biliary tree stem cell niche within PBG) and hHPSCs within canals of Herring (26, 27). These findings suggest that CCA has more than one type of cell-of-origin and the differences can be looked at to develop a treatment strategy(s) that is personified from an anatomical point of view (34).

FACTORS INFLUENCING THE INFLAMMATORY TUMOR MICROENVIRONMENT OF CCA

CCA is one of the most desmoplastic tumors and the tumor microenvironment of CCA is characterized by a dense bed of connective tissue intertwining the tumor cells. This dense stroma is composed of a contiguously activated subset of fibroblasts called CAFs that play key roles in modulating several aspects of CCA progression (35). Further during tumor development and progression and resulting increase in cellular and metabolic demands there is often restricted access to nutrients and oxygen supply. This results in regions of the solid tumor having permanent or transient hypoxia, due to alterations in the tumor associated vasculature (36). The expanding vascular network is unable to meet up with the growing demands of the tumor and hypoxic regions persist and induce cellular pathways that promote more malignant phenotypes. In addition, there are immune cells, blood vessels, and lymphatic vessels that contribute to tumor progression which will be discussed in the following sections.

Role of Cancer Associated Fibroblasts

CAFs release a number of molecules functioning as extracellular matrix proteins (ECM) such as collagen I and fibronectin (35). In CCA, CAFs typically infiltrate the tumor stroma, and are differentially stimulated by a variety of molecular factors released by CCA tumor cells as well as hypoxia. The CAFs population in CCA thus is heterogenous in origin (37). Two of the main sources of these CAFs are liver (hepatic stellate cells, HSCs) and portal vein (portal fibroblasts), while bone marrow derived MSCs also serve as a source of CAFs to a minor extent (37). CCA tumor cells and other immune cells such as macrophages secrete inflammatory chemokines, cytokines and growth factors that not only signal fibroblasts from liver and portal vein to infiltrate the tumor microenvironment but also result in constitutive activation of fibroblasts (35). Platelet derived growth factor (PDGF-DD) overexpressed by CCA cells under hypoxic condition has been shown to be an important CAF infiltrating factor. Binding of PDGF-DD to its receptor PDGFRβ activates Cdc42, Rac1, and Rho GTPases and JNK pathways (38). PDGF-DD binding Cdc42 induces the formation of filopodia and Rac1 induces the formation of lamellipoda, thus ensuring the migration of CAFs to CCA tumor stroma. In addition to PDGF-DD, a number of other growth factors such as FGF (fibroblast growth factor), numerous factors belonging to PDGF family and TGF-β also aid CAF infiltration (39).

Alpha-smooth muscle actin-positive (α-SMA) fibroblasts promote biliary cell proliferation and correlate with poor survival in CCA. CCA fibroblasts have proliferative effects that enhance tumor promotion and progression of CCA (40). CCA patients with a high population of CAFs have poorer prognosis than patients with low number of CAFs (41). Consequently, CAF-specific α-SMA is a prognostic factor of CCA patient survival (42). The tumor boosting ability of stromal CAFs was also shown using a 3D collagen matrix-based co-culturing system, in which CCA cells and CAFs isolated from a syngeneic orthotopic rat model of CCA showed a corresponding increase in the formation of structures resembling ducts from CCA cells with the increase in CAF plating density (43). Interestingly, hepatic stellate cells (HSCs) under the influence of CCA cells can also transform into CAFs and support CCA growth (44, 45). These findings were further corroborated by studies in a syngeneic rat CCA model with selective stromal CAF depletion that exhibited improved host survival and decreased tumor growth (46).

Factors Supporting CAF-CCA Cross-Talk

CAFs in CCA show unique characteristics and gene signatures (47). Gene expression studies with human CCA sample derived CAFs showed significant differences between normal liver fibroblasts and CAFs. Most of the genes that were induced in CAFs were involved in controlling cellular metabolism, a prerequisite for the active production of cellular proteins to support the tumor microenvironment and promote tumorigenesis (47). In addition, exosomes also serve as important vessels for transporting regulatory molecular factors (between CAFs and CCA cells) thus supporting cross-talk between CCA cells and CAFs. While studies characterizing the exosomal cargo involved in CAF-CCA crosstalk has been relatively limited (48, 49), it has been shown that exosomes shuttle miR-195 between CAFs and CCA (50). Stimulation of MSCs to CCA cell-derived exosomes lead to increased migration and production of inflammatory tumor promoting cytokines as CXCL1, CCL2, and IL-6 (51). In addition, several growth factors contribute to the inflammatory microenvironment.

EGFA/EGFR binding has been shown to promote tumorigenesis and metastasis in CCA, another important EGFR ligand, HB-EGF was found to be highly expressed in myofibroblasts. HB-EGF activated EGF signaling promotes proliferation of CCA cells and also induces epithelial-mesenchymal (EMT) changes as well as invasion. HB-EGF secretion from fibroblasts is also activated by the pro-tumorigenic growth factor TGF-β secreted by tumor cells that in turn favors CCA growth (52).

Stromal cell derived factor 1 or SDF-1 has previously been reported to be involved in promoting cancer growth as a ligand for CXCR4/CXCR7 (53). In CCA, SDF-1 expression is only produced by the stromal CAF, possibly as a result of the HSC infiltration under stimulatory signals derived from angiotensin-II secreted by cancer cells (54). *In vitro* studies indicate that when SDF-1 is expressed by HSCs, a number of pro-tumorigenic responses are induced such Bcl-2, and activation of PI3K/Akt pathway. These responses initiate increased CCA cell invasion and prolonged survival in addition to inducing epithelial-mesenchymal transition (45, 55). Tumor associated macrophages were shown to produce TNF-α that induces CXCR4 expression, thus promoting SDF-1 mediated pro-tumorigenic effects (54). CAFs are also shown to release high levels of HGF (hepatocyte growth factor) that might mediate high expression of CXCR4 (43).

Role of Mesenchymal Stem Cells (MSCs)

One of the most important cellular components of CCA stroma are MSCs. MSCs may activate a series of tumor signaling pathways through the release of cytokines and that may either promote or inhibit tumor development and progression (56). The function of MSCs in tissue repair is similar to the homing of MSCs to sites of tissue damage and to sites of tumor microenvironment (51). Injured tissues secrete a wide variety of inflammatory chemokines that sends signals to MSCs for repair. It has been seen in a number of studies that tumor cells too, while modulating several other factors in their microenvironment that foster a metastatic condition, secrete inflammatory chemokines that result in MSC infiltration (51). CCA cells also secrete exosomal vesicles that are shown to enhance expression of IL-6, CXCL-1, and CCL2 by MSCs. Further, conditioned medium from MSCs exposed to tumor cell-derived extracellular vesicles (EVs) caused an upregulation in STAT3 phosphorylation and proliferation of CCA cells, possibly by secretion of CCL2/MCP1, CXCL1/GRO-α, CXC3CL1/Fractalkine, IL-6, and PDGF-AA (51). Conditioned media from MSCs also has been found to upregulate the Wnt signaling pathway in CCA cells and increased nuclear translocation of ß-catenin (57). Further, coculture studies of CCA and MSCs have shown that increased CCR5 expression by tumor cells upregulates metalloproteinases MMP-2 and MMP-9 in CCA cells and thereby promoted angiogenesis and CCA metastasis (58).

Role of Macrophages

The CCA stroma is densely populated by different infiltrating immune cells among which tumor associated macrophages (TAMs) play an important role by regulating angiogenesis, lymphangiogenesis, tumor proliferation and also modulating matrix related changes (59, 60). In a study by Wongkham et al. more than half of CCA tumor samples showed high macrophage infiltration in CCA (61). It has also been seen that $CD14^+/CD16^+$ monocyte cells which are precursors of tissue resident macrophages are present in an increased number in CCA patients. It is significant that these circulating $CD14^+/CD16^+$ monocytes have high VEGF and CXCL3 expression that promote tumor angiogenesis (62). In a correlation study it was seen that $CD163^+$ M2 macrophages were associated with $FOXP3^+$ regulatory T cell-related infiltration. Additionally, this study also showed that CCA conditioned media treatment of macrophages led to polarization bias toward M2 macrophages along with secretion of TGFβ, IL10, and VEGF-A (63). A high density of the M2-TAMs in patients is significantly associated with increased extrahepatic metastases possibly due to the effects on EMT pathways (41).

ROLE OF INFLAMMATORY CYTOKINES

The association between chronic inflammation and the development and progression of malignancy is significantly pronounced in onset and development of CCA (64). Inflammation in the tumor microenvironment of CCA is promoted by a number of cytokines and chemokines that further enhance tumor progression and aid pathways involved in distant metastasis (47). Below, we discuss several inflammatory cytokines that contribute to an inflammatory tumor microenvironment and enhance CCA progression.

Tumor Necrosis Factor-Alpha (TNF-α)

TNF-α is one of the most well-known mediators of inflammatory stimuli in the tumor microenvironment (65). Although TNF-α is involved in cancer progression, its more prominent pro-tumoral effects have been seen in angiogenesis and invasion of cancer cells (66, 67). During pathogenesis, TNF-α elicits an immune response at tissue injury locations. TNF-α also induces hepatic stellate cells (HSCs) so that they secrete oxidative radicals such as hydroxyl radical, nitic oxide (NO), and superoxide anion and is associated with aggressive development of CCA (68). Suksawat et al. showed that CCA cells express very high levels of eNOS and phosphorylated eNOS that correlate with poor prognosis in CCA patients. This phosphorylation mediated activation of eNOS by VEGF-C is through activation of PI3K/AKT pathway. The downstream effects of eNOS/peNOS/iNOS is thought to originate from VEGF-C pathway activation (69). TNF-α has been shown to promote migration of CCA cells by upregulating expression of S100A4, vimentin and ZEB2, molecules involved in EMT transition. In neoplastic bile ducts, these molecules have been seen to be associated with upregulation of TGF-β and downregulation of E-cadherin expression, an observation that has been correlated to poor prognosis in CCA patients (70).

Interleukin 1β (IL-1β)

Classified as one of the most important pro-inflammatory cytokines, IL-1β has been shown to be highly expressed from HSCs. The autocrine signaling mediated by CCA cells also becomes prominent in this regard as CCA cells have been shown to produce high levels of IL-1β that further enhances the CXCL5/CXCR2 pathway that in turn activates AKT/PI3K or ERK1/2 pathways. In fact, heightened CXCL5 expression has been seen to indicate poor rates of survival in CCA patients (71, 72).

Interleukin 6 (IL-6)

Bone marrow derived MSCs (BM-MSC) when exposed to tumor conditioned medium can transform into CAFs and stimulate tumor growth via secretion of inflammatory cytokine IL-6 in the tumor stroma. In CCA, this IL-6 overexpression was found to decrease the methylation of the EGFR promoter and enhance EGFR expression that in turn is associated with poor prognosis and overall survival (64, 73). IL-6 also mediates its tumorigenic effects by causing hypermethylation based silencing of tumor suppressor genes (74). In CCA, IL-6 has been shown to activate the p38 pathway and consequently downregulate $p21^{WAF/CIP1}$ a cyclin dependent kinase inhibitor, involved in cell cycle regulation (75). IL-6 also induces upregulation of STAT3 and Mcl-1 (myeloid cell leukemia-1) genes that mediate an anti-apoptotic response in neoplastic cholangiocytes (76). In addition, IL-6 also induces EMT by increasing expression of Snail and JAK/STAT and a resulting downregulation of E-cadherin and promotes CCA progression (77).

Transforming Growth Factor (TGF-β)

TGF-β plays dual roles in cancer progression and inhibits cell proliferation, regulates anti-inflammatory, and pro-apoptotic effects in cells under normal physiological conditions (78). It also actively promotes tumor progression and most cancer cells are resistant to its anti-proliferative effects. TGF-β activates the expression of its downstream genes (such as Bim) through differential phosphorylation and nuclear translocation of SMAD transcription factors (79). Mutational changes in the TGF-β receptor resulting in changes in Smad4 phosphorylation, increased cyclin D1 levels activate pathways that make CCA cells resistant to the tumor suppressive effects of TGF-β (80). Mouse model-based studies have shown that loss of expression of PTEN and SMAD4 gives rise to CCA (81). Correlation studies have shown that high levels of TGF- β is related to CCA metastasis to lymph nodes and distant sites as well as CCA recurrence (82). Consequently, inhibition of TGF-β resulted in significant reduction of CCA cell invasion (83). Further, altered TGF-β signaling in CCA cells also causes EMT-driven changes in cytoskeletal structure and CCA cell motility thus influencing cancer cell invasion through upregulation of EMT genes (84).

Overall, inflammatory cytokines set the stage for CCA growth by enhancing proliferation, activation of tumor promoting mechanisms such as EMT, activation of signaling pathways that promote tumor growth and loss of cell cycle checkpoints. However, the major cause for the high mortality associated with these cancers is its ability to metastasize, that is aided by the activation of lymphangiogenic (growth of new lymphatic vessels) and angiogenic (growth of new blood vessels). The various growth factors secreted by CCA cells into their stroma and other components of the tumor microenvironment foster the development of new lymphatic and blood vessels that in turn promote tumor growth and dissemination to distant organs.

LYMPHANGIOGENESIS AND ANGIOGENIC MECHANISMS IN CCA PROGRESSION AND METASTASIS

Tumor cells employ several mechanisms to establish a functional and integrated vascular system comprised of both blood and lymphatic vessels to promote cellular growth and metabolism. Expansion of these vascular networks is key to migration of the tumor cells to distant sites where they establish tumor niches. A surge of recent data has implicated the roles of both lymphatic and the blood vascular in promoting CCA metastasis.

Lymphangiogenesis and Lymph Node Remodeling

Tumor-associated lymphangiogenesis, or the sprouting of new lymphatic vessels in the tumor microenvironment is a form of tumor-associated neovascularization that has been the focus of studies concerning the metastatic spread of highly aggressive form of cancers (85). Lymphatic involvement has emerged as a hallmark of CAA with significant lymphatic invasion or lymph node metastasis implicated with poor disease prognosis (86, 87). Early metastatic CCA is characterized by a striking expansion of the intratumoral and peritumoral lymphatic vessels, which represents a key determinant of the early metastasis to the regional lymph nodes in patients rendering patients unable to opt for surgical resection. Post-surgical resection period is characterized by an increase in lymphangiogenesis and lymphatic vessel remodeling that correlates with poor post-surgical survival (86). Hence, it is critical to look at the elements in the tumor microenvironment of CCA that cause lymphangiogenesis and lymph node remodeling.

As discussed above, the tumor microenvironment of CCA is enriched with abundant cytokines and chemokines necessary for paracrine signaling that promotes development of a lymphatic bed dedicated to sustaining the growth of tumor. CAFs actively crosstalk with CCA cells in driving the development of a rich lymphatic vasculature within a pro-lymphangiogenic tumor stroma (35). High expression of VEGF-C and VEGFR-3 has been observed in the tumor microenvironment of intrahepatic CCA patients (iCCA), that also correlated with poor prognosis in patients (88–90). VEGF-C is required for the growth of small (or intial) lymphatic vessels whereas angiopoietin 1 & 2 are need by VEGF-C to form terminal lymphatic vessels in the adult body (91, 92). The dense network of lymphatic vessels and a reduced number of blood vessels, in the CCA tumor stroma also creates a hypoxic microenvironment (93). Hypoxia inducible factor-1 (HIF-1α) is known to induce lymphangiogenesis in several cancers (94). In CCA, high expression of HIF-1α promotes tumor progression and metastasis and is associated with poor patient survival (95). Interestingly, HIF-1α has also been shown to support cancer related lymphangiogenesis by upregulating the expression and subsequent secretion of Ang1/2, VEGF-C/D and PDGF-B from neoplastic cells into the tumor stroma, in several cancers as breast cancer, esophageal cancer, and oral squamous carcinoma (96–98). PDGF-D secreted from neoplastic CCA cells binds PDGFRβ on CAFs resulting in activation of ERK/NF-kB and JNK signaling networks that in turn secretes VEGF-C and promotes expansion of the lymphatic vasculature and tumor cell intravasation. Pharmacological depletion of CAFs in a CCA *in vivo* however, significantly reduced lymphatic vascularization and reduced lymph node metastases (99). VEGF-C expression in CCA is also mediated by M2 macrophages (63). Further, overexpression of Nerve Growth Factor Beta (NGF-B) overexpression correlated with VEGF-C overexpression, lymphatic vessel density and lymph node metastasis along with nerve cell invasion in patients of hilar CCA (100). Different correlation studies have established lymphatic vessel density (LVD) and expression of several lymphatic specific markers such as podoplanin and VEGFR-3 as prognostic biomarkers of CCA (101, 102). Podoplanin is highly expressed on the surface of CAFs as well as LECs and emerged to be a prognostic biomarker in human perihilar CCA (101). Lymph node metastasis has also been correlated with a high podoplanin expression on activated CAFs in intrahepatic CCA (90). Further studies are needed to determine the role of podoplanin in tumor lymphangiogenesis in CCA. However, podoplanin mediated regulation of small GTPases as Cdc42 induces capillary morphogenesis, polarized migration, and invasiveness of LECs (103, 104).

Thelen et al. have demonstrated that a high lymphatic vessel density or existence of lymphangiogenesis significantly correlates with poor prognosis in patients with hilar CCA. This observation adds to the role of lymphatic vessel remodeling in cancer progression, specifically the migration of cancer cells via lymphatic vessels (104, 105). In CCA, a "high" LVD is associated with increased nodal spread, and "high" LVD tumors more frequently develop recurrence (105). Indeed recent studies have shown that both peritumoral as well as intratumoral lymphatic bed is composed of capillaries that lack organization and/or drainage function thus favoring neoplastic cell infiltration because of the differential permeability or leaky nature of these vessels (106). In this regard, LECs lining these vessels also interact with tumor cells to transport them through endothelium, an event mediated by the CCL1-CCR8 chemokine axis. CC-type chemokine ligand 1 (CCL1) is expressed on the surface of LECs which bind CC-type chemokine receptor 8 (CCR8) on the surface of tumor cells and thus help in their trans-endothelial migration (107). Tumor lymphangiogenesis, which results in proliferation of LECs also functions in immune-evasion of the cancer cells. LECs in draining lymph nodes express on their surface the well-known antigen PD-L1 which binds to PD-1 on the surface of cancer specific CD 8^{+} cells and induces their apoptosis (108). However, there is a need to study the mechanisms of lymph node remodeling and lymphatic metastasis in CCA, that would further establish the link between lymphatic vessel remodeling, tumor stroma, tumor lymphangiogenesis and CCA metastasis.

Angiogenesis

Tumor related angiogenesis, or the sprouting of new blood vessels is one of the key mechanisms for tumor metastasis that is promoted by angiogenic factors actively secreted by tumor cells (109). Tumor angiogenesis is pronounced in CCA, one of the most aggressive and metastatic cancers. Cholangiocytes promote neo-vascularization by enhanced expression of pro-angiogenic growth factors both at the site of primary tumor as well as in the tumor stroma of distant sites where these cholangiocytes have metastasized. Thus, a sprawling network of blood vessels created by secreted factors from cholangiocytes supports the growth and spread of cholangiocytes (110). Critical mediators and activators of angiogenesis include the growth hormones VEGF, EGF, and NGF, FGF, placental growth factor, the angiopoietins and their receptors, Tiel and Tie2. Further, neuropilin, ephrin, and leptin are being recognized as key mediators of angiogenesis and tumor growth (111). These pro-angiogenic factors play important roles both in maintenance and growth of the primary tumor as well as neo-vascularization during CCA metastasis (111). In normal tissues, following induction of angiogenesis by pro-angiogenic factors such as the VEGF factor family proteins (VEGF-A, VEGF-B, VEGF-C), remodeling of the newly formed vessel wall takes place where intercellular tight junctions and adherens junctions are created between vascular endothelial cells (BECs), that brings about permeability and elasticity in the vessel (110). After vessel remodeling is completed in normal tissues the ensuing blood flow and establishment of normoxia (normal/physiological

O_2 concentration) results in the inhibition of angiogenesis inhibition. In tumor cells however, hypoxia or a low oxygen environment in the region of the tumor induces expression of VEGF hormones. Cholangiocytes, accordingly, have been found to secrete high levels of both VEGF-A in the tumor stroma and VEGFR-2 during cholangiocyte hyperplasia (112). This suggests an autocrine mechanism by which cholangiocytes regulate their own growth. Similar to the studies in CCA lymphangiogenesis where high VEGFR-3 expression is enhanced under the influence of CAFs and tumor cells on the surface of LECs, it has been shown that a similar paracrine signaling mechanism exists in BECs where high levels of VEGFR-2 are expressed on its surface (112). Enhanced expression of VEGF-A and other members of the VEGF family such as VEGF-C cause BECs to secrete MMP-9 and MMP-7 which help in remodeling of the basement membrane and surrounding ECM and promotes tumor metastasis. Interestingly, it has been shown that TGF-β and VEGF are co-expressed in human CCA and that overexpression and functional interaction of TGF-β and VEGF could potentially contribute to the "angiogenic switch" and the malignant phenotype in human CCC (113). In addition to hypoxia stimulating production of VEGF, additional factors such as estrogen along with IGF1 (insulin like growth factor 1) and IGFR (IGF1 receptor) synergistically increases the expression of VEGFs such as VEGF-A, VEGF-C and their corresponding receptors in cultured CCA cells (114). In addition, metastasis-associated in colon cancer-1 (MACC1) protein upregulates VEGF-A thus favoring the growth of CCA (115). Overexpression of histidine decarboxylase (HDC) enzyme correlated with that of VEGF-A/C expression. HDC knockdown/inhibition significantly reduced tumor growth by reducing tumor cell proliferation and VEGF expression (109).

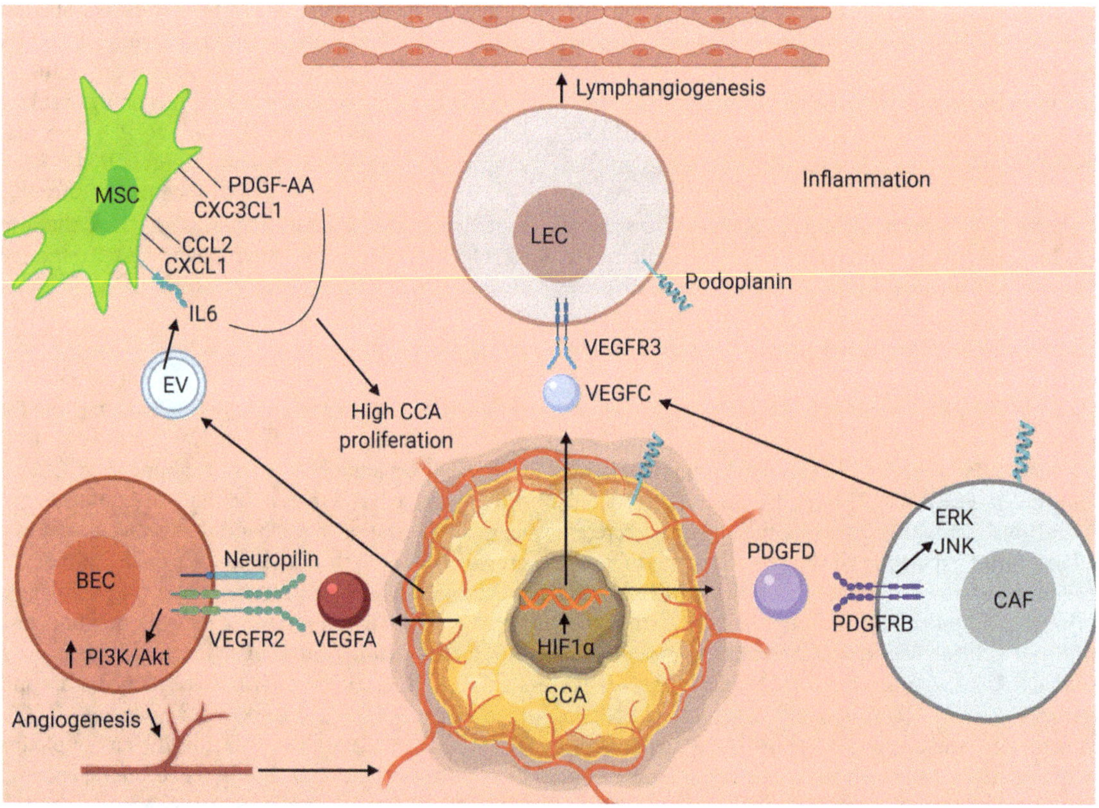

FIGURE 1 | Schematic illustrating interaction of key elements in the tumor stroma in CCA progression. Several components of the CCA tumor microenvironment activate mechanisms that promote tumor growth, migration and activation of tumor associated angiogenesis and lymphangiogenesis. Interaction between VEC and CCA cell via VEGFR2-VEGFA assisted by neuropilin leads to tumor angiogenesis via upregulation of PI3K/Akt pathway. HIF1α activated by an inflamed tumor microenvironment stimulates CCA progression. VEGFC secreted by CCA as well by CAF (via PDGFD stimulation of tumor cells) aids in the process of lymphangiogenesis by stimulating LECs to divide via VEGFR3 engagement and upregulation of ERK/JNK pathway. Further contributing to the surrounding milieu, exosomal vesicles secreted by CCA triggers production of IL6, CCL2, CXCL1, CXC3CL1, and PDGF-AA which in turn when secreted in the tumor stroma induces CCA proliferation and growth pathways. CCA, Cholangiocarcinoma; MSC, Mesenchymal Stem Cell; LEC, Lymphatic Endothelial Cell; CAF, Cancer Associated Fibroblast; VEC, Vascular Endothelial Cell; PDGF-AA, Platelet Derived Growth Factor-AA; CXC3CL1, Chemokine Ligand 1 (Fractalkine); CCL2, C-C Motif Chemokine Ligand 2; CXCL1, C-X-C Motif Chemokine Ligand 1; IL6, Interleukin 6; VEGFR3, Vascular Endothelial Growth Factor Receptor 3; VEGFC, Vascular Endothelial Growth Factor C; VEGFA, Vascular Endothelial Growth Factor A; VEGFR2, Vascular Endothelial Growth Factor 2; PI3K, Phosphoinositide 3-kinase; Akt, Protein Kinase B; HIF1α, Hypoxia Inducible Factor 1 α; PDGFD, Platelet Derived Growth Factor D; PDGFRB, Platelet Derived Growth Factor Receptor B; ERK, Extracellular Receptor Kinase; JNK, c-Jun N-terminal Kinase.

microRNA Regulation of Lymphangiogenesis and Angiogenesis in CCA

Growing evidence from literature suggests that microRNAs (miRNA), endogenous small non-coding RNAs (19–24 nucleotides) regulate various aspects of cholangiopathies including CCA and has been extensively reviewed elsewhere (116, 117). However, studies evaluating their role in regulation of lymphangiogenesis associated with CCA is very limited. The miRNAs involved in CCA associated angiogenesis have been more extensively investigated and miR-92a, miR-126, miR-132, and miR-296 regulate several key pathways that enhance CCA associated angiogenesis (118). Overexpression of miR 16 and miR-424 has been shown to regulate the VEGF-A/FGF signaling cascades and reduce tumor cell proliferation and migration (119). miR-101, an miRNA highly expressed in liver was found to inhibit the growth of CCA by inhibiting VEGF expression (120). Understanding how miRNA regulate different molecular players involved at different levels of CCA progression also will help design better therapeutic interventions for arresting tumor progression. Further these miRNAs have the potential of being diagnostic biomarkers for CCA metastasis.

CONCLUSION AND FUTURE DIRECTIONS

The epidemiology of CCA varies across different regions owing to the differences in the number and intensity of the risk factors present in each place, the malignancy also varies in terms of the epidemiology of its types (iCCA, pCCA, dCCA), however based on the data above it can be postulated that inflammation of the tumor microenvironment and its associated players have a crucial role in shaping the response of the CCA cells to therapeutic strategies, their growth and progression. To this end, the early metastatic events of CCA is an area that can be pursued in the future to look for new therapeutic targets as well as to unravel the intricacies of the inflammatory tumor microenvironment-CCA crosstalk. While therapies targeting specific molecules and signaling pathways have shown promise, combinatorial therapies as a whole have come up to be effective in different cancer types. Hence, a better understanding of the different components of the tumor stroma that the CCA cells modulate and exploit in order to give rise to a pro-inflammatory and pro-tumorigenic environment can lead to a holistic understanding and approach toward treating CCA. Some of these key mechanisms that interact and promote the onset and progression and subsequent metastasis of CCA is shown in **Figure 1**. It is also evident that the aggressiveness of this cancer is directly related to its ability to metastasize and hence understanding key events that promote lymphatic metastasis in the early stages of the cancer will be critical for development of targeted therapies. Specific traits of CCA such as the high rate of lymphangiogenesis vs. the low rate of angiogenesis, deserve special research focus to unravel some of the underlying molecular pathways that mediate disease progression.

AUTHOR CONTRIBUTIONS

SR, SG, and SC planned and wrote the manuscript and approved the final submitted version. SR made the figure.

REFERENCES

1. Banales JM, Cardinale V, Carpino G, Marzioni M, Andersen JB, Invernizzi P, et al. Expert consensus document: Cholangiocarcinoma: current knowledge and future perspectives consensus statement from the European Network for the Study of Cholangiocarcinoma (ENS-CCA). *Nat Rev Gastroenterol Hepatol.* (2016) 13:261–80. doi: 10.1038/nrgastro.2016.51
2. Sriputtha S, Khuntikeo N, Promthet S, Kamsa-Ard S. Survival rate of intrahepatic cholangiocarcinoma patients after surgical treatment in Thailand. *Asian Pac J Cancer Prev.* (2013) 14:1107–10. doi: 10.7314/APJCP.2013.14.2.1107
3. Rizvi S, Gores GJ. Pathogenesis, diagnosis, and management of cholangiocarcinoma. *Gastroenterology.* (2013) 145:1215–29. doi: 10.1053/j.gastro.2013.10.013
4. Rizvi S, Khan SA, Hallemeier CL, Kelley RK, Gores GJ. Cholangiocarcinoma - evolving concepts and therapeutic strategies. *Nat Rev Clin Oncol.* (2018) 15:95–111. doi: 10.1038/nrclinonc.2017.157
5. Ghouri YA, Mian I, Blechacz B. Cancer review: cholangiocarcinoma. *J Carcinog.* (2015) 14:1. doi: 10.4103/1477-3163.151940
6. Everhart JE, Ruhl CE. Burden of digestive diseases in the United States Part III: Liver, biliary tract, and pancreas. *Gastroenterology.* (2009) 136:1134–44. doi: 10.1053/j.gastro.2009.02.038
7. Khan SA, Taylor-Robinson SD, Toledano MB, Beck A, Elliott P, Thomas HC. Changing international trends in mortality rates for liver, biliary and pancreatic tumours. *J Hepatol.* (2002) 37:806–13. doi: 10.1016/S0168-8278(02)00297-0
8. Endo I, Gonen M, Yopp AC, Dalal KM, Zhou Q, Klimstra D, et al. Intrahepatic cholangiocarcinoma: rising frequency, improved survival, and determinants of outcome after resection. *Ann Surg.* (2008) 248:84–96. doi: 10.1097/SLA.0b013e318176c4d3
9. Boonstra K, Weersma RK, van Erpecum KJ, Rauws EA, Spanier BW, Poen AC, et al. Population-based epidemiology, malignancy risk, and outcome of primary sclerosing cholangitis. *Hepatology.* (2013) 58:2045–55. doi: 10.1002/hep.26565
10. Tyson GL, El-Serag HB. Risk factors for cholangiocarcinoma. *Hepatology.* (2011) 54:173–84. doi: 10.1002/hep.24351
11. Patel T. Cholangiocarcinoma. *Nat Clin Pract Gastroenterol Hepatol.* (2006) 3:33–42. doi: 10.1038/ncpgasthep0389
12. Erichsen R, Jepsen P, Vilstrup H, Ekbom A, Sørensen HT, Incidence and prognosis of cholangiocarcinoma in Danish patients with and without inflammatory bowel disease: a national cohort study, 1978-2003. *Eur J Epidemiol.* (2009) 24:513–20. doi: 10.1007/s10654-009-9365-4
13. Sørensen JØ, Nielsen OH, Andersson M, Ainsworth MA, Ytting H, Bélard E, et al. Inflammatory bowel disease with primary sclerosing cholangitis: a

Danish population-based cohort study 1977-2011. *Liver Int.* (2018) 38:532–541. doi: 10.1111/liv.13548
14. Palmer WC, Patel T. Are common factors involved in the pathogenesis of primary liver cancers? A meta-analysis of risk factors for intrahepatic cholangiocarcinoma. *J Hepatol.* (2012) 57:69–76. doi: 10.1016/j.jhep.2012.02.022
15. Chang JS, Tsai CR, Chen LT. Medical risk factors associated with cholangiocarcinoma in Taiwan: a population-based case-control study. *PLoS ONE.* (2013) 8:e69981. doi: 10.1371/journal.pone.0069981
16. Sithithaworn P, Yongvanit P, Duenngai K, Kiatsopit N, Pairojkul C. Roles of liver fluke infection as risk factor for cholangiocarcinoma. *J Hepatobil Pancreat Sci.* (2014) 21:301–8. doi: 10.1002/jhbp.62
17. Honjo S, Srivatanakul P, Sriplung H, Kikukawa H, Hanai S, Uchida K, et al. Genetic and environmental determinants of risk for cholangiocarcinoma via Opisthorchis viverrini in a densely infested area in Nakhon Phanom, northeast Thailand. *Int J Cancer.* (2005) 117:854–60. doi: 10.1002/ijc.21146
18. Brindley PJ, Loukas A. Helminth infection-induced malignancy. *PLoS Pathog.* (2017) 13:e1006393. doi: 10.1371/journal.ppat.1006393
19. Li H, Hu B, Zhou Z-Q, Guan J, Zhang Z-Y, Zhou G-W. Hepatitis C virus infection and the risk of intrahepatic cholangiocarcinoma and extrahepatic cholangiocarcinoma: evidence from a systematic review and meta-analysis of 16 case-control studies. *World J Surg Oncol.* (2015) 13:161. doi: 10.1186/s12957-015-0583-9
20. Matsumoto K, Onoyama T, Kawata S, Takeda Y, Harada K, Ikebuchi Y, et al. Hepatitis B and C virus infection is a risk factor for the development of cholangiocarcinoma. *Intern Med.* (2014) 53:651–4. doi: 10.2169/internalmedicine.53.1410
21. Ralphs S, Khan SA. The role of the hepatitis viruses in cholangiocarcinoma. *J Viral Hepat.* (2013) 20:297–305. doi: 10.1111/jvh.12093
22. Schottenfeld D, Beebe-Dimmer J. Chronic inflammation: a common and important factor in the pathogenesis of neoplasia. *CA Cancer J Clin.* (2006) 56:69–83. doi: 10.3322/canjclin.56.2.69
23. Kim HJ, Kim JS, Joo MK, Lee BJ, Kim JH, Yeon JE, et al. Hepatolithiasis and intrahepatic cholangiocarcinoma: a review. *World J Gastroenterol.* (2015) 21:13418–31. doi: 10.3748/wjg.v21.i48.13418
24. Petrick JL, Yang B, Altekruse SF, Van Dyke AL, Koshiol J, Graubard BI, et al. Risk factors for intrahepatic and extrahepatic cholangiocarcinoma in the United States: a population-based study in SEER-Medicare. *PLoS ONE.* (2017) 12:e0186643. doi: 10.1371/journal.pone.0186643
25. Abdalla EK, Forsmark CE, Lauwers GY, Vauthey JN, Monolobar Caroli's Disease and cholangiocarcinoma. *HPB Surg.* (1999) 11:271–6; discussion: 276–7. doi: 10.1155/1999/70985
26. Komuta M, Govaere O, Vandecaveye V, Akiba J, Van Steenbergen W, Verslype C, et al. Histological diversity in cholangiocellular carcinoma reflects the different cholangiocyte phenotypes. *Hepatology.* (2012) 55:1876–88. doi: 10.1002/hep.25595
27. Nakanuma Y, Sato Y, Harada K, Sasaki M, Xu J, Ikeda H. Pathological classification of intrahepatic cholangiocarcinoma based on a new concept. *World J Hepatol.* (2010) 2:419–27. doi: 10.4254/wjh.v2.i12.419
28. Roskams T. Liver stem cells and their implication in hepatocellular and cholangiocarcinoma. *Oncogene.* (2006) 25:3818–22. doi: 10.1038/sj.onc.1209558
29. Aishima S, Oda Y. Pathogenesis and classification of intrahepatic cholangiocarcinoma: different characters of perihilar large duct type versus peripheral small duct type. *J Hepatobiliary Pancreat Sci.* (2015) 22:94–100. doi: 10.1002/jhbp.154
30. Liau JY, Tsai JH, Yuan RH, Chang CN, Lee HJ, Jeng YM. Morphological subclassification of intrahepatic cholangiocarcinoma: etiological, clinicopathological, and molecular features. *Mod Pathol.* (2014) 27:1163–73. doi: 10.1038/modpathol.2013.241
31. Cardinale V, Wang Y, Carpino G, Cui CB, Gatto M, Rossi M, et al. Multipotent stem/progenitor cells in human biliary tree give rise to hepatocytes, cholangiocytes, and pancreatic islets. *Hepatology.* (2011) 54:2159–72. doi: 10.1002/hep.24590
32. Carpino G, Cardinale V, Onori P, Franchitto A, Berloco PB, Rossi M, et al. Biliary tree stem/progenitor cells in glands of extrahepatic and intraheptic bile ducts: an anatomical in situ study yielding evidence of maturational lineages. *J Anat.* (2012) 220:186–99. doi: 10.1111/j.1469-7580.2011.01462.x
33. Visvader JE, Lindeman GJ. Cancer stem cells in solid tumours: accumulating evidence and unresolved questions. *Nat Rev Cancer.* (2008) 8:755–68. doi: 10.1038/nrc2499
34. Cardinale V, Carpino G, Reid L, Gaudio E, Alvaro D. Multiple cells of origin in cholangiocarcinoma underlie biological, epidemiological and clinical heterogeneity. *World J Gastrointest Oncol.* (2012) 4:94–102. doi: 10.4251/wjgo.v4.i5.94
35. Cadamuro M, Morton SD, Strazzabosco M, Fabris L. Unveiling the role of tumor reactive stroma in cholangiocarcinoma: an opportunity for new therapeutic strategies. *Transl Gastrointest Cancer.* (2013) 2:130–44. doi: 10.3978/j.issn.2224-4778.2013.04.02
36. Brivio S, Cadamuro M, Fabris L, Strazzabosco M. Epithelial-to-mesenchymal transition and cancer invasiveness: what can we learn from cholangiocarcinoma? *J Clin Med.* (2015) 4:2028–41. doi: 10.3390/jcm4121958
37. Leyva-Illades D, McMillin M, Quinn M, Demorrow S. Cholangiocarcinoma pathogenesis: role of the tumor microenvironment. *Transl Gastrointest Cancer.* (2012) 1:71–80. doi: 10.3978/j.issn.2224-4778.2011.11.05
38. Cadamuro M, Nardo G, Indraccolo S, Dall'olmo L, Sambado L, Moserle L, et al. Platelet-derived growth factor-D and Rho GTPases regulate recruitment of cancer-associated fibroblasts in cholangiocarcinoma. *Hepatology.* (2013) 58:1042–53. doi: 10.1002/hep.26384
39. Quail DF, Joyce JA. Microenvironmental regulation of tumor progression and metastasis. *Nat Med.* (2013) 19:1423–37. doi: 10.1038/nm.3394
40. Chuaysri C, Thuwajit P, Paupairoj A, Chau-In S, Suthiphongchai T, Thuwajit C. Alpha-smooth muscle actin-positive fibroblasts promote biliary cell proliferation and correlate with poor survival in cholangiocarcinoma. *Oncol Rep.* (2009) 21:957–69. doi: 10.3892/or_00000309
41. Thanee M, Loilome W, Techasen A, Namwat N, Boonmars T, Pairojkul C, et al. Quantitative changes in tumor-associated M2 macrophages characterize cholangiocarcinoma and their association with metastasis. *Asian Pac J Cancer Prev.* (2015) 16:3043–50. doi: 10.7314/APJCP.2015.16.7.3043
42. Okabe H, Beppu T, Hayashi H, Horino K, Masuda T, Komori H, et al. Hepatic stellate cells may relate to progression of intrahepatic cholangiocarcinoma. *Ann Surg Oncol.* (2009) 16:2555–64. doi: 10.1245/s10434-009-0568-4
43. Campbell DJ, Dumur CI, Lamour NF, Dewitt JL, Sirica AE. Novel organotypic culture model of cholangiocarcinoma progression. *Hepatol Res.* (2012) 42:1119–30. doi: 10.1111/j.1872-034X.2012.01026.x
44. Okabe H, Beppu T, Hayashi H, Ishiko T, Masuda T, Otao R, et al. Hepatic stellate cells accelerate the malignant behavior of cholangiocarcinoma cells. *Ann Surg Oncol.* (2011) 18:1175–84. doi: 10.1245/s10434-010-1391-7
45. Gentilini A, Rombouts K, Galastri S, Caligiuri A, Mingarelli E, Mello T, et al. Role of the stromal-derived factor-1 (SDF-1)-CXCR4 axis in the interaction between hepatic stellate cells and cholangiocarcinoma. *J Hepatol.* (2012) 57:813–20. doi: 10.1016/j.jhep.2012.06.012
46. Mertens JC, Fingas CD, Christensen JD, Smoot RL, Bronk SF, Werneburg NW, et al. Therapeutic effects of deleting cancer-associated fibroblasts in cholangiocarcinoma. *Cancer Res.* (2013) 73:897–907. doi: 10.1158/0008-5472.CAN-12-2130
47. Utispan K, Thuwajit P, Abiko Y, Charngkaew K, Paupairoj A, Chau-in S, et al. Gene expression profiling of cholangiocarcinoma-derived fibroblast reveals alterations related to tumor progression and indicates periostin as a poor prognostic marker. *Mol Cancer.* (2010) 9:13. doi: 10.1186/1476-4598-9-13
48. Dutta S, Reamtong O, Panvongsa W, Kitdumrongthum S, Janpipatkul K, Sangvanich P, et al. Proteomics profiling of cholangiocarcinoma exosomes: a potential role of oncogenic protein transferring in cancer progression. *Biochim Biophys Acta.* (2015) 1852:1989–99. doi: 10.1016/j.bbadis.2015.06.024
49. Kitdumrongthum S, Metheetrairut C, Charoensawan V, Ounjai P, Janpipatkul K, Panvongsa W, et al. Dysregulated microRNA expression profiles in cholangiocarcinoma cell-derived exosomes. *Life Sci.* (2018) 210:65–75. doi: 10.1016/j.lfs.2018.08.058

50. Li L, Piontek K, Ishida M, Fausther M, Dranoff JA, Fu R, et al. Extracellular vesicles carry microRNA-195 to intrahepatic cholangiocarcinoma and improve survival in a rat model. *Hepatology.* (2017) 65:501–14. doi: 10.1002/hep.28735
51. Haga H, Yan IK, Takahashi K, Wood J, Zubair A, Patel T. Tumour cell-derived extracellular vesicles interact with mesenchymal stem cells to modulate the microenvironment and enhance cholangiocarcinoma growth. *J Extracell Vesicles.* (2015) 4:24900. doi: 10.3402/jev.v4.24900
52. Clapéron A, Mergey M, Aoudjehane L, Ho-Bouldoires TH, Wendum D, Prignon A, et al. Hepatic myofibroblasts promote the progression of human cholangiocarcinoma through activation of epidermal growth factor receptor. *Hepatology.* (2013) 58:2001–11. doi: 10.1002/hep.26585
53. Chatterjee S, Behnam Azad B, Nimmagadda S. The intricate role of CXCR4 in cancer. *Adv Cancer Res.* (2014) 124:31–82. doi: 10.1016/B978-0-12-411638-2.00002-1
54. Ohira S, Sasaki M, Harada K, Sato Y, Zen Y, Isse K, et al. Possible regulation of migration of intrahepatic cholangiocarcinoma cells by interaction of CXCR4 expressed in carcinoma cells with tumor necrosis factor-alpha and stromal-derived factor-1 released in stroma. *Am J Pathol.* (2006) 168:1155–68. doi: 10.2353/ajpath.2006.050204
55. Okamoto K, Tajima H, Nakanuma S, Sakai S, Makino I, Kinoshita J, et al. Angiotensin II enhances epithelial-to-mesenchymal transition through the interaction between activated hepatic stellate cells and the stromal cell-derived factor-1/CXCR4 axis in intrahepatic cholangiocarcinoma. *Int J Oncol.* (2012) 41:573–82. doi: 10.3892/ijo.2012.1499
56. Chang AI, Schwertschkow AH, Nolta JA, Wu J, Involvement of mesenchymal stem cells in cancer progression and metastases. *Curr Cancer Drug Targets.* (2015) 15:88–98. doi: 10.2174/1568009615666150126154151
57. Wang W, Zhong W, Yuan J, Yan C, Hu S, Tong Y, et al. Involvement of Wnt/beta-catenin signaling in the mesenchymal stem cells promote metastatic growth and chemoresistance of cholangiocarcinoma. *Oncotarget.* (2015) 6:42276–89. doi: 10.18632/oncotarget.5514
58. Zhong W, Tong Y, Li Y, Yuan J, Hu S, Hu T, et al. Mesenchymal stem cells in inflammatory microenvironment potently promote metastatic growth of cholangiocarcinoma via activating Akt/NF-kappaB signaling by paracrine CCL5. *Oncotarget.* (2017) 8:73693–704. doi: 10.18632/oncotarget.17793
59. Gentilini A, Pastore M, Marra F, Raggi C. The role of stroma in cholangiocarcinoma: the intriguing interplay between fibroblastic component, immune cell subsets and tumor epithelium. *Int J Mol Sci.* (2018) 19:2885. doi: 10.3390/ijms19102885
60. Brivio S, Cadamuro M, Strazzabosco M, Fabris L. Tumor reactive stroma in cholangiocarcinoma: the fuel behind cancer aggressiveness. *World J Hepatol.* (2017) 9:455–68. doi: 10.4254/wjh.v9.i9.455
61. Subimerb C, Pinlaor S, Khuntikeo N, Leelayuwat C, Morris A, McGrath MS, et al. Tissue invasive macrophage density is correlated with prognosis in cholangiocarcinoma. *Mol Med Rep.* (2010) 3:597–605. doi: 10.3892/mmr_00000303
62. Subimerb C, Pinlaor S, Lulitanond V, Khuntikeo N, Okada S, McGrath MS, et al. Circulating CD14(+) CD16(+) monocyte levels predict tissue invasive character of cholangiocarcinoma. *Clin Exp Immunol.* (2010) 161:471–9. doi: 10.1111/j.1365-2249.2010.04200.x
63. Hasita H, Komohara Y, Okabe H, Masuda T, Ohnishi K, Lei XF, et al. Significance of alternatively activated macrophages in patients with intrahepatic cholangiocarcinoma. *Cancer Sci.* (2010) 101:1913–9. doi: 10.1111/j.1349-7006.2010.01614.x
64. Wehbe H, Henson R, Meng F, Mize-Berge J, Patel T. Interleukin-6 contributes to growth in cholangiocarcinoma cells by aberrant promoter methylation and gene expression. *Cancer Res.* (2006) 66:10517–24. doi: 10.1158/0008-5472.CAN-06-2130
65. Popa C, Netea MG, van Riel PL, van der Meer JW, Stalenhoef AF. The role of TNF-alpha in chronic inflammatory conditions, intermediary metabolism, and cardiovascular risk. *J Lipid Res.* (2007) 48:751–62. doi: 10.1194/jlr.R600021-JLR200
66. Moore RJ, Owens DM, Stamp G, Arnott C, Burke F, East N, et al. Mice deficient in tumor necrosis factor-alpha are resistant to skin carcinogenesis. *Nat Med.* (1999) 5:828–31. doi: 10.1038/10552
67. Balkwill F. TNF-alpha in promotion and progression of cancer. *Cancer Metastasis Rev.* (2006) 25:409–16. doi: 10.1007/s10555-006-9005-3
68. Jaiswal M, LaRusso NF, Burgart LJ, Gores GJ. Inflammatory cytokines induce DNA damage and inhibit DNA repair in cholangiocarcinoma cells by a nitric oxide-dependent mechanism. *Cancer Res.* (2000) 60:184–90. Available online at: https://cancerres.aacrjournals.org
69. Suksawat M, Techasen A, Namwat N, Boonsong T, Titapun A, Ungarreevittaya P, et al. Inhibition of endothelial nitric oxide synthase in cholangiocarcinoma cell lines - a new strategy for therapy. *FEBS Open Bio.* (2018) 8:513–22. doi: 10.1002/2211-5463.12388
70. Techasen A, Loilome W, Namwat N, Khuntikeo N, Puapairoj A, Jearanaikoon P, et al. Loss of E-cadherin promotes migration and invasion of cholangiocarcinoma cells and serves as a potential marker of metastasis. *Tumour Biol.* (2014) 35:8645–52. doi: 10.1007/s13277-014-2087-6
71. Okabe H, Beppu T, Ueda M, Hayashi H, Ishiko T, Masuda T, et al. Identification of CXCL5/ENA-78 as a factor involved in the interaction between cholangiocarcinoma cells and cancer-associated fibroblasts. *Int J Cancer.* (2012) 131:2234–41. doi: 10.1002/ijc.27496
72. Zhou SL, Dai Z, Zhou ZJ, Chen Q, Wang Z, Xiao YS, et al. CXCL5 contributes to tumor metastasis and recurrence of intrahepatic cholangiocarcinoma by recruiting infiltrative intratumoral neutrophils. *Carcinogenesis.* (2014) 35:597–605. doi: 10.1093/carcin/bgt397
73. Mishra PJ, Mishra PJ, Humeniuk R, Medina DJ, Alexe G, Mesirov JP, et al. Carcinoma-associated fibroblast-like differentiation of human mesenchymal stem cells. *Cancer Res.* (2008) 68:4331–9. doi: 10.1158/0008-5472.CAN-08-0943
74. Gasche JA, Hoffmann J, Boland CR, Goel A, Interleukin-6 promotes tumorigenesis by altering DNA methylation in oral cancer cells. *Int J Cancer.* (2011) 129:1053–63. doi: 10.1002/ijc.25764
75. Tadlock L, Patel T. Involvement of p38 mitogen-activated protein kinase signaling in transformed growth of a cholangiocarcinoma cell line. *Hepatology.* (2001) 33:43–51. doi: 10.1053/jhep.2001.20676
76. Yu C, Bruzek LM, Meng XW, Gores GJ, Carter CA, Kaufmann SH, et al. The role of Mcl-1 downregulation in the proapoptotic activity of the multikinase inhibitor BAY 43-9006. *Oncogene.* (2005) 24:6861–9. doi: 10.1038/sj.onc.1208841
77. Yadav A, Kumar B, Datta J, Teknos TN, Kumar P, IL-6 promotes head and neck tumor metastasis by inducing epithelial-mesenchymal transition via the JAK-STAT3-SNAIL signaling pathway. *Mol Cancer Res.* (2011) 9:1658–67. doi: 10.1158/1541-7786.MCR-11-0271
78. Santibanez JF, Quintanilla M, Bernabeu C. TGF-beta/TGF-beta receptor system and its role in physiological and pathological conditions. *Clin Sci.* (2011) 121:233–51. doi: 10.1042/CS20110086
79. Massague J. TGFbeta in cancer. *Cell.* (2008) 134:215–30. doi: 10.1016/j.cell.2008.07.001
80. Zen Y, Harada K, Sasaki M, Chen TC, Chen MF, Yeh TS, et al. Intrahepatic cholangiocarcinoma escapes from growth inhibitory effect of transforming growth factor-beta1 by overexpression of cyclin D1. *Lab Invest.* (2005) 85:572–81. doi: 10.1038/labinvest.3700236
81. Xu X, Ehdaie B, Ohara N, Yoshino T, Deng CX. Synergistic action of Smad4 and Pten in suppressing pancreatic ductal adenocarcinoma formation in mice. *Oncogene.* (2010) 29:674–86. doi: 10.1038/onc.2009.375
82. Chen Y, Ma L, He Q, Zhang S, Zhang C, Jia W, TGF-beta1 expression is associated with invasion and metastasis of intrahepatic cholangiocarcinoma. *Biol Res.* (2015) 48:26. doi: 10.1186/s40659-015-0016-9
83. Sato Y, Harada K, Itatsu K, Ikeda H, Kakuda Y, Shimomura S, et al. Epithelial-mesenchymal transition induced by transforming growth factor-{beta}1/Snail activation aggravates invasive growth of cholangiocarcinoma. *Am J Pathol.* (2010) 177:141–52. doi: 10.2353/ajpath.2010.090747

84. Araki K, Shimura T, Suzuki H, Tsutsumi S, Wada W, Yajima T, et al. E/N-cadherin switch mediates cancer progression via TGF-beta-induced epithelial-to-mesenchymal transition in extrahepatic cholangiocarcinoma. *Br J Cancer.* (2011) 105:1885–93. doi: 10.1038/bjc.2011.452
85. Inoue K, Makuuchi M, Takayama T, Torzilli G, Yamamoto J, Shimada K, et al. Long-term survival and prognostic factors in the surgical treatment of mass-forming type cholangiocarcinoma. *Surgery.* (2000) 127:498–505. doi: 10.1067/msy.2000.104673
86. Fabris L, Alvaro D. The prognosis of perihilar cholangiocarcinoma after radical treatments. *Hepatology.* (2012) 56:800–2. doi: 10.1002/hep.25808
87. Sha M, Jeong S, Wang X, Tong Y, Cao J, Sun HY, et al. Tumor-associated lymphangiogenesis predicts unfavorable prognosis of intrahepatic cholangiocarcinoma. *BMC Cancer.* (2019) 19:208. doi: 10.1186/s12885-019-5420-z
88. Fava G, Demorrow S, Gaudio E, Franchitto A, Onori P, Carpino G, et al. Endothelin inhibits cholangiocarcinoma growth by a decrease in the vascular endothelial growth factor expression. *Liver Int.* (2009) 29:1031–42. doi: 10.1111/j.1478-3231.2009.01997.x
89. Augustin HG, Koh GY, Thurston G, Alitalo K, Control of vascular morphogenesis and homeostasis through the angiopoietin-Tie system. *Nat Rev Mol Cell Biol.* (2009) 10:165–77. doi: 10.1038/nrm2639
90. Aishima S, Nishihara Y, Iguchi T, Taguchi K, Taketomi A, Maehara Y, et al. Lymphatic spread is related to VEGF-C expression and D2-40-positive myofibroblasts in intrahepatic cholangiocarcinoma. *Mod Pathol.* (2008) 21:256–64. doi: 10.1038/modpathol.3800985
91. Xu Y, Yuan L, Mak J, Pardanaud L, Caunt M, Kasman I, et al. Neuropilin-2 mediates VEGF-C-induced lymphatic sprouting together with VEGFR3. *J Cell Biol.* (2010) 188:115–30. doi: 10.1083/jcb.200903137
92. Okada K, Osaki M, Araki K, Ishiguro K, Ito H, Ohgi S. Expression of hypoxia-inducible factor (HIF-1alpha), VEGF-C and VEGF-D in non-invasive and invasive breast ductal carcinomas. *Anticancer Res.* (2005) 25:3003–9. Available online at: http://ar.iiarjournals.org
93. Park BK, Paik YH, Park JY, Park KH, Bang S, Park SW, et al. The clinicopathologic significance of the expression of vascular endothelial growth factor-C in intrahepatic cholangiocarcinoma. *Am J Clin Oncol.* (2006) 29:138–42. doi: 10.1097/01.coc.0000204402.29830.08
94. Pezzuto A, Carico E. Role of HIF-1 in cancer progression: novel insights. A review. *Curr Mol Med.* (2018) 18:343–51. doi: 10.2174/1566524018666181109121849
95. Thongchot S, Yongvanit P, Loilome W, Seubwai W, Phunicom K, Tassaneeyakul W, et al. High expression of HIF-1alpha, BNIP3 and PI3KC3: hypoxia-induced autophagy predicts cholangiocarcinoma survival and metastasis. *Asian Pac J Cancer Prev.* (2014) 15:5873–8. doi: 10.7314/APJCP.2014.15.14.5873
96. Mills CN, Joshi SS, Niles RM. Expression and function of hypoxia inducible factor-1 alpha in human melanoma under non-hypoxic conditions. *Mol Cancer.* (2009) 8:104. doi: 10.1186/1476-4598-8-104
97. Currie MJ, Hanrahan V, Gunningham SP, Morrin HR, Frampton C, Han C, et al. Expression of vascular endothelial growth factor D is associated with hypoxia inducible factor (HIF-1alpha) and the HIF-1alpha target gene DEC1, but not lymph node metastasis in primary human breast carcinomas. *J Clin Pathol.* (2004) 57:829–34. doi: 10.1136/jcp.2003.015644
98. Liang X, Yang D, Hu J, Hao X, Gao J, Mao Z. Hypoxia inducible factor-alpha expression correlates with vascular endothelial growth factor-C expression and lymphangiogenesis/angiogenesis in oral squamous cell carcinoma. *Anticancer Res.* (2008) 28:1659–66. Available online at: http://ar.iiarjournals.org
99. M. Cadamuro, M. Vismara, S. Brivio, A. Furlanetto, M. Strazzabosco, L. Fabris, JNK signaling activated by Platelet-Derived Growth Factor D (PDGF-D) stimulates secretion of Vascular Endothelial Growth Factor-C (VEGF-C) by cancer-associated fibroblasts to promote lymphangiogenesis and early metastatization in cholangiocarcinoma. *Digest Liver Dis.* (2015) 47:e22–3. doi: 10.1016/j.dld.2015.01.052
100. Xu LB, Liu C, Gao GQ, Yu XH, Zhang R, Wang J. Nerve growth factor-beta expression is associated with lymph node metastasis and nerve infiltration in human hilar cholangiocarcinoma. *World J Surg.* (2010) 34:1039–45. doi: 10.1007/s00268-010-0417-4
101. Obulkasim H, Shi X, Wang J, Li J, Dai B, Wu P, et al. Podoplanin is an important stromal prognostic marker in perihilar cholangiocarcinoma. *Oncol Lett.* (2018) 15:137–46. doi: 10.3892/ol.2017.7335
102. Sha M, Jeong S, Chen XS, Tong Y, Cao J, Sun HY, et al. Expression of VEGFR-3 in intrahepatic cholangiocarcinoma correlates with unfavorable prognosis through lymphangiogenesis. *Int J Biol Sci.* (2018) 14:1333–42. doi: 10.7150/ijbs.26045
103. Cueni LN, Hegyi I, Shin JW, Albinger-Hegyi A, Gruber S, Kunstfeld R, et al. Tumor lymphangiogenesis and metastasis to lymph nodes induced by cancer cell expression of podoplanin. *Am J Pathol.* (2010) 177:1004–16. doi: 10.2353/ajpath.2010.090703
104. Navarro A, Perez RE, Rezaiekhaligh M, Mabry SM, Ekekezie II, et al. T1alpha/podoplanin is essential for capillary morphogenesis in lymphatic endothelial cells. *Am J Physiol Lung Cell Mol Physiol.* (2008) 295:L543–51. doi: 10.1152/ajplung.90262.2008
105. Thelen A, Scholz A, Benckert C, Schröder M, Weichert W, Wiedenmann B, et al. Microvessel density correlates with lymph node metastases and prognosis in hilar cholangiocarcinoma. *J Gastroenterol.* (2008) 43:959–66. doi: 10.1007/s00535-008-2255-9
106. Padera TP, Kadambi A, di Tomaso E, Carreira CM, Brown EB, Boucher Y, et al. Lymphatic metastasis in the absence of functional intratumor lymphatics. *Science.* (2002) 296:1883–6. doi: 10.1126/science.1071420
107. Alitalo K, Mohla S, Ruoslahti E. Lymphangiogenesis and cancer: meeting report. *Cancer Res.* (2004) 64:9225–9. doi: 10.1158/0008-5472.CAN-04-2475
108. Tewalt EF, Cohen JN, Rouhani SJ, Guidi CJ, Qiao H, Fahl SP, et al. Lymphatic endothelial cells induce tolerance via PD-L1 and lack of costimulation leading to high-level PD-1 expression on CD8 T cells. *Blood.* (2012) 120:4772–82. doi: 10.1182/blood-2012-04-427013
109. Francis H, DeMorrow S, Venter J, Onori P, White M, Gaudio E, et al. Inhibition of histidine decarboxylase ablates the autocrine tumorigenic effects of histamine in human cholangiocarcinoma. *Gut.* (2012) 61:753–64. doi: 10.1136/gutjnl-2011-300007
110. Leite de Oliveira R, Hamm A, Mazzone M. Growing tumor vessels: more than one way to skin a cat - implications for angiogenesis targeted cancer therapies. *Mol Aspects Med.* (2011) 32:71–87. doi: 10.1016/j.mam.2011.04.001
111. Cherry-Bohannan J, Baker K, Francis HJ. VEGF and cholangiocarcinoma: feeding the tumor. *Transl Gastrointest Cancer.* (2012) 1:95–102. doi: 10.3978/j.issn.2224-4778.2011.12.06
112. Gaudio E, Barbaro B, Alvaro D, Glaser S, Francis H, Ueno Y, et al. Vascular endothelial growth factor stimulates rat cholangiocyte proliferation via an autocrine mechanism. *Gastroenterology.* (2006) 130:1270–82. doi: 10.1053/j.gastro.2005.12.034
113. Benckert C, Jonas S, Cramer T, Von Marschall Z, Schäfer G, Peters M, et al. Transforming growth factor beta 1 stimulates vascular endothelial growth factor gene transcription in human cholangiocellular carcinoma cells. *Cancer Res.* (2003) 63:1083–92. Available online at: https://cancerres.aacrjournals.org
114. Mancino A, Mancino MG, Glaser SS, Alpini G, Bolognese A, Izzo L, et al. Estrogens stimulate the proliferation of human cholangiocarcinoma by inducing the expression and secretion of vascular endothelial growth factor. *Dig Liver Dis.* (2009) 41:156–63. doi: 10.1016/j.dld.2008.02.015
115. Peng T, Li Z, Li D, Wang S. MACC1 promotes angiogenesis in cholangiocarcinoma by upregulating VEGFA. *Onco Targets Ther.* (2019) 12:1893–903. doi: 10.2147/OTT.S197319
116. Zheng B, Jeong S, Zhu Y, Chen L, Xia Q, miRNA and lncRNA as biomarkers in cholangiocarcinoma(CCA). *Oncotarget.* (2017) 8:100819–30. doi: 10.18632/oncotarget.19044
117. Meadows V, Francis H. MicroRNAs and cholangiocarcinoma: elucidating the effects of tiny giants. *AME Med J.* (2018) 3:98. doi: 10.21037/amj.2018.09.10

118. Anand S, Cheresh DA. MicroRNA-mediated regulation of the angiogenic switch. *Curr Opin Hematol.* (2011) 18:171–6. doi: 10.1097/MOH.0b013e328345a180
119. Qu KZ, Zhang K, Li H, Afdhal NH, Albitar M, Circulating microRNAs as biomarkers for hepatocellular carcinoma. *J Clin Gastroenterol.* (2011) 45:355–60. doi: 10.1097/MCG.0b013e3181f18ac2
120. Fu Y, Wei X, Tang C, Li J, Liu R, Shen A, et al. Circulating microRNA-101 as a potential biomarker for hepatitis B virus-related hepatocellular carcinoma. *Oncol Lett.* (2013) 6:1811–5. doi: 10.3892/ol.2013.1638

20

Role of Glucose Metabolism Reprogramming in the Pathogenesis of Cholangiocarcinoma

Kishor Pant[1], *Seth Richard*[1], *Estanislao Peixoto*[1] *and Sergio A Gradilone*[1,2*]

[1] *The Hormel Institute, University of Minnesota, Austin, MN, United States,*

[2] *Masonic Cancer Center, University of Minnesota, Minneapolis, MN, United States*

Correspondence:
Sergio A Gradilone
sgradilo@umn.edu

Cholangiocarcinoma (CCA) is one of the most lethal cancers, and its rate of occurrence is increasing annually. The diagnoses of CCA patients remain elusive due to the lack of early symptoms and is misdiagnosed as HCC in a considerable percentage of patients. It is crucial to explore the underlying mechanisms of CCA carcinogenesis and development to find out specific biomarkers for early diagnosis of CCA and new promising therapeutic targets. In recent times, the reprogramming of tumor cells metabolism has been recognized as a hallmark of cancer. The modification from the oxidative phosphorylation metabolic pathway to the glycolysis pathway in CCA meets the demands of cancer cell proliferation and provides a favorable environment for tumor development. The alteration of metabolic programming in cancer cells is complex and may occur via mutations and epigenetic modifications within oncogenes, tumor suppressor genes, signaling pathways, and glycolytic enzymes. Herein we review the altered metabolism in cancer and the signaling pathways involved in this phenomena as they may affect CCA development. Understanding the regulatory pathways of glucose metabolism such as Akt/mTOR, HIF1α, and cMyc in CCA may further develop our knowledge of this devastating disease and may offer relevant information in the exploration of new diagnostic biomarkers and targeted therapeutic approaches for CCA.

Keywords: cholangiocarcinoma, metabolic reprogramming, aerobic glycolysis, glucose metabolism, warburg effect

INTRODUCTION

Cholangiocarcinoma (CCA) is a primary malignancy that originates from the cholangiocytes lining the biliary tree, also known as bile duct cancer. CCA is classified according to anatomical position, as either intrahepatic (iCCA), arising in the liver, and extrahepatic (eCCA), arising outside the liver. Extrahepatic cholangiocarcinoma can then be further classified as perihilar (pCCA) and distal cholangiocarcinoma (dCCA). The majority of CCA tumors are found in the perihilar and distal region, whereas only 10% are reported as intrahepatic, although responsible for 10–20% of all hepatic tumors (1–3). CCA characteristically manifests late with non-specific symptoms. Due to an insufficient knowledge of risk factors, coupled with inaccurate screenings, dependable early diagnosis has proven problematic. Diagnosed at late stages, CCA is among the most deadly cancers with an ~5% 5-year survival rate in patients (3).

EPIDEMIOLOGY

The incidence of CCA varies considerably between East-West dichotomy, reflecting variations in genetic and environmental risk factors. The highest incidence of CCA is reported in the north-east part of Thailand with rates of (113/100,000) in men and (50/100,000) in women; which is almost 100 fold more than Europe and North America (1-2/100,000), whereas Australia has the lowest number of CCA incidence (with 0.4/100,000). The prevalence of CCA is increasing worldwide for unknown reasons (4). The on-going overall increase in the rate of CCA makes it imperative to understand the disease's etiology and risk factors.

RISK FACTORS AND PATHOGENESIS OF CCA

Eighty percent of CCA cases in the western world are periodic and have no identifiable risk factor (4, 5). Smoking, alcohol abuse, obesity, and diabetes have not been consistently linked to higher risk, though a small involvement cannot be ruled out (6). Chronic biliary inflammation is another risk factor that has been generally associated with CCA. For instance, in the western world, primary sclerosing cholangitis (PSC) is associated with 10% of CCA cases (6, 7). Because of the often desmoplastic nature of CCA, it is challenging to discriminate between malignant and the benign characteristic of PSC. Liver cirrhosis of mixed etiology conveys a ten-fold relative risk (7). Uncommon defects of biliary anatomies, such as choledochal cysts (bile duct cyst), Caroli's syndrome (intrahepatic biliary cysts), biliary papillomatosis or adenoma, are linked with a high risk (6–30%) of CCA development. The high frequency of malignant transformation of the cells promotes prophylactic resection (6–8). Inborn or acquired defects of the biliary duct in pancreaticobiliary junction allows pancreatic reflux and subsequently leads to chronic cholangitis and increasing risk of CCA. Hepatolithiasis and chronic intraductal gallstones are also predominantly linked to CCA in Asia, as more than 10% of these patients develop CCA (5, 6).

ALTERED METABOLISM IN CANCER

Transformed metabolism is a common property of most cancer cells, including cholangiocarcinoma (9). The most common and one of the first identified biochemical features of cancer cells is uncharacteristic glucose metabolism. Glucose is known as a primary energy and carbon source for the cells, providing not only energy in form of ATP but also metabolites for several anabolic pathways (8, 9). Glucose transporters help the cells uptake glucose, and when in the cytosol, it is metabolized to pyruvate to yield a small amount of ATP by a multi-step path known as glycolysis. In normal healthy cells, the pyruvate derived from glycolysis is mainly transported into the mitochondrial matrix where the pyruvate dehydrogenase (PDH) enzyme complex oxidizes it into acetyl coenzyme A (CoA). Acetyl CoA further participates in the tricarboxylic acid (TCA) cycle, followed by a high-efficiency ATP generation process known as oxidative phosphorylation (OXPHOS). The full oxidation of one glucose molecule can produce up to 38 molecules of ATP (10).

On the contrary, cancer cells show changes in glucose metabolism. As shown in **Figure 1**: (i) Comparison between normal healthy cells, cancer cells characteristically show increased glucose uptake and glycolytic rates. Increased consumption of glucose produces more glycolytic intermediate metabolites and a substantial amount of ATP from glycolysis. (ii) Additionally, instead of generating pyruvate, a large fraction of carbon from glucose is moved into multiple biosynthetic pathways. (iii) Finally, in the cytoplasm maximum amount of pyruvate is converted to lactate by the action of lactate dehydrogenase (LDH) and secreted out instead of being oxidized in the mitochondria. This process is aerobic glycolysis as it occurs even in the presence of adequate oxygen to maintain mitochondrial respiration. This phenomenon of cancer cells was first observed by Otto Warburg in 1920s; therefore, it is also referred to as the "Warburg effect" (8, 9). Though cancer cells exhibit various kinds of metabolic profiles, the Warburg effect is a widespread cancer-associated characteristic. Interestingly, higher levels of LDHA have been reported in CCA patients (11, 12).

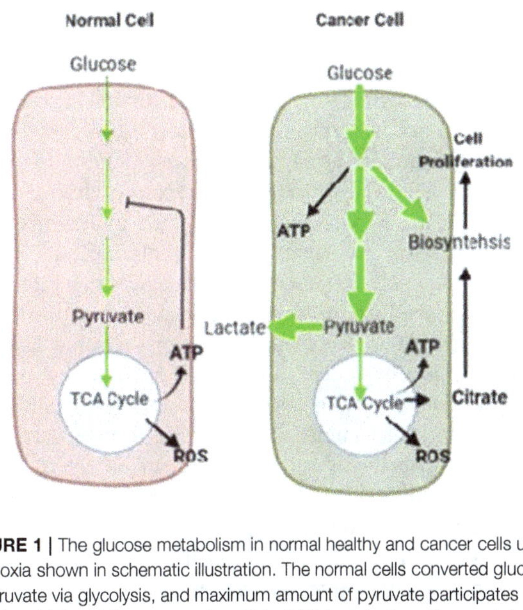

FIGURE 1 | The glucose metabolism in normal healthy and cancer cells under normoxia shown in schematic illustration. The normal cells converted glucose to pyruvate via glycolysis, and maximum amount of pyruvate participates in mitochondrial oxidative process for efficient ATP production. Glucose is largely used for cellular energy requirements. In healthy cells high levels of ATP mitigate glycolysis by feedback inhibition. In cancer cells Glucose uptake increased and thereby glycolysis. A substantial part of glucose is used to biosynthetic pathways to support cell proliferation. Pyruvate is mainly used in lactate production. Oxidative phosphorylation exists, but is separated from augmented glycolysis. The amount of glucose carbon flux is indicated by relative thickness of green arrows. Key mitochondrial metabolism by-products are shown in red and the metabolic effects on cancer are in indicated in bold black arrows.

GLYCOLYSIS PROVIDES BIOSYNTHETIC PRECURSORS

The mitochondrial function in cancer cells is mostly unchanged, in opposition to the original Warburg hypothesis. Warburg also witnessed that the rate of mitochondrial respiration in cancer cells remains almost similar to that of normal cells (13). Oxidative metabolism is also present in the majority of cancers and the main source for ATP generation (10, 13). However, the elevated glucose flux in cancer cells predominantly leads to lactate fermentation, and the flow to oxidative metabolism does not change. In summary, augmented glucose intake in cancer cells leads to lactate formation and it is uncoupled from oxidative metabolism in mitochondria. Higher uptake of glucose by cancer cells is also the basis for positron emission tomography (PET) with 18-fluorodeoxyglucose, which particularly accumulate in cancer cells. Due to the prevalence of this phenotype, PET is an effective clinical imaging method to diagnose most cancers and monitor therapeutic approaches (4). This technique has been useful in the clinical diagnosis of CCA in patients (14, 15).

The Warburg effect has been the canter of metabolism research in cancer cells. Genetic and epigenetic alterations in oncogenes and tumor suppressor genes may affect cancer metabolism. Thus, the variations in metabolic activities in the cancer cells are considered as a secondary effect on the cancer development process. Though tumor cell growth requires more production of the basic cellular macromolecules and metabolites for new cell development and it is well known that changes in tumor cell metabolism aid in cell growth by substantially producing biomolecules (16). Glycolytic metabolism of glucose yields several metabolites, which may act as precursors for anabolic pathways including the triacylglycerol and serine biosynthesis pathways for the production of amino acids, nucleotides, and lipids (8, 16). Whereas normal healthy cells utilize glucose almost entirely for energy, cancer cells increase glucose intake mainly to produce a persistent source of glycolytic intermediate products to fulfill the anabolic requirement of proliferating cells. Thus, intermediate product of glycolysis play a very important role as compared to pyruvate. In tumor cells the last steps of glycolysis is slow down, which is controlled by pyruvate kinase (13, 16), permitting glycolytic intermediates build-up for biosynthesis of macromolecules. The transformed metabolism of glucose consequently supports the alteration of glucose into biomass and withstands the rapid growth of cancer cells (9). Modifications in oncogenes and tumor suppressors drive unfavorable cell proliferation, and concurrently maintain cellular metabolism to satisfy the biosynthetic burdens of constant cell proliferation.

THE REGULATORY MECHANISM IN GLUCOSE METABOLISM

Oncogenes are an important set of genes found to be either mutated or over-expressed in cancer cells, which may elicit tumor initiation and continuous cell growth. Healthy cells do not grow independently, but rather go in the cell cycle only after prompted for it via signaling pathways, and growth factors, that may affect the cell morphology and gene expression (13, 17). Given that cell growth depends on many events of metabolic pathways, it is also known that these activities also regulated by the growth factors. The metabolism intermediates regulates metabolic functions that are mostly controlled via the intermediate metabolites on rate-limiting enzymes, providing self-regulatory capability in pathways and gives control at starting points of intersecting pathways (18). A number of these mechanisms in dividing cancer cells help to recognize the influence of signal activities on cell growth and it has shown a range of effects focused on metabolic fluxes (**Figure 2**).

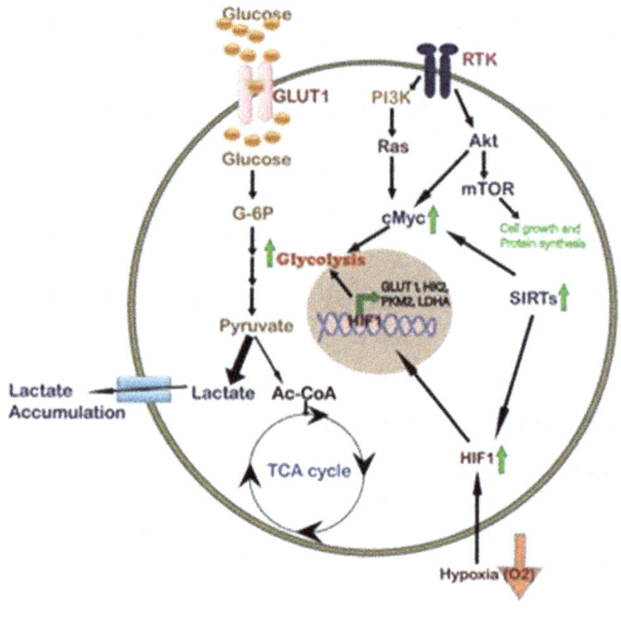

FIGURE 2 | Cellular pathways regulating the cancer cell metabolism. Different signaling pathways affected in tumor cells like Akt/mTOR, KRAS, and SIRTs activate the transcription factor cMyc which in turn, together with HIF1 induced by hypoxia and/or Sirtuins, promotes the expression of glycolytic proteins such as GLUT1, HK2, PKM2, and LDHA to regulate cancer cell metabolism. In CCA activation of HIF1, SIRTs, and cMyc inducing glycolysis has been described (Green Arrows).

THE Akt/mTOR PATHWAY REGULATES AEROBIC GLYCOLYSIS IN CANCER CELLS

The Akt/mTOR regulatory axis is a highly conserved and commonly expressed system in cells regulated by the growth factors (19). Coupling of growth factors (EGF, IGF, VEGF and cytokines) to cell surface receptors triggers PI3K activation, causing the phosphatidylinositol lipids phosphorylation at the plasma membrane. This process is involved in the activation of downstream pathways, mainly the serine/threonine kinases like Akt/mTOR pathway. Stimulation of the PI3K/Akt/mTOR regulatory axis by the growth factors in cancer cells, augments many of the metabolic processes that support cell growth. Mainly, it allows cells to increases nutrient transporters expression at the cell surface, enabling enhanced nutrient uptake, including, glucose and amino acids (20–22). The Akt/mTOR pathway may affect gene expression and enzyme activity, increase glycolysis and lactate accumulation in the cells, and to prompt aerobic glycolysis (Warburg effect) in either cancer cells or normal cells (22–24). Additionally, initiation of this pathway may enhance the macromolecule biosynthesis. PI3K/Akt encourage expression of lipogenesis genes in various cell types (25), while mTOR is a key controller of protein synthesis in cancer cells (26).

Irrespective of mutation, Akt initiation is among the main signaling events in cancer cell metabolism, for the reason that Akt can initiate aerobic glycolysis and lactate assembly and inhibit degradation of macromolecules in tumor cells including CCA (27). Similarly, CCA cells have been reported to resist the chemotherapy treatment via Akt/mTOR pathway (27).

HIF1 MODULATE THE CANCER CELL METABOLISM

Hypoxia (decreased oxygen condition) can stimulate increased glucose consumption and lactate production in the cells. This process is regulated by hypoxia-inducible factor 1 (HIF-1), is a transcription factor complex (28, 29). HIF-1 targets genes for glucose transporters, glycolytic enzymes, and LDHA (14, 30). HIF-1 can also expressed in the influence of growth factor signaling, and the Akt/mTOR axis in particular (31–34). During normal oxygen conditions PHD2 induce the posttranslational modification of HIF-1 by prolyl hydroxylation that encourages its interaction with a tumor suppressor called von Hippel-Lindau (VHL), which induces HIF-1 ubiquitination followed by degradation. During hypoxia, prolyl hydroxylation of HIF is withdrawn, resulting in stability and transcriptional activity of the HIF-1 protein complex (35, 36). Cellular stabilization of HIF-1 in normoxia occurs in tumors as an outcome of mutations in the VHL (37, 38).

An interesting study of Xu et al. showed that decreased expression of SIRT3 was correlated with high rate of glycolysis in CCA. Consistently, changes in glucose metabolism were observed in SIRT3 knockout mice. Furthermore, the authors also confirmed that SIRT3 prevents the Warburg effect in CCA cells and a xenograft mouse model by inhibiting the HIF1α/PDK1/PDHA1 pathway. Collectively, this study suggests that SIRT3 shows anti-Warburg effect activity via regulating the HIF1α/PDK1/PDHA1 pathway and may be a potential therapeutic intervention to impair CCA progression (39).

cMyC

Many previous studies have shown that some glucose metabolism genes are directly regulated by cMyc (40). These genes include Hexokinase 2 (HK2), glucose transporter GLUT1, phosphofructokinase, and enolase 1 (ENO1) (41–43). In addition, cMyc also has been reported to decrease pyruvate levels by stimulating LDHA and PKM2 levels, which can decrease the inhibition of HDAC3 and protect CCA from apoptosis (44). Augmented expression of these genes by cMyc induces the Warburg effect and the capacity of cancer cells to metabolize glucose to pyruvate even in inadequate oxygen availability. Animal models overexpressing cMyc in the liver demonstrated increased glycolytic enzymatic activity and up-regulated lactic acid production. Conversely, rodent fibroblasts cells overexpressing LDHA alone, or cMyc increased the lactate production. This study suggests that LDHA is a downstream target of cMyc, and can induce the Warburg effect (45, 46).

In CCA cells, the SIRT2/cMYC pathway was reported to play a critical role in modulating glucose oxidative metabolism to serine anabolic metabolism. Furthermore, the high level of SIRT2/cMYC pathway not only converts glucose to serine, but also provides antioxidants for oxidative stress resistance in CCA cells. Therefore, the metabolic reprogramming induced by SIRT2/cMYC pathway may provide a new therapeutic target for CCA (47).

THERAPEUTIC INTERVENTIONS RELATED TO REPROGRAMMED METABOLISM

Targeting cancer cell metabolism has become a significant emerging field to address effective cancer therapies, including tumor relapse and drug-resistance. To inhibit glucose metabolism in cancer cells, glycolytic enzymes (Pyruvate kinase M2, Hexokinase 1-2, and lactate dehydrogenase) and glucose transporter (GLUT 1-4) have been considered as therapeutic targets (9). GLUT1, found overexpressed in a varity of cancers including CCA (48, 49), helps in rapid uptake of glucose and its expression associates with anaerobic glycolysis in the cells (50). Targeting GLUT1 by WZB117 induced breast cancer cell sensitivity for radiation therapy (51), inhibited cancer cell growth and proliferation in nude mouse (52) and inhibited cancer stem cells self-renewal and tumor development capacity (53). MiR-218, miR-132 and miR-148a have been reported to inhibit cancer cell proliferation via targeting GLUT1 in bladder, prostate and pancreatic cancer respectively (54–56). Therefore, the use of GLUT1 inhibitors in CCA may shed light on the pathogenesis of CCA and may provide novel tools in clinical prognosis and treatment.

Alternative potential target is the adaptive characteristic of cancer cells inside the tumor microenvironment. A cancer cell can transmit its metabolism in heterogeneous environmental conditions, glucose deficiency, hypoxia, and acidic environment; this adaptation to metabolic response by cancer cells plays an essential role in cell metastasis or chemotherapy resistance (16). HIF1α is an important enzyme for metabolic adjustment during hypoxia and is involved in cancer cell survival, angiogenesis, and metastasis (28, 37, 57). CCA patients showed a higher level of Pyruvate dehydrogenase kinase 1 (PDK1) (58), which has been known to control the metabolic shift during hypoxia via regulating the acetyl-coA production to yield energy in the TCA cycle by mitochondria oxidation (59, 60). The mTOR pathway regulates energy homeostasis and engages in cancer cell survival in cellular metabolic stress such as depletion in nutrients and energy (23, 24). The downregulation of mTOR pathway signaling reduces cancer growth and has therapeutic potential for CCA (61–64). CCA cells which need OXPHOS for energy requirements can be targeted by impairing mitochondrial energy metabolism. Targeting the Peroxisome proliferator-activated receptor-γ coactivator (PGC1α) can inhibit the Warburg effect and cause cell death in CCA (65). Inhibition of mitochondrial protein UCP2 can block mitochondrial OXPHOS by the inhibition of mitochondrial function using a UCP2 inhibitor (genipin), which has toxicity against CCA (66). In the same way, TRAP1 a mitochondrial chaperone inhibitor prompts the diminishing of protein folding in mitochondria, also targeting mitochondrial metabolism (67–69). Many studies strongly advocate that targeting OXPHOS in cancer cell mitochondria could be an effective approach to against CCA and to decrease tumor growth and chemotherapy-resistance (70, 71). Therefore, it is crucial to develop the specific therapeutic targets to inhibit mitochondrial OXPHOS only in CCA and for the metabolic alteration of cancer cells with no negative effect in the normal cells that generally use OXPHOS for energy requirements.

CONCLUSION

The reprogramming of glucose metabolism in malignant cells is a multi-factor and multi-step route that can be controlled by carcinogenic signaling processes, and by epigenetic modulations. The advancement in cancer metabolism research significantly improved our knowledge of carcinogenesis and gave several potential targets for cancer. The drug that targets glycolytic enzymes or glycolysis pathways revealed several encouraging effects in cancer prevention and therapy (72). The cause and consequences of metabolism reprogramming in CCA is understudied, therefore further efforts to understand how the Warburg effect is regulated are warranted. A better understanding of this topic in CCA might help in the development of novel therapeutic approaches. Nevertheless, the drawback of anti-cancer remedy targeting glycolysis should also be explored further. As several enzymes catalyze this multistep process of cancer metabolism, here is a characteristic compensatory routes in cell metabolism. Thus, drug candidate may not have a prominent effect on cancer metabolism targeting specially only one modulator of glycolysis. In future, The impact of treatments and drug therapies in combination need to be assessed in CCA. In addition, drugs, which can target several pathways like Akt/mTOR and HIF1, are also required to be considered in future studies.

AUTHOR CONTRIBUTIONS

KP wrote the first draft of the manuscript. SR, EP, and SG critically revised the manuscript. All authors contributed to manuscript revision, read, and approved the submitted version.

REFERENCES

1. Galassi M, Iavarone M, Rossi S, Bota S, Vavassori S, Rosa L, et al. Patterns of appearance and risk of misdiagnosis of intrahepatic cholangiocarcinoma in cirrhosis at contrast enhanced ultrasound. *Liver Int.* (2013) 33:771-9. doi: 10.1111/liv.12124
2. Blechacz B, Gores GJ. Cholangiocarcinoma: advances in pathogenesis, diagnosis, and treatment. *Hepatol Baltim Md.* (2008) 48:308-21. doi: 10.1002/hep.22310
3. Rizvi S, Khan SA, Hallemeier CL, Kelley RK, Gores GJ. Cholangiocarcinoma — evolving concepts and therapeutic strategies. *Nat Rev Clin Oncol.* (2018) 15:95–111. doi: 10.1038/nrclinonc.2017.157
4. Khan SA, Davidson BR, Goldin RD, Heaton N, Karani J, Pereira SP, et al. Guidelines for the diagnosis and treatment of cholangiocarcinoma: an update. *Gut.* (2012) 61:1657–69. doi: 10.1136/gutjnl-2011-301748
5. Razumilava N, Gores GJ. Cholangiocarcinoma. *Lancet.* (2014) 383:2168-79. doi: 10.1016/S0140-6736(13)61903-0
6. Clements O, Eliahoo J, Kim JU, Taylor-Robinson SD, Khan SA. Risk factors for intrahepatic and extrahepatic cholangiocarcinoma: a systematic review and meta-analysis. *J Hepatol.* (2019) 72:95–103. doi: 10.1016/j.jhep.2019.09.007
7. Tyson GL, El-Serag HB. Risk factors for cholangiocarcinoma. *Hepatology.* (2011) 54:173–84. doi: 10.1002/hep.24351
8. Potter M, Newport E, Morten KJ. The warburg effect: 80 years on. *Biochem Soc Trans.* (2016) 44:1499–505. doi: 10.1042/BST20160094
9. Hsu PP, Sabatini DM. Cancer cell metabolism: warburg and beyond. *Cell.* (2008) 134:703–7. doi: 10.1016/j.cell.2008.08.021
10. Zheng J. Energy metabolism of cancer: Glycolysis versus oxidative phosphorylation (Review). *Oncol Lett.* (2012) 4:1151-7. doi: 10.3892/ol.2012.928
11. Yu Y, Liao M, Liu R, Chen J, Feng H, Fu Z. Overexpression of lactate dehydrogenase-A in human intrahepatic cholangiocarcinoma: its implication for treatment. *World J Surg Oncol.* (2014) 12:78. doi: 10.1186/1477-78 19-12-78
12. Thonsri U, Seubwai W, Waraasawapati S, Sawanyawisuth K, Vaeteewoottacharn K, Boonmars T, et al. Overexpression of lactate dehydrogenase a in cholangiocarcinoma is correlated with poor prognosis. *Histol Histopathol.* (2017) 32:503–10. doi: 10.14670/HH-11-819
13. Jose C, Bellance N, Rossignol R. Choosing between glycolysis and oxidative phosphorylation: a tumor's dilemma? *Biochim Biophys Acta BBA.* (2011) 1807:552–61. doi: 10.1016/j.bbabio.2010.10.012
14. Suzuki H, Komuta M, Bolog A, Yokobori T, Wada S, Araki K, et al. Relationship between 18-F-fluoro-deoxy-d-glucose uptake and expression of glucose transporter 1 and pyruvate kinase m2 in intrahepatic cholangiocarcinoma. *Dig Liver Dis.* (2015) 47:590–6. doi: 10.1016/j.dld.2015.03.017
15. Paudyal B, Oriuchi N, Paudyal P, Tsushima Y, Higuchi T, Miyakubo M, et al. Clinicopathological presentation of varying 18F-FDG uptake and expression of glucose transporter 1 and hexokinase iI in cases of hepatocellular carcinoma and cholangiocellular carcinoma. *Ann Nucl Med.* (2008) 22:83-6. doi: 10.1007/s12149-007-0076-1
16. Vander Heiden MG, DeBerardinis RJ. Understanding the intersections between metabolism and cancer biology. *Cell.* (2017) 168:657–69. doi: 10.1016/j.cell.2016.12.039
17. Solaini G, Sgarbi G, Baracca A. Oxidative phosphorylation in cancer cells. *Biochim Biophys Acta BBA.* (2011) 1807:534-42. doi: 10.1016/j.bbabio.2010.09.003
18. Witsch E, Sela M, Yarden Y. Roles for growth factors in cancer progression. *Physiol Bethesda Md.* (2010) 25:85–101. doi: 10.1152/physiol.00045.2009
19. Simons AL, Orcutt KP, Madsen JM, Scarbrough PM, Spitz DR. The role of Akt pathway signaling in glucose metabolism metabolic oxidative stress. In: Spitz DR, Dornfeld KJ, Krishnan K, Gius D. *Oxidative Stress in Cancer Biology Therapy Oxidative Stress in Applied Basic Research Clinical Practice.* Totowa, NJ: Humana Press (2012). p. 21–46. doi: 10.1007/978-1-61779-397-4_2
20. Zhao Y, Hu X, Liu Y, Dong S, Wen Z, He W, et al. ROS signaling under metabolic stress: cross-talk between aMPK and aKT pathway. *Mol Cancer.* (2017) 16:1. doi: 10.1186/s12943-017-0648-1

21. Koundouros N, Poulogiannis G. Phosphoinositide 3-Kinase/Akt signaling and redox metabolism in cancer. *Front Oncol.* (2018) 8:160. doi: 10.3389/fonc.2018.00160
22. Coloff JL, Rathmell JC. Metabolic regulation of akt: roles reversed: figure 1. *J Cell Biol.* (2006) 175:845–7. doi: 10.1083/jcb.200610119
23. Conciatori F, Bazzichetto C, Falcone I, Pilotto S, Bria E, Cognetti F, et al. Role of mTOR signaling in tumor microenvironment: an overview. *Int J Mol Sci.* (2018) 19:2453. doi: 10.3390/ijms19082453
24. Lien EC, Lyssiotis CA, Cantley LC. Metabolic reprogramming by the pI3K-Akt-mTOR pathway in cancer. *Recent Results Cancer Res Fortschritte Krebsforsch Progres Dans Rech Sur Cancer.* (2016) 207:39–72. doi: 10.1007/978-3-319-42118-6_3
25. Luo X, Zhao X, Cheng C, Li N, Liu Y, Cao Y. The implications of signaling lipids in cancer metastasis. *Exp Mol Med.* (2018) 50. doi: 10.1038/s12276-018-0150-x
26. Gingras AC, Raught B, Sonenberg N. Regulation of translation initiation by fRAP/mTOR. *Genes Dev.* (2001) 15:807–26. doi: 10.1101/gad.887201
27. Yokoi K, Kobayashi A, Motoyama H, Kitazawa M, Shimizu A, Notake T, et al. Survival pathway of cholangiocarcinoma via aKT/mTOR signaling to escape rAF/MEK/ERK pathway inhibition by sorafenib. *Oncol Rep.* (2018) 39:843–50. doi: 10.3892/or.2017.6153
28. Morine Y, Shimada M, Utsunomiya T, Imura S, Ikemoto T, Mori H, et al. Hypoxia inducible factor expression in intrahepatic cholangiocarcinoma. *Hepatogastroenterology.* (2011) 58:1439–44. doi: 10.5754/hge11156
29. Gordan JD, Simon MC. Hypoxia-inducible factors: central regulators of the tumor phenotype. *Curr Opin Genet Dev.* (2007) 17:71–7. doi: 10.1016/j.gde.2006.12.006
30. Sadlecki P, Bodnar M, Grabiec M, Marszalek A, Walentowicz P, Sokup A, et al. The role of hypoxia-Inducible factor-1α, glucose transporter-1, (GLUT-1) and carbon anhydrase iX in endometrial cancer patients. *BioMed Res Int.* (2014) 2014:616850. doi: 10.1155/2014/616850
31. Cramer T, Yamanishi Y, Clausen BE, Förster I, Pawlinski R, Mackman N, et al. HIF-1alpha is essential for myeloid cell-mediated inflammation. *Cell.* (2003) 112:645–57. doi: 10.1016/s0092-8674(03)00154-5
32. Majumder PK, Febbo PG, Bikoff R, Berger R, Xue Q, McMahon LM, et al. mTOR inhibition reverses akt-dependent prostate intraepithelial neoplasia through regulation of apoptotic and hIF-1-dependent pathways. *Nat Med.* (2004) 10:594–601. doi: 10.1038/nm1052
33. Xie Y, Shi X, Sheng K, Han G, Li W, Zhao Q, et al. PI3K/Akt signaling transduction pathway, erythropoiesis and glycolysis in hypoxia (Review). *Mol Med Rep.* (2019) 19:783–91. doi: 10.3892/mmr.2018.9713
34. Courtnay R, Ngo DC, Malik N, Ververis K, Tortorella SM, Karagiannis TC. Cancer metabolism and the warburg effect: the role of hIF-1 and pI3K. *Mol Biol Rep.* (2015) 42:841–51. doi: 10.1007/s11033-015-3858-x
35. Soni S, Padwad YS. HIF-1 in cancer therapy: two decade long story of a transcription factor. *Acta Oncol Stockh Swed.* (2017) 56:503–15. doi: 10.1080/0284186X.2017.1301680
36. Pezzuto A, Carico E. Role of hIF-1 in cancer progression: novel insights. A review. *Curr Mol Med.* (2018) 18:343–51. doi: 10.2174/1566524018666181109121849
37. Agani F, Jiang B-H. Oxygen-independent regulation of hIF-1: novel involvement of pI3K/AKT/mTOR pathway in cancer. *Curr Cancer Drug Targets.* (2013) 13:245–51. doi: 10.2174/1568009611313030003
38. Yu L, Chen X, Wang L, Chen S. The sweet trap in tumors: aerobic glycolysis and potential targets for therapy. *Oncotarget.* (2016) 7:38908–26. doi: 10.18632/oncotarget.7676
39. Xu L, Li Y, Zhou L, Dorfman RG, Liu L, Cai R, et al. SIRT3 elicited an anti-Warburg effect through hIF1α/PDK1/PDHA1 to inhibit cholangiocarcinoma tumorigenesis. *Cancer Med.* (2019) 8:2380–91. doi: 10.1002/cam4.2089
40. Miller DM, Thomas SD, Islam A, Muench D, Sedoris K. c-Myc and cancer metabolism. *Clin Cancer Res Off J Am Assoc Cancer Res.* (2012) 18:5546–53. doi: 10.1158/1078-0432.CCR-12-0977
41. Osthus RC, Shim H, Kim S, Li Q, Reddy R, Mukherjee M, et al. Deregulation of glucose transporter 1 and glycolytic gene expression by c-Myc. *J Biol Chem.* (2000) 275:21797–800. doi: 10.1074/jbc.C000023200
42. Dang CV, Le A, Gao P. MYC-induced cancer cell energy metabolism and therapeutic opportunities. *Clin Cancer Res Off J Am Assoc Cancer Res.* (2009) 15:6479–83. doi: 10.1158/1078-0432.CCR-09-0889
43. Wu S, Yin X, Fang X, Zheng J, Li L, Liu X, et al. c-MYC responds to glucose deprivation in a cell-type-dependent manner. *Cell Death Discov.* (2015) 1:15057. doi: 10.1038/cddiscovery.2015.57
44. Zhang M, Pan Y, Tang D, Dorfman RG, Xu L, Zhou Q, et al. Low levels of pyruvate induced by a positive feedback loop protects cholangiocarcinoma cells from apoptosis. *Cell Commun Signal CCS.* (2019) 17:23. doi: 10.1186/s12964-019-0332-8
45. Lewis BC, Prescott JE, Campbell SE, Shim H, Orlowski RZ, Dang CV. Tumor induction by the c-Myc target genes RCL and lactate dehydrogenase a. *Cancer Res.* (2000) 60:6178–6183.
46. Shim H, Dolde C, Lewis BC, Wu CS, Dang G, Jungmann RA, et al. c-Myc transactivation of lDH-A: implications for tumor metabolism and growth. *Proc Natl Acad Sci USA.* (1997) 94:6658–63. doi: 10.1073/pnas.94.13.6658
47. Xu L, Wang L, Zhou L, Dorfman RG, Pan Y, Tang D, et al. The sIRT2/cMYC pathway inhibits peroxidation-Related apoptosis in cholangiocarcinoma through metabolic reprogramming. *Neoplasia NYN.* (2019) 21:429–41. doi: 10.1016/j.neo.2019.03.002
48. Kubo Y, Aishima S, Tanaka Y, Shindo K, Mizuuchi Y, Abe K, et al. Different expression of glucose transporters in the progression of intrahepatic cholangiocarcinoma. *Hum Pathol.* (2014) 45:1610–7. doi: 10.1016/j.humpath.2014.03.008
49. Amann T, Hellerbrand C. GLUT1 as a therapeutic target in hepatocellular carcinoma. *Expert Opin Ther Targets.* (2009) 13:1411–27. doi: 10.1517/14728220903307509
50. Adekola K, Rosen ST, Shanmugam M. Glucose transporters in cancer metabolism. *Curr Opin Oncol.* (2012) 24:650–4. doi: 10.1097/CCO.0b013e328356da72
51. Zhao F, Ming J, Zhou Y, Fan L. Inhibition of glut1 by wZB117 sensitizes radioresistant breast cancer cells to irradiation. *Cancer Chemother Pharmacol.* (2016) 77:963–72. doi: 10.1007/s00280-016-3007-9
52. Liu Y, Cao Y, Zhang W, Bergmeier S, Qian Y, Akbar H, et al. A small-molecule inhibitor of glucose transporter 1 downregulates glycolysis, induces cell-cycle arrest, and inhibits cancer cell growth *in vitro* and *in vivo*. *Mol Cancer Ther.* (2012) 11:1672–82. doi: 10.1158/1535-7163.MCT-12-0131
53. Shibuya K, Okada M, Suzuki S, Seino M, Seino S, Takeda H, et al. Targeting the facilitative glucose transporter gLUT1 inhibits the self-renewal and tumor-initiating capacity of cancer stem cells. *Oncotarget.* (2015) 6:651–61. doi: 10.18632/oncotarget.2892
54. Li P, Yang X, Cheng Y, Zhang X, Yang C, Deng X, et al. MicroRNA-218 increases the sensitivity of bladder cancer to cisplatin by targeting glut1. *Cell Physiol Biochem.* (2017) 41:921–32. doi: 10.1159/000460505
55. Qu W, Ding S, Cao G, Wang S, Zheng X, Li G. miR-132 mediates a metabolic shift in prostate cancer cells by targeting glut1. *FEBS Open Bio.* (2016) 6:735–41. doi: 10.1002/2211-5463.12086
56. Wu L, Qiu W, Sun J. Down regulation of miR-148a is related to enhanced pancreatic cancer pathogenesis through targeting gLUT1. *Int J Clin Exp Pathol.* (2018) 11:4950–6.
57. Vanichapol T, Leelawat K, Hongeng S. Hypoxia enhances cholangiocarcinoma invasion through activation of hepatocyte growth factor receptor and the extracellular signal-regulated kinase signaling pathway. *Mol Med Rep.* (2015) 12:3265–72. doi: 10.3892/mmr.2015.3865
58. Sanmai S, Proungvitaya T, Limpaiboon T, Chua-On D, Seubwai W, Roytrakul S, et al. Serum pyruvate dehydrogenase kinase as a prognostic marker for cholangiocarcinoma. *Oncol Lett.* (2019) 17:5275–82. doi: 10.3892/ol.2019.10185
59. Stacpoole PW. Therapeutic targeting of the pyruvate dehydrogenase complex/Pyruvate dehydrogenase kinase (PDC/PDK) axis in cancer. *J Natl Cancer Inst.* (2017) 109. doi: 10.1093/jnci/djx071
60. Sradhanjali S, Reddy MM. Inhibition of pyruvate dehydrogenase kinase as a therapeutic strategy against cancer. *Curr Top Med Chem.* (2018) 18:444–53. doi: 10.2174/1568026618666180523105756
61. Corti F, Nichetti F, Raimondi A, Niger M, Prinzi N, Torchio M, et al. Targeting the pI3K/AKT/mTOR pathway in biliary tract cancers: a review of current evidences and future perspectives. *Cancer Treat Rev.* (2019) 72:45–55. doi: 10.1016/j.ctrv.2018.11.001
62. Zuo M, Rashid A, Churi C, Vauthey J-N, Chang P, Li Y, et al. Novel therapeutic

strategy targeting the hedgehog signalling and mTOR pathways in biliary tract cancer. *Br J Cancer.* (2015) 112:1042–51. doi: 10.1038/bjc.2014.625
63. Zhang S, Song X, Cao D, Xu Z, Fan B, Che L, et al. Pan-mTOR inhibitor mLN0128 is effective against intrahepatic cholangiocarcinoma in mice. *J Hepatol.* (2017) 67:1194–203. doi: 10.1016/j.jhep.2017.07.006
64. Song X, Liu X, Wang H, Wang J, Qiao Y, Cigliano A, et al. Combined cDK4/6 and pan-mTOR inhibition is synergistic against intrahepatic cholangiocarcinoma. *Clin Cancer Res Off J Am Assoc Cancer Res.* (2019) 25:403–13. doi: 10.1158/1078-0432.CCR-18-0284
65. Li D, Wang C, Ma P, Yu Q, Gu M, Dong L, et al. PGC1α promotes cholangiocarcinoma metastasis by upregulating pDHA1 and mPC1 expression to reverse the warburg effect. *Cell Death Dis.* (2018) 9:1–15. doi: 10.1038/s41419-018-0494-0
66. Yu J, Shi L, Shen X, Zhao Y. UCP2 regulates cholangiocarcinoma cell plasticity via mitochondria-to-AMPK signals. *Biochem Pharmacol.* (2019) 166:174–84. doi: 10.1016/j.bcp.2019.05.017
67. Masgras I, Sanchez-Martin C, Colombo G, Rasola A. The chaperone tRAP1 as a modulator of the mitochondrial adaptations in cancer cells. *Front Oncol.* (2017) 7:58. doi: 10.3389/fonc.2017.00058
68. Im C-N. Past, present, and emerging roles of mitochondrial heat shock protein tRAP1 in the metabolism and regulation of cancer stem cells. *Cell Stress Chaperones.* (2016) 21:553–62. doi: 10.1007/s12192-016-0687-3
69. Kim H, Yang J, Kim MJ, Choi S, Chung J-R, Kim J-M, et al. Tumor necrosis factor receptor-associated protein 1 (TRAP1) mutation and tRAP1 inhibitor gamitrinib-triphenylphosphonium (G-TPP) induce a forkhead box o (FOXO)-dependent cell protective signal from mitochondria. *J Biol Chem.* (2016) 291:1841–1853. doi: 10.1074/jbc.M115.656934
70. Porporato PE, Filigheddu N, Pedro JMB-S, Kroemer G, Galluzzi L. Mitochondrial metabolism and cancer. *Cell Res.* (2018) 28:265–80. doi: 10.1038/cr.2017.155
71. Guerra F, Arbini AA, Moro L. Mitochondria and cancer chemoresistance. *Biochim Biophys Acta Bioenerg.* (2017) 1858:686–99. doi: 10.1016/j.bbabio.2017.01.012
72. Zabron A, Edwards RJ, Khan SA. The challenge of cholangiocarcinoma: dissecting the molecular mechanisms of an insidious cancer. *Dis Model Mech.* (2013) 6:281–92. doi: 10.1242/dmm.010561

21

Disturbances in Cholesterol Homeostasis and Non-alcoholic Fatty Liver Diseases

*Pooja Malhotra [1], Ravinder K. Gill [1], Seema Saksena [1,2] and Waddah A. Alrefai [1,2]**

[1] *Division of Gastroenterology and Hepatology, Department of Medicine, University of Illinois at Chicago, Chicago, IL, United States,*
[2] *Jesse Brown VA Medical Center, Chicago, IL, United States*

***Correspondence:**
Waddah A. Alrefai
walrefai@uic.edu

Non-alcoholic fatty liver disease (NAFLD) is a major health problem associated with obesity and other features of the metabolic syndrome including insulin resistance and dyslipidemia. The accumulation of lipids in hepatocytes causes liver damage and triggers inflammation, fibrosis, and cirrhosis. Beside fatty acids and triglycerides, evidence showed an increased accumulation of free cholesterol in the liver with subsequent toxic effects contributing to liver damage. The maintenance of cholesterol homeostasis in the body requires a balance between several pathways responsible for cholesterol synthesis, transport and conversion into bile acids. Intestinal absorption is also one of the major determinants of cholesterol homeostasis. The nature of changes in cholesterol homeostasis associated with NAFLD has been a subject of extensive investigations. In this article, we will attempt to provide a brief overview of the current knowledge about the disturbances in cholesterol metabolism associated with NAFLD and discuss how certain molecular targets of these pathways could be exploited for the treatment of this multifactorial disease.

Keywords: NPC1L1, ezetimibe, statins, bile acids, fatty liver

INTRODUCTION

Non-alcoholic fatty liver disease (NAFLD) is a common chronic hepatic disorder associated with obesity and metabolic syndrome (1, 2). Histologically, NAFLD encompasses a broad range of liver injury including simple steatosis or non-alcoholic fatty liver (NAFL), non-alcoholic steatohepatitis (NASH) and subsequent fibrosis as well as cirrhosis (3). The key feature is lipid accumulation in the liver that is not related to alcohol in hepatocytes (4). The accumulation of lipids in hepatocytes as a result of dyslipidemia and insulin resistance leads to liver damage and triggers elaborate response causing hepatic inflammation and fibrosis (2). It is widely accepted that increased flux of fatty acids associated with insulin resistance and/or increased *de novo* lipogenesis in the liver lead to fatty acid accumulation in the liver with associated lipotoxicity (5). However, emerging evidence also suggested that the increased level of cellular cholesterol contributes to the development of NAFLD and the progression of the disease (6). Understanding the roles of cholesterol in the pathophysiology of NAFLD is of a particular importance as it may unravel novel molecular targets for effective therapeutic interventions for NAFLD. In this review, we will give a brief summary about processes involved in the maintenance of cholesterol homeostasis and discuss their potential roles in NAFLD. A synopsis of current knowledge regarding the benefits of cholesterol lowering drugs in the management of patients with NAFLD is also included.

CHOLESTEROL HOMEOSTASIS

Maintaining cholesterol pool in the body is achieved by balancing between input and output pathways of cholesterol metabolism (7). Components of input pathways include endogenous *de novo* synthesis and intestinal absorption of cholesterol, whereas the output pathways include the excretion of free cholesterol in bile, the conversion into bile acids, and the non-biliary trans-epithelial cholesterol efflux (TICE) in the intestine (8, 9). Cholesterol is secreted into the circulation in the very low-density lipoprotein (VLDL) from the liver, and its clearance from the blood involves the uptake of low-density lipoprotein (LDL) by the LDL receptor (LDLr). Cholesterol is transported from the peripheral tissues to liver in the high-density lipoproteins (HDL) particles by the process of reverse cholesterol transport (8).

Intestinal cholesterol absorption represents one of the major determinants of cholesterol homeostasis. The total amount of cholesterol in the intestinal lumen is derived from multiple sources including diet (~300–500 mg/day from western-type of diet) as well as the epithelial cells that are shed into the lumen (~300 mg/day) and biliary cholesterol (~800–1,200 mg/day). A total amount of ~1,400–1,700 mg of cholesterol is presented in the intestine on a daily basis for absorption (10). The efficiency of cholesterol absorption exhibits wide inter-individual variations (28–80%) and depends on several luminal (emulsifiers: bile acids, phospholipids) and epithelial factors (10). Cholesterol uptake by enterocytes is mainly mediated by the specific transporter protein Niemann-Pick C1 Like 1 (NPC1L1), which is abundantly expressed on the brush-border membrane of small-intestinal enterocytes (8, 11) (**Figure 1**). Cholesterol is esterified by acetyl-CoA cholesterol acyltransferase 2 (ACAT-2) and incorporated along with triglycerides and apolipoprotein B-48 into chylomicrons. Triglycerides are hydrolyzed by lipoprotein lipase and chylomicrons are transformed into chylomicron remnants that are taken up by the liver (10).

The *de novo* synthesis of cholesterol occurs in all cells in the body. However, the liver represents the main site for cholesterol synthesis and storage (8). Cholesterol synthesis starts with acetyl-CoA and involves multiple reactions. The two rate-limiting steps in this complex process are mediated by 3-hydroxy-3-methyl-glutaryl CoA reductase (HMGCoAr) and squalene monooxygenase. Cholesterol, the newly synthesized in the liver and the one derived from the intestinal absorption, is then packaged along with triglycerides and apolipoprotein B-100 into the VLDL particles that are assembled by the microsomal transfer protein. The VLDL loses its load of triglycerides while circulating in the tissues by lipoprotein lipase and transforms into LDL that represents the main vehicle of cholesterol transport to the peripheral tissues. Other processes involving cholesterol in the liver include esterification by ACAT2 for storage, excretion into bile by the function of heterodimer of ATP-binding cassette transporters ABCG5/G8 found on the canalicular membrane of hepatocytes, or the conversion to bile acids by a complex process in which the cytochrome P450 7A1 (CYP7A1) enzyme mediates the rate-limiting reaction (8). The expression of CYP7A1 is mainly regulated by a signal generated from the ileum represented by fibroblast growth factor 19 in human and 15 in rodents (FGF19/15) (12). The synthesis and secretion of FGF19/15 are induced by the uptake of bile acids by enterocytes in the distal ileum that is mediated by the action of the apical sodium dependent bile acid transporter ASBT. The inhibition of ASBT reduces FGF19/15 expression and promotes hepatic bile acid synthesis and therefore, decreases levels of hepatic cholesterol (**Figure 1**).

The transport of cholesterol from the peripheral tissues back to liver is initiated by cholesterol efflux from cells via the ATP-binding cassette transporter ABCA1 to the nascent apolipoprotein A containing HDL particles. Cholesterol could be transferred from HDL in the circulation to LDL by cholesterol-ester transfer protein (CETP). HDL is taken up by hepatocytes via the scavenger receptor B1 (SR-B1) (8) (**Figure 1**).

The expression of genes responsible for cholesterol transport and metabolism are tightly regulated by coordinated actions of transcription factors. For example, the decrease in the level of cellular cholesterol activates the ER membrane-bound transcription factor Sterol regulatory element-binding protein isoform 2 (SREBP-2) that induces the expression of HMGCoAr and LDLr (8). On the other hand, the increase in cellular cholesterol elevates the levels of the oxygenated cholesterol intermediates oxysterols that trigger Liver X receptors (LXRs) transcription factors to stimulate the pathways of cholesterol efflux and to promote cholesterol elimination from the liver (8).

CHOLESTEROL AND THE PATHOPHYSIOLOGY OF NAFLD

The interest in understanding the relationship between cholesterol metabolism and the development of NAFLD and NASH was incited by observational studies linking liver damage with the risk for the development of cardiovascular disease (CVD) (13). In fact, the increased prevalence of metabolic syndrome in patients with NAFLD was to such an extent that some authors suggested that NALFD represents the hepatic manifestation in a spectrum of metabolic disorders (14). The metabolic syndrome refers to a cluster of metabolic disturbances including obesity, insulin resistance, hypertension, and atherogenic dyslipidemia that increase the risk for cardiovascular disease, stroke and diabetes mellitus (14). Meta-analysis of observational retrospective and prospective studies demonstrated an increased risk for CVD of both fatal and non-fatal events of CVD in patients with NAFLD as compared to patients without NAFLD (15). Such a link between NAFLD and CVD provided a compelling rationale to closely examine cholesterol metabolism in patients with NAFLD. The features of dyslipidemia associated with NALFD include hypertriglyceridemia and a decrease in HDL cholesterol (2). Although there is no evidence for an increase in total LDL cholesterol, patients with NAFLD were shown to have elevated levels of highly atherogenic subpopulations of LDL such as the oxidized particles (2). Furthermore, feeding high cholesterol atherogenic diets was able to induce lesions of early NAFLD as well as atherosclerosis in several animal models.

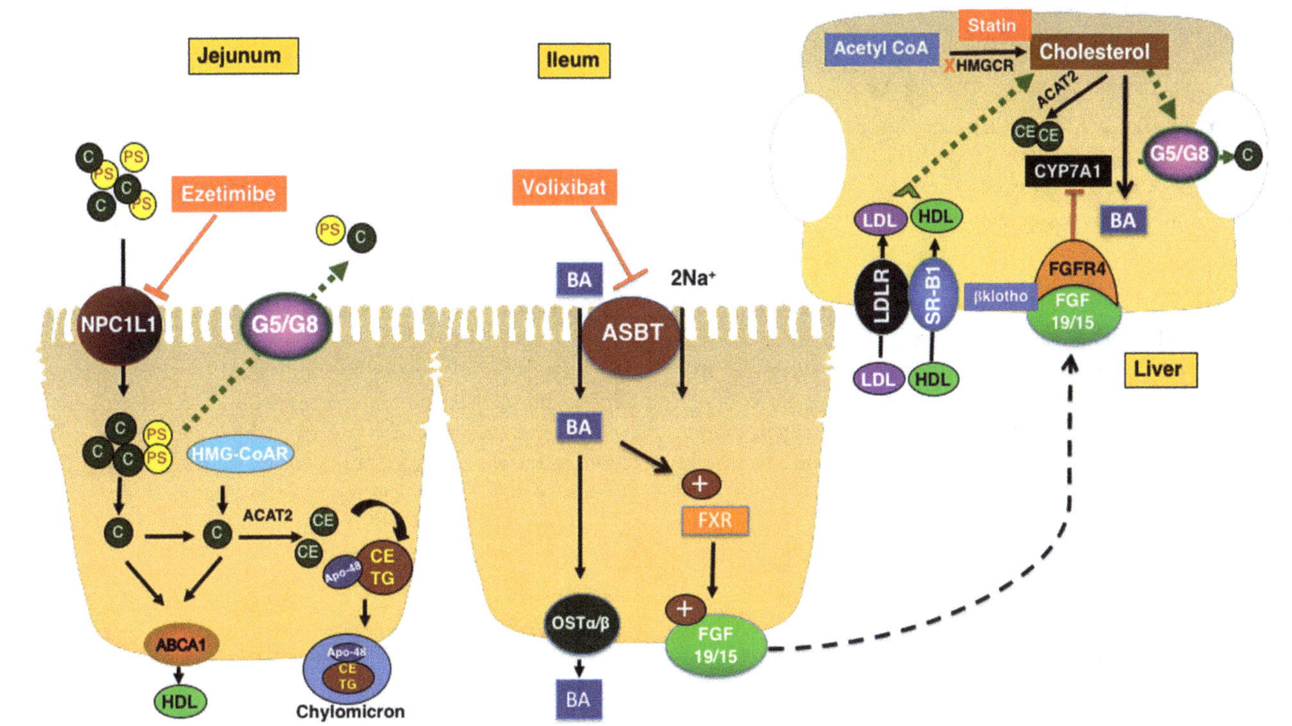

FIGURE 1 | Cholesterol metabolism and transport. NPC1L1 mediates the uptake of cholesterol and plant sterols into small intestinal epithelial cells. The majority of plant sterols are secreted back into the lumen by the action of ABCG5/G8 heterodimer. Cholesterol is esterified and packaged into chylomicrons along with triglycerides. Ezetimibe inhibits NPC1L1 and decreases the intestinal cholesterol absorption. Cholesterol is synthesized in the liver and intestine. ABCA1 transporter mediates the efflux of cholesterol to a nascent HDL particle. Cholesterol enters the hepatocytes via LDLr or the HDL receptor SR-B1. In hepatocytes, cholesterol is esterified, secreted as free cholesterol into bile via ABCG5/G8 transporters, or converted to bile acids with a process in which CYP7A1 mediates the rate-limiting step. Bile acids are reabsorbed by ASBT in the ileum and activate FXR which increased the expression and secretion of FGF19 in humans (15 is rodents). FGF19/15 circulates back to the liver to inhibit CYP7A1 via FGF4 receptor and β-klotho co-receptor. ASBT, apical sodium-dependent bile acid transporter; BA, bile acid; CYP7A1, cytochrome P450 7A1; FGF15/19, fibroblast growth factor 15/19; FXR, farnesoid X receptor; Ost a & β, organic solute transporter alpha and beta; HMGCR, 3-Hydroxy-3-methylglutaryl-CoA Reductase; C, cholesterol; PS, plant sterols; NPC1L1, Niemann-pick C1 Like 1; G5/G8, ATP binding casette transporter G5 and G8; SR-B1, scavenger receptor B1; ABCA1, ATP-binding cassette transporter ABCA1; ACAT2, Acetyl-Coenzyme A Acetyltransferase 2; HDL, High density lipoprotein; CE, cholesterol ester; TG, triglyceride; FGFR4, fibroblast growth factor receptor 4; LDLR, Low density lipoprotein receptor; LDL, low density lipoprotein.

It should be noted that animal species have remarkable differences in cholesterol metabolism and respond differently to cholesterol rich diet. In this regard, it is well-established that rabbits have features of cholesterol metabolism that are closer to those in humans (16). For example, the predominant plasma lipoproteins in both rabbits and humans is LDL whereas it the HDL in mice. This difference is due to the fact that the CETP is lacking in the plasma of mice (17). More importantly, rabbits are sensitive to dietary cholesterol and develop severe hypercholesterolemia in response to high dietary cholesterol with prominent atherosclerosis (16). A recent study showed that diet-induced hypercholesterolemia in rabbits fed with diet containing 1% cholesterol caused liver injury that resembles early lesions of NAFLD (changes in fatty acid and sporadic fibrosis) concomitant with the development of atherosclerosis in the aorta (18). This study generated evidence linking blood cholesterol with NAFLD and provided novel insights into the roles of free cholesterol in inducing liver damage. In the mouse model, hypercholesterolemia and atherosclerosis can be produced only in genetically modified animals such as apoE and LDLr knockout mice (19). In this regard, steatohepatitis was shown in apoE knockout mice in response to high fat high cholesterol feeding (20). Combined transcriptomics and metabolomics analysis demonstrated that high dose of dietary cholesterol in apoE knockout mice triggered hepatic inflammation (21).

An interesting observation was made in wildtype mice (but not in the transgenic mice models of hypercholesterolemia) showing that high cholesterol in the diet was essential to elicit steatohepatitis and fibrosis after 30 weeks of feeding, whereas high fat diet alone failed to produce the same degree of liver injury (22). This role of high dose of dietary cholesterol in the induction of liver damage in wildtype mice was also illustrated in other species. For example, a study showed that feeding Ossabaw pigs atherogenic diet containing high fat along with 2% cholesterol caused severe metabolic syndrome along with lesions in the liver with features resembling human steatohepatitis including microvesicular and macrovesicular steatosis, fatty Kupffer cells, hepatocyte ballooning and fibrosis (23). Collectively, the evidence from preclinical animal models strongly indicate that a high dose of cholesterol is an independent risk factor for liver damage and the development of atherosclerosis. A conclusion can be drawn from these studies linking NAFLD with atherosclerosis implicating the accumulation of cholesterol in the liver and arteries as a trigger for inflammation and subsequent manifestations of liver disease and CVD.

Beside the studies in animal models, the results of a landmark study in humans also supported the role of cholesterol in NAFLD/NASH. Puri et al. (24) showed high levels of free cholesterol in patients with NAFLD (simple steatosis) that were more pronounced in cases with progressive form of the disease, NASH. Cholesterol esters remained unchanged despite the increase in free cholesterol suggesting an impaired function and/or expression of the enzyme responsible for cholesterol esterification (ACAT). Collectively, the evidence from animal models and humans indicates that cholesterol is one of the toxic lipids that accumulates in the liver contributing to liver damage during the course of NAFLD and the progression to NASH.

Recent studies investigated the molecular mechanisms underlying the toxic effects of high cholesterol in the liver. The findings of Mari et al. (25) provided evidence showing that accumulation of free cholesterol but not triglycerides or fatty acids makes hepatocytes more sensitive to TNFa and Fas-mediated apoptosis due to depletion of mitochondrial glutathione. Other studies suggested that the accumulated free cholesterol in damaged hepatocytes precipitates as crystals which in turn induce inflammatory response by interacting with NLRP3 inflammasomes of Kupffer cells (26). Free cholesterol was shown also to directly accumulates in lysosomes of Kupffer cells triggering an inflammatory response (27). Such inflammatory cascade was blocked by 27-hyroxycholesterol that prevented the accumulation of cholesterol in Kupffer cells and reduced NASH. The accumulation of cholesterol in hepatic stellate cells (HSCs) was also implicated in the progression to NASH and fibrosis (28). For example, studies provided evidence showing that the accumulation of free cholesterol in HSCs resulted in an increase in the expression of TLR4 receptor and an increase in the sensitivity of HSCs to TGFb with subsequent fibrosis (29). It is apparent therefore, that increased cellular levels of cholesterol in different cell types in the liver may be responsible for liver damage and the progression from simple steatosis to NASH.

MOLECULAR PATHWAYS UNDERLYING CHOLESTEROL ACCUMULATION IN NAFLD

The accumulation of free cholesterol in NAFLD may occur due to an upregulation in the input pathways or a decrease in the elimination of cholesterol. Studies showed that the expression of HMGCoAr are increased in patients with NAFLD/NASH (30). There is evidence to suggest that changes in microRNAs (miRs) might be responsible for the observed increase in HMGCoAr. Several studies demonstrated the roles of several miRs in the development of liver diseases including NAFLD. The roles of these miRs including miR-122, miR-33, and miR-24a are discussed in details in other excellent review articles (31, 32). Studies have also demonstrated the regulation of several genes involved in cholesterol metabolism such as HMGCoAr by miRs and these findings are nicely summarized in other review articles (33, 34).

With respect to cholesterol metabolism as it relates to NAFLD/NASH, miR-34a levels were shown to be elevated in patients with NAFLD/NASH causing a decrease in hepatic NAD-dependent deacetylase Sirtuin1 with subsequent dephosphorylation and an increase in HMGCoAr (30). The roles of miR-29a was also suggested by a supporting evidence showing a negative correlation between miR-29a and HMGCoAr expression after 3 weeks feeding of methionine-choline deficient diet (MCD) to mice (35). The study revealed that 3′ un-translated region (3′UTR) of HMGCoAr was targeted by miR-29a (35). The decrease in miR-29a was concomitant with a decrease in hepatic Dicer1 enzyme that is essential for the maturation of microRNAs. In fact, liver-specific knockout of Dicer1 enzyme resulted in an increase in HMGCoAr associated with accumulation of free cholesterol in the liver (35). These findings revealed an important molecular pathway involving hepatic Dicer1 and microRNAs in the increase in cholesterol synthesis and accumulation of free cholesterol in the liver contributing to the development of NAFLD/NASH.

The expression of SREBP2 transcription factor was also increased in patients with NAFLD/NASH (30). Since SREBP2 induces the expression HMGCoAr, the observed increase in active SERBP2 represents an additional molecular pathway that might be responsible for the increases in hepatic levels of free cholesterol. Mari et al. (25) demonstrated that SREBP2 overexpression was not found in obese patients and patients with other chronic liver diseases such as hepatitis C, but was rather a specific feature associated with NAFLD/NASH. It should be noted that the accumulation of free cholesterol in hepatocytes is expected to inhibit the activation of SREBP2 (36). It is possible that SREBP2 is activated in NAFLD/NASH by a mechanism independent from the canonical pathway related to changes in cellular cholesterol (37). Indeed, a previous study showed that the injection of cytokines in C57BL mice resulted in an increase in hepatic SREBP2 and HMGCoAr expression (38). Similar findings were obtained in response to incubation of human hepatic HepG2 cells with cytokines. Although loading of HepG2 cells with cholesterol inhibited the SREBP2 pathways as expected, such a negative feedback inhibition was overridden by inflammatory stress caused by the cytokines (38). It is also reported that miR-122 stabilizes the inactive form of SREBP2 (39). Interestingly, miR-122 was shown to be significantly decreased in patients with NASH, thus providing a potential explanation for the increase in SREBP2 (39). It is possible also that hyperinsulinemia resulted from increased insulin resistance may also cause an increase in the active form of SREBP2 (40). Collectively, the inflammatory stress, the decrease in miR-122 and associated hyperinsulinemia in NASH presents a reasonable explanation for the constant activation of SREBP2 bypassing the canonical negative feedback inhibitory effect of high levels of cellular cholesterol (37). Beside the role of hepatic SREBP2 in the pathophysiology of NAFLD/NASH, our studies in transgenic mouse model of intestine-specific overactivation of SREBP2, demonstrated hepatic steatosis, and increased susceptibility of the animals to severe liver damage and profound inflammation and fibrosis in response to a high fat/high cholesterol diet (41). These observations strongly suggest that the activation of SREBP2 not only in the liver but also in the intestine plays a critical role in the development of NAFLD/NASH.

Beside the increase in cholesterol synthesis, changes in the pathways involved in the elimination of cholesterol were also noted in patients with NASH. Among these observations is the decrease in the expression of CYP7A1 implicating reduced bile acid synthesis from cholesterol (30). Also, a decrease in the expression of cholesterol transporters ABCG5/G8 responsible for cholesterol excretion into bile was reported (30). It is clear therefore, that the accumulation of hepatic free cholesterol in NAFLD/NASH patients is multifactorial with underlying increase in synthesis and decrease in the elimination of cholesterol.

With respect to dietary cholesterol and liver disease in humans, an epidemiological study suggested that dietary cholesterol is an independent risk factor for liver cirrhosis and hepatic cancer (42). These studies provide support to the observations made in animal models demonstrating the role of cholesterol in the induction of liver damage (43, 44). Since dietary cholesterol represents only a small portion of the total amount of luminal cholesterol presented for absorption (10), one could argue that the relation between the efficiency of cholesterol absorption and the development of liver diseases including NALFD/NASH should be carefully investigated. One study by Simonen et al. (45) evaluated serum surrogate markers for cholesterol synthesis (cholestenol, desmosterol, and lathosterol) and absorption (plant sterols). Individuals with NALFD were identified as those having liver fat $\geq$ 5.56% as judged by with proton magnetic resonance spectroscopy. The authors found that the content of liver fat was positively correlated with markers of cholesterol synthesis and inversely correlated with markers of cholesterol absorption (45). It is possible that there is an interrelationship between these two processes so that the decrease in cholesterol absorption may represent a homeostatic response to an increase in cholesterol synthesis (45). It will be important to investigate a possible difference in the efficiency of cholesterol absorption in patients with NASH as compared to those with NAFLD. With respect to the expression of intestinal NPC1L1, previous studies showed an increase in the expression of this intestinal in patients with diabetes mellitus (46). It is of central importance to investigate the expression of NPC1L1 in patients with NAFLD and NASH to a make a conclusion regarding potential changes in cholesterol absorption. Also, the studies mentioned above assessed the efficiency of cholesterol absorption indirectly by measuring serum plant sterols as surrogate markers. A direct measurement of cholesterol absorption in patients with NAFLD/NASH is warranted.

CHOLESTEROL LOWERING DRUGS IN THE MANAGEMENT OF NAFLD/NASH

According to current guidelines, decreasing the levels of plasma cholesterol to stringent low levels is highly recommended in patients with high risk for CVD (47, 48). Patients with NAFLD/NASH have high risk of developing CVD (15, 49). Therefore, it is of central importance to address treatment options available to lower plasma cholesterol in this patient population. **Table 1** summarizes the results of selected studies related to cholesterol-based therapy for NAFLD.

Inhibitors of Cholesterol Synthesis

Statins, the inhibitors of HMGCoAr, are the widely used drugs to lower plasma cholesterol (61). It is well-established that statins reduce LDL cholesterol and significantly decrease the risk for CVD. Thus, it is logical to use statins in NAFLD patients who are at risk for CVD (62). The use of statins was noted to be associated with an increase in the levels of serum transaminases raising concerns about their safety especially in patients with NAFLD/NASH (63). However, recent studies in a cohort of ~1,200 European patients provided strong evidence demonstrating the beneficial effects of statins in the protection against steatosis, steatohepatitis, and fibrosis as assessed by liver biopsies (50). Several other meta-analysis of available data suggested that atorvastatin improved liver injury in NAFLD/NASH patients and was more potent in decreasing CVD risk as compared to individuals with normal liver function (64).

The effects of statins on several aspects of liver injury was shown in animal models (51). Statins were shown to decrease experimentally induced fibrosis in rats by inhibiting the activation of hepatic stellate cells (52). Recent study also showed that simvastatin reduced liver inflammation and fibrosis in ApoE knockout mice fed with western-type of diet (53). These effects were attributed to the inhibition of RhoA and Ras signaling (53). It is possible therefore, that the amelioration of liver injury by statins is due to other effects beside the inhibition of cholesterol synthesis (65). Statins may also affect cholesterol metabolism in other organs and indirectly influence liver function. For example, it was shown that statin treatment in humans increased the expression of intestinal SREBP2 (66). In this regard, our studies demonstrated that the intestine-specific overexpression of SREBP2 caused hepatic steatosis and profound diet-induced liver injury in mice (41). It is possible therefore, that statins may negatively affect liver function by increasing intestinal SREBP2 expression. In light of the complexity underlying the global effects of statins, comprehensive studies are warranted to delineate the molecular pathways involved in the effects of statins on NAFLD/NASH.

Inhibitors of Bile Acid Absorption

Blocking the absorption of bile acids eliminates the negative feedback inhibition on their hepatic synthesis and promotes cholesterol degradation (12). ASBT mediates the first and rate limiting step in bile acid absorption and its inhibition represents an attractive therapeutic target to reduce hepatic cholesterol toxicity in NAFLD/NASH (12). Recent studies provided a

TABLE 1 | Therapeutic interventions for NAFLD/NASH.

Therapeutic intervention	Therapeutic agent	Molecular target	Effect on NALFD/NASH	Model	Ref
Inhibition of cholesterol synthesis	Statins	HMGCoAr	Protection against steatosis, steatohepatitis and fibrosis [assessed by liver biopsies]	Retrospective study-humans	(50)
	Simvastatin	HMGCoAr	Protects parenchymal and endothelial components of the liver after warm reperfusion.	Rat model of steatotic graft	(51)
	Fluvastatin	HMGCoAr	Reduced hepatic steatosis and fibrosis scores, α-SMA protein expression, mRNA expression of pro-inflammatory, and pro-fibrogenic genes	Choline-deficient L-amino acid-defined diet-induced Rat NASH model	(52)
	Simvastatin	RhoA and Ras signaling	Decreased hepatic inflammation and fibrosis. No effect on steatosis	Diet-induced NASH in apo$E^{-/-}$ mice	(53)
Inhibition of bile acid absorption	SC-435	ASBT	Restored glucose tolerance, reduced hepatic triglyceride and total cholesterol, improved NAFLD activity score	High fat diet-induced NAFLD in C57BL mice	(54)
	Volixibat	ASBT	Attenuated the hepatocyte hypertrophy, reduced hepatic triglyceride and cholesteryl ester levels, decreased NAFLD activity score	Diet-induced NASH in LDLr–/–/ Leiden mice	(55)
	Volixibat	ASBT	Interim-endpoint was not met and the study was terminated owing to lack of efficacy	Clinical trial-humans	(56)
Inhibition of cholesterol absorption	Ezetimibe	NPC1L1	Decreased hepatic cholesterol content and increased the hepatic total bile acid content, ameliorated hepatic insulin resistance	C57BL mice fed with high fat diet	(57)
	Ezetimibe	NPC1L1	Fibrosis stage and ballooning score were significantly improved with ezetimibe treatment [Histological evaluation]	Clinical trial-humans	(58)
	Ezetimibe	NPC1L1	Failed to reduce liver fat assessed by MRI-PDFF imaging	Clinical trial-humans	(59)
	Ezetimibe	NPC1L1	Decreased NAFLD activity score (NAS) but not hepatic steatosis	Meta-analysis of RCTs-humans	(60)

compelling evidence showing that the lack of ASBT in knockout mice protected against diet-induced liver injury and steatosis (54). Further, these studies showed that the pharmacological inhibition of ASBT significantly decreased hepatic triglycerides and total cholesterol and improved NAFLD activity score (54). Additional studies using the ASBT inhibitor volixibat in LDLr leiden knockout mice supported that conclusion and demonstrated a significant decrease in diet-induced Non-alcoholic fatty liver disease activity score by the inhibition of ASBT (55). In humans however, a phase 2 clinical trial to assess the effects of 48 weeks treatment with the ASBT inhibitor, volixibat, was terminated after mid-term assessment due to lack of improvement in NASH score as judged by MRI-PDFF imaging (56). It should be noted that the histological evaluations including the scores for ballooning and inflammation in this clinical trial were lacking. Such histological analysis in response to treatment with volixibat is crucial as it may provide more insights on the potential effects of inhibiting bile acid absorption on liver injury in NAFLD/NASH. Also, additional studies in preclinical models seem essential to unravel the molecular basis for the observed improvement of NAFLD/NASH in the animal models. Enhanced understanding of these pathways at the molecular level may unravel novel targets that could be more efficacious in the treatment of NALFD/NASH in humans.

Inhibitors of Cholesterol Absorption

Studies showed that the inhibitor of cholesterol absorption ezetimibe reduces plasma cholesterol and decreases the risk of CVD when used alone or in combination with statins (67, 68). Earlier studies in animal models showed that ezetimibe alleviated liver steatosis in mice fed with high fat diet and had promising effects on NAFLD/NASH (57). However, the studies about the beneficial effects of ezetimibe in patients with NAFLD/NASH generated conflicting results (69). Takeshita et al. (58) showed in a randomized clinical trial in a cohort of 32 patients with NAFLD that ezetimibe improved hepatic fibrosis. However, the clinical trial by Loomba et al. (59) with 50 patients showed that ezetimibe failed to significantly reduce liver fat in NAFLD as assessed by MRI-PDDF imaging. A recent meta-analysis, which exclusively included studies assessing NAFLD/NASH based on biopsy, with only one study that was based MRI-PDFF imaging, showed that ezetimibe decreased NAFLD activity score (NAS) but not hepatic steatosis (60). It was noted that current available data about ezetimibe and NAFLD/NASH were generated from limited number of clinical trials with small sample size (69). Large scale randomized clinical trials are needed for better assessment of the outcome of ezetimibe on the disease activity in patients with NAFLD/NASH. It is noteworthy to mention that the inter-individual variations in the efficiency in cholesterol absorption may influence the results of these studies. We suggest that this potential confounding factor be taken into consideration when assessing the effects of ezetimibe on NAFLD/NASH.

CONCLUSION

Disturbances in cholesterol metabolism contribute to the pathophysiology of NAFLD/NASH. An increase in cholesterol synthesis and a decrease in the pathways responsible for the elimination of cholesterol lead to accumulation of free cholesterol in the liver. The toxicity of high cellular levels of cholesterol in hepatocytes is one of the major factors causing inflammation and fibrosis leading to liver damage. The pathways involved in cholesterol metabolism are potential targets for the treatment of NAFLD/NASH. One challenging area is the complex nature of the processes involved in cholesterol homeostasis. For example, cholesterol absorption exhibits wide interindividual variations that may explain the conflicting results when evaluating the efficacy of cholesterol lowering drugs in the treatment of NAFLD/NASH. Such variations evoke the need for precision medicine approaches and individualized treatment. It is possible that individuals with naturally occurring low efficiency of cholesterol absorption may not benefit from the use of cholesterol absorption blocker ezetimibe. It will be interesting in future studies to stratify patients into relevant subgroups in a rigorous manner and take into consideration the inter-individual variations in cholesterol metabolism when assessing the outcome of cholesterol lowering drugs in the treatment of NAFLD/NASH. Precision medicine approaches necessitate the development of novel and simple methods to directly measure dynamic processes such as cholesterol absorption when individualized therapeutic interventions are to be considered for NAFLD/NASH treatment.

AUTHOR CONTRIBUTIONS

WA and PM wrote the initial draft. RG and SS edited the initial manuscript. PM and RG made the figure. RG and WA made the table. PM, RG, SS, and WA edited and approved the final draft. All authors contributed to the article and approved the submitted version.

REFERENCES

1. Huang PL. A comprehensive definition for metabolic syndrome. *Dis Model Mech.* (2009) 2:231–7. doi: 10.1242/dmm.001180
2. Chatrath H, Vuppalanchi R, Chalasani N. Dyslipidemia in patients with nonalcoholic fatty liver disease. *Semin Liver Dis.* (2012) 32:22–9. doi: 10.1055/s-0032-1306423
3. Kerr TA, Davidson NO. Cholesterol and NAFLD: renewed focus on an old villain. *Hepatol Baltim Md.* (2012) 56:1995–8. doi: 10.1002/hep.26088
4. Zhang QQ, Lu LG. Nonalcoholic fatty liver disease: dyslipidemia, risk for cardiovascular complications, and treatment strategy. *J Clin Transl Hepatol.* (2015) 3:78–84. doi: 10.14218/JCTH.2014.00037
5. Ipsen DH, Lykkesfeldt J, Tveden-Nyborg P. Molecular mechanisms of hepatic lipid accumulation in non-alcoholic fatty liver disease. *Cell Mol Life Sci.* (2018) 75:3313–27. doi: 10.1007/s00018-018-2860-6
6. Ioannou GN. The role of cholesterol in the pathogenesis of NASH. *Trends Endocrinol Metab.* (2016) 27:84–95. doi: 10.1016/j.tem.2015.11.008
7. Cook RP. *Cholesterol, Chemistry, Biochemistry And Pathology.* New York, NY: Academic Press, Inc. (1958) p. xii+542.
8. Luo J, Yang H, Song BL. Mechanisms and regulation of cholesterol homeostasis. *Nat Rev Mol Cell Biol.* (2020) 21:225–45. doi: 10.1038/s41580-019-0190-7
9. Nemes K, Åberg F, Gylling H, Isoniemi H. Cholesterol metabolism in cholestatic liver disease and liver transplantation: from molecular mechanisms to clinical implications. *World J Hepatol.* (2016) 8:924–32. doi: 10.4254/wjh.v8.i22.924
10. Wang DQH. Regulation of intestinal cholesterol absorption. *Annu Rev Physiol.* (2007) 69:221–48. doi: 10.1146/annurev.physiol.69.031905.160725
11. Alrefai WA, Annaba F, Sarwar Z, Dwivedi A, Saksena S, Singla A, et al. Modulation of human niemann-Pick C1-like 1 gene expression by sterol: role of sterol regulatory element binding protein 2. *Am J Physiol Gastrointest Liver Physiol.* (2007) 292:G369–76. doi: 10.1152/ajpgi.00306.2006
12. Ticho AL, Malhotra P, Dudeja PK, Gill RK, Alrefai WA. Intestinal absorption of bile acids in health and disease. *Compr Physiol.* (2019) 10:21–56. doi: 10.1002/cphy.c190007
13. Mantovani A, Ballestri S, Lonardo A, Targher G. Cardiovascular disease and myocardial abnormalities in nonalcoholic fatty liver disease. *Dig Dis Sci.* (2016) 61:1246–67. doi: 10.1007/s10620-016-4040-6
14. Neuschwander-Tetri BA. Nonalcoholic steatohepatitis and the metabolic syndrome. *Am J Med Sci.* (2005) 330:326–35. doi: 10.1097/00000441-200512000-00011
15. Targher G, Byrne CD, Lonardo A, Zoppini G, Barbui C. Non-alcoholic fatty liver disease and risk of incident cardiovascular disease: a meta-analysis. *J Hepatol.* (2016) 65:589–600. doi: 10.1016/j.jhep.2016.05.013
16. Fan J, Kitajima S, Watanabe T, Xu J, Zhang J, Liu E, et al. Rabbit models for the study of human atherosclerosis: from pathophysiological mechanisms to translational medicine. *Pharmacol Ther.* (2015) 146:104–19. doi: 10.1016/j.pharmthera.2014.09.009
17. Tall AR. Plasma cholesteryl ester transfer protein. *J Lipid Res.* (1993) 34:1255–74.
18. Kim EJ, Kim B, Seo HS, Lee YJ, Kim HH, Son HH, et al. Cholesterol-induced non-alcoholic fatty liver disease and atherosclerosis aggravated by systemic inflammation. *PLoS ONE.* (2014) 9:e97841. doi: 10.1371/journal.pone.0097841
19. Knowles JW, Maeda N. Genetic modifiers of atherosclerosis in mice. *Arterioscler Thromb Vasc Biol.* (2000) 20:2336–45. doi: 10.1161/01.ATV.20.11.2336
20. Schierwagen R, Maybüchen L, Zimmer S, Hittatiya K, Bäck C, Klein S, et al. Seven weeks of western diet in apolipoprotein-E-deficient mice induce metabolic syndrome and non-alcoholic steatohepatitis with liver fibrosis. *Sci Rep.* (2015) 5:12931. doi: 10.1038/srep12931
21. Kleemann R, Verschuren L, van Erk MJ, Nikolsky Y, Cnubben NH, Verheij ER, et al. Atherosclerosis and liver inflammation induced by increased dietary cholesterol intake: a combined transcriptomics and metabolomics analysis. *Genome Biol.* (2007) 8:R200. doi: 10.1186/gb-2007-8-9-r200
22. Savard C, Tartaglione EV, Kuver R, Haigh WG, Farrell GC, Subramanian S, et al. Synergistic interaction of dietary cholesterol and dietary fat in inducing experimental steatohepatitis. *Hepatol Baltim Md.* (2013) 57:81–92. doi: 10.1002/hep.25789
23. Lee L, Alloosh M, Saxena R, Van Alstine W, Watkins BA, Klaunig JE, et al. Nutritional model of steatohepatitis and metabolic syndrome in the ossabaw miniature swine. *Hepatol Baltim Md.* (2009) 50:56–67. doi: 10.1002/hep.22904
24. Puri P, Baillie RA, Wiest MM, Mirshahi F, Choudhury J, Cheung O, et al. A lipidomic analysis of nonalcoholic fatty liver disease. *Hepatol Baltim Md.* (2007) 46:1081–90. doi: 10.1002/hep.21763
25. Marí M, Caballero F, Colell A, Morales A, Caballeria J, Fernandez A, et al. Mitochondrial free cholesterol loading sensitizes to TNF- and fas-mediated steatohepatitis. *Cell Metab.* (2006) 4:185–98. doi: 10.1016/j.cmet.2006.07.006
26. Ioannou GN, Subramanian S, Chait A, Haigh WG, Yeh MM, Farrell GC, et al. Cholesterol crystallization within hepatocyte lipid droplets and its role in murine NASH. *J Lipid Res.* (2017) 58:1067–79. doi: 10.1194/jlr.M072454

27. Bieghs V, Hendrikx T, van Gorp PJ, Verheyen F, Guichot YD, Walenbergh SMA, et al. The cholesterol derivative 27-hydroxycholesterol reduces steatohepatitis in mice. *Gastroenterology.* (2013) 144:167–78.e1. doi: 10.1053/j.gastro.2012.09.062
28. Tirosh O. Hypoxic signaling and cholesterol lipotoxicity in fatty liver disease progression. *Oxid Med Cell Longev.* (2018) 2018:2548154. doi: 10.1155/2018/2548154
29. Tomita K, Teratani T, Suzuki T, Shimizu M, Sato H, Narimatsu K, et al. Acyl-CoA:cholesterol acyltransferase 1 mediates liver fibrosis by regulating free cholesterol accumulation in hepatic stellate cells. *J Hepatol.* (2014) 61:98–106. doi: 10.1016/j.jhep.2014.03.018
30. Min HK, Kapoor A, Fuchs M, Mirshahi F, Zhou H, Maher J, et al. Increased hepatic synthesis and dysregulation of cholesterol metabolism is associated with the severity of nonalcoholic fatty liver disease. *Cell Metab.* (2012) 15:665–74. doi: 10.1016/j.cmet.2012.04.004
31. McDaniel K, Herrera L, Zhou T, Francis H, Han Y, Levine P, et al. The functional role of microRNAs in alcoholic liver injury. *J Cell Mol Med.* (2014) 18:197–207. doi: 10.1111/jcmm.12223
32. Kerr TA, Korenblat KM, Davidson NO. MicroRNAs and liver disease. *Transl Res.* (2011) 157:241–52. doi: 10.1016/j.trsl.2011.01.008
33. Aryal B, Singh AK, Rotllan N, Price N, Fernández-Hernando C. microRNAs and lipid metabolism. *Curr Opin Lipidol.* (2017) 28:273–80. doi: 10.1097/MOL.0000000000000420
34. Moore KJ, Rayner KJ, Suárez Y, Fernández-Hernando C. The role of microRNAs in cholesterol efflux and hepatic lipid metabolism. *Annu Rev Nutr.* (2011) 31:49–63. doi: 10.1146/annurev-nutr-081810-160756
35. Liu M, Gao M, Li C, Yu C, Yan H, Peng C, et al. Dicer 1 /miR-29/HMGCR axis contributes to hepatic free cholesterol accumulation in mouse non-alcoholic steatohepatitis. *Acta Pharmacol Sin.* (2017) 38:660–71. doi: 10.1038/aps.2016.158
36. Brown MS, Radhakrishnan A, Goldstein JL. Retrospective on cholesterol homeostasis: the central role of scap. *Annu Rev Biochem.* (2018) 87:783–807. doi: 10.1146/annurev-biochem-062917-011852
37. Rooyen DMV, Farrell GC. SREBP-2: a link between insulin resistance, hepatic cholesterol, and inflammation in NASH. *J Gastroenterol Hepatol.* (2011) 26:789–92. doi: 10.1111/j.1440-1746.2011.06704.x
38. Zhao L, Chen Y, Tang R, Chen Y, Li Q, Gong J, et al. Inflammatory stress exacerbates hepatic cholesterol accumulation via increasing cholesterol uptake and *de novo* synthesis. *J Gastroenterol Hepatol.* (2011) 26:875–83. doi: 10.1111/j.1440-1746.2010.06560.x
39. Cheung O, Puri P, Eicken C, Contos MJ, Mirshahi F, Maher JW, et al. Nonalcoholic steatohepatitis is associated with altered hepatic microRNA expression. *Hepatol Baltim Md.* (2008) 48:1810–20. doi: 10.1002/hep.22569
40. Xie X, Liao H, Dang H, Pang W, Guan Y, Wang X, et al. Down-regulation of hepatic HNF4alpha gene expression during hyperinsulinemia via SREBPs. *Mol Endocrinol Baltim Md.* (2009) 23:434–43. doi: 10.1210/me.2007-0531
41. Malhotra P, Aloman C, Ankireddy A, Khadra H, Ooka K, Gill RK, et al. Overactivation of intestinal sterol response element-binding protein 2 promotes diet-induced nonalcoholic steatohepatitis. *Am J Physiol Gastrointest Liver Physiol.* (2017) 313:G376–85. doi: 10.1152/ajpgi.00174.2017
42. Ioannou GN, Morrow OB, Connole ML, Lee SP. Association between dietary nutrient composition and the incidence of cirrhosis or liver cancer in the United States population. *Hepatol Baltim Md.* (2009) 50:175–84. doi: 10.1002/hep.22941
43. Subramanian S, Goodspeed L, Wang S, Kim J, Zeng L, Ioannou GN, et al. Dietary cholesterol exacerbates hepatic steatosis and inflammation in obese LDL receptor-deficient mice. *J Lipid Res.* (2011) 52:1626–35. doi: 10.1194/jlr.M016246
44. Van Rooyen DM, Larter CZ, Haigh WG, Yeh MM, Ioannou G, Kuver R, et al. Hepatic free cholesterol accumulates in obese, diabetic mice and causes nonalcoholic steatohepatitis. *Gastroenterology.* (2011) 141:1393–403. doi: 10.1053/j.gastro.2011.06.040
45. Simonen P, Kotronen A, Hallikainen M, Sevastianova K, Makkonen J, Hakkarainen A, et al. Cholesterol synthesis is increased and absorption decreased in non-alcoholic fatty liver disease independent of obesity. *J Hepatol.* (2011) 54:153–59. doi: 10.1016/j.jhep.2010.05.037
46. Lally S, Tan CY, Owens D, Tomkin GH. Messenger RNA levels of genes involved in dysregulation of postprandial lipoproteins in type 2 diabetes: the role of niemann-pick C1-like 1, ATP-binding cassette, transporters G5 and G8, and of microsomal triglyceride transfer protein. *Diabetologia.* (2006) 49:1008–16. doi: 10.1007/s00125-006-0177-8
47. Jarcho JA, Keaney JF. Proof that lower is better — ldl cholesterol and IMPROVE-IT. *N Engl J Med.* (2015) 372:2448–50. doi: 10.1056/NEJMe1507041
48. Kastelein JJP, Akdim F, Stroes ESG, Zwinderman AH, Bots ML, Stalenhoef AFH, et al. Simvastatin with or without ezetimibe in familial hypercholesterolemia. *N Engl J Med.* (2008) 358:1431–43. doi: 10.1056/NEJMoa0800742
49. Munteanu MA, Mircea PA. From NAFLD to cardiovascular disease. Is it (still) the metabolic syndrome? *Clujul Med.* (2014) 87:80–6. doi: 10.15386/cjmed-277
50. Dongiovanni P, Petta S, Mannisto V, Mancina RM, Pipitone R, Karja V, et al. Statin use and non-alcoholic steatohepatitis in at risk individuals. *J Hepatol.* (2015) 63:705–12. doi: 10.1016/j.jhep.2015.05.006
51. Gracia-Sancho J, García-Calderó H, Hide D, Marrone G, Guixé-Muntet S, Peralta C, et al. Simvastatin maintains function and viability of steatotic rat livers procured for transplantation. *J Hepatol.* (2013) 58:1140–6. doi: 10.1016/j.jhep.2013.02.005
52. Chong LW, Hsu YC, Lee TF, Lin Y, Chiu YT, Yang KC, et al. Fluvastatin attenuates hepatic steatosis-induced fibrogenesis in rats through inhibiting paracrine effect of hepatocyte on hepatic stellate cells. *BMC Gastroenterol.* (2015) 15:22. doi: 10.1186/s12876-015-0248-8
53. Schierwagen R, Maybüchen L, Hittatiya K, Klein S, Uschner FE, Braga TT, et al. Statins improve NASH via inhibition of RhoA and Ras. *Am J Physiol Gastrointest Liver Physiol.* (2016) 311:G724–33. doi: 10.1152/ajpgi.00063.2016
54. Rao A, Kosters A, Mells JE, Zhang W, Setchell KDR, Amanso AM, et al. Inhibition of ileal bile acid uptake protects against non-alcoholic fatty liver disease in high fat diet-fed mice. *Sci Transl Med.* (2016) 8:357ra122. doi: 10.1126/scitranslmed.aaf4823
55. Salic K, Kleemann R, Wilkins-Port C, McNulty J, Verschuren L, Palmer M. Apical sodium-dependent bile acid transporter inhibition with volixibat improves metabolic aspects and components of non-alcoholic steatohepatitis in Ldlr-/-.Leiden mice. *PLoS ONE.* (2019) 14:e0218459. doi: 10.1371/journal.pone.0218459
56. Newsome PN, Palmer M, Freilich B, Sheikh MY, Sheikh A, Sarles H, et al. Volixibat in adults with non-alcoholic steatohepatitis: 24-week interim analysis from a randomized, phase II study. *J Hepatol.* (2020) 73:231–40. doi: 10.1016/j.jhep.2020.03.024
57. Muraoka T, Aoki K, Iwasaki T, Shinoda K, Nakamura A, Aburatani H, et al. Ezetimibe decreases SREBP-1c expression in liver and reverses hepatic insulin resistance in mice fed a high-fat diet. *Metabolism.* (2011) 60:617–28. doi: 10.1016/j.metabol.2010.06.008
58. Takeshita Y, Takamura T, Honda M, Kita Y, Zen Y, Kato K, et al. The effects of ezetimibe on non-alcoholic fatty liver disease and glucose metabolism: a randomised controlled trial. *Diabetologia.* (2014) 57:878–90. doi: 10.1007/s00125-013-3149-9
59. Loomba R, Sirlin CB, Ang B, Bettencourt R, Jain R, Salotti J, et al. Ezetimibe for the treatment of nonalcoholic steatohepatitis: assessment by novel magnetic resonance imaging and magnetic resonance elastography in a randomized trial (MOZART trial). *Hepatol Baltim Md.* (2015) 61:1239–50. doi: 10.1002/hep.27647
60. Lee HY, Jun DW, Kim HJ, Oh H, Saeed WK, Ahn H, et al. Ezetimibe decreased nonalcoholic fatty liver disease activity score but not hepatic steatosis. *Korean J Intern Med.* (2019) 34:296–304. doi: 10.3904/kjim.2017.194
61. Kreisberg RA, Oberman A. Medical management of hyperlipidemia/dyslipidemia. *J Clin Endocrinol Metab.* (2003) 88:2445–61. doi: 10.1210/jc.2003-030388
62. Vuppalanchi R, Chalasani N. Statins for hyperlipidemia in patients with chronic liver disease: are they safe? *Clin Gastroenterol Hepatol.* (2006) 4:838–9. doi: 10.1016/j.cgh.2006.04.020
63. Chalasani N. Statins and hepatotoxicity: focus on patients with fatty liver. *Hepatol Baltim Md.* (2005) 41:690–5. doi: 10.1002/hep.20671
64. Athyros VG, Boutari C, Stavropoulos K, Anagnostis P, Imprialos KP, Doumas M, et al. Statins: an under-appreciated asset for the prevention and the treatment of NAFLD or NASH and the related cardiovascular risk. *Curr Vasc Pharmacol.* (2018) 16:246–53. doi: 10.2174/1570161115666170621082910

65. Pose E, Trebicka J, Mookerjee RP, Angeli P, Ginès P. Statins: old drugs as new therapy for liver diseases? *J Hepatol.* (2019) 70:194–202. doi: 10.1016/j.jhep.2018.07.019
66. Tremblay AJ, Lamarche B, Lemelin V, Hoos L, Benjannet S, Seidah NG, et al. Atorvastatin increases intestinal expression of NPC1L1 in hyperlipidemic men. *J Lipid Res.* (2011) 52:558–65. doi: 10.1194/jlr.M011080
67. Bohula EA, Giugliano RP, Cannon CP, Zhou J, Murphy SA, White JA, et al. Achievement of dual low-density lipoprotein cholesterol and high-sensitivity C-reactive protein targets more frequent with the addition of ezetimibe to simvastatin and associated with better outcomes in IMPROVE-IT. *Circulation.* (2015) 132:1224–33. doi: 10.1161/CIRCULATIONAHA.115.018381
68. Assmann G, Kannenberg F, Ramey DR, Musliner TA, Gutkin SW, Veltri EP. Effects of ezetimibe, simvastatin, atorvastatin, and ezetimibe-statin therapies on non-cholesterol sterols in patients with primary hypercholesterolemia. *Curr Med Res Opin.* (2008) 24:249–59. doi: 10.1185/030079908X253663
69. Jun BG, Cheon GJ. The utility of ezetimibe therapy in nonalcoholic fatty liver disease. *Korean J Intern Med.* (2019) 34:284–5. doi: 10.3904/kjim.2019.043

Permissions

All chapters in this book were first published by Frontiers; hereby published with permission under the Creative Commons Attribution License or equivalent. Every chapter published in this book has been scrutinized by our experts. Their significance has been extensively debated. The topics covered herein carry significant findings which will fuel the growth of the discipline. They may even be implemented as practical applications or may be referred to as a beginning point for another development.

The contributors of this book come from diverse backgrounds, making this book a truly international effort. This book will bring forth new frontiers with its revolutionizing research information and detailed analysis of the nascent developments around the world.

We would like to thank all the contributing authors for lending their expertise to make the book truly unique. They have played a crucial role in the development of this book. Without their invaluable contributions this book wouldn't have been possible. They have made vital efforts to compile up to date information on the varied aspects of this subject to make this book a valuable addition to the collection of many professionals and students.

This book was conceptualized with the vision of imparting up-to-date information and advanced data in this field. To ensure the same, a matchless editorial board was set up. Every individual on the board went through rigorous rounds of assessment to prove their worth. After which they invested a large part of their time researching and compiling the most relevant data for our readers.

The editorial board has been involved in producing this book since its inception. They have spent rigorous hours researching and exploring the diverse topics which have resulted in the successful publishing of this book. They have passed on their knowledge of decades through this book. To expedite this challenging task, the publisher supported the team at every step. A small team of assistant editors was also appointed to further simplify the editing procedure and attain best results for the readers.

Apart from the editorial board, the designing team has also invested a significant amount of their time in understanding the subject and creating the most relevant covers. They scrutinized every image to scout for the most suitable representation of the subject and create an appropriate cover for the book.

The publishing team has been an ardent support to the editorial, designing and production team. Their endless efforts to recruit the best for this project, has resulted in the accomplishment of this book. They are a veteran in the field of academics and their pool of knowledge is as vast as their experience in printing. Their expertise and guidance has proved useful at every step. Their uncompromising quality standards have made this book an exceptional effort. Their encouragement from time to time has been an inspiration for everyone.

The publisher and the editorial board hope that this book will prove to be a valuable piece of knowledge for researchers, students, practitioners and scholars across the globe.

List of Contributors

Alessio Gerussi, Martina Lucà, Laura Cristoferi, Clara Mancuso, Chiara Milani, Daphne D'Amato, Sarah Elizabeth O'Donnell, Marco Carbone and Pietro Invernizzi
Division of Gastroenterology and Center for Autoimmune Liver Diseases, Department of Medicine and Surgery, University of Milano-Bicocca, Monza, Italy
European Reference Network on Hepatological Diseases (ERN RARE-LIVER), San Gerardo Hospital, Monza, Italy

Vincenzo Ronca
Division of Gastroenterology and Center for Autoimmune Liver Diseases, Department of Medicine and Surgery, University of Milano-Bicocca, Monza, Italy
European Reference Network on Hepatological Diseases (ERN RARE-LIVER), San Gerardo Hospital, Monza, Italy
National Institute of Health Research Liver Biomedical Research Centre Birmingham, Centre for Liver Research, Institute of Immunology and Immunotherapy, University of Birmingham, Birmingham, United Kingdom

Ju Zou, Ling Wang and Ruo-Chan Chen
Department of Infectious Disease, Xiangya Hospital, Central South University, Changsha, China
Hunan Key Laboratory of Viral Hepatitis, Xiangya Hospital, Central South University, Changsha, China

Ying-Hao Wang
Department of Ophthalmology, The Second Xiangya Hospital, Central South University, Changsha, China

Lei Zhang
The First Clinical Medical College, Lanzhou University, Lanzhou, China
Department of General Surgery, The First Hospital of Lanzhou University, Lanzhou, China
Key Laboratory of Biological Therapy and Regenerative Medicine Transformation Gansu Province, Lanzhou, China

Ke Pu, Suyang Bai and Yi Li
Department of Gastroenterology, The First Hospital of Lanzhou University, Lanzhou, China
Key Laboratory for Gastrointestinal Diseases of Gansu Province, Lanzhou University, Lanzhou, China

Xiaojun Liu
Department of Medical Oncology, The First Hospital of Lanzhou University, Lanzhou, China

Sarah Da Won Bae, Romario Nguyen and Liang Qiao
Storr Liver Centre, Westmead Institute for Medical Research, University of Sydney at Westmead Clinical School, Westmead, NSW, Australia

Anuradha Rao, Saul J. Karpen and Paul A. Dawson
Department of Pediatrics, Emory University School of Medicine, Atlanta, GA, United States

Ivo P. van de Peppel
Section of Molecular Metabolism and Nutrition, Department of Pediatrics, University Medical Center Groningen, University of Groningen, Groningen, Netherlands

Sanjeev Gumber
Division of Pathology, Yerkes National Primate Research Center, Emory University, Atlanta, GA, United States

Xiaofan Jiang, Shixiu Zhang, Baozhen Wang and Xin Guo
Department of Nutrition and Food Hygiene, School of Public Health, Cheeloo College of Medicine, Shandong University, Jinan, China

Juan Zheng
Department of Endocrinology, Union Hospital, Tongji Medical College, Huazhong University of Science and Technology, Wuhan, China
Hubei Provincial Clinical Research Center for Diabetes and Metabolic Disorders, Wuhan, China

Chaodong Wu
Department of Nutrition, Texas A&M University, College Station, TX, United States

Chandrashekhar R. Gandhi
Divisions of Gastroenterology, Hepatology and Nutrition, Department of Pediatrics, Cincinnati Children's Hospital Medical Center, Cincinnati, OH, United States
Cincinnati VA Medical Center, Cincinnati, OH, United States

Hai-zhu Zhang
School of Pharmacy and Chemistry, Dali University, Dali, China

Xian He
School of Pharmacy and Chemistry, Dali University, Dali, China
Department of Liver Diseases, Fifth Medical Center of Chinese PLA General Hospital, Beijing, China

Jing Jing, Ying Huang and Ge-zi Shi
Department of Liver Diseases, Fifth Medical Center of Chinese PLA General Hospital, Beijing, China

Zi-teng Zhang
Department of Liver Diseases, Fifth Medical Center of Chinese PLA General Hospital, Beijing, China
China Military Institute of Chinese Medicine, Fifth Medical Center of Chinese PLA General Hospital, Beijing, China

Yue-cheng Yu
Liver Diseases Center of General Hospital of PLA Eastern Theater Command, Bayi Hospital Affiliated to Nanjing University of Chinese Medicine, Nanjing, China

Jia-bo Wang
Department of Liver Diseases, Fifth Medical Center of Chinese PLA General Hospital, Beijing, China
School of Traditional Chinese Medicine, Capital Medical University, Beijing, China
China Military Institute of Chinese Medicine, Fifth Medical Center of Chinese PLA General Hospital, Beijing, China

Thit Mynster Kronborg, Henriette Ytting and Lise Hobolth
Gastro Unit, Medical Division, Amager-Hvidovre University Hospital, Hvidovre, Denmark

Søren Møller
Department of Clinical Physiology and Nuclear Medicine 260, Center for Functional and Diagnostic Imaging and Research, Amager-Hvidovre Hospital, Hvidovre, Denmark
Department of Clinical Medicine, Faculty of Health Sciences, University of Copenhagen, Copenhagen, Denmark

Nina Kimer
Gastro Unit, Medical Division, Amager-Hvidovre University Hospital, Hvidovre, Denmark
Novo Nordisk Foundation Centre for Basic Metabolic Research, Faculty of Health Sciences, University of Copenhagen, Copenhagen, Denmark

Massimiliano Cadamuro and Noemi Girardi
Department of Molecular Medicine, University of Padua, Padua, Italy

Gregory J. Gores
Division of Gastroenterology and Hepatology and the Mayo Clinic Center for Cell Signaling in Gastroenterology, Mayo Clinic, Rochester, NY, United States

Luca Fabris
Department of Molecular Medicine, University of Padua, Padua, Italy
Liver Center, Department of Medicine, Yale University, New Haven, CT, United States

Mario Strazzabosco
Liver Center, Department of Medicine, Yale University, New Haven, CT, United States

Ying Huang
College of Pharmacy, Hunan University of Chinese Medicine, Changsha, China
China Military Institute of Chinese Medicine, Fifth Medical Center of Chinese PLA General Hospital, Beijing, China

Xu Zhao, Jing Jing and Zhao-fang Bai
China Military Institute of Chinese Medicine, Fifth Medical Center of Chinese PLA General Hospital, Beijing, China

Zhuo Shi
China Military Institute of Chinese Medicine, Fifth Medical Center of Chinese PLA General Hospital, Beijing, China
Department of Liver Diseases, The Fifth Medical Center of Chinese People's Liberation Army General Hospital, Beijing, China

Yu-ming Guo
China Military Institute of Chinese Medicine, Fifth Medical Center of Chinese PLA General Hospital, Beijing, China
Department of Liver Diseases, The Fifth Medical Center of Chinese People's Liberation Army General Hospital, Beijing, China

Ang Huang
Center for Non-Infectious Liver Disease, Fifth Medical Center of Chinese PLA General Hospital, Beijing, China

Zheng-sheng Zou
Center for Non-Infectious Liver Disease, Fifth Medical Center of Chinese PLA General Hospital, Beijing, China
Department of Liver Diseases, Fifth Medical Center of Chinese PLA General Hospital, Beijing, China

Ming Niu
China Military Institute of Chinese Medicine, Fifth Medical Center of Chinese PLA General Hospital, Beijing, China
Department of Poisoning Treatment, Fifth Medical Center of Chinese PLA General Hospital, Beijing, China

Mary Stofan
Department of Pharmacology and Toxicology, Ernest Mario School of Pharmacy, Rutgers University, Piscataway, NJ, United States

Grace L. Guo
Department of Pharmacology and Toxicology, Ernest Mario School of Pharmacy, Rutgers University, Piscataway, NJ, United States
Environmental and Occupational Health Sciences Institute, Rutgers, The State University of New Jersey, Piscataway, NJ, United States
VA New Jersey Health Care System, Veterans Administration Medical Center, East Orange, NJ, United States

Shuai-shuai Chen
School of Pharmacy, Chengdu University of Traditional Chinese Medicine, Chengdu, China
Department of Liver Diseases, The Fifth Medical Center of Chinese People's Liberation Army General Hospital, Beijing, China
China Military Institute of Chinese Medicine, Fifth Medical Center of Chinese PLA General Hospital, Beijing, China

Ying Huang
Department of Liver Diseases, The Fifth Medical Center of Chinese People's Liberation Army General Hospital, Beijing, China

Shan-shan Li
Department of Liver Diseases, The Fifth Medical Center of Chinese People's Liberation Army General Hospital, Beijing, China
China Military Institute of Chinese Medicine, Fifth Medical Center of Chinese PLA General Hospital, Beijing, China

Xiao-he Xiao
Department of Liver Diseases, The Fifth Medical Center of Chinese People's Liberation Army General Hospital, Beijing, China
China Military Institute of Chinese Medicine, Fifth Medical Center of Chinese PLA General Hospital, Beijing, China

Claudio Pinto, Elisabetta Ninfole, Antonio Benedetti, Luca Maroni and Marco Marzioni
Department of Gastroenterology and Hepatology, Università Politecnica delle Marche, Ancona, Italy

Muhammad Amir and Peijian He
Division of Digestive Diseases, Department of Medicine, Emory University School of Medicine, Atlanta, GA, United States

Michael Yu
Department of Medicine, Emory University School of Medicine, Atlanta, GA, United States

Shanthi Srinivasan
Division of Digestive Diseases, Department of Medicine, Emory University School of Medicine, Atlanta, GA, United States
Research-Gastroenterology, Atlanta VA Health Care System, Decatur, GA, United States

Samira Safarikia, Rosanna Venere and Domenico Alvaro
Department of Precision and Translational Medicine, Sapienza University of Rome, Rome, Italy

Guido Carpino
Department of Movement, Human and Health Sciences, Division of Health Sciences, University of Rome "Foro Italico," Rome, Italy

Diletta Overi, Antonio Franchitto, Paolo Onori and Eugenio Gaudio
Department of Anatomical, Histological, Forensic Medicine and Orthopedic Sciences, Sapienza University of Rome, Rome, Italy

Vincenzo Cardinale
Department of Medico-Surgical Sciences and Biotechnologies, Sapienza University of Rome, Latina, Italy

Jiping Yao, Xue Liang, Yanning Liu and Min Zheng
The State Key Laboratory for Diagnosis and Treatment of Infectious Diseases, National Clinical Research Center for Infectious Diseases, Collaborative Innovation Center for Diagnosis and Treatment of Infectious Diseases, The First Affiliated Hospital, College of Medicine, Zhejiang University, Hangzhou, China

Sumeyye Soydemir and Olivia Comella
Department of Life Sciences, Faculty of Science and Engineering, Manchester Metropolitan University, Manchester, United Kingdom

Dina Abdelmottaleb and James Pritchett
Department of Life Sciences, Faculty of Science and Engineering, Manchester Metropolitan University, Manchester, United Kingdom
Centre for Bioscience, Faculty of Science and Engineering, Manchester Metropolitan University, Manchester, United Kingdom

Sukanya Roy, Shannon Glaser and Sanjukta Chakraborty
Department of Medical Physiology, Texas A&M Health Science Center College of Medicine, Bryan, TX, United States

Kishor Pant, Seth Richard and Estanislao Peixoto
The Hormel Institute, University of Minnesota, Austin, MN, United States

Sergio A Gradilone
The Hormel Institute, University of Minnesota, Austin, MN, United States
Masonic Cancer Center, University of Minnesota, Minneapolis, MN, United States

Pooja Malhotra and Ravinder K. Gill
Division of Gastroenterology and Hepatology, Department of Medicine, University of Illinois at Chicago, Chicago, IL, United States

Seema Saksena and Waddah A. Alrefai
Division of Gastroenterology and Hepatology, Department of Medicine, University of Illinois at Chicago, Chicago, IL, United States
Jesse Brown VA Medical Center, Chicago, IL, United States

Index

www.ingramcontent.com/pod-product-compliance
Lightning Source LLC
LaVergne TN
LVHW081024210926
848485LV00004B/946